Physiotherapy with Older Pe

PAHC Library

University of Plymouth

(01752) 588 588

LibraryandITenquiries@plymouth.ac.uk

Physiotherapy with Older People

Edited by

BARRIE PICKLES
Professor, School of Rehabilitation Therapy,
Queen's University, Kingston, Canada

ANN COMPTON
Physiotherapy Consultant,
Formerly Course Leader,
Diploma in Community Physiotherapy,
Southampton Institute of Higher Education,
Southampton, UK

JANET M SIMPSON
Lady Youde Lecturer in the Rehabilitation
of Elderly People,
St George's Hospital Medical School, London, UK

CHERYL A COTT
Assistant Professor, Department of Physical
Therapy/Centre for Studies of Aging,
University of Toronto, Toronto, Canada

ANTHONY A VANDERVOORT
Associate Professor, Department of Physical Therapy,
University of Western Ontario, London, Canada

Foreword by

HANA M HERMANOVA
Regional Advisor for Elderly, Disability and
Rehabilitation, World Health Organization
Regional Office for Europe,
Copenhagen, Denmark

WB Saunders Company Ltd
London • Philadelphia • Toronto • Sydney • Tokyo

WB Saunders Company

An imprint of Harcourt Publishers Ltd

© 1995 WB Saunders Company Ltd
© 2000 Harcourt Publishers Ltd

This book is printed on acid free paper

A catalogue record for this book is available from the British Library

ISBN 0-7020-1931-3

Design by Landmark Design Associates

Editorial and Production Services by Fisher Duncan
10 Barley Mow Passage, London W4 4PH

Typeset by J&L Composition Ltd, Filey, North Yorkshire

Printed and bound in Great Britain by Redwood Books, Trowbridge

Contents

A   BACKGROUND TO AGEING

Section Editor: B Pickles

B   THE AGEING PROCESS

Section Editor: AA Vandervoort

Contents

E   HANDICAPS OF AGEING

Section Editor: B Pickles

Contributors

April D'Aubin
Research Officer, Council of Canadians with Disabilities,
Winnipeg, Manitoba, Canada

Lesley A Bainbridge BSR (PT), MEd
Acting Head, Division of Physical Therapy,
University of British Columbia, Vancouver,
Canada

Jerome E Bickenbach Ph D
Professor, Department of Philosophy,
Queen's University, Kingston, Ontario, Canada

Karen Brunton BSc, PT
Senior Physiotherapist,
The Queen Elizabeth Hospital, Toronto, Ontario,
Canada

Ann Compton MCSP
Physiotherapy Consultant,
Southampton, UK

Cheryl A Cott BPT, Dip Ger, PhD
Assistant Professor (Tenure-stream),
Department of Physical
Therapy/Centre for Studies of Aging,
University of Toronto, Ontario, Canada

Elsie G Culham PhD, PT
Assistant Professor and Head, Division of
Physical Therapy,
Queen's University, Kingston, Ontario, Canada

Geoffrey R Fernie PhD
Director of Centre for Studies in Aging,
Sunnybrook Hospital, and
Professor, Department of Surgery,
University of Toronto, Toronto, Ontario, Canada

Olwen E Finlay FCSP, HT, DMS, SRP
Superintendent Physiotherapist, Department of
Health Care for Elderly People,
The Royal Hospitals, Belfast, Northern Ireland,
UK

Nancy M Gerein PhD
Associate Professor, School of Rehabilitation
Therapy,
Queen's University, Kingston, Ontario, Canada

Lydia Gillham BA, MCSP, DipTP, SRP
Senior Physiotherapist and Director of
Educational Development,
St Oswald's Hospice, Gosforth, UK

Dorothy Hammond MEd, RN
Coordinator, Regional Geriatric Assessment
Program,
St Mary's of the Lake Hospital, Kingston,
Ontario, Canada

Elizabeth C Henley BSc, BPT, MCISc
Senior Lecturer, Department of Physiotherapy,
Cumberland College,
University of Sydney, New South Wales,
Australia

Edith Herman PhD, MHSc, MCSP, PT
*Assistant Professor (Ret), School of
Occupational Therapy and Physiotherapy,
McMaster University, Hamilton, Ontario,
Canada*

Gaye DM Hill MEd, MPA, RN
*Nursing Supervisor, Kingston Psychiatric
Hospital, and
Assistant Professor, School of Nursing,
Queen's University, Kingston, Ontario, Canada*

Pamela J Holliday MSc, BSc
*Research Associate, Centre for Studies in Aging,
Sunnybrook Hospital, Toronto, Ontario, Canada*

Susan M Johnson BA, MCSP
*Private Practitioner,
Boston, Lincolnshire, UK*

Linda Kremer BSc(PT)
*Supervisor, Education and Health Promotion,
Baycrest Centre for Geriatric Care, Toronto,
Ontario, Canada*

Sandra Kunanec BSc
*Physiotherapist,
Queen Street Mental Health Centre, Toronto,
Ontario, Canada*

Hok-Lin Leung PhD
*Professor, School of Urban and Regional
Planning,
Queen's University, Kingston, Ontario, Canada*

MaryAnn McColl PhD
*Associate Professor and Head, Division of
Occupational Therapy,
Queen's University, Kingston, Ontario, Canada*

Carolyn McCullough BSc, PT
*Senior Physiotherapist,
Baycrest Centre for Geriatric Care, Toronto,
Ontario, Canada*

Eric G Moore PhD
*Professor, Department of Geography,
Queen's University, Kingston, Ontario, Canada*

Kelli A O'Brien MSc, BSc(PT)
*Senior Physiotherapist,
Western Memorial Hospital, Corner Brook,
Newfoundland, Canada*

Sandra J Olney PhD, MEd, BSc(P&OT)
*Professor, School of Rehabilitation Therapy,
Queen's University, Kingston, Ontario, Canada*

JB Orange PhD, SLP(C)
*Associate Professor, Department of
Communicative Disorders,
University of Western Ontario, London,
Ontario, Canada*

Barrie Pickles MS, BPT, MCSP, DipTP
*Professor, School of Rehabilitation Therapy,
Queen's University, Kingston, Ontario, Canada*

John AH Puxty MD
*Associate Professor and Head, Division of
Geriatric Medicine,
Queen's University, Kingston, Ontario, Canada*

Mark W Rosenberg PhD
*Associate Professor, Department of Geography,
Queen's University, Kingston, Ontario, Canada*

Carolyn Rosenthal PhD
*Associate Professor, School of Occupational
Therapy and Physiotherapy,
McMaster University, Hamilton, Ontario,
Canada*

W Kirby Rowe
*Senior Rehabilitation Consultant,
Government of Ontario,
Inverary, Ontario, Canada*

Ellen B Ryan PhD
*Professor, Department of Psychology, and
Director, Office for Gerontological Studies,
McMaster University, Hamilton, Ontario,
Canada*

Julie A Sanford MHSc
*Lecturer, School of Occupational Therapy
and Physiotherapy,
McMaster University, Hamilton, Ontario,
Canada*

Roger Scudds PhD
*Assistant Professor, Department of Physical
Therapy,
University of Western Ontario, London,
Ontario, Canada*

Michelle Shilton BSc, BHSc(PT)
*Senior Physiotherapist,
St Peter's Hospital, Hamilton, Ontario, Canada*

Janet M Simpson PhD, MSc, BSc, MCSP, AFBPsS
*Lady Youde Lecturer in the Rehabilitation of
Elderly People,
St George's Hospital Medical School, London,
UK*

Amanda Squires MSc, FCSP, SRP
*Quality Assurance Officer, Barking and Havering
Health Authority,
and President, Association of Chartered
Physiotherapists with a Special Interest
in Elderly People,
Romford, Essex, UK*

Robin L Stadnyk MEd, OT(C)
*Research Associate, Kingston, Frontenac,
Lennox and Addington Health Unit,
Kingston, Ontario, Canada*

Laurie R Swanson PhD
*Assistant Professor, School of Occupational
Therapy and Physiotherapy,
McMaster University, Hamilton, Ontario,
Canada*

G Elizabeth Tata BSc, MClSc(PT)
*Assistant Professor, Division of Physical Therapy,
Queen's University, Kingston, Ontario, Canada*

Scott G Thomas PhD
*Assistant Professor, Department of Physical
Therapy,
University of Toronto, Ontario, Canada*

Angela U Topping MSc, BSc, OT(C)
*Canadian Association of Occupational
Therapists,
Toronto, Ontario, Canada*

Robyn L Twible MA, DipOT
*Senior Lecturer, Department of Occupational
Therapy, Cumberland College,
University of Sydney, New South Wales,
Australia*

Anthony A Vandervoort PhD
*Associate Professor and Chair of Graduate
Studies,
Department of Physical Therapy,
University of Western Ontario, London,
Ontario, Canada*

Sarita Verma BA, LlB, MD, CCFP
*Assistant Professor, Department of Family
Medicine,
Queen's University, Kingston, Ontario, Canada*

Leah E Weinberg BPT, MSc
*PhD candidate,
University of Manitoba, Winnipeg, Manitoba,
Canada*

Foreword

HANA M HERMANOVA

The world is greying. Demographic forecasts for both developed and developing countries confirm the same trend for the next decades. Multiple diseases that result in frailty or long-term disability are increasing among the old-old, creating more pressure on available health and social services. To these problems must be added environmental, economic and social difficulties. Together, these may create a situation of dependence that the health services are left to deal with, because there is no other option in many places.

The world has changed dramatically in the past few years and so has the face of health care. Emphasis on cost-effectiveness has led to shorter periods of hospitalization for the elderly, and this has increased the demand for both publicly-funded and privately-operated home care and community based programmes, to meet the expanding needs of physically and mentally disabled older people. Programmes that focus on the long-term disabling conditions of the elderly must be acceptable to formal and informal caregivers and to the taxpaying public, as well as the elderly clients.

Studies have shown the benefits of rehabilitation in old age: the functioning improves, the need for drug prescriptions can be reduced, and the well-being of old people increases. Yet, rehabilitation of elderly people has not become a standard practice in many hospitals, long-term care institutions and communities. The attitude of some health care providers is still sceptical, the scientific basis for rehabilitation of older people is still greatly underestimated, the rehabilitation methodologies are not well known and the results of rehabilitation may not be appropriately evaluated and reported. It is vital that rehabilitation be recognized as an important and efficient intervention for elderly people with dysfunctions.

Physiotherapy with Older People helps to bridge these gaps. It is an excellent textbook that provides many valuable insights and a great deal of up-to-date information. Professor Pickles and his colleagues have produced a major contribution to physiotherapy in old age, that should lead towards better acute and long-term care of the elderly, and enhance the quality of their lives.

Copenhagen,
March 1995

Hana M Hermanova
*Regional Advisor for
Elderly, Disability and
Rehabilitation,
World Health Organization,
Regional Office for Europe*

Preface

Physiotherapy with Older People is primarily intended for use by undergraduate physiotherapy students, although clinicians and students should also find the material useful. It provides a conceptual model for working with healthy older people, as well as elderly patients in both institutional and community settings.

The book first provides background information on the demography of ageing and disability, attitudes towards ageing and older people, cultural differences, and the development of health and social policies for older members of society. Second, the biological and physiological changes during the human ageing process are summarized and strategies for reducing the effects of these changes to a minimum are discussed. Third, consideration is given to a range of clinical problems frequently presented by older people, but often given little consideration in other parts of the physiotherapy curriculum. Fourth, attention is paid to many of the social considerations affecting the well-being of older people, especially those with increasing disabilities. Finally, various approaches to the delivery of care and treatment services to older persons with multiple clinical, rehabilitative, and social problems are explored. Previous knowledge of anatomy, histology, physiology, psychology and basic pathology is assumed.

The book does not attempt to deal with many of the social aspects of ageing. The many differences that exist as people age in various societies go beyond the planned scope of this text. However, students should consult and study appropriate sources on social gerontology, in parallel with their reading of this text.

In those parts of the book that deal with clinical care, emphasis is on the management of disabilities and handicaps, rather than of the underlying impairments. In other words, the focus is on the role and activities of physiotherapists, rather than being a book on geriatric medicine, simplified for use by a non-medical readership.

Physiotherapy with Older People benefits greatly from the contributions of a large international authorship, most of whom are physiotherapists. Each was invited to author or co-author a particular chapter on the basis of their special interest and expertise in that field. At my request, each agreed to strictly limit the length of their chapter and the number of references cited, in order to allow space for discussion of a wide range of topics; and to provide both a short review of the major literature on that subject, and a discussion of the practical clinical implications, where appropriate. The book, it was emphasized, was intended to meet the needs of undergraduate students preparing for careers as clinicians, rather than being a handbook for researchers or specialists in the field. Over forty people agreed to contribute, despite these restrictive conditions. I thank each and every member of this large group of authors for their outstanding cooperation in meeting the many requests of the editors.

The Editorial Group comprises two long-time friends, Cheryl Cott and Tony Vandervoort, from other Ontario universities and two colleagues from the United Kingdom, Ann Compton and Janet Simpson, in addition to myself. Cheryl, Tony and I have worked together on the Rehabilitation Professions Committee of the Ontario University Coalition for Education in Ageing and Health since 1989. This committee developed recommendations for an 'ideal' curriculum in gerontology and geriatric rehabilitation for physiotherapy and occupational therapy programmes in the five Ontario Health Science Centres. After a great deal of trial and error in attempting to introduce these recommendations into our own courses it was natural to want to share our experiences with others. The addition of Ann and Janet to our discussions provided just the stimulus needed to translate a thought that 'we must do something someday' into 'let's start now'. I am pleased to have this opportunity to thank these friends publicly for all the work they have done to bring this book into being. They are recognized in alphabetical order for their editorial contributions; it would have been impossible to list them in order according to the value and extent of their individual contributions.

During this process we did discover that sometimes Canada and the United Kingdom were indeed 'two nations separated by a common language'. Terminology on three points was particularly difficult to resolve:

1. Terms such as 'old', 'senior', 'aged', 'elderly' and 'geriatric' had different meanings. To some, 'senior' was patronizing, while 'aged', 'elderly' and 'geriatric' might infer a degree of frailty that did not really exist. 'Old' was difficult to define. We decided to use the term 'older people' wherever possible; to restrict the terms 'aged' and 'elderly' to be synonymous with 'frail elderly' and to confine the use of 'geriatric' to describe the multidisciplinary team approach to management of multiple clinical, psychological, rehabilitative and social problems in older people.

2. Although many problems can be recognized in the WHO's definitions of 'impairment', disability and 'handicap' these definitions are retained. Also, the terms 'person with a disability' or 'person with a handicap' is preferred to 'disabled person' and 'handicapped person'. Use of terms such as 'the disabled' or 'the handicapped' are avoided.

3. 'Person', 'patient', and 'client' should not be used interchangeably. Each indicates a different type of relationship between the physiotherapist and the older person – a human relationship, a dependent relationship for the older individual and an empowering relationship, respectively.

We have not been hesitant to seek advice from students, patients and colleagues during the book's gestation period, and so many have provided guidance that there just is no space to thank each person individually. It would be remiss of me, however, if I failed to mention the especially valuable insights of my colleagues on the Ontario University Coalition for Education in Ageing and Health, and in the Queen's Gerontology Group. My special appreciation, too, to Dr Hana Hermanova of the WHO for contributing the Foreword, as well as her counsel and friendship.

Financial support for this project has come from a number of sources – the Educational Council for Ageing and Health in Ontario at McMaster University, the University of Toronto, the University of Western Ontario, the School of Rehabilitation Therapy at Queen's University and the British Council. Without this financial support, it is difficult to imagine how the venture could have occurred at all.

Last, but not least, to Gill Robinson, Rosa-Maria Gane and Carol Parr at WB Saunders goes my gratitude for their unfailing help and endless patience, in finding new ways to translate my vague ideas into tangible reality.

Barrie Pickles

1

Physiotherapy with Older People: A Conceptual Framework

BARRIE PICKLES, ANN COMPTON

Impairments, Disabilities and Handicaps in Older People
•
Increase in the Prevalence of Chronic Diseases and Multiple Pathologies in Older People
•
Inpact of Biological Changes of Ageing on the Physiological Responses of Older People
•
Professional Relationships Between Physiotherapists and Older People
•
Building a Rapport with Older People
•
The Step-by-step Development of a Conceptual Framework for Physiotherapy with Older People
•
Conclusion

Seven key points have been identified as determinants of good practice for physiotherapists when working with elderly patients.

1. Accurate examination, assessment and recording of each patient's physical state, taking into account individual psychosocial and environmental needs; this must be followed by continued reassessment and review.
2. Cooperation with other team members. These will include all those concerned with the patient's management and support.
3. Recognition of the patient's need to regain or maintain personal autonomy and to aim for increasing personal responsibility for recovery.
4. The establishment with each patient of agreed individual goals both short-term and long-term. Goals should be realistic, subject to ongoing review, discussion and modifica-

tion. A specified end result needs to be identified, and priorities established.
5. The need for the highest standards of physiotherapy and the importance of sharing these skills and knowledge with others involved with the patient. The importance for the patient of teaching, followed by regular practice and feedback information.
6. The provision of advice on prevention of unnecessary problems and encouraging the patient to achieve optimum levels of independence and health.
7. Evaluation of treatments and patterns of management to check whether the previous key points have been effective.

(ACP, 1985)

The ACP guidelines provide a wide range of insights and a wealth of practical suggestions for effective implementation of these seven key points. This list might be criticized on the grounds that these key points really address determinants of good practice for physiotherapists when working with most adult patients, not only those who are elderly.

Pfeiffer (1985) has produced another list that more closely considers the special needs of older patients:

1. Older patients are treatable.
2. Not only are older patients treatable, they are also teachable.
3. Older people can teach us about ageing.
4. Intervention in the life of an older patient should always be preceded by a comprehensive assessment of that patient's functioning.
5. Care of the elderly patient requires a new kind of service – coordination of services, or case management.
6. Care of the elderly requires a multidisciplinary approach.
7. The role of the family is critically important in the care of older patients.
8. Care of the elderly requires special training in gerontology and geriatrics.

Accepting these two sets of principles, this chapter will first consider a number of general issues of considerable relevance to physiotherapists and then follow this with a series of illustrative case studies in an attempt to build a conceptual framework for physiotherapy with older people.

Impairments, Disabilities and Handicaps in Older People

The International Classification of Impairments, Disabilities and Handicaps (WHO, 1980) describes itself as a manual of classification relating to the consequences of disease. It offers the following definitions:

> Impairment – any loss or abnormality of psychological, physiological or anatomical structure or function. Impairment represents exteriorization of a pathological state and in principle it reflects disturbances at the level of the organ.
> Disability – any restriction or lack (resulting from an impairment) of ability to perform an activity in the manner or within the range considered normal for a human being. Disability reflects disturbances at the level of the person.
> Handicap – any disadvantage for a given individual, resulting from an impairment or a disability, that limits or prevents the fulfilment of a role that is normal (depending on age, sex and social and cultural factors) for that individual. Handicap reflects the consequences for the individual – cultural, social, economic and environmental – that stem from the presence of impairment or disability.

There has been extensive discussion about the appropriateness of these definitions since they were first formulated. Considerable difficulty, and an occasional impossibility, was found of translating many of the terms into languages other than English. However, by providing a distinction between impairments, disabilities and handicaps, the Classification clearly exposes the multi-faceted character of disablement, and the need for a coordinated multidisciplinary approach in its management. Although there will be considerable overlap between them, the major responsibility for treatment of impairments is handled by physicians, disability management is the responsibility of the rehabilitation therapy professions, while social workers take responsibility for dealing with handicaps. However, physiotherapists deal with older people who have problems in each of the three categories – attention to impairments such as weakened muscles, locomotor disabilities and physical independence handicaps.

Impairments are caused by disease and injury; they may also be the result of general deconditioning or ageing changes; in most older persons seen by physiotherapists a mixture of all three types of problem usually exists. It is important for the physiotherapist to attempt to distinguish between impairments from these three different causes. Diseases are treatable; deconditioning can be reduced or overcome; while the irreversible changes of ageing are fewer than generally supposed.

In younger people, impairments are usually treatable and temporary, and any consequent disability or handicap is equally transient. For example, after a fracture of the shaft of his femur, a young man would have a temporary mobility disability for some months and may have an accompanying temporary vocational handicap until his mobility disability is resolved. However, once the impairments (broken bone, damaged thigh muscles, reduced range of movement in the knee, pain, general deconditioning etc) have been dealt with, there should be no residual mobility disability (the man should be able to walk normally without a limp, use stairs easily and run and jump without discomfort or hesitation) and no continuing vocational handicap (he should expect to return to his previous occupation, even if this entails heavy physical work).

With an older person, the same impairment is less likely to clear up completely, leaving the older person with some residual ongoing disability and possibly some degree of permanent handicap. Also, due to reduction in the older person's reserve capacity caused by the ageing process, the severity of disability that results from a measurable impairment is likely to be greater than in a younger subject.

Although they are more prevalent, most impairments in older people can be treated effectively, most disabilities can be reduced, and most handicaps alleviated.

Increase in the Prevalence of Chronic Diseases and Multiple Pathologies in Older People

The prevalence of chronic diseases increases with age. In chronic diseases there is a progressive degree of impairment in the affected tissues that results from successive exacerbations of the disease. Increased impairment usually produces increased disability.

Not only are older people more likely than younger persons to have a chronic disease, they are also more likely to have problems resulting from two or more concurrent conditions. The presence of two or more diseases at the same time does not mean that the disabilities created by their combined presence will be a simple summation of those that would have resulted from each disease separately. In most cases, an interaction between the two results in greater disability and possibly increased handicap.

With age, in addition to the increased prevalence of disease and the greater likelihood of injury, there is also an increase in personal problems, family difficulties, emotional crises, economic worries and concerns about living arrangements. When multiple problems exist, no one person, whether a health care professional, a family member or the affected older person, can be expected to shoulder sole responsibility for all aspects of the care, advice, treatment and rehabilitation that will be required. Considerable effort and ingenuity are often necessary to provide effective coordination between the many services required to deal with the complex mixture of impairments, disabilities and handicaps that are present.

In complex cases, where a number of impairments, several disabilities and some handicaps are discovered through the assessment process, the problems are often too numerous for all to be given adequate attention at the start of the rehabilitation programme. It is usually necessary for the various problems to be ranked in order of priority, with attention being concentrated initially only on the more critical items at the head of the priority list. It is perhaps better to develop a treatment programme that will deal effectively with a small number of critical objectives, rather than one that spreads its efforts too thinly across a wider range of problems. As each of the more critical problems is overcome, attention can be extended to those of lower priority, always providing that the patient is agreeable and has the ability and motivation to begin to address the new challenge.

Impact of Biological Changes of Ageing on the Physiological Responses of Older People

The physiological responses of older people are more varied than those of younger individuals, due to age-related changes in the tissues, and in the neurological and endocrinal control mechanisms.

Age-related changes in the tissues are largely degenerative in character; thus, the tissues of older people are generally less able to respond to stimulation than those of younger persons. Although it is possible to document the nature and sequence of age-related changes that occur in each type of cell and tissue separately, there is no consistency between older people regarding which cells or tissue will be affected first, the order in which each different type of cell or tissue

will be affected, how rapidly the degeneration will progress at each site, or how severe the changes at a particular site might eventually become. Thus, the development of age-related changes in each person tends to follow a pattern that is unique for that individual. It would be wrong to consider the ageing process as being a simple reversal of the predictable sequence of events that occurred during development and maturation earlier in life. An appreciation of this uniqueness in the pattern of changes in each person as they become older is vital.

Because of degenerative changes in the neurological system in older people, a higher threshold level of stimulation is required to produce any physiological response; the range of stimulation that produces a beneficial response is narrowed; a given level of stimulation produces a lower physiological response; the maximum possible (peak) response is produced by a lower level of stimulation; and a strong stimulus, that in a younger person would be beneficial, may have a destructive effect. In addition, as the location and extent of the neurological degeneration varies between individuals, physiological responses become increasingly more varied, and therefore less predictable.

Changes in the endocrinal homeostatic control mechanisms also lead to an increased variability of response. As fine endocrinal control is lost through the ageing process, the concentration of hormones in the blood stream is less carefully regulated, and homeostatic control reactions become more erratic. If stimuli are applied at times when the level of function is already high, the response may be small, and conversely, if stimulation is applied when the level of function is low, the response will be greater. This phenomenon is known as the Law of Initial Values. Responses of an individual to similar stimuli at different times of the day tend to vary; these variations increase with age, as ongoing degeneration of the homeostatic mechanisms continues.

One endocrinal mechanism, the Stress Response, becomes increasingly active as people age, due to increasing exposure of the older person to physical and psychological stress. This response is triggered by factors that require a tissue, organ, system or the total person to function at, or close to, maximum capacity. The degenerative biological changes of ageing progressively lower maximum capacity levels, and therefore reduce the amount of available reserve. When older people perform any activity or function they are working closer to their personal maximum capacity than a younger person would do in similar circumstances. Thus, the stress response is likely to be triggered off more easily and more often as people age. If the stress response is small or moderate, this may increase the speed and effectiveness of neuromuscular and cognitive activity, but if the stress response is excessive or unusually prolonged, the ability to function may be either reduced or completely abolished.

For a variety of reasons, therefore, physiotherapists should expect to find great variability among their older patients and clients insofar as their responses to both testing and treatment procedures are concerned, and recognize that these responses may also be quite different from those of younger persons. Physiotherapy programmes designed for older people must take these differences into account if they are to produce the maximum effect.

Professional Relationships Between Physiotherapists and Older People

Physiotherapists work with older people in a number of situations. They may work with healthy older people in health promotion and disability prevention programmes; they may treat older people who are in hospital, or who attend ambulatory clinics; they may provide services to older people in their homes or in other community settings. Their work may include assessment, treatment, teaching, counselling and advocacy.

Older people are variously referred to as 'persons', 'patients', 'clients', 'residents' or 'consumers'. Each of these terms indicates a quite different type of relationship between the older individual and the physiotherapist, although in everyday usage the terms may tend to be used interchangably.

Not all older individuals who seek the help of a physiotherapist should be considered to be 'patients'. Legally, a person only becomes a patient, when, after an appropriate assessment, there is an informed consent to the physiotherapist proceeding with an agreed treatment procedure or programme. The agreement to proceed places a legal obligation on both parties — an obligation on the part of the physiotherapist to provide that treatment as effectively as possible, and to keep the patient's best interests paramount in all aspects of the professional relationship, together with an expectation or obligation on the part of the patient to follow the instructions and advice provided within that relationship to the best of his/her ability. In the physiotherapist—patient relationship, decisions regarding treatment are made by the physiotherapist, with the patient's best interest in mind, because the patient lacks the technical knowledge to make the decision on his own behalf.

The 'patient' relationship pervades work in Hospitals and in institutionally-based Geriatric Assessment Units, Geriatric Medicine programmes, Geriatric Rehabilitation facilities and Geriatric Day Hospitals, where the major purpose is the medical management of 'impairment' problems. This medical model presumes acquiescence, and indeed some degree of passivity, on the part of the recipient of treatment services. It is natural that physiotherapists working in acute care hospitals, who view their responsibilities primarily as assisting the medical team in the management of impairments, will consider the people they treat to be 'patients'. In physiotherapy clinics specializing in treatment of impairments that result from injury, this view would be equally appropriate.

In community-based or home care settings the priorities are usually different. The major thrust of these programmes is directed at care rather than cure, and at the management of disabilities and handicaps rather than the treatment of disease. Rehabilitation is a process to enable persons with disabilities and handicaps to improve their ability to function as members of society. Successful rehabilitation involves the transference of responsibility for achieving this maximum functional capacity from the professional to the disabled person. Part of this involves the transfer of responsibility for decision making. It is essential that physiotherapists who work with older disabled people in community and home care settings should design their approach so that, whenever possible, it facilitates an increasing acceptance of responsibility by the disabled individual. Alternative priorities and alternative approaches to deal with the problems that have been identified need to be discussed, with the final decision on the preferred course of action being made by the disabled individual. The nature of this interaction is obviously very different from that in the 'patient' relationship. In this context it is preferable to consider the disabled individual as a 'client', rather than a 'patient'.

Physiotherapists involved in health promotion or disability prevention programmes for older people would be similarly advised to consider this group as 'clients' rather than as 'patients'. They are not sick; they may have no disabilities or handicaps; and they may lead very active lifestyles. It would be inappropriate and indeed counterproductive for the physiotherapist to approach them as compliant and subservient 'patients'.

Definition of the role of physiotherapists working in nursing homes is often more difficult. Here, the role is usually to provide assistance to maintain function, rather than improve it. Here again, the rehabilitation approach that regards the elderly nursing home resident as a 'client' rather than as a 'patient' should be preferred, although this may not be appropriate in palliative care or terminal care situations. What is sometimes overlooked is that those who live in nursing homes (unless they have been legally committed there) are 'residents' in that home, not 'patients'. It is unfortunate that sometimes administrative policies exist in nursing homes that do not readily acknowledge the right of residents to make decisions on matters that affect their lives. A rejection of this right creates unnecessary handicaps. It would be equally unfortunate if physiotherapists failed to understand the impact that such restrictive practices can have on nursing home residents.

Whether it is appropriate for older persons to make decisions about their own circumstances depends not only on the physical setting, but also on the older person's physical and mental condition at the time. The appearance of an intercurrent illness, a sudden flare-up of a long dormant chronic condition, the loss of a spouse or other close relative, or a financial emergency may result in a temporary incapacity to cope and make decisions, whatever the location. In these situations it would be appropriate for the physiotherapist to make decisions temporarily on behalf of older people until they recover the capacity to make decisions for themselves. The ability of a person to make decisions does not follow the 'all or none' principle; physiotherapists will often be confronted with situations where the capacity to make certain kinds of decision is retained, while the ability to make proper judgements in other areas is lacking. Considerable skill and careful judgement is required by the physiotherapist to deal with such situations.

Building a Rapport with Older People

Building a rapport or relationship with a client requires effective communication based on an awareness of the cultural background and an understanding of the attitudes, beliefs and behaviours of the person. Failure to properly appreciate these factors will render communication difficult or impossible. This applies particularly if the older person is now living in a culture very different in its values from the one into which they were born, or in which they grew up.

The likelihood today of people growing old in a culture different from the one in which they were raised continues to increase. In part, this is due to high migration rates between countries for most of the present century. While some groups of immigrants are assimilated easily into the main-

stream culture of their new homeland, in most cases assimilation is less than complete. In some countries immigrants are encouraged to retain many of the cultural values of the society from which they came and sometimes an immigrant group will continue as a cohesive sub-culture almost independent of the wider society. Working immigrants may sponsor elderly parents to come and live with them in their new country; these elderly people usually live closely within the confines of their family, and make little effort to learn the language or customs of their new hosts.

Physiotherapists will often work in settings where the cultural values of some of their clients will differ significantly from their own; they will often have very different perspectives on health, the causes of health problems, the likely effectiveness of various approaches to treatment, the impact of disabilities and the appropriate role for the family in helping to deal with the problems of ageing.

The differences in culture between people from different generations in a single society is also worth noting. As the rate of technological and social change continues to accelerate, the gap between attitudes, beliefs and expectations of the older and younger generations becomes wider. Younger physiotherapists may need to give conscious consideration as to how their own values, personal and professional, may differ from those of their older clients and how these differences may create misunderstandings that will hamper communication and disrupt the rehabilitation process.

Communication is most effective when there is a sense of trust between people, and when tension is absent. It has already been noted that as people age, the stresses of life tend to increase relentlessly, and result in increased levels of anxiety and even panic. Elderly patients who appear withdrawn and uncooperative may be unresponsive because of high anxiety. It is no wonder that this possibility becomes more prevalent if the older person has multiple and worsening difficulties, and regards these as requiring unwanted lifestyle changes to be made, or even to be life-threatening. In these kinds of situations it is particularly challenging to find a way of achieving effective communication.

The Step-by-step Development of a Conceptual Framework for Physiotherapy with Older People

As the problems of impairments, disabilities and handicaps of older people are not exclusive to this age group, some consider that it is inappropriate to regard work with older people as a valid area of clinical specialization in physiotherapy. However, while these problems may not be exclusive to older people, some may predominate. The presentation of disease and the response to treatment are frequently different in older people, due to the age-related degenerative biological and physiological changes that have occurred. It is also true that, as people age, these problems are increasingly associated with chronic, rather than acute disorders. Furthermore, the problems of the elderly usually tend to be multiple, rather than single and often comprise a complex interlinking pattern of biological, psychological, psychosocial, economic and environmental factors; in these situations physiotherapy will need to be highly coordinated with a wide range of other health and social services.

To illustrate the special considerations that need to be addressed when working with older people, five case studies will be considered. Each of these will focus on one major theme; each will add a number of extra items to the factors considered in the previous case(s).

These cases will illustrate:

1. Working with healthy older people.
2. Working with an older patient who has a single clinical problem.
3. Working with an older client who has multiple clinical problems.
4. Working with an older client and his caregiver, when both have clinical problems.
5. Working with an older client who has multiple clinical and social problems.

From these five case studies, some 24 separate concepts are identified. Each of these concepts relates to issues discussed elsewhere in the book. Taken together, they may provide a useful frame of reference for physiotherapy with older people.

Case Study 1
Working with Healthy Older People

The Health Promotion Coordinator at your hospital recently received the following letter from a local group of older people:

> *We (the local Senior Citizens Club) had a talk from one of your staff recently. Our members were interested in the heart programme that is being developed. Some have a family member with heart disease, and others are just interested in the topic. About 20 people have indicated that they would like to be involved in the 'Healthy Heart' programme, which we understand includes lectures, discussions and a physical activity programme. We are all over 70 but get ourselves to the club, although some of us are not very fit or too good on our feet. Could you help us please?*

As the Senior Physiotherapist in the Cardiovascular Service at your hospital, you have been asked to take responsibility for planning and conducting the exercise component of this programme.

Some general questions should be addressed when trying to deal with these problems:

1. What are the cultural norms of society regarding participation in the kind of programme? Do the perspectives of the group reflect these norms? Is the group culturally homogeneous? (Chapters 4, 5).

2. What attitude(s) of individual members of this group of older people might affect their willingness to participate in this kind of activity? (Chapter 3).

3. What ethical and/or legal issues have to be considered in developing and implementing this type of programme with older people? (Chapter 27).

4. How can you communicate more effectively with older people? (Chapter 10).

5. Taking into account how older people learn, what teaching strategies are most likely to be successful in assisting cognitive learning (Chapter 8), and motor learning (Chapter 9).

6. How can you increase the possibility that ongoing changes in the lifestyle of older people may result from participation in your programme? (Chapter 13).

7. Do you have a knowledge and understanding of the biological and physiological changes of both ageing and inactivity? (Chapters 6, 7).

8. Are you familiar with the principles of design of exercise and activity programmes for older people, and how these principles may differ from those designed for younger persons? (Chapter 12).

Case Study 2
Working with an Older Patient who has a Single Clinical Problem

You are an employee in a private physiotherapy clinic located in a suburb of a large (1 000 000 population) city. Although the clinic specializes in the treatment of patients with industrial injuries, during the past year an increasing number of older patients have been referred by physicians in the building, and other older people come directly to your clinic as the result of recommendations from their friends. You have taken a particular interest in increasing the number of older persons among your caseload, as this increases the variety of problems with which you have to deal.

Earlier today a woman came to the clinic, bringing with her a referral note from Dr X, whose office is on the same floor of your building.

I am referring to you Mrs A of No. 4, 22 Side Street, Mainsville, aged 71.

Mrs A attended my office this morning with her husband. She has an acute inflammation of her left knee, and some wasting of her quadriceps. She is complaining of generalized pain in her left leg, for which naproxen has been prescribed. She has had difficulty walking for the past two days. There is a past history of skiing injuries that required a menisectomy at age 32 and a cruciate ligament repair at age 50. She tells me that she tripped over a stone when she and her husband were out for their daily walk yesterday, but did not fall as they were walking arm in arm.

On questioning her she admits that there has been some occasional slight swelling in her left calf and foot on and off for years, and occasional aching and stiffness, particularly after playing golf. She recently gave up golf because of the problems it seemed to cause in her left leg.

X-Rays indicate narrowing of the joint space with some flattening of the lateral margins.

All the general questions (1–8) raised in Case Study No. 1 will also apply in this situation, but the following considerations need to be added:

9. What treatment goals need to be set for each of the impairments, disabilities and handicaps that are identified in this older patient? (Chapter 14).

10. Is there any evidence of unusual presentation of signs and symptoms in this older patient that might lead to an expectation of altered response to any treatment you might consider? (Chapter 1).

11. Do any special considerations need to be given to the fact that in this older patient some problems are of long duration? (Chapter 22).

12. What adjustments are necessary to treatment programmes for older peo-

ple, to take into account that changes resulting from ageing and disuse are always superimposed on the impairments of disease and injury, and increase the resulting disabilities? (Chapter 12).

13. Is any assistive device likely to help the older person decrease or overcome a disability or handicap that may be present? (Chapters 25, 26).

14. Would a referral to any other health care professional be in the best interests of the patient? (Chapter 28).

Case Study 3
Working with an Older Client who has Multiple Clinical Problems

You work in the out-patient service of the physiotherapy department at a medium sized general hospital (175 beds) in a town of 65 000 people. You have received the following referral from a family doctor in the town, who has asked for your help to see what might be done to deal with Mr Black's incontinence, and set up a realistic programme of general reactivation and rehabilitation for him. You are given the following summary of Mr Black's case notes:

Mr Black, a 75-year-old carpenter, had a stroke five years ago. This left him with a spastic hemiparesis affecting his right arm and leg, and a slight speech impediment. Until three months ago, however, he had continued to take his daily walk outside his home, whenever the weather permitted.

One day a couple of months ago he was

out walking alone, when a sudden pain developed in his left calf; the pain did not disappear when he stopped to rest, and he was forced to get help from a passer-by to call for a taxi home. As the pain and swelling had increased by the following morning his wife insisted that he should be checked over at the Emergency Department of the local hospital. A diagnosis of deep venous thrombosis was confirmed. A programme of anticoagulant therapy was instituted, that is still being continued. Tests revealed that the DVT was probably caused by the presence of a carcinoma in his prostate gland. This was removed by surgery one week after Mr Brown's admission to hospital. He was discharged home a week after his surgery. He had lost some weight before his admission to hospital, and lost a further 6 kg during his hospital stay.

He has tolerated a follow-up course of chemotherapy for his cancer surprisingly well, without any untoward side-effects. Although his wife insists that he is out of bed and properly dressed during the day, he remains weak and lethargic and hardly moves from his chair. Mrs Black does give him some assistance with dressing, and with his toilet needs. He remains occasionally incontinent of urine.

Fortunately, Mrs Black, who is five years younger than her husband, remains in excellent health, and continues to have a very positive attitude towards life. She claims it is no problem to provide this extra care for her husband, and that she can continue to manage their two-bedroomed apartment (on the second floor of a custom-built block) without assistance.

In this case all the considerations (1–14) raised in Case Study No. 2 will apply, with the addition of:

15. The reduced energy capacity in older people may make it necessary to prioritize the multiple impairments and disabilities that are present in order of precedence. What priorities would you set, and how would you establish these? (Chapter 14).

16. In situations where more than one problem exists it may not always be possible to provide comprehensive treatment for each. The presence of one problem may mean that some aspects of treatment for another may not be possible or may be contraindicated. Is this a difficulty in the case under review? (There can be no general reference given to this question. Each case is different, and the physiotherapist will need to decide each situation on its individual merits.)

17. Are any of the problems that have been identified likely to be iatrogenic i.e. created or worsened by the physiotherapy, or by drugs the older patient may be taking? (Consult standard texts about these various possibilities.)

18. To what extent is it appropriate for the older person to make their own decisions regarding the physiotherapy interventions and their rehabilitation? (Chapter 11). Is the older person a patient, client or consumer? (Chapter 1). What is the importance of independence to the older person with disabilities? (Chapters 22, 23).

19. Severe, multiple and long-standing problems in older people often place severe strain and hardship on their primary caregiver. Is there any

evidence of this, and if so, what forms of support that are available might be appropriate? (Chapter 31).

Case Study 4
Working with an Older Client and his Caregiver When Both Have Clinical Problems

Mr Clark was referred by his family physician to the Geriatric Day Hospital where you are the Senior Physiotherapist, for assessment and treatment. The following unusually detailed report was provided:

Mr Clark is a 74-year-old man who retired from the Navy in 1969 with the rank of Lieutenant Commander. He had been attached to the Administrative Branch of the service and had qualified some years before as a Chartered Accountant. He established an accountancy practice in the city upon his retirement from the service; until last year he continued as senior managing partner in this flourishing business with five other partners and two associates. A year ago he handed over control to one of the junior partners, in order to be able to spend more time with his wife.

For the past ten years Mr Clark has had problems associated with a late-developing rheumatoid arthritis. Initially, only his hands and shoulders were involved, but since his 70th birthday the disease has also affected his knees and ankles. For some months Mr Clark did not feel well; he seemed to lose his natural energy and drive about six months ago and suffered a series of colds and coughs. Last month Mr Clark developed a lung infection that progressed to lobar pneumonia. A routine chest X-ray taken at the time revealed the presence of a bronchial carcinoma in his left lower lobe bronchus, with some infiltration into the hilar lymph glands. A lobar resection was performed four weeks ago; the post-operative period has been routine and without complications. Mr Clark has remained in hospital since his surgery. Mr Clark, who was somewhat weak and debilitated at the time of his admission, has continued to lose weight since then. He is able to walk around the ward slowly without assistance, although he quickly tires. When attempting to go upstairs yesterday in the company of a nurse he became dyspnoeic and complained of pain on the left side of his chest; he insisted on walking back to his room after taking a short rest.

On examination, Mr Clark's breathing pattern at rest does not appear to be particularly laboured. There is, of course, unequal expansion on the two sides of his chest. You observe that when he is walking at his own pace his accessory muscles of respiration are brought into action. Exertion may still trigger off a bout of coughing, particularly early in the day, when a progressively reducing amount of clear, viscous sputum may be expectorated.

Mr Clark will tell you that his muscles seem stiff, and that it takes him quite some time each morning before he can move about fairly easily. There appears to be a generalized soreness in his muscles, and he complains of mild discomfort in his right wrist, although none of his other joints are giving him trouble at this time. There is no evidence of freshly active neurological or vascular complications from his arthritis, although he gives a history of rheumatoid-related angiopathy in the small blood vessels in his right calf and foot on two previous occasions.

Mr Clark is a thin man, of above average height. He is pale and tense. His usual posture is somewhat bowed, mostly due to a slight flexion deformity of his hips, plus an inability to straighten out his right leg fully due to his long standing arthritis. He leans a little to the left while standing; when he knows he is being observed his naval pride still causes him to straighten up a little further. He walks slowly but his stride length is equal on the two sides, and his stride cadence is even.

Mr and Mrs Clark have lived in their 3-bedroomed penthouse condominium for the past ten years. Mr Clark has expressed some concern about his wife to one of the nurses. He explained that, although she continues to enjoy good physical health, during the past 18 months his wife appeared to have become increasingly forgetful and careless. She would forget to buy items she had gone out to buy, she misplaced articles around the home and would spend long periods of time searching for these. Occasionally, she would be less careful than she had always been about her dress and appearance. It was after these changes were diagnosed as symptoms of Alzheimer's disease a year ago, that Mr Clark resigned his position as managing partner.

The Clark's two sons are both in Asia. Mrs Clark's younger sister lives close by; they have seen her two or three times a week since the death of her own husband two years ago. Since Mr Clark was admitted to hospital she has spent considerable time each day looking after Mrs Clark's needs. In addition, the Clarks have a large circle of friends and business acquaintances in the city. They continued to lead a busy, indeed hectic, social life until Mr Clark was admitted to hospital last month. Mr Clark continues to have many visitors each day at the hospital.

The Clarks have no financial problems. Mr Clark has an income from his accounting practice that is well into six figures and considerable investment income, in addition to his naval and government pensions. Mrs Clark shared a large inheritance with her sister from their wealthy parents.

Here, all considerations (1–19) raised in Case Study No. 3 will apply, with the addition of:

20. Are the present housing arrangements the most satisfactory? What alternatives might be considered? (Chapter 24).

21. How can the efforts of the physiotherapist be linked most effectively with those of other members of the Day Hospital team? (Chapter 28).

Case Study No. 5
Working with an Older Person who has Multiple Clinical and Social Problems

You were recently appointed as a physiotherapist to the Regional Geriatric Assessment and Treatment Service, located in a large teaching hospital. The service provides multidisciplinary assessment in the homes of elderly people, or in the hospital, as appropriate. In some cases, the team provides treatment for the problems that are discovered. In other cases, the problems are dealt with on an outpatient basis, usually through the Day Hospital programme. Continuity of care is ensured through effective liaison with family doctors and the wide range of community health and social services that are available.

This morning you received a summary report from the Head of your Service (a physician with specialist qualifications in Geriatric Medicine) following a home visit he had made yesterday.

Mrs Williams is a 76-year-old woman who had a below-knee amputation of her left leg three years ago, because of gangrenous toes and poor circulation in her lower leg resulting from a long standing diabetes. Since that time she has used a PTB prosthesis to which she is well adapted, her stump is well shaped, and is perfectly healed.

Six weeks ago she accidentally scraped the skin off her right lateral malleolus and subsequently this developed into a 3 cm diameter ulcer which is not healing. Since this accident she experiences pain in her right calf when attempting to walk more than 100 metres without stopping. Consequently, she has adopted the use of a cane, which she feels helps her to walk for longer distances before needing to stop. She also finds this steadies her — she had noticed her gait was becoming a little less steady for some time.

Last week Mrs Williams tripped when walking outside. She was admitted to hospital suffering from concussion, but after overnight observation was allowed to return home, as no other signs of serious injury were found.

Mrs Williams agreed with her family doctor that it would be a good idea to have a complete review of her situation through the Regional Geriatric Programme.

Mrs Williams' right foot is markedly discoloured, the skin is shiny and smooth, and there is no growth of hair on the skin below her knee. The discolouration (with some pigmentation) extends up the lateral side of her leg to mid-tibial level. She has a noticeable oedema around both malleoli and on the dorsum of her foot, but none higher up the calf. The lower leg feels cool to the touch, and Mrs Williams says it has been rather numb and cold since last winter.

For years she has had to take great care to trim her toenails properly, to keep the skin in the affected area dry through regular use of talcum powder, and she always wears loose-fitting woollen socks to bed. She applies a fresh dry dressing over the ulcer each day before putting on her night socks. The ulcer is not infected, but is draining slightly. Around the ulcer is an elevated, thickened dark purple area approximately 4 cm in width.

Mrs Williams' eyesight, that has never been very good, has deteriorated considerably during the past year, to the point where she was recently refused renewal of her drivers permit. Mr Williams, who is two years older than his wife, still continues to drive their 15-year-old car.

Mrs Williams is a rather obese woman, who seems pale and tense. She fidgets nervously both during the examination and treatment sessions and when she is alone. She says that she is not in the least worried about her right leg, because she knows it will get better, and that things will be alright. She has been on a diet to lose weight, but finds it difficult to stick to it. She takes insulin regularly for her diabetes, and has never had a hyper- or hypo-glycaemic coma.

Mr Williams is naturally anxious about his wife. Although his general health remains fair, he does have increasing problems with an osteoarthritis in his right hip, that have forced him to reduce his mobility, especially during the past two years. Mr Williams' last job had been as the Manager of a privately owned men's clothing store in the city for almost ten years, before he became unemployed at the age of 63, when the business was forced into bankruptcy. He has no pension from his previous employment; the Williams' only income comes from their government pensions.

Their only daughter lives with her husband and two teenage children some 300 miles away. Mrs Williams' sister lives close by, and visits them at least weekly. In contrast, the Williams seem to have few friends in the city; Mr Williams did not maintain contact with his previous work *colleagues after his forced early retirement.*

The Williams' small bungalow has always been important to them. In their earlier years they had sacrificed many other things in order to be able to purchase it. They were able to finally pay off their mortgage a year or so before Mr Williams was forced to stop work. Their home is their only remaining investment; their previous savings have been progressively depleted since Mr Williams stopped working. One of Mr Williams' worries is that some major repair might be needed to either their house or their car, and he knows there is no money available for either of these.

In this situation, all considerations (1–21) raised in Case Study No. 4 will apply, with the addition of:

22. *How should a comprehensive assessment be done to identify and prioritize the many medical, rehabilitative, economic and social needs of an elderly person with multiple problems? (Chapter 29).*

23. *What range of services is available in the community that enable older people with multiple problems to continue to live in their own homes? (Chapter 31).*

24. *In those cases where it is no longer feasible for older persons to remain in their own home, what alternative type of institutional care would be most appropriate? (Chapter 30).*

Conclusion

Working with older people can present the physiotherapist with a set of challenges unparalleled in other areas of practice. The caseload is very mixed; patients with musculoskeletal, neurological and cardiovascular problems may all be found in a single caseload and often in the same patient. Interlinking between medical, psychological, rehabilitative, economic and social problems that all need attention is the norm, rather than the exception. Add to these the differences in presentation of disease, the unique pattern of ageing in each individual, and the varying responses that older people may demonstrate, and the complexity of the challenge is obvious.

The framework outlined in this chapter should help the physiotherapist give systematic consideration to the wide range of issues involved, and so improve the quality of help they are able to offer to their elderly clients.

References

Association of Chartered Physiotherapists in Geriatric Medicine (1985) *Physiotherapy with elderly patients.* London: Chartered Society of Physiotherapy.

Pfeiffer E (1985) Some basic principles of working with older patients. *Journal of the American Geriatrics Society* 33: 44–47.

World Health Organization (1980) *International Classification of Impairments, Disabilities and Handicaps.* Geneva: WHO.

A

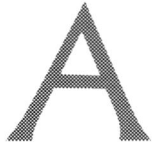

Background to Ageing

SECTION EDITOR: BARRIE PICKLES

2

Demography of Ageing and Disability

MARK W ROSENBERG, ERIC G MOORE

Introduction
•
The Present Older Population
•
Ageing and Disability
•
Future Trends

Introduction

The demography of ageing and disability is a fundamental component to understanding how to plan services for an older population. For example, when choosing the level and mix of rehabilitation services for an older population (see Section E), health planners need to take into consideration the proportion of the older population who are part of the young-old versus the old-old, those with mild disabilities versus those with severe disabilities and those with single impairments versus multiple impairments (see Section C). These and other demographic factors are described in this chapter.

While there is no scientific definition of old age, most researchers have tended to use age 65 as a convenient, if arbitrary, division between the working age population and the older population in Canada, Australia and the UK (McCracken, 1985; Norland, 1994). In Canada and Australia, age 65 is also the age when individuals generally become eligible for government transfer payments. In the UK, the Office of Population Censuses and Surveys (OPCS) often reports the older population based on males aged 65 and over and females aged 60 and over, reflecting the differences in age when men and women become eligible for state pensions.

It is important to distinguish between the *young-old* (those between the ages of 65 and 74) and the *old-old* (those aged 75 and over). Generally, it is only after the age of 75 that rates of disability increase rapidly, thus reducing the ability of the older population to live independently and increasing the probability that formal services such as physiotherapy or even institutional care will be required (see Sections D and E, especially Chapter 24).

This chapter reflects three key themes of the demography of ageing and disability in Canada, Australia and the UK: (1) the present size of the older population in all three countries; (2) the links between ageing and disability; (3) the future growth of the ageing population. Running throughout the chapter will be a fourth theme which is the gendered nature of ageing and disability.

The Present Older Population

In 1991, the population aged 65 and over represented 11.6% of the total population of Canada, 11.3% of the total population of Australia and 15.9% of the total population of the UK (Table 1). The higher percentage of older persons in the UK indicates that its age profile is characteristic of a more demographically mature society compared with Canada and Australia. In 1991, about 60% of the older population in Canada and Australia were between the ages of 65 and 74 or part of the young-old. In the UK, only 56% of the older population could claim to be part of the young-old.

The growing size of the older population in each

Table 1
The demography of ageing in Canada, Australia and the UK in 1991

Population		Canada[a]		Australia[b]		UK[c]	
		('000s)	(%)	('000s)	(%)	('000s)	(%)
15 to 64 ('000s)	M	10 170.2	75.6	5 885.6	68.0	18 231.0	66.7
	F	10 142.3	73.3	5 718.0	65.9	18 481.0	63.5
	T	20 312.5	74.4	11 603.6	66.9	36 712.0	65.0
65+ ('000s)	M	1 330.4	9.9	840.0	9.7	3 604.0	13.2
	F	1 839.5	13.3	1 126.4	13.0	5 395.0	18.5
	T	3 169.9	11.6	1 966.8	11.3	8 999.0	15.9
65 to 74 ('000s)	M	851.5	6.3	549.2	6.3	2 266.0	8.3
	F	1 043.6	7.5	637.2	7.3	2 796.0	9.6
	T	1 895.1	6.9	1 186.4	6.8	5 062.0	9.0
75+ ('000s)	M	479.0	3.6	291.2	3.4	1 338.0	4.9
	F	795.9	5.7	489.2	5.6	2 598.0	8.9
	T	1 274.9	4.7	780.4	4.5	3 936.0	7.0
Total ('000s)	M	13 454.6		8 655.7		27 344.0	
	F	13 842.3		8 679.2		29 123.0	
	T	27 296.9		17 334.9		56 467.0	

[a] Based on Statistics Canada 1991 Census (Statistics Canada, 1993).
[b] Based on Australian Bureau of Statistics 1991 population estimates using Series D (Australian Bureau of Statistics 1990).
[c] Based on Central Statistical Office 1991 Census (Central Statistical Office, 1994).

Figure 1   Growth in older populations compared, 1981–91. Note: Data not available for Aus-75+.

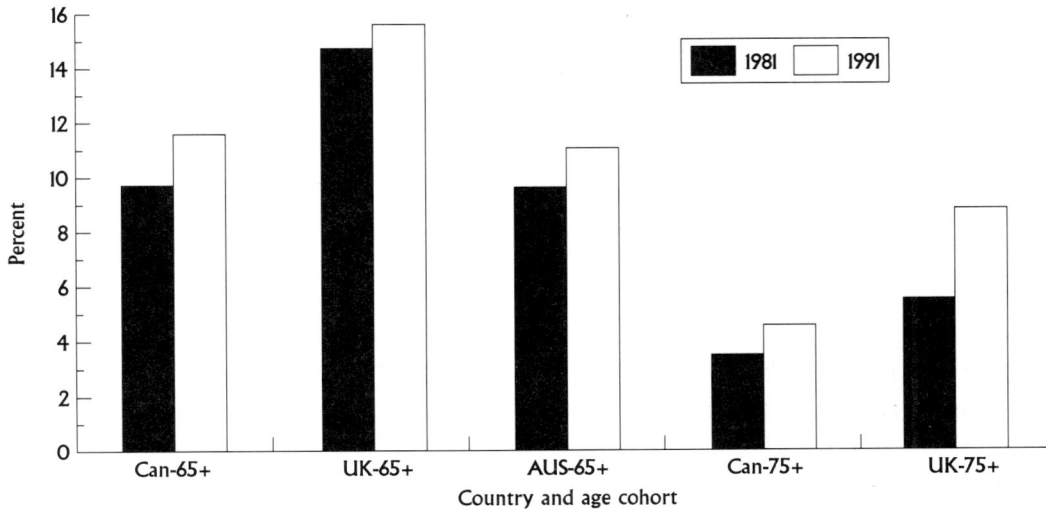

country represents a trend which has its origins at the beginning of the twentieth century. The 'flattening out' of the growth of the older population in each country between 1951 and 1971 was the result of the 'baby boom' which took place after World War II. With declining fertility rates, the older population is now growing in all three countries (Figure 1).

The relative size of the old-old population has grown much more rapidly than the young-old in the UK since 1971. The same trend is now becoming apparent in Canada. Shu et al. (1994, p. 8) have also noted a similar trend in Australia for the old-old, albeit with slightly different age categories: 'In 1992 there were 164 000 persons aged 80 years and older compared with 71 300 persons in 1972, an increase of 130 per cent.'

In all three countries, hidden within these aggregate figures are important differences in the population of older males compared with older females. The male to female sex ratios in the population aged 65 and over are 723 males per 1000 females in Canada, 746 males per 1000

females in Australia and 668 males per 1000 females in the UK (based on Table 1). In the population aged 75 and over this difference is even more apparent. In Canada, the sex ratio for the population aged 75 and over is 602 males per 1000 females, in Australia the ratio is 595 males per 1000 females and in the UK, the ratio is 515 males per 1000 females. The differences in the sex ratios mainly reflect the differences in life expectancy between men and women in the three countries.

Another way of thinking about the older population in demographic terms is to examine dependency ratios. A dependency ratio is a measure of the size of an age cohort compared to the size of the working age population (persons aged 15 to 64). The 'old component' of the dependency ratio or the 'older population dependency ratio' is found by dividing the population aged 65 and over by the working age population and multiplying by 100. Higher dependency ratios are crude indicators of the potential difficulty societies will have because of the relative lack of a working age population and al that this entails for income generation and the provision of formal and informal support. Using information from Table 1, the older population's dependency ratio for Canada is about 16%, for Australia it is about 17% and for the UK it is about 25%.

The distribution of older people may vary considerably among communities in each country. Just prior to retirement, on retirement, or as the result of a life course change (e.g. the death of a spouse), many older people relocate. The result is that in some parts of Canada, Australia and the UK, the percentage of the o der population will be well above, while in other parts the percentages will be below, the figures given above.

In Canada, in the areas surrounding Victoria and Vancouver, in the Okanagan Valley of British Columbia and around Niagara-on-the-Lake and Kingston in Ontario, there has been unprece-

dented growth in older populations as the result of immigration (Moore et al., 1989). In Australia, the Gold and Sunshine Coasts of Queensland and northern New South Wales have been the recipients of older people seeking high-amenity retirement locations (Maher, 1993), while other older people have moved inland seeking other locational needs (Drysdale, 1991). In the UK, the older population is increasingly concentrating in coastal areas in the southwest and southeast and 'selected attractive rural areas' in other parts of England and Scotland (Rees, 1992).

While the migration of the older population to high-amenity, recreational areas has received considerable attention because of the impact it is having on the receiving communities, the great majority of the older population age in place. In the future, the relative size of the older population in most communities is likely to depend most on

Table 2

The demography of disability in Canada, Australia and Great Britain

		% of population 65 to 74	% of population 75+
Canada[a]			
• With disabilities	M	35.8	53.0
	F	35.9	58.1
• With severe disabilities	M	5.7	16.8
	F	6.6	22.2
Australia[b]			
• With severe handicaps	M	9.5	20.8
	F	11.4	38.1
Great Britain[c]			
• With a longstanding illness	M	61.0	40.0
	F	55.0	34.0
• With a limiting longstanding illness	M	63.0	46.0
	F	65.0	51.0

[a] Based on Statistics Canada (n.d.). Unpublished data from the 1991 Health and Activity Limitations Survey.
[b] Based on the Australian Institute of Health (1990), p. 21.
[c] Based on Thomas et al. (1994), p. 31.

the size of the current working age population. In some places the relative size of the older population is growing as a result of the outmigration of young, working age persons, as in southern Saskatchewan and Manitoba in Canada (Moore *et al.*, 1989).

Ageing and Disability

Linked to these basic demographic measures are measures of disability (see also Sections C and D). With the growth in the older population, governments in all three countries have become increasingly interested in the health status of their older citizens. Surveys have been carried out in all three countries to measure the size of the population who live disability-free, and those with disabilities but who live independently within the community or in institutional settings (see Section D). In these surveys, disability is determined through self-assessment in response to a series of questions

reflecting the World Health Organization's definition of the 'continuum of disability'.

In Canada, about 1.2 million older people living in households reported disabling conditions in 1991 (Health and Activity Limitations Survey (HALS), 1991, unpublished data) (see Chapter 22). The proportion of older females with disabilities is greater than the proportion of older males; the difference between the sexes increases with age (Table 2 and Figure 2).

The severity and number of disabilities largely determine an individual's ability to live independently. There are distinctly different severity profiles between people living in households and those living in institutions (see Chapter 24 and Section F). Among the older population living in households, 40% had disabilities categorized as mild, 35% as moderate and 25% as severe. In the institutional population, only 10% were mildly disabled, 17% were moderately disabled,

Figure 2   Disability rates compared by age and sex, Canada, 1991.
Source: 1991 HALS unpublished data, adults residing in households only.

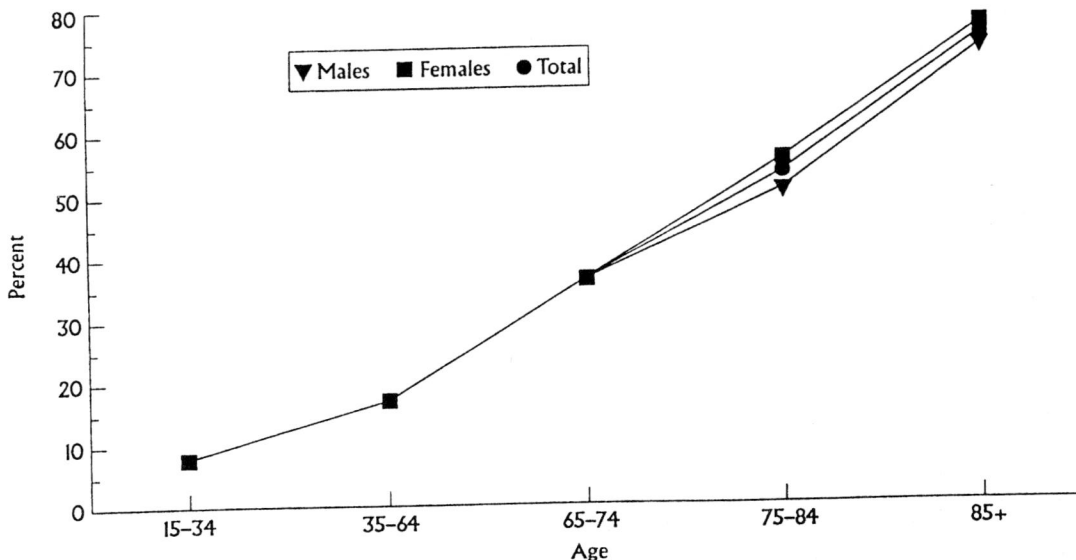

while 73% were severely disabled (HALS, 1991, unpublished data).

Among the Canadian older population living in households, the most likely disabilities to be reported are mobility, followed by agility, then hearing, seeing and speaking (Chapters 22, 23; see also Section F). Multiple disabilities are much higher among the older population and a very high proportion of those with multiple disabilities are mobility disabled, which means that access to services can often be a problem. Among the older population living in households, the average number of disabilities reported by those aged 65 to 74 was 1.87 (Chapter 11; see also Section F). The average number of disabilities increases to 2.19 among those between the ages of 75 and 84 and then to 2.72 among those 85 and over (calculated from Dunn, 1990, p. 9).

Slightly more than half of older Canadians with disabilities living in households were married in 1986, almost 38% were widowed and the remainder were separated, divorced or never married. Almost 81% of this group reported total annual incomes of less than Can $15 000 (HALS, 1986).

In comparison, 63.2% of all adults and 57.2% of all older people were married in 1991, while 6.2% of all adults and 32.5% of older people were divorced (Norland, 1994, p. 22). Only 46.9% of all adults and 59.4% of all older people reported incomes of less than Can $15 000 in 1991 (Norland, 1994, p. 44).

In Australia, the most comprehensive picture of disability comes from the 1988 Disabled and Aged Persons Survey. In this survey, a distinction is made between disabled persons and handicapped persons:

> A disabled person is defined as a person who has one or more of a group of selected impairments and disabilities which have lasted or are likely to last, for six months or more . . . A handicapped person is defined as a disabled person aged 5 years or over who is limited to some degree in his/her ability to perform certain tasks in relation to one or more of the following five areas:
>
> - self care
> - mobility
> - verbal communication
> - schooling
> - employment
>
> (Australian Institute of Health, 1990, p. 20).

Figure 3 Prevalence of severe handicap by age and sex, Australia, 1988. Source: Australian Institute of Health (1990), p. 21.

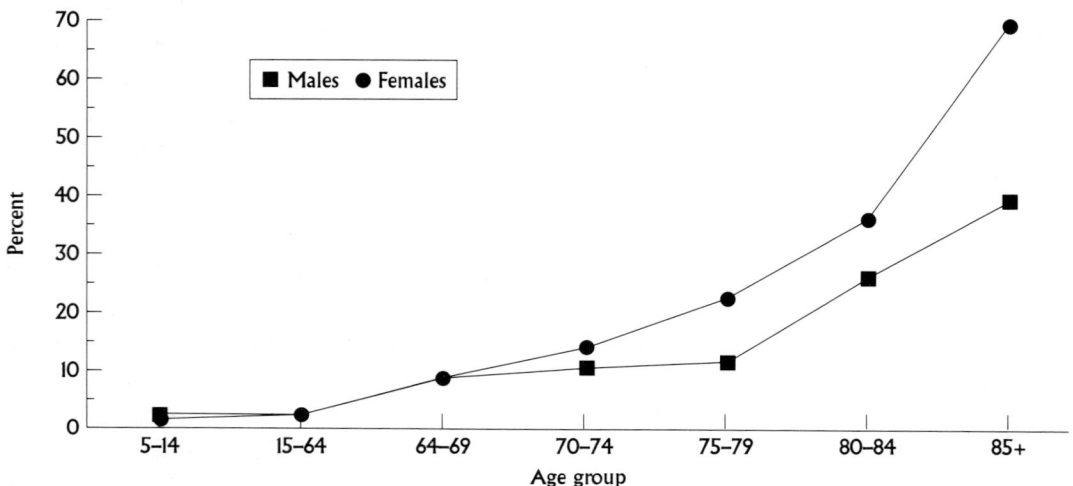

In the age group 65 to 74, almost 10% of males and 11.4% of females reported having severe handicaps (Table 2), while in those 75 years and over, the percentages increase to slightly over 20% for males and 38% for females. Figure 3 shows that the prevalence of severe handicap increases with age and increases more rapidly for females than males (see Chapter 22).

In the 1988 Australian survey, *disabling conditions* are reported in contrast to the Canadian practice of reporting *disabilities*. The five most prevalent disabling conditions were circulatory diseases (Chapter 6), hearing loss, musculoskeletal diseases (Chapter 6), sight loss and mental disorders (Chapter 8). Rates increase with age and generally female rates are higher than male rates (Australian Institute of Health, 1990, p. 219).

In the UK, the older population with disabilities can be examined in a limited way through the General Household Survey (GHS). The GHS is an annual survey of a sample of individuals living in households in Great Britain. Within the GHS chronic sickness is distinguished from acute sickness, and a distinction is also made between longstanding illnesses that do or do not limit activities in any way.

As in Canada and Australia, the young-old and the old-old both report much higher rates of longstanding illness and limiting longstanding illness than the total population, although the old-old report lower rates than the young-old. In contrast to Canada and Australia, in Great Britain the higher rates for older females are only seen among the old-old (Table 2).

While the trend over time shows an increase in the percentage of the older population with a longstanding illness, the percentage of the older population with a limiting longstanding illness has decreased (Thomas *et al.*, 1994, p. 31). A

possible interpretation of these findings is that with a growing older population, more individuals are likely to report a longstanding illness, but the young-old in each time period are likely to have improved overall health as the result of the improving socioeconomic conditions under which they live.

The UK 1991 Census shows that only a very small percentage of the older population live in communal establishments (Charlton *et al.*, 1994); most of those who do indicated that they have long-term illnesses. Although based on slightly different age cohorts, definitions of establishments, and long-term illness, these findings can be compared with those in Canada where a much higher percentage of the older population live in institutional settings, although the rates of disability are similar to those in Great Britain.

For a 65-year-old male in Canada in 1986, life expectancy was 14.9 years and for 8.1 years of this period he could expect to live disability-free (Wilkins and Adams, 1992, p. 60). The comparable numbers for a 65-year-old male living in Australia in 1988 were 14.8 years and 8.0 years, respectively (Australian Institute of Health, 1990, p. 214). A 65-year-old female in Canada in 1986 had a life expectancy of 19.2 years, of which she could expect to live 9.4 years disability-free (Wilkins and Adams, 1992, p. 60). The comparable numbers for a 65-year-old female in Australia in 1988 were 18.7 years and 9.6 years, respectively (Australian Institute of Health, 1990, p. 214).

A slightly different measure is used to compare disability-free life expectancy between Canada and the UK. A male born in Canada in 1986 would have a total life expectancy of 73.0 years, of which 61.3 years would be disability-free (Wilkins and Adams, 1992, p. 60). A male born in England or Wales in 1985 would have a total life expectancy of 71.8 years, of which 58.7 years would be disability-free (Bebbington, 1988, as cited in van Ginneken *et al.*, 1992, p. 39). For a female born in Canada in 1986, total life expectancy would be 79.8 years, of which 64.9 years would be disability-free (Wilkins and Adams, 1992, p. 60), while for a female born in England or Wales in 1985, total life expectancy would be 77.7 years, of which 61.5 years would be disability-free (Bebbington, 1988, as cited in van Ginneken *et al.*, 1992, p. 39). These numbers indicate that the Canadian older population lives longer and with fewer years of disability than the Australian older population. In contrast, the Canadian older population lives longer but with more years of disability compared to the older population in the UK.

Future Trends

The analysis of life expectancy is also a good place to start an examination of future trends. Life expectancy in all three countries has been increasing since the end of World War II as the result of a complex combination of socioeconomic, medical and environmental improvements. While there is an ongoing debate about whether the rate of increase in life expectancy is now beginning to slow and whether there is a limit on life expectancy, Table 3 shows that between 1981 and 1990, life expectancy continued to increase in all three countries, and that, although the life expectancy of females is greater than that of males, the difference appears to be decreasing. Those born in 1990 can expect to live until somewhere around 2065 or 2070 if they experience today's age-specific mortality during their lifetimes.

How large will the older population be in the next century? In all three countries, population projections are made on the basis of assumptions about fertility, mortality and net migration (immigration minus emigration). Projections based on low fertility, low net migration and constant mortality assumptions that have the effect of accentuating the growth of the older population relative to the young and working age populations appear to be most likely.

By 2031 under these assumptions, the population of Canada is projected to be about 28.4 million, of whom 7.8 million or about 27% will be 65 years of age or older and 3.7 million or about 13% will be above 75 years of age. The size of the older population will grow almost 150% and the old-old population will grow almost 190% between 1991 and 2031 (Figure 4). The increase in the

Table 3

Life expectancy in Canada, Australia and the UK (1981 and 1990 compared)

Life expectancy in years		Canada		Australia		UK	
		1981	1990	1981	1990	1981	1990
At birth	M	71.9	73.8	71.4	73.9	70.8	73.0
	F	79.1	80.4	78.4	80.0	76.8	78.5
At age 60	M	18.0	18.9	17.3	18.8	16.3	17.5
	F	22.9	23.7	22.1	23.1	20.8	21.8
At age 80	M	6.9	7.1	6.3	6.8	5.7	6.2
	F	8.8	9.3	8.1	8.6	7.5	8.2

Source: OECD Health Data, version 1.5 (1993) as cited in Nair and Karim (1993).

number of older females will be greater than the increase in older males, especially in the over 75 group.

Assuming the 1991 rate of disability (Chapter 22) for the population aged 65 and over remains constant, in 2031 approximately 3 million older people in Canada are expected to report some form of disability, with 25% of these having a severe disability.

In Australia, the total population is expected to be about 23.3 million in 2031. Of this population, about 5.1 million or almost 27% will be aged 65 and over, and 2.4 million or 10% of the total population will be over 75. These projections represent a growth of almost 160% in the older population and 206% in the old-old group between 1991 and 2031. As in Canada, the increase in the number of older women, and especially in women aged 75 and over, will be even greater than in men. Using the disability rate of 40% of the population aged 60 to 84 as

a crude estimator of rates in the year 2031, over 2 million older Australians are likely to be disabled in 2031.

In the case of the UK, only population projections for England for the much shorter time period of 1989 to 2011 are available. In 2011, almost 8.2 million or 16.2% of the population are expected to be over 65 in England, 3.8 million or 7.5% of these over 75. The rate of growth in both these groups during this period is projected to be much slower than in Canada or Australia. Applying the rates of limiting longstanding illness in 1991 to the over 65 population in 2011, almost 3.5 million older people in England are expected to report limiting longstanding illnesses in 2011.

In all three countries the older population will make up a substantial and increasing proportion of the total population, especially in Canada and Australia, during the next century. Beyond this, even with improving socioeconomic conditions, health and diet, increasingly large numbers of

Figure 4   Future older populations in Canada, Australia and England. Sources: Canada — Perreault *et al.* (1990), Projection Series No. 1; Australia — Australian Bureau of Statistics (1990), Series D; England — Office of Population Censuses and Surveys (1991), Series PP3, No. 8.

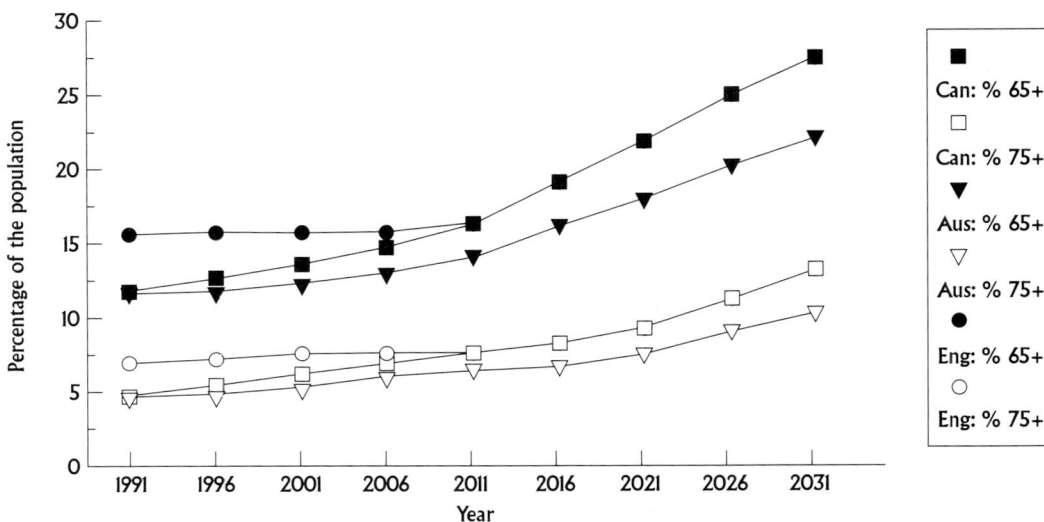

older people are likely to live at least part of their lives with disabling conditions that require health and social service interventions.

In summary, in all three countries, older people represent a growing proportion of the population. They are not uniformly distributed geographically, but concentrate in high-amenity recreational areas. The old-old part of the older population is growing more rapidly than the young-old. The proportion of older women is greater than the proportion of older men, and the older population's dependency ratio is increasing. The challenge will be to provide services that properly meet their needs.

References

Australian Bureau of Statistics (1990) Projections of the Populations of Australia, States and Territories 1989 to 2031, 127 pp. Canberra: Commonwealth Government Printer.

Australian Institute of Health (1990) Australia's Health 1990, 291 pp. Canberra: Australian Government Publishing Service.

Bebbington, AC (1988) The expectation of life without disability in England and Wales. Social Science and Medicine 27: 321–326.

Central Statistical Office (1994) Annual Abstract of Statistics. London: HMSO.

Charlton, J, Wallace, M, White, I (1994) Long-term illness: results from the 1991 Census. Population Trends 75: 18–25.

Drysdale, R (1991) Aged migration to coastal and inland centres in NSW. Australian Geographical Studies 29: 268–284.

Dunn, PA (1990) Barriers Confronting Seniors with Disabilities in Canada, 33 pp. Ottawa: Minister of Supply and Services.

Maher, C (1993) Recent trends in Australian urban development: locational change and policy quandary. Urban Studies 30: 791–825.

McCracken, KWJ (1985) Disaggregating the elderly. Australian Geographer 16: 218–224.

Moore, EG, Rosenberg, MW, Bekkering, MH (1989) Atlases of the Elderly Population of Canada. Kingston, Canada: Department of Geography, Queen's University.

Nair, C, Karim, R (1993) An overview of health care systems: Canada and selected OECD countries. Health Reports 5: 259–279.

Norland, JA (1994) Profile of Canada's Seniors, 112 pp. Ottawa: Statistics Canada.

Office of Population Censuses and Surveys (1991) 1989-based Sub-National Population Projections, 117 pp. London: HMSO.

Perreault, J, Declos, M, Costa, R, Larrivée, D, Loh, S (1990) Population Projections for Canada, Provinces and Territories 1989–2011, 192 pp. Ottawa: Statistics Canada.

Rees, P (1992) Elderly migration and population redistribution in the United Kingdom. In Rogers, A (ed.) Elderly Migration and Population Redistribution, pp. 203–225. London: Bellhaven Press.

Shu, J, Khoo, SE, Struik, A, McKenzie, F (1994) Australia's Population Trends and Prospects 1993, 111 pp. Canberra: Australian Government Publishing Service.

Statistics Canada (1993) 1991 Census of Canada. Ottawa: Canadian Government Publishing Centre.

Thomas, M, Goddard, E, Hickman, M, Hunter, P (1994) General Household Survey 1992, 207 pp. London: HMSO.

van Ginneken, JKS, Dissevelt, AG, Bonte, JTP (1992) Summary of results of calculation of life expectancy free of disability in the Netherlands in 1981–85. In Robine, J-M, Blanchet, M, Dowd, JE (eds) Health Expectancy: First Workshop of the International Healthy Life Expectancy Network (REVES), pp. 35–40. London: HMSO.

Wilkins, R, Adams, O (1992) Health expectancy in Canada, 1986. In Robine, J-M, Blanchet, M, Dowd, JE (eds) Health Expectancy: First Workshop of the International Healthy Life Expectancy Network (REVES), pp. 57–60. London: HMSO.

3

Attitudes Towards Ageing and Older People

MICHELLE SHILTON

Introduction

Attitudes are universal. They pervade all aspects of our daily lives. They influence the simplest decisions and our most complex behaviours. 'Do you agree with the political stand of your governing party?' 'How do you feel about the state of our environment?' 'Do you enjoy football or hockey?' 'Do you like coffee or tea?' As physiotherapists, our attitudes will shape our patient interactions, choice of treatment and ultimately, our daily practice when working with older people.

This chapter will begin with a definition of 'attitude' and a description of the theories of attitude development. Throughout our lifetime each of us will undergo role changes. The issues related to role transitions for the older adult will be reviewed with respect to their impact on the individual and their familial relations. Factors that have an influence on attitude formation will be considered and several programmes that have been developed to promote attitudinal change will be examined. Finally, the impact on social policies and our professional organizations will be discussed (see also Chapters 8, 11, 27 and Section F).

Defining Attitudes

In 1935 Gordon W Allport, a social psychologist, provided the following definition:

> An attitude is a mental or neural state of readiness, organized through experience, exerting a directive or dynamic influence upon the individual's response to all objects and situations with which it is related.

In a review of this definition Rajecki (1990) noted first, that attitudes reside in the personal experiences of the individual and we cannot directly experience the attitudes of another individual. Second, individuals are not born with a pre-existing set of attitudes, but rather acquire them through experience and direct and indirect interactions. For health care professionals such interactions include clinical placements, academic education and the opinions of others. Third, attitudes motivate us into action and influence us to do things in an orderly fashion. For example, Mr Jones is interested in Alzheimer's disease because his wife has this condition. As a result, it is not hard to imagine him volunteering to work with these patients, raising donations for research on Alzheimer's disease or starting a support group for spouses. Each of these situations is different, but is based upon a single positive attitude toward the treatment of patients with Alzheimer's disease.

Three Components of Attitudes

The most common definitions of attitudes attempt to combine cognitive, affective and behavioural components. Attitudes may be positive, negative or neutral (Rajecki, 1990; Worchel *et al.*, 1991).

The cognitive component consists of all the thoughts that the person has about a particular object in relation to society. For example, if we consider the issue of smoking, some of the cognitive elements might be the taste and smell of a cigarette as well as thoughts about treating those patients who smoke. Other elements might be impersonal such as the workplace regulations on smoking.

The affective or evaluative component consists of all the emotions that a person expresses toward an object. These may be positive, negative or neutral. Elder abuse, institutionalization of the elderly, long-term care reform and the provision of services for the elderly will evoke varying emotions.

The behavioural component consists of a person's response or readiness to respond to that object. For instance, an elderly gentleman may write to a local politician in response to the government's proposed decrease in the old age pension.

Negative attitudes include stereotyping, prejudice and discrimination. Stereotyping, the cognitive component, consists of beliefs about the typical characteristics of members of a particular group. For instance, stereotyping characterizes older adults as slow, feeble-minded and white-haired. Prejudice is the affective component. It is the evaluation of an individual based on their group membership and is exhibited when members of one group (the ingroup) hold negative attitudes towards members of another group (the outgroup). Negative beliefs or prejudgement based on ethnicity or race are examples of prejudice. Discrimination is the overt behaviour or actions resulting from stereotyping and prejudice. Racial slurs, jokes based on age and ethnicity are examples of discriminatory behaviour.

Theories of Attitude Development

Our attitudes are formed early in life. Our parents serve as important forces in their development. Through information sharing, new concepts are integrated or assimilated with existing knowledge. For instance, children who learn from their parents that the elderly are slow and forgetful will likely attempt to integrate this information into their developing opinion of the older people they have encountered. Later, parental influences are supplemented by those of teachers, peers, friends and relatives, all serving as reference groups against which personal attitudes and values are compared.

Attitudes have been studied through three principal frameworks. They include the learning, cognitive and behavioural theories (Chapters 8 and 11).

Learning theorists believe that attitudes are a learned response. Basically, if a behaviour occurs in a particular situation, and is given positive reinforcement, it is likely to be repeated. This is known as classical conditioning. For instance, if teenagers who volunteer at a retirement home are given praise or rewards by their parents and the community, they are more likely to volunteer again. Hence, learning theorists believe that attitude formation is based upon the sum of all of the positive and negative associations that have been gathered. The strength of an attitude will vary according to the number of positive and negative responses that it evokes as well as its importance to the individual.

Cognitive theories of attitudes include the balance and cognitive dissonance theories. The basic premise behind the balance theory is one's desire for coherence and meaning. This system is usually based on (1) the first person's evaluation of the other person; (2) the first person's evaluation of the object; and (3) the other person's evaluation of the object. The assumption underlying this theory is that each individual holds several beliefs and attitudes, and will strive to maintain a consistency among those beliefs.

This theory can be used to determine whether an interpersonal system is balanced. For instance, if John and Edith hold the same opinion toward a retirement residence, then the system is balanced. If they do not share the same attitude, the system becomes imbalanced and a motivational force to restore balance is established. For example, suppose John is helping Edith look for residence at his retirement home. Edith likes John but dislikes his selection of residence. The inconsistency is that we expect people similar to ourselves to hold the same opinions. The other assumption is that an imbalanced system will attempt to restore balance, through a change in attitudes or by some cognitive distortion. In this instance, Edith might decide she really dislikes both John and the retirement home or she might attempt to alter the information and perceive that John is not very happy with his current residence after all.

The cognitive dissonance theory examines attitude—behaviour inconsistency — the effects of making decisions or engaging in behaviour that is inconsistent with one's attitude. For example, Ken is a physiotherapist who dislikes working with elderly patients. Upon graduation, he takes a job in a nursing home. Ken's behaviour is inconsistent with his attitude. In order to restore harmony, Ken has two courses of action: (1) he can identify all the positive qualities of the job; or (2) he can quit the job. Therefore, cognitive dissonance theory espouses the belief that a tension results from inconsistencies between attitude and behaviour. This can be resolved by either a change in cognition or behaviour.

Behaviourists have criticized the cognitive theories of attitude, particularly the cognitive dissonance theory, because the theories are not measurable or directly observable states. The self-perception theory claims that individuals will often look to external environmental forces to explain their behaviour, and in the absence of such forces, the behaviour is thought to be a true reflection of their attitude. For example, Donald was trying to decide whether to sell his home and enter a retirement residence. If his daughters were present when he made the decision, he may conclude that they forced or coerced his decision. His behaviour (moving to the residence) can be explained by external forces and may not be a true reflection of his attitude. However, if he made the decision on his own, without family members present, he may conclude that he really wants to move to the residence.

Behaviour and Attitude Change

Attitudes serve as powerful energizers for behaviour. Frequently, the assumption is made that attitudes provide accurate indicators for our actions. To a significant extent, however, this assumption has not been supported in the literature; many studies have revealed a limited correlation between expressed attitudes and behaviour (Worchel *et al.*, 1991). Various researchers have attempted to resolve this matter by suggesting that behaviour is a function of at least two attitudes – those toward the object and those toward the situation.

A further refinement of the complex relationship between attitude and behaviour suggests that our attitudes influence our overall response to the object, but do not predict a specific behaviour pattern. The behavioural intentions that underlie our actions are shaped by three factors: our attitude toward the action; the belief others have about us performing the action; and our motivation to comply with these beliefs.

The Process of Attitude Change

Attitude change involves three elements: the communicator, the message and the recipient of the message (Worchel *et al.*, 1991). The communicator's role is to convey the message. In an attempt to change an attitude, a highly credible source is preferable to someone with little or no credibility. Traits such as expertise and trustworthiness have been found in effective communicators. These are evidenced by the individual's level of education, social status and professional attainment. It is helpful if the speaker possesses similar characteristics to those of the message recipient. Multiple sources each conveying the same message can be helpful.

Central to the process is the message. If the communicator wishes to encourage an attitude change, it is necessary to convey the idea in a form that can be readily transmitted. The more details the message includes, the more the listener will assume that the speaker knows what he or she is talking about. Pleasurable emotions can enhance the effectiveness of communications, while those associated with fear may be effective if the fear is not unmanageable or if the audience is taught how to reduce the fear. The effectiveness of one- or two-sided communication will vary according to the target. One-sided communication has been shown to be effective if the audience already agrees with or supports the message, whereas if the audience is well informed or opposed to the message, two-sided communication will be more useful. Finally, the personal characteristics of the recipient will influence the effects of any communication; factors such as persuasibility, gender and race all influence the process.

Attitudes Towards Older People: A Historical Perspective

'Ageism' is a term that has been used to describe prejudice against an individual or group of individuals because of their age. It has been described as a 'deep seated uneasiness on the part of the young and middle-aged; a personal revulsion to distaste for growing old, disease, disability; and a fear of powerlessness, uselessness and death' (Butler, 1969). According to Guccione (1993) ageist attitudes foster beliefs about the capabilities, intelligence and physical skills of our elders; they support judgements about a person on the basis of age and negate the concept of the individual approach to patient care. Much of the history of attitudes towards the older adult is based upon the work of Binstock and Shanas (1985).

Perception of Age in Ancient Culture

In the Old Testament, a variety of positive images are presented about old age. Proverbs 16:31 says 'A hoary head is a crown of glory; it is gained in a righteous life'. Longevity was seen as a reward for prior service (Deuteronomy 4:40) and adherence to the commandments (Deuteronomy 5:33). Respect for age was also seen to govern parent–child relations: 'Honour your father and your mother as the Lord your God commands you' (Deuteronomy 5:16). However, not all the images presented are positive. Ecclesiastes (12:1–8) describes some of the physical manifestations of growing old: trembling arms, stooping legs, missing teeth, failing vision and swollen stomachs.

The ancient Greek myths provided similar points of view about ageing and old age. Throughout these ancient myths and folklore, there was a sense of vulnerability about the older adult. Acts of strength and victories were frequently ascribed to younger men. In fact, generational conflict frequently arose when elders did not make way for the younger generation. Once again, older adults were frequently portrayed as gruesome figures. Geras, the god who typified old age, was described as a dreadful monster, with wrinkles, thinning hair and an emaciated body.

Mediaeval literature and society are filled with both positive and negative images. Shakespeare has provided several conflicting images of old age. Doddering old women and foolish men are recurrent characters in his works. King Lear, a dispossessed father who is ill-treated by his heirs, serves as one example which illustrates the difficulties encountered by the elderly. Folk artists and painters of the time depicted power as the result of societal rank rather than the cumulative effects of a long life.

Modernization

Advances in science and technology in more recent times have resulted in a re-examination of old age. With improved living conditions, improved longevity and decreased mortality rates (Chapter 2), older adults should have held a uniquely beneficial position. Instead, they became the victims of a society that had begun to deny death and old age.

Older workers came to be viewed as less competent than their younger counterparts. As a result, a new practice of retiring after the attainment of a certain age was developed and represented to society that the older employee was less useful. Evaluations of cost and efficiency and the development of new technologies also helped to hasten the rapid departure of the older worker as younger workers were seen to be faster learners who were easier to train.

Ageism Today

Negative attitudes toward older people today can be found in both cultural and societal forces (Chapters 4 and 5, respectively). The words used to describe older adults provide a basis for the formation of ageist attitudes. Nussel (1982), who studied the language of ageing, found very few age-specific terms such as "mature', 'venerable' and 'veteran' that refer positively to older people. Most of the ageist terms are used to demean people according to age and gender. 'Biddy', 'granny' and 'hag' are used to describe older women. Similarly, 'coot', 'geezer' and 'codger' are used to describe older males. According to Guccione (1993), elders themselves are often guilty of ageism through their acceptance of these negative perceptions. The use of this negative terminology is more than a choice of words; it is a verbalization of negatively held beliefs which, if left over time, will become less offensive and more acceptable.

The media, which can reflect as well as shape society's views, have also had a strong impact on the images of the older adult. Older adults are given limited television roles and their representation is inconsistent with current day societal norms. Older adults are frequently portrayed as financially secure and in good health, except in commercials, where they are portrayed as deprived and suffering. During prime time viewing, elderly characters are seen as more comical, stubborn and foolish than the other characters. Older male characters are likely to appear as powerful, active and in productive roles. On the other hand, older females are given limited screen time and are frequently seen as useful assistants to the male characters.

Advertising on television and in magazines frequently denounce the signs of ageing. Commercial messages indicate that older adults are preoccupied with constipation, irregularity and incontinence. Younger adults are urged to erase any signs of ageing by 'washing away the grey' and using creams to 'soften tiny lines and wrinkles'.

Ageing: Personal and Family Perspectives

Personal Perspectives

During their lifetime, each person undergoes a series of role changes and developments. Pivotal transitions occur upon entering school and the workforce, marriage, parenthood, retirement and spousal death. Some of these transitions are voluntary, expected and planned for, as in marriage and parenthood. Others such as spousal death are unplanned, occur more suddenly, and as a result, are often more traumatic. Role transitions are based on chronological age and societal norms. Timing of these transitions varies slightly between individuals and societies.

Although it is impossible for us to experience directly these transitions and their impact on our elderly clients, Laurence (1964) has attempted to provide us with a personalized perspective. In her novel *The Stone Angel*, Hagar Shipley reminisces about her earlier years as she nears the end of her life. Three passages graphically depict reactions to some of the role changes faced by people as they age:

1. Hagar's feelings about a visit to her doctor's office with her daughter-in-law, Doris:

> Finally I'm called (into the office). Doris comes in as well, and speaks to Doctor Corby as though she'd left me at home.
> 'Her bowels haven't improved one bit . . . the other evening she threw up. She's fallen a lot – '
> And so on and so on . . . Why doesn't she let me tell him? Whose symptoms are they, anyhow?

2. Hagar's reaction to being supervized when her son and daughter-in-law wish to go out:

> 'We thought we might go to a movie', Doris says . . . 'I've asked the girl next door if she'll come in, in case there's anything you want. Is that okay?'
> (Hagar) stiffens. 'You think I need a sitter, like a child?'
> 'It's not that at all,' Doris says quickly. 'But what would happen if you fell, Mother . . .'
> 'I'm sorry if I tie you down,' (Hagar says). 'I'm sorry to be a – '

3. Hagar's feelings on being a hospital patient:

> This ward must have thirty beds or more. It's bedlam. I lie here on my slab of a bed, the sheet drawn under my chin, my belly like a hill of gelatine under the covers, quivering a little with each breath. My feet are stuck straight up to ward off cramps. I'm like an exhibition in a museum. Anyone may saunter past and pause to peer at me. Admission free.

A model of role transition for older adults has been developed that considers the individual's status prior to the role change; the components of the new role that are stress producing; the amount or degree to which the individual perceives the situation as stressful (degree of change, impact on current life routine); their response to stress (amount of social or familial support, type of coping methods); and the outcome or adjustment to the role change. The entire process is influenced by personal resources (personality, methods of coping) (Chapters 4, 8 and 11); socialization experiences and social status (marital status, gender, race and ethnicity).

The transition from middle age to old age has been depicted by many as a period of role loss or weakening. For the older adult, retirement, spousal death and a decrease in functional and/or financial independence often result in a loss of what was once a source of power, status and prestige. Older adults may be so conditioned to losing control, due in part to society's ageist attitudes, that they begin voluntarily to give up control over their lives, which results in even further role loss (Guccione, 1993).

The loss is further heightened by physical changes (Chapter 6). White hair, wrinkles, glasses, hearing aids and mobility devices are just some of the examples. The appearance of these age-related physical changes may generate some of the negative attitudes and behaviours associated with older people. Consequently, the older adult often begins to act 'old' because of society's expectations.

It is important for health care professionals to remember that the elderly are not a homogenous group. Differences in ethnicity (Chapter 4), social status, education, personality and life experiences serve to heighten the diversity within this group.

Family Perspectives

The family provides the basic unit of socialization throughout the life cycle. It transcends all emotional, social and economic spheres. Until recently, ageing research examined the older adult as an individual with little interest in their dynamic interactions as a family member during their lifetime.

With the increase in life expectancy, the appearance of three-, four- and five-generation families is not uncommon. Socially, the timing of these events has also been altered. People marry at an older age. There has been a decline in the number of children. The onset of empty-nesting and widowhood is occurring even later in life. Increased rates of divorce and separation combined with remarriage have resulted in reconstituted families. All of these have affected not only the individual and their familial structure, but also their relations across the life cycle. Role transitions for the older adult can involve a change in structure and dynamics of both nuclear and extended families. Thus the family has an important part to play in assisting their older adults in adjusting to their changing identities and status.

The parent–child relationship is one of most stable bonds within our society. This relationship can vary in frequency, type and quality, according to the needs of both individuals. During early childhood, the relationship s essentially unidirectional, with parents providing care, nurture and support for their dependent children. During adolescence, the relationship becomes more reciprocal and independent, and at times conflicts may occur between the generations based on differences in values and beliefs. When children leave home and develop nuclear families of their own, they begin to realize and understand the parental perspective. At this time, the nature of the interaction may vary according to the conflicting demands of work and family faced by the child. As parents grow older and their children enter middle adulthood, the relationship may

once again become unidirectional, with children providing care and assistance to their ageing parent. As children enter older adulthood many of them will continue to be responsible for the care and assistance of an ageing parent.

Most older adults continue to see their children on a regular basis. Primary contact with parents is frequently through the daughter. Geographic distance remains the primary factor which influences the frequency and nature of interactions between parents and their adult children. The second major influence is the health status of the older adult. With a decline in physical and functional independence, the relationship with the child changes to that of caregiver. For some children, it is an opportunity to give back or reward a parent for their years of nurturance. For others, it is a time to seek justice or revenge for past or perceived inequities.

Stressful transitions such as death of a spouse, illness or changes in financial status can result in intergenerational conflict (McPherson, 1990). These conflicts usually take one of three forms: (1) continuing conflict – this is a conflict that was present between the parent and child prior to the child's departure from home; (2) new conflict – this is a type of conflict that has not been previously experienced; and (3) reactivated conflict – this is conflict that was present during childhood and returns again in later life. Although role conflict occurs from time to time, most older adults report that their relationship with their children is satisfying and that their family remains a supportive environment for the provision of their physical and emotional needs.

Unlike most other familial roles, the role of grandparent is acquired involuntarily and may vary across families. The quality and type of interaction will vary according to several features, such as: residential proximity; the support and attitude of the parents toward the child–grandparent relationship; the lifestyle, personality and employment status of the grandparents; and the age of the grandchildren.

In recent years, the relationship of grandparents and grandchildren has been examined. Children who interact frequently with grandparents have fewer negative attitudes toward older people in general. The relationship goes through similar role transitions to that of the children of older adults. Initially the grandparent is viewed as a babysitter or giftgiver, whereas in later years, the child often may come to view the grandparent as either a companion or someone for whom they are responsible.

Health care professionals should consider the older client holistically. This includes biological, psychological and social spheres. Within the social perspective, as well as within the context of their family, the older adult needs to be considered as an individual. For the older adult, advancing age is often seen as a time of role loss and fragmentation, during which time the family can play an integral part in maintaining the health and emotional well-being of their older relative. However, the presence of intergenerational conflict and ageist attitudes may serve to impact negatively on the process. For the physiotherapist, the family can be an important source of information on the care needs of the client, as they are frequently involved in the client's day to day management. Frequently, the family are called upon to assist in treatment interventions or to provide continuing support within the home environment. If they are to succeed, it is essential that the plan of care be developed through the collective and coordinated efforts of the physiotherapist, client and family.

Factors That Influence Attitudes of Health Care Professionals Towards Older People

The factors that influence the attitudes of health care professionals, including physiotherapists, towards older people include: age; ethnicity; relationship with grandparents; educational level; prior experience with older people; academic education; clinical education; and the work environment. Other factors, such as gender, social class and marital status, produce inconsistent results (see also Chapters 3, 23 and Section F).

Age

The age of the health care provider has been found to be a significant determinant of attitude and willingness to work with older clients. Brower (1985) analysed the relationship between age, educational level and the degree of exposure to elders in four work environments and found that age was a significant variable, but only when coupled with the work setting. Older nurses who worked in nursing homes had more favourable attitudes toward the elderly than younger nurses or older nurses who worked in other settings (see Chapter 24 and Section F).

Ethnicity

Health care providers who are members of minority ethnic groups (such as Asian, Hispanic or Italian) have been shown to have more positive attitudes towards older people. Shimamoto and Rose (1987) (Chapter 4) examined the attitudes of 188 nursing students at the University of Hawaii. They found that only 50% of the Caucasians were interested in gerontology, in comparison to 71% of the non-Caucasians (Pacific–Asians). This interest may well be a reflection of the greater reverence for the aged found in Pacific–Asian culture. This trend was also found by Feldbaum and Feldbaum (1981) in their study of Asian and Hispanic students.

Relationship with Grandparents

Shimamoto and Rose (1987) reported that having had a positive personal experience with an older person, such as a grandparent, also correlated with an interest in working with older adults.

Educational Level

Brower (1985) found that higher professional educational levels such as a bachelor's or master's degree were associated with more favourable attitudes towards older people.

Prior Experience with Older People

Coren et al. (1987) conducted a survey with master's-level physiotherapy students, from which they concluded that previous experiences such as a job, volunteer work, course work or clinical placements with older people all increased the likelihood of a decision to work with the elderly.

Academic Education

Attitude formation in health care professionals is influenced by the academic or educational environment. Collins and Brown (1989) suggested that negative attitudes to gerontology and working with older clients exist for several reasons. First of all, most curricula remain weak in this area with few programmes allocating enough time to this specialty. Second, as this is a new area, there are very few faculty, researchers or clinicians trained in gerontological content and who are able to provide a positive role model. In practical classes, students are frequently assigned to older, more chronic patients and as a result, they often feel overwhelmed by their complexity. Consequently, as new graduates, they will often choose to work in specialty areas where their educational preparation has been more complete and more positive.

Clinical Education

Clinical placements and internships in a specialty area can help to improve interest levels. Clinical placements result in more positive attitudes when the exposure occurs early in clinical training. Attitudinal changes have been more apparent in junior level rather than senior level students. Exposure to well elderly clients as opposed to chronic and complex patients can result in more positive attitudinal change. The type of placement can also have an influence on students' attitudes; students who work in an ambulatory care wing or nursing home setting show less favourable attitudes than classmates who work with older people in a home care programme. Finally, the presence of positive supervising physiotherapists who can act as role models remains essential.

Work Environment

The type of work environment has a strong influence on attitudes towards older people. Health care professionals who work in home care (Section F) or a hospital tend to have more favourable attitudes than those employed in nursing homes (Chapter 24 and Section F) or other chronic care facilities. The type of client can also influence attitudes. Brower (1985) found that staff who worked with older patients who had multiple physical and/or emotional problems tended to have more negative attitudes. Conversely, those who worked with healthy older people were generally found to have strongly positive attitudes. The presence of staff members with positive attitudes who can act as a support or mentor to a new graduate has been linked with high job satisfaction. Occupational therapy students considered work in geriatrics in situations where they felt that they were effective in their treatment, and that the care setting philosophy was consistent with their own personal values. Less important reasons cited were employment availability, salaries, the opportunity for advancement into supervisory or administrative areas and the availability of part-time work.

Attitudes of Health Care Professionals

A critical review of the research examining attitudes of health care professionals has revealed several studies that demonstrate negative attitudes toward providing care for the older adult (Feldbaum and Feldbaum, 1981) (see Section F). In general, the findings illustrate a reluctance to work with older people, and the perception of such negative characteristics as isolation, loneliness, irritability and anger as being associated with the older adult. Others have demonstrated that health professionals set less aggressive treatment goals for their older patients in order that they can spend less time in direct patient care. Among new graduates, geriatric care is frequently found to be the least favoured specialty, with this trend being mirrored across the health disciplines (Coren *et al.*, 1987). Some health care professionals view older people as less physically

capable and, when combined with the functional impairments of a stroke or fracture, they are often seen as having even less potential for improvement. It is a matter of special concern that those charged with the responsibility for care hold such negative attitudes.

It is essential that health care professionals look at the older adult as a person, who deserves to be treated with dignity and respect. Health care professionals need to view each client as an individual first, regardless of their physical and mental impairments (Guccione, 1993). Some physiotherapists get caught in the trap of viewing clients according to their disabilities – the 'stroke' or the 'fracture'. They may be so concerned as to whether the older adult is ambulatory or wheelchair-bound; cognitively intact or impaired; or whether they live independently or reside in a nursing home, that they forget about the person who is seeking care. All of our client interactions need to be governed by dignity and respect. Respect implies giving our older people the opportunity to participate in the decision-making processes surrounding their treatment, irrespective of their chronological age.

Programmes to Promote Attitudinal Change

Several workers have attempted to modify the attitudes of these health care professionals towards older people through various programmes and educational strategies; these programmes have produced mixed results.

Huber *et al.* (1992) studied staff attitudes and knowledge about ageing before and after attendance at three formal educational sessions. All the participants were involved in direct patient contact, including staff from physiotherapy, nursing, recreation, administration, housekeeping and dietary services. The educational programme included three 1-hour classes consisting of a simulation of handicaps, normal age-related changes and myths and realities of ageing. Overall, the results showed a significant increase in knowledge scores from pre-test to post-test. Upon completion of the study, an improvement in attitude towards older people was noted; however, a slightly negative attitude continued to exist among the participants. This study demonstrates that continuing education programmes can be used to improve attitudes.

Role playing exercises have been used to develop effective therapeutic behaviours. Brown *et al.* (1992) developed a mock geriatric clinic to assist physiotherapy students to develop positive behaviours. During their regular clerkship programme, students spent three 4-hour sessions in the mock clinic. Within each session the students had a 30-minute orientation to the clinic. The next 2.5 hours were spent treating patients. Each student had contact with three elderly volunteer patients. Each student simulated the role of student-therapist and student-Clinical Instructor (CI). During session one, one student was the student-therapist while their partner was the student-CI. In session two, the roles were reversed. In the third session, the students saw patients independently. Feedback was given during the last hour of each session. The authors claimed that the orientation allowed students to discuss their feelings in an honest and non-threatening manner. The clinic allowed the students access to patients in a controlled setting while at the same time allowing them to solve problems during difficult patient interactions. The debriefing session allowed for feedback and reinforcement about treatment skills. Brown *et al.* (1992)

believed that each of these components had contributed to the success of the experience. The impact of the change over time was not examined.

Games and simulations may also be effective in changing attitudes. The game 'Into Ageing' allows the individual to step into the ageing role. Players begin at the identity table where they select an age, lifestyle and identity. Sensory deficits are simulated using ear plugs and eye patches. Physical impairments can be simulated with weighted limbs. Throughout the game, the players experience role losses through dependency and restraint (Samter and Voss, 1992). More formalized studies are indicated to evaluate their effectiveness.

Gillis (1991) suggested that role modelling can also be used to improve clinical expertise and problem solving. Grand rounds, patient conferences and regular inservice training may also provide physiotherapists with an opportunity for support in which to gain new skills.

Smith and Wattis (1989) examined the attitudes of two cohorts of medical students at Nottingham University during the years 1983–84 and 1986–87. They used a before–after type of design methodology. They hypothesized that: (1) attitudes toward the older adult would remain stable over time; (2) attitudes toward their medical care for older people would change positively; and (3) the likelihood of considering a career in geriatric psychiatry or geriatrics would increase after a 1-month placement on these services. Using the Rosencrantz–McNevin semantic differential scale to measure attitudes, the authors found no significant changes in attitudes, although knowledge scores about the ageing process showed statistically significant improvements. A questionnaire on career aspirations was also administered to the students. The 1983–84 group had 8 students at the beginning of the study expressing a 'definitely interested' or 'ranks high' response about working with geriatrics, compared to 11 students at the completion of the study. For the 1986–87 cohort this went from 1 to 9 students for the same period.

Currently, a large number of programmes to promote attitude change are in existence. Role playing, games, and educational sessions have all been attempted with varying success. More long-term programmes are needed as well as follow-up studies to determine the consistency of attitudinal changes over time. In addition, the relationship between attitudinal change and its impact on the behaviour of the health professional requires further research.

Attitudes and Social Policy

With the growth of our ageing population, the social and political structure has changed. Senior citizens have become better informed about their needs and concerns, and are more active in the development of policies to address those needs (see also Chapter 5). As a result, governments at the local, provincial and federal levels are now responsible for the development and administration of policies directed specifically for the elderly in such areas as social services, recreation, health, and housing among others (Chapter 24).

It is beyond the scope of this chapter to address all of the policies directed towards our older adults. Therefore, the following sections will examine some of the issues associated with the development and implementation of social policy related to our ageing population. This information is drawn from the research of McPherson (1990) and Marshall (1980).

Underlying the development of public policies for the aged is an ongoing debate as to whether the individual or society is ultimately responsible to meet the needs of the elderly. Some central issues are (1) how should resources be rationed; (2) who should be responsible for the allocation of resources; and (3) how scarce resources should be allocated. Clearly the issues related to the development of social policy remain complex with no easy answers. Variability in policy implementation will be affected by political, economical and social influences.

As we have seen, our ageing population is a heterogenous group with diversified needs. As a result, policy development must attempt to address some of these needs. One of the major challenges of policymakers is to encourage older adults to take responsibility for their own care needs; to integrate services to meet these needs and to provide a continuum of services for the older client throughout their lifetime. Part of the problem with the current system is that older people often lack the knowledge of the availability of existing services, or they are unable to gain access to a specific service due to financial or environmental barriers. For other programmes there are often long waiting lists or stringent programme requirements. Where policies do exist, the problem is often one of inadequate service delivery. Policymakers are also continuing to address some of the other inequities within the system. The effects of social class, ethnicity and race have been shown to further compound and heighten the inequality within the system.

Our growing elderly population has resulted in changes in social policy related to the elderly. As attitudes change there is a growing concern for the patients' rights. More than ever before, physiotherapists are charged with the responsibility of informing patients of their rights. The medical arena is shifting away from a paternalistic role to giving patients more responsibility and freedom to direct their care. For the older adult, who grew up with the traditional type of care, this new role is often disconcerting and even threatening. Our older clients are consumers of health care. As physiotherapists, it is our responsibility to provide assistance in guiding these choices.

The Future

As the average age of the population continues to rise (Chapter 2), and the numbers of older adults continues to increase, there is a need to address the impact of changing societal structure. Health care professionals, policymakers, social scientists and researchers continue to be concerned about the lack of knowledge about the processes of ageing, needs of the aged and the ageist attitudes that pervade our society.

Knowledge about these issues must continue to grow if we are to meet the needs of our expanding ageing population. Our educational settings must strive to address some of the issues and care needs of our ageing clients through coursework at the undergraduate and post graduate levels. Early exposure to the older adult through clinical placements is needed to dispel some of the negative attitudes and stereotypes as well as to illuminate the rehabilitation potential of this group of individuals. Professional associations need to heighten awareness of the difficulties created by ageist attitudes. Beyond this, ongoing research in the area of ageism, as well as programmes to promote more positive attitudes, continue to be required.

Acknowledgements

This research was funded by the Physiotherapy Foundation of Canada and the Education Centre for Aging and Health at McMaster University.

References

Binstock, RH, Shanas, E (1985) *Handbook of Aging and the Social Sciences*, 809 pp. New York: Van Nostrand Reinhold Company.

Brower, HT (1985) Do nurses stereotype the aged? *Journal of Gerontological Nursing* 11: 17–20, 26–28.

Brown, DS, Gardner, DL, Perritt, L, Kelly, DG (1992) Improvement in attitudes toward the elderly following traditional and geriatric mock clinics for physical therapy students. *Physical Therapy* 72: 251–259.

Butler, R (1969) Ageism: another form of bigotry. *The Gerontologist* 9: 243–246.

Collins, DL, Brown, VM (1989) Learning to care about gerontological nursing. *Journal of Gerontological Nursing* 15: 8–14.

Coren, A, Andreassi, A, Blood, H, Kent, B (1987) Factors related to physical therapy students' decision to work with elderly patients. *Physical Therapy* 67: 60–65.

Feldbaum, E, Feldbaum, M (1981) Caring for the elderly: who dislikes it least? *Journal of Health Politics, Policy and Law* 5: 62–72.

Gillis, DM (1991) Strategies to promote positive behaviour toward elderly patients. *Clinical Nurse Specialist* 5: 165–168.

Guccione, AA (ed.) (1993) *Geriatric Physical Therapy*, 444 pp. St Louis, MO: CV Mosby.

Huber, M, Reno, B, McKenney, J (1992) Long-term care personnel assess their attitudes and knowledge of the older adult. *Journal of Advanced Nursing* 17: 1114–1121.

Laurence, M (1964) *The Stone Angel*, 316 pp. Canada: McClelland & Stewart.

Marshall, VM (1980) *Aging in Canada*, 314 pp. Canada: Fitzhenry & Whiteside.

McPherson, BD (1990) *Aging As a Social Process*, 473 pp. Canada: Butterworth.

Noessel, FH (1982) The language of ageism. *The Gerontologist* 22(3): 273–276.

Rajecki, DW (1990) *Attitudes*, 522 pp. Massachusetts: Sinauer Associates.

Samter, J, Voss, BJ (1992) Challenging the myths of aging. *Geriatric Nursing* 13: 17–21.

Shimamoto, Y, Rose, CL (1987) Identifying interest in gerontology. *Journal of Gerontological Nursing* 13: 8–13.

Smith, CW, Wattis, JP (1989) Medical students' attitudes to old people and career preference: the case of Nottingham medical school. *Medical Education* 23: 81–85.

Worchel, S, Cooper, J, Goethals, GR (1991) *Understanding Social Psychology*, 585 pp. California: Wadsworth Inc.

4

Cultural Differences in Ageing

GAYE DM HILL

Introduction
•
Background
•
Culture
•
Ethnicity
•
Communication
•
Other Factors to be Considered in Health and Culture
•
Conclusions

Introduction

Over the past decade, health care professionals and students of physiotherapy have become increasingly aware of the need to gain a better understanding of the racial and cultural dimensions of health care. There is also a growing recognition amongst health educators and health policy makers that without this knowledge and understanding, health programmes, services, and indeed, care, are less effective, and those engaged in the delivery of these services are less satisfied with their work. Physiotherapists with different insights and deeper appreciation of human life and values are developing a sensitivity for culturally appropriate, individualized clinical approaches when working with the older people from cultures different to their own.

Background

The demographic shifts throughout the world clearly show a change in population composition from a monolithic towards a pluralistic society brought about in part through immigration patterns in countries like Australia, the UK and Canada — to name a few. The initial disruption of life associated with immigration is commonly seen in terms of losses of family ties. Unplanned changes, such as revolutions, wars, and cultural and religious deprivation are reasons for geographical relocation of many older people from different cultures. Refugees have the additional problems of living in fear and uncertainty while awaiting decisions regarding their status in a new country. While all immigrant groups may encounter similar problems, older immigrants usually experience greater difficulties during the period of resettlement. For them, the new culture rarely becomes familiar, and the stresses of their loss of independence may lead to physical and mental health problems. The unfamiliar language, geography and climatic conditions (temperatures too warm or too cold) also increase the risk of sickness in older people, who are more prone to multiple illnesses than any other age group.

Different climatic conditions may call for adaptation to new styles of clothing and housing. Foods may also be dissimilar to those in their native country. Customs relating to when and how to eat may be confusing. During the ageing process, many previously discarded rituals surrounding dress, traditions, lifestyles, freedom etc., resurface with increased rigidity. In order to cope with resettlement and the novelty of a different culture, some immigrants establish their own community of members who share the same cultural identity. This may create an added problem of social isolation as many older people develop new group memberships at a much slower rate than younger members of their families. Thus, pluralism in itself, with its potential for added stress and ill health for those elderly from marginalized cultures, presents a challenge for health professionals to develop a better understanding of the principles involved in effective and empathic cross-cultural care.

This chapter aims to assist the physiotherapist to develop some awareness regarding the knowledge, skills and attitudes necessary to better respond to the health needs of older people in racially and culturally diverse populations. Significantly, the emphasis will be on the fundamental importance of a cross-cultural approach to health care, rather than diagnostic and prescriptive solutions for members of cultural or racial groups. The emphasis will be on culture and communication as they impact on the health issues of the elderly. Case studies will highlight the impact of culture and communication on health issues affecting the life of older people.

Culture

Culture is a complex, integrated system that includes knowledge, beliefs, skills, art, morals, laws, customs and any other acquired habits and capabilities of a group of people. Culture is characterized by being learned, shared with others, and adapted to the environment. As a learned set of traits, culture is transformed from one generation to the next by both formal education and imitation.

Every society has a culture, and every cultural group has beliefs and practices related to health and illness (Helman, 1990). Beliefs include opinions, knowledge, and faith about various aspects of the world. Beliefs of particular concern to health care providers are those related to illness, causation, preferred methods of treatment, expected outcomes, and fears about the illness. How an individual defines illness is based on his or her belief system and is largely determined by the culture. Decisions about wellness and illness are derived from experiences of biological, sociological, psychological and cultural influences of daily life. Although many meanings have been assigned to the word 'culture', Ishawaran (1990) asserts that there is no universally accepted definition; culture involves 'rules of conduct and tacit laws (often unwritten) that occasionally overlap with the organizational requirements of society'. Health care that is acceptable to members of specific groups requires understanding of and respect for life-style, community, and sociocultural orientations as they relate to health promotion, maintenance and restoration (Leininger, 1989b).

Immigrant women who cannot speak English feel especially isolated from the larger community, and have problems understanding their new environment and culture and adapting effectively to it. This is particularly so in the case of women from rural India, who are brought up to think of their families before they think of themselves, and so neglect themselves, consciously or unconsciously. Cultural isolation and the absence of social support have a major impact on the health of Indo-Canadian women who do not speak English and may be unfamiliar with or hesitant to use existing health services. Since cultures are not static, norms and values that are acceptable in one generation may not be acceptable in the next, nor in the country to which the refugee or immigrant has taken up residence.

Ethnicity

A popular definition of 'ethnicity', is 'a sense of peoplehood, a shared history, a common place of origin, shared language, food preferences' etc., as it relates to everyday living (Coutu-Wakulczyk and Beckingham, 1993). Thus, ethnicity refers to a personally accepted state of one's mind, a conscious state of inner identity. It also implies a sense of community transmitted over generations by families. Culture and ethnicity should not be confused. Two people may share the same

cultural background without having the same ethnic group membership. Ethnicity also differs from race, in that racial background refers to a person's specific biological characteristics such as colour of skin, texture of hair and facial features. Ethnic groups share traits such as a common national or regional origin and linguistic, ancestral, and physical characteristics.

For some older adults, ethnicity is seen as both a blessing and curse. Although many older immigrants have been sponsored by their children to a new and different country, they have left their peers behind. They often experience continuing ambivalence about living in a new country even if they understand the language of the dominant society. They may feel marginalized from the mainstream cultures because of the social, economic and racial context of their lives. Depending on where they live, many are invisible members of the society because they do not represent large numbers of consumers, or voters, nor hold positions in the workforce, nor are they very vocal in articulating their needs. Often, they must rely on their children to be 'brokers' for them in the community. They may use their own culturally specific medicine before accessing the local health care system, either because of their own cultural expectations and values or their understanding of health, caring, illness and death, which may be incongruent to that of the host country. Care that emphasizes cultural preservation or maintenance facilitates the inclusion or incorporation of helpful and/or harmless health and illness beliefs from folk medical systems into biomedical treatment programmes. For example, encouraging the use of herbal teas or ethnic foods may facilitate acceptance of less familiar aspects of care or treatment plans as well as other nutritional needs. Because many ethnic older people view visits to hospitals as a social isolation from their immediate families, the health care system is often used on an emergency basis only, thus compounding their fear and reluctance to access the system fully.

In addition, many older immigrants are female, poor and widowed and require more family support than do seniors of the dominant culture. According to MacLean and Bonar (1983) this support is even more critical for ethnic elderly persons entering a long-term facility of the dominant culture who face several challenges from being a minority group member. Loss of daily contact with family members is problematic in such institutions because the ethnic individual experiences a great sense of family loss by being institutionalized. This loss is more severe and more difficult to adjust to than that experienced by those who have socialized their children to lead more independent lives. Thus, when an ethnic elderly person enters a long-term care facility he or she may have to cope with feelings of shame, disrespect and dishonour as well as the normal feelings of anxiety related to the institutionalized process. Furthermore, many of these institutions lack staff or volunteers who speak the language, or understand the cultural values of the diverse groups for whom they provide care.

Ethnic older women, like women of the majority culture, act as caregivers for their grandchildren and other family members and also play an active role in defining illness and managing it. For instance, it is not uncommon for family members to introduce traditional medicine or treatment based on the advice of grandparents at the same time the family is engaged in the 'health culture' of the new country, because older women are seen as the fountains of cultural heritage.

The aged have been equated with minority groups and this presents further difficulties in the context of ageing and ethnicity. The problem becomes clear as one analyses the double and multiple jeopardy hypotheses, which states that there is interaction between two or more factors such as ageing and ethnicity. Many researchers believe that occupying two or more stigmatized statuses has greater negative consequences for the occupants than if they held one negative status alone. Thus being old, female and a member of a minority group (in this case, ethnic) is worse than being old, female and a member of the dominant group. An opposing argument is that age is a leveller which equates everyone's experience to a common low denominator. From this perspective being old is just as bad for a man as a woman, whether the individual is Australian, British or Canadian.

Communication

Communication, in this context, may be seen as a continuous process whereby one person may affect another through verbal (words) or non-verbal (gestures, facial expressions, body language) ways. When caregiver and client have different communication styles, or if communication is blocked for some other reason, e.g. both do not speak the same language, or a barrier exists even during the use of an interpreter, both the healthcare provider and the client may feel alienated and helpless. A client who feels misunderstood may appear angry, non-compliant or withdrawn, or may express feelings of discrimination, prejudice or racism. Likewise, a physiotherapist may feel angry and helpless if misunderstood. Without the ability to communicate effectively, the healing process can be delayed as the result of inadequate care, unnecessary treatment, or ethical problems. It becomes essential for the health care provider to develop a broad understanding of the client from a cultural perspective in order to understand thoroughly the racial, cultural and social factors that may affect communication. Indeed, in many cases, knowledge about cultural health issues is as important as knowing about sex, age and mental state of the patient. It remains relevant even when cultural groups have been well integrated and speak the same language as the physiotherapist, since variances may continue to occur in the definitions of 'illness', i.e. in the dietary habits, ways of dealing with mental illness, rituals surrounding specific events like illness and dying, and use of traditional remedies. Therefore, health care professionals need to be constantly aware that errors in judgement can occur because of miscommunication patterns and misunderstandings due to differences in cultural orientation. Errors may also occur if service providers base their assessments on their perceptions and stereotyping of persons from other cultures.

Communication and culture are closely intertwined; communication is the means by which culture is transmitted and preserved. Improved communication strategies can help reduce or avoid an imposition of the physiotherapist's values. Culture influences how feelings are expressed and what verbal and non-verbal expressions are appropriate. Since cultural patterns of communication are learned early during childhood, health care providers engaged in cross-cultural care and treatment need to be constantly aware of the difficulty elderly patients may encounter when listening to or speaking with a physiotherapist from a different culture. The challenge is for the physiotherapist to bear in mind common cultural patterns, while approaching patients as individuals who should not be categorized because of their cultural heritage, and avoid projecting their own values and behaviours on their clients. A projection of values, as well as hindering care, may contribute to non-compliance.

A common strategy when dealing with ethnic older people who lack language fluency is to make use of an interpreter. While an interpreter may be extremely helpful, there is the danger that there might be a social misfit between client and interpreter, or interpreter and physiotherapist. Interpreters may have difficulty requesting clinical information from an older person of their own ethnic group, or may refrain from revealing some belief system such as folk medicine to the physiotherapist. The interpreter should recognize that the physiotherapist is genuinely interested in the client and views the inquiry process as important to the treatment plan. There should also be thorough preliminary discussions between the physiotherapist and the interpreter to clarify their roles during the interview; a follow-up session is also invaluble for evaluation purposes. Family members may be useful as interpreters, although the use of young children should be avoided. When an interpreter is used, the dialogue should be between the physiotherapist and the patient, with the interpreter occupying a background position; at no time should the patient be ignored. This arrangement maintains trust and rapport even if the verbal communication from the patient is inadequate.

Case Study 1

Danny, a 78-year-old Algonquin Indian hunter who had lived all his life in solitary existence in a Northern Canadian forest was found by another trapper in an incoherent and semiconscious state and rushed by air ambulance to a large 1500-bed teaching hospital, 500 miles to the south, where he was initially assessed as suffering from intense fatigue, gross weight loss, an injured right leg and dehydration. Prompt laboratory and X-ray investigations revealed kidney failure and a fractured right leg. He was placed on peritoneal dialysis and a cast was applied to his right leg. The goal of the health care interdisciplinary team was to assist in the restoration of self-care by Danny.

His only personal belongings were the overalls he wore and a hunting knife which was in his pocket. He communicated by using facial expressions, a few hand gestures, and high-pitched groans.

After being hospitalized for 3 days, it was obvious that Danny was experiencing great difficulty in having his needs understood. The hospital environment and routine were so foreign to him that he removed his cast by soaking his leg in the toilet bowl; he was suspicious of the medication and diet that were prepared for him and was uncooperative with any attempts to assist him with his personal care.

On the fourth day, he used his familiar hunting knife to disconnect the plastic tubing from his abdomen, thus discontinuing his treatment for his kidney failure. Health care workers discovered him checking his belongings, fingering his touchstones, and chanting a song while alternatively lying and sitting on the floor; he refused to use the bed.

Danny's physiotherapist, who had some knowledge of cultural underpinnings and cultural assessment, interpreted the patient's behaviour and explained that this 78-year-old gentleman was experiencing not only culture shock, but a transformation of his body image — he was now connected to a machine, which he did not understand to be an aid to his recovery. While his goals and that of the health care team were similar, in that the outcome was directed towards optimum health recovery and self-care, the two cultures collided in that both he and the health care workers could not and did not agree on the method. The technology was unfamiliar to him. He yearned for the elders of his community and his familiar geographical locale with the foods he had enjoyed all his life. The team saw him initially as non-compliant, but later felt helpless as he was unable to acknowledge their good medical intentions. His touchstones and hunting knife were the only familiar objects in a place where people in his village went for help and never returned because they died there. Thus, his external environment conflicted with his internal perception of himself as he knew it.

In order to regain some degree of control, he used his familiar hunting knife to disengage himself from the machine by cutting the plastic tubing from his body, and to remove the cast from his leg. Although by this time he was in physiological shock, his facial expression was calm and peaceful as he lay on the floor, which provided him with a more customary and comfortable position than a hospital bed.

The physiotherapist, who was aware of the need for cross-cultural communication, began to build upon the awareness, sensi-

tivity and knowledge which he previously learned about effective cross-cultural communication and quickly recognized that both his colleagues and Danny were misunderstood and misinterpreted.

Recovery skills are necessary when the health care provider has said or done something that has aroused the client's anger or suspicion, or otherwise distanced the patient, or realizes that the resources available in that setting are not meeting the client's needs (Kavanagh and Kennedy, 1992). Communication recovery is a three-stage strategy used after a misunderstanding has arisen. The physiotherapist, therefore, first articulated and presented the problem as it was being perceived by Danny and advocated on Danny's behalf to reduce the risk of imposition of values that were not familiar to him. He communicated non-verbally to Danny that he recognized and valued his dignity and respected his decision to lie on the floor by offering him an extra sheet and blanket; Danny accepted the sheet but refused the blanket. The physiotherapist also non-verbally modelled for Danny how a fibreglass cast would enable him to wear his own clothing and promote healing in his leg.

Second, the physiotherapist acknowledged that everyone makes interactive mistakes. He risked disapproval of his peers on the interdisciplinary team as well as the anger and hostility of the patient by doing so.

The third stage involved recognizing and reducing Danny's resistance and defensiveness, since such behaviour can hinder productive relationships between care providers and patients. In attempting to *decrease this resistance the physiotherapist altered his manner of non-verbal communication through changing his body language, i.e. he altered his position to that of Danny's by also sitting on the floor near Danny and returning his approval smiles. His ultimate goal was the restoration of the integrity of the patient as well as his peers.*

Other Factors To Be Considered in Health and Culture

Many older people from a culturally diverse background are accustomed to receiving their health care from a single physician or nurse; the idea of sharing personal information with a social worker or physiotherapist or other health care professionals may be alien to them. They are usually unfamiliar with detailed history taking and lengthy procedures, and the notion of health promotion and follow-up care. Lengthy interrogations and tests, although routine to the practitioner, may be viewed as incompetence by the patient who may expect the physiotherapist to 'know' what is wrong without questioning. Circumstances other than ethnicity may interfere with the physiotherapist/client relationship even when they both share the same ethnicity. Even when ethnicity is the same, practitioners need to evaluate how class, religious affiliation, gender, age and other differences may make it particularly difficult for them to work with their own clients. Indeed, practitioners need to evaluate their own cultural biases and values especially when engaged in cross-cultural care (Special Issue on Women's Health, 1987).

Many ethnic elderly fail to seek explanations from practitioners and appear to agree with prescribed medication and treatment without questions. If in doubt, the practitioner should take the time to understand the cultural factors which may influence compliance and medical regimens.

Some biological variances are ethnically determined. For example, Asians respond to neuroleptics at a lower dosage than others; sickle-cell anaemia and hypertension are more commonly diagnosed among Black people than in the general population; lactose intolerance is found more frequently in South and South East Asians than amongst other ethnic groups. An understanding of the biological variations between various cultural groups is important if health care is to be effective.

Any discussion about cultural differences in ageing would be incomplete without reference to the theories of ageing. While several prominent theories on this subject have been debated over the years, for the purposes of this chapter, two will be mentioned. The activity theory argues that optimum activity during the middle years guarantees similar activity levels in old age. It further suggests that a high level of social activity is a key ingredient to successful ageing (Maddox, 1968; Havighurst et al., 1968). The disengagement theorists contend that mutual withdrawal by society and the elderly occurs; that there is a tendency not to replace broken ties as well as conscious disengagement from previous roles as one enters old age. Factors like health and socioeconomic status are not discussed within the framework of these theories, which suggest that disengagement results in negative life satisfaction while activity in itself forms the basis for life satisfaction in old age. Critics of the activity theory suggest that the theory was based on studies on a sample of elderly who were in good health and financially independent.

Case Study 2

An 85-year-old Vietnamese lady was admitted to hospital for congestive heart failure and abnormally high blood sugar. Several family members and extended kin visited her throughout the days and early evenings following her hospital stay. One such regular visitor, her first-born daughter, was reported to make frequent requests from staff to receive information from her mother's doctor. The staff felt that she was demanding and ignoring their professional capabilities by seeking information from the doctor personally.

Becoming increasingly defensive, the staff reminded the daughter that her mother was only one of several patients on the doctor's busy caseload. They began to set limits on the family's visiting hours and went out of their way to avoid the daughter, as well as becoming increasingly suspicious of the type of foods that the daughter was bringing to her mother as they felt these treats were in opposition to the goals of the dietary therapy prescribed for their patient. They believed that the daughter was physically abusing the mother and feared that they would be blamed for the skin abrasions discovered on the patient's body after the daughter's visit.

The staff invited the family to an interdisciplinary meeting to discuss the family's needs, to share their feelings of dissatisfaction with the family's requests, to set limits to prevent further manipulation by the family, and to restore respect for the staff. During the meeting, mixed feelings were expressed by different staff members. Some excused the Vietnamese patient and daughter through a lack of familiarity with the hospital etiquette and protocol; others expressed deep resentment that 'those little foreigners are bossing us around and telling us what to do!' Although the head nurse explained to the family that their mother was getting the best health care possible and was physically improving, the relationship between the staff and the family did not change. Finally, Tess, a health care professional with cross-cultural training was asked to consult with the staff and family.

Tess understood that the transition period for East Asian immigrant families can be very difficult and that language, customs, religious beliefs and values, family organization and processes within the context of a specific culture all have a great impact on the situation. She met alone with the family and learned some of the dynamics within the family, including the fact that their only brother had died in hospital shortly upon arrival to the new country, and that they and their mother were becoming increasingly worried that their mother may die also.

Tess learned from the daughter that their concerns to see the doctor were legitimate. In Vietnam the doctor is the sole authority in health care and speaks directly with the family. They were also concerned that their mother was not given any herbal medicine, an important healing practice in Vietnam since it is considered 'cool medicine' while Western medicine is 'hot'. The daughter requested that the doctor prescribe medicine to restore the normal Yin—Yang balance and stressed the need for other types

of treatment including acupuncture, massage, and abrasive practices such as cupping, rubbing and scratching the wind. Tess was aware of the South East Asian belief that illness needs to be drawn out of the body, and that this may be accomplished through coin rubbing, in which a heated coin or one smeared with oil is vigorously rubbed over the body, sometimes producing red welts. In accordance with other health beliefs, the resulting red marks are evidence of the illness being brought to the surface of the body. The mother complained to the daughter that the signal to beckon another with the finger or the palm of the hand was used toward her by the nurse and this was offensive to her mother; this is the motion used to call a dog in the home country.

On meeting with the staff, Tess explained to them the strong group ties of the Vietnamese culture and that daughters have proscribed obligations, both spoken and unspoken, to care for their elderly mother. As she was more fluent in English than their mother, the eldest daughter believed it was her role to be the advocate and spokesperson for her ailing mother and her extended kin. Tess also explained that, in Vietnam, health professionals are considered authority figures and experts; patients expect to be informed and instructed without being asked, and asking questions is considered impolite. Hence, the daughter's reluctance to ask direct questions of the staff whom she sees every day, but by presenting herself to them frequently she gives them the opportunity to offer information without being asked. She also explained how uncomfortable it *was for the family to make eye contact, as looking directly into another's eyes when speaking is considered disrespectful in Vietnam.*

Conclusions

In summary, it is imperative for health care providers to have a conceptual framework of wellness. Cross-cultural sensitivity is the core ingredient in practising culturally appropriate healthcare; without it there can be no cross-cultural caring. A good foundation in these principles is essential for the physiotherapist, since it provides a conceptual framework for holistic patient care and a variety of clinical settings. Several countries have recognized the need to change their health care policies to impact positively on the needs of their immigrants and refugees.

From a cross-cultural perspective the Dutch government is engaged in the development of teaching materials which would provide occupational therapy students with the cultural skills they need to meet the expectations of immigrant patients who come to the Netherlands from all over the world but mainly from Indonesia, Vietnam, the middle East, the Mediterranean, Surinam, China and Sri Lanka. Kinebanian and Stomph (1992) reported that in a survey of 24 clinics selected from 134 occupational therapy clinics which treated immigrants in the Netherlands, only one had a policy regarding treatment directed towards specific groups of immigrants, although most of those interviewed, stressed the importance of being experienced in cross-cultural care to provide adequate health care.

Kanitsaki (1993) has questioned whether the unique needs of Australia's culturally diverse people are being met since the mainstream health services available to the community are essentially monocultural (i.e. reflect the domination of Anglo-Australian cultural values). To compound this problem some professions, like nursing, rigorously defend the notions of holistic and morally accountable practice. Whitehead *et al.* (1993) have documented how federal and state governments in Australia have confronted inequalities in health by allocating resources to implement the National Aboriginal Health Strategy.

In Canada, the federal and provincial governments have advocated a change in the unilateral approach to health care to one that is culturally sensitive. Colleges and universities have implemented curriculum changes that will better prepare students to meet the needs of a multicultural society. Health care professionals are being encouraged to recognize human differences, confront their own biases, acknowledge their own deficits, and develop the awareness, sensitivity, knowledge and skills required to provide validation within their own practice.

In the USA an increasing number of states now require that teachers become multiculturally prepared (Pedersen, 1988). The question has been asked whether health care practitioners are in any way less responsible for provision of culturally appropriate care (Sedlacek, 1988; Leininger, 1989a, 1991). It may be that legal requirements will eventually demand demonstration of understanding of the contributions of lifestyles of members of various racial, cultural and economic groups in society; of recognitions and the ability to cope with dehumanizing biases, discrimination and prejudices; and of respect for human diversity and personal rights. Because health care providers learn primarily through role modelling (Helman, 1990), it is important that practitioners, medical faculties in the field, as well as students be prepared through their curriculum and inservice training to facilitate effective handling of inter-cultural competence, whether encountered in the classroom or clinical setting.

Researchers in London, UK, have examined the use of its health services by older people from ethnic minorities, particularly those who are Jewish. Jewish respondents were more likely than other older people to report problems with emotional well-being, mental and physical health problems and problems with functional ability, and they were also more likely to use health services than other respondents (Bowling et al., 1992).

In contrast, in an analysis of the needs of other British ethnic minority groups, Bhopal (1992) pointed out that there is as much variation between ethnic minority groups as between them and the Anglo-Saxon community; the common experience is one of family migration, the struggle for respect, well-being and social position, and evidence of alienation from White society, discrimination and relative poverty. Dif-ferences in health of ethnic minority groups were considered to be mainly due to current and past social and environmental deprivation.

References

Bhopal, R (1992) Needs of black and ethnic minorities. *British Medical Journal* 305: 1156–1157.

Bowling, A, Farquhar, M, Leaver, J (1992) Jewish people and ageing: their emotional well-being, physical health status and use of services. *Nursing Practice* 5: 5–16.

Coutu-Wakulczyk, G, Beckingham, AG (1993) Ethnicity and aging. In Beckingham, A, Witter DuGas, B (eds) *Promoting Healthy Aging*, pp. 370–394. Toronto: CV Mosby.

Havighurst, RJ, Neugarten, BL, Tobin, SS (1968) Disengagement and patterns of aging. In Neugarten BL (ed.) *Middle Age and Aging*, pp. 161–172. Chicago: University of Chicago Press.

Helman, CG (1990) *Culture, Health and Illness: An Introduction for Health Professionals.* London: Wright.

Ishawaran, K (1990) *Sociology: An Introduction.* Toronto: Addison-Wesley.

Kanitsaki, O (1993) Acute health care and Australia's ethnic people. *Contemporary Nurse* 2: 122–127.

Kavanagh, KH, Kennedy, PH (1992) *Promoting Cultural Diversity: Strategies for Health and Health Care Professionals*, 160 pp. London: Sage.

Kinebanian, I, Stomph, M (1992) Cross-cultural occupational therapy: Critical reflection. *American Journal of Occupational Therapy* 46: 751–756.

Leininger, MM (1989a) The transcultural nurse specialist: Imperative in today's world. *Nursing and Health Care* 10: 251–256.

Leininger, MM (1989b) Lenninger's theory of nursing: Cultural care diversity and universality. *Nursing Science Quarterly* 1: 152–160.

Leininger, MM (1991) Transcultural nursing: The study and practice field. *Imprint* 38: 55–66.

Maddox, GL (1968) Persistence of life style among the elderly: A longitudinal study of patterns of social activity in relation to life satisfaction. In Neugarten, BL (ed.) *Middle Age and Aging*, pp. 181–183. Chicago: University of Chicago Press.

MacLean, ML, Bonar, R (1983) Ethnic elderly in a dominant culture long term care facility. *Canadian Ethnic Studies* 15: 51–59.

Pedersen, P (1988) The three stages of multicultural development: Awareness, knowledge, and skill. In Pedersen, P (ed.) *A Handbook for Developing Multicultural Awareness*, pp. 3–18. Alexandria, VA: American Association for Counseling and Development.

Sedlacek, WE (1988) Institutional racism and how to handle it. *Health Pathways* 10: 4–6.

Special Issue on Women's Health (1987) *Health Promotion* 25(4). Health & Welfare. Canada.

Whitehead, M, Judge, K, Hunter, DJ, Maxwell, R (1993) Tackling inequalities in health: the Australian experience. *British Medical Journal* 306: 783–787.

5

Health and Social Policies

NANCY M GEREIN, JEROME E BICKENBACH

Social policy shapes both the form and the content of all human services in a country. Although the physiotherapist provides professional services that greatly enhance the quality of life of the population as a whole, these services form a relatively small part of what countries provide for their citizens. Still, the social role played by the profession of physiotherapy can only properly be understood by noting how these services fit into the much larger picture of all human services. This is especially true for services that are designed to meet the needs of a specific, and permanent, subpopulation, such as the elderly (see also Chapter 27).

The Nature of Social Policy

Social, or public, policy is a network of decisions that create responsibilities on the part of governments and their agencies to act, or refrain from acting, in certain ways, as well as defining processes for fulfilling those responsibilities (Armitage, 1988). The aim of social policy is to set out the legal and administrative machinery necessary to resolve social problems that have been identified through the political process. This may either result in universal programmes that ignore differences between individuals, or targeted programmes directed to an identifiable segment of the population with similar needs or difficulties.

Here, the target population is characterized by

age, although over the years the boundaries of what counts as 'elderly' have shifted somewhat. Social policy for older people arises from the perceived, unmet and ongoing needs of this population, so that the first task of decision-makers is to identify these, and organize them into existing policy categories, such as health, income security, housing, transportation and recreation. Usually, these categories are associated with specific governmental agencies, which themselves do not focus on any specific target population, but are concerned, for example, with health or housing needs across the board. There are, though, some populations which are thought to have such unique problems that government agencies have been created to look after their needs, e.g. people with intellectual disabilities. The elderly have not as yet been brought under the umbrella of a single government agency in Canada, UK or Australia, but that is certainly a future possibility.

Social policy decisions aimed at a targeted population are put into effect through statutory law or legislation – an Act of Parliament or Provincial or State Legislature. Statutes set out the general structure for policy in an area and articulate the political values that are to govern. The details of putting these values into practice are then incorporated into regulations or guidelines; thus, later decision-makers, empowered by the statute to make these decisions, are free to respond to changes in needs or economic conditions. (Regulations have the force of law, whereas guidelines are recommendations for implementing policy.)

Policy changes are most often incremental and provide for slight adjustments to existing policies in order to further their objectives more effectively. More rarely, there may be major, ideological changes in policy direction, such as the abandonment of universality in health care services, or a shift away from income security provisions or social assistance to mandatory training programmes.

All changes to existing social policy affect the population the policy serves. Closing a regional office that delivers a service to a rural elderly population may have devastating consequences to these people, even though, as a policy shift, it is minor. The forces and people that create changes and reforms to policy are centrally important players. At the highest level, shifts in political ideologies may take the lead in altering policy from the top down. Public pressure on legislators and bureaucrats may also result in policy shifts, by forcing the government to investigate perceived problems or, if the issue is sensitive enough, to create standing committees or Royal Commissions to recommend reforms. Increasingly, organized advocacy or consumer groups influence policy changes at all levels. Less publicly, professional organizations and well-funded business interests use the power of direct lobbying to influence politicians to make legislative or other policy changes.

Guiding Principles of Social Policy

The dominant political ideology in most developed countries is one of liberalism, characterized by an adherence to the rule of law, democratic institutions, legal protection of individual liberties, and a recognized role for the state in regulating an otherwise open, capitalistic economic market for private exchanges. The principal debate within liberalism is the degree to which state intrusion into the economy is justified on grounds of the other values of liberalism, namely individual liberty and democracy. During the period of 1940–1980, several countries put into place universal, publicly administered programmes in health, education, and a variety of social service programmes; including income support, unemployment, worker's compensation, and pension programmes. Less buoyant economies in the 1990s and fiscal crises brought on by international economic restructuring have encouraged a rethinking of the welfare state, cuts in government programmes and bureaucracy, and the privatization of some human and social services.

In addition, there are a number of background principles which, though rarely expressed, implicitly guide policy formation and implementation for both health and general social policy. These principles include autonomy, democracy, respect for diversity, equality, universal access and de-medicalization of health.

The principle of autonomy presumes that individuals have the right to make informed decisions concerning issues pertaining to their lives. In legal terms, this principle is captured by the doctrine of informed consent that requires that health interventions are based on a full disclosure of all relevant information and the consent of the individual, otherwise a charge of negligence or malpractice may be laid.

There are some well-known and widely accepted circumstances in which autonomy is overruled by social policy. Where personal decisions adversely affect the welfare of others, as in criminal law or in self-harming activity (such as smoking, drug use and dangerous driving), the actual or potential harm to others caused by these activities – including the additional burdens on the health care system – is judged to outweigh the value of autonomy.

With older people, the principle of autonomy may depend on the competency of the individual to understand the nature of the decisions being made. Emergency decisions are made for people who are unconscious, since in that state they cannot exercise their autonomy. By the same token, people suffering from extreme cases of dementia, or severe mental illness, may not be fully competent to make some personal decisions. The guardianship, or substitute decision-making, law in Canada, Australia and UK, in slightly different ways, provides for personal decision in the case of incapacity as well as safeguards against the manipulation of this licence to override the principle of autonomy.

Another principle guiding social policy might be called the principle of democracy, requiring that consumers of services must always be involved, to the greatest degree possible, in the development and implementation of policy regarding those services. This also reflects the concept that those who govern or set out the rules should respect the views of those who will be subject to those rules. With the recent growth of consumer and advocacy groups, policy-makers rely increasingly on public hearings, forums and town hall meetings to involve people in policy debates.

Changes in the ethnic and cultural composition of many countries have highlighted the importance of a third guiding principle, namely respect for diversity (see Chapter 4). Policy-makers can no longer assume that their targeted populations are homogeneous and culturally uniform. The difficulty here is that a policy that may be appropriate and beneficial to one group of seniors may, because of cultural, religious or ethnic differences, be quite inappropriate for another group.

Lastly, social policy is guided by the principle of equality. To some, equality merely involves treating people the same, but this approach often results in those with fewer needs benefiting most. Equality of opportunity, another version of the value of equality, requires that the state ensure that no one is disadvantaged by the denial of an opportunity that is available to others to develop talents or abilities. Lastly, equality of result requires the state to guarantee that all disadvantageous differences – for example, differences in income, social position, or even happiness – be eliminated, or compensated. In this wide spectrum of possible versions of equality lie the various political positions that characterize our era.

The political processes of policy-making differ from country to country since these more directly involve basic political structures. As a rule, unitary systems, such as in the UK, are able to implement ideological changes in policy much more quickly than non-unitary, or federal systems, as in Canada and Australia. In federal systems, there is a constitutional division of policy-making powers between the federal and provincial or state governments. In theory, responsibilities for programming are neatly divided; in practice, because of differences between responsibilities and tax-raising powers, policy for the elderly has had to be administered jointly, particularly pension and income security programmes. The inevitable conflict between the two levels of government has greatly hindered the prospects of meaningful reform in this area (Banting, 1987). On the other hand, federal systems allow for the input of regional and local differences in the shaping of social policy. The outcome is programmes which vary widely between states and provinces, with federal policies (and funding) attempting to create some uniformity.

The presence of a written constitutional protection of rights and freedoms is also significant. In Canada, the Charter of Rights and Freedoms makes it possible for an individual to launch a legal challenge to the validity of legislation, or any action of government, on the grounds that it violates basic rights. If, for example, revisions to health care policies have the effect of adversely affecting the elderly, then an action might be brought under the equality rights provisions. In neither Australia nor the UK is it possible to challenge directly the legal validity of policy in this manner, although it is always possible to argue that the procedures set in place for determining the impact of policy changes were not followed, or were inadequate.

Older people benefit from a wide range of social policies, but, other than pensions, there is no social policy for older people as such. As a rule, health and social policies are not coordinated, so that legislation designed to improve programming for older people is usually cobbled onto existing programmes, leading to the provision of uncoordinated services that are not geared precisely to the needs of this older group.

Health Care Policy Development

These four principles guide all social policy. Another more specific and contentious principle relating to health care policy is that of universal access – that access to all levels of health care should be available to everyone with health needs, irrespective of their ability to pay. This principle, needless to say, has been under recent threat in Canada, Australia and UK because, with escalating health costs, there is always the temptation for governments to return to a system in which services depend on ability to pay. Nonetheless, universal access remains a guide to health policy development.

Health care policy has undergone profound changes in recent years as a result of a new understanding of what health entails. Policy-makers increasingly aim at health promotion as well as treatment of illness, and recognize that far more is involved in the creation of a healthy population than provision of medical treatment. Creating healthy social environments, eliminating child poverty, unemployment and family violence, increasing the levels of self-managed health care — these are all health policy objectives that only tangentially involve the traditional health professions. They draw our attention to an ecological approach to health. Indeed, the guiding principle here might be called the de-medicalization of health.

This new understanding of the nature of health has consequences for policy for the elderly. It is now increasingly common for policy-makers to argue that ageing should not be seen as a pathology or disease condition, calling upon the resources of health professions, but as a natural process of human development (see Chapter 6). This means, from a policy point of view, that seniors are not 'medical problems', they are citizens who are justifiably calling upon the state and its agencies to design policy that meets their needs. The needs of seniors, in other words, are in no sense 'special'; they are needs that human beings have as a consequence of age.

Parallel to this policy shift is the move to see physical and mental disabilities not as medical problems needing cures, but as limitations of functional capacity requiring rehabilitation. Increasingly too, functional incapacity is distinguished from handicaps, understood as socially created (and so, socially remediable) disadvantages that people with disabilities are forced to confront (see Section E). Handicaps are the various ways in which people with disabilities are denied full participation in society: an elderly person in a wheelchair has a disability of mobility, but the lack of ramps or elevators is the handicap he or she must confront. Understanding disability and handicap in this manner, the policy-maker can then seek ways of accommodating these limitations so that the elderly and others with disabilities can fully participate in all aspects of social life.

Policy Challenges in Health Care for Older People

Contrary to common belief, the majority of older people are not chronically ill, disabled, or living in nursing homes (see Chapter 24). Although 75% of older people have suffered from at least one chronic health problem, according to a national health survey conducted in Canada in 1978, 80% were capable of living independently and caring for themselves (McDaniel, 1986). Only 6–10% of the elderly received institutional care in the early 1980s in Canada, although this number rises with age. In 1988, the nursing home participation rate in Australia for those 70 and over was 53 per 1000, increasing to 440 per 1000 for those aged 95–99 (Andrews and Carr, 1990). The majority of elderly people are living longer, healthier lives free of major disability (see also Chapter 2).

Nonetheless, the demographic fact of an increasingly older population structure raises concerns about burdens on health care and pensions in all three countries (Chapter 2). Accommodation for the elderly, enforced retirement, the possibility of voluntary work in retirement, and availability of family members for care of the elderly are also major areas of policy debate. That debate should heat up when consumer and advocacy groups representing the elderly (the grey power movement) move from the current strategy of defending existing programmes to a more aggressive strategy of demanding new programmes. Whatever form this policy debate takes, though, it will inevitably involve the application to the elderly population of basic principles of social policy that are held in common in the UK, Canada and Australia.

In the case of health policy, it remains true that older people use more health services, particularly for chronic care. The predictable future ageing of the population is expected to increase the overall costs of health care. Many of the challenges posed are due to problems inherent in the organization of the health delivery system, and, arguably, increases in health care costs are more a function of new technologies and existing inefficiencies. For example, there is no adequate coordination or continuity of care between primary medical services, acute care hospitals, community care settings, rehabilitation services, and informal caregivers (Section E). Historically, health care systems are more oriented to acute care for disease than to rehabilitation of disability. Most rehabilitation services focus on work-life potential and a younger clientele, while geriatric medicine focuses more on acute care rather than on rehabilitation (see also Chapter 3). The traditional view has been that older people are both difficult and expensive to rehabilitate, yet recent research shows that many disabling conditions can be prevented or improved with a combination of rehabilitation, medical and lifestyle interventions (Wray and Torres-Gil, 1992). Such weaknesses point to the need for knowledgeable physiotherapists to be involved in initiatives to redirect and expand rehabilitation services at local and national levels.

A change to a more ecological approach to health would recognize the role of housing, family structures, income security, workplace health, stress and lifestyle on the maintenance of health, as individuals age. Programmes to promote health and prevent illness have been aimed at younger groups, but more and more older people are taking advantage of health promotion programmes, such as fitness programmes, that can postpone the onset of disability and enhance their independence (Chapter 13).

Concerns about long-term care needs in the future, and the realization that families provide most of this care, have suggested the need to seek a balance between family support and institutional or community service options. The challenge is to design policies that offer a continuum of care, from minimal to maximal support environments, including the family home (Chapter 24), community settings, multifunction living and care complexes, congregate or sheltered housing, all the way to long-term care facilities and hospice and palliative care (Driedger and Chappell, 1987) (see Section F).

One clear trend has been a move away from residential homes for older people to medically oriented long-term care facilities. This is a reflection both of the rapid increase in the number of the very old with their higher incidence of dementia and severe medical problems, and the expansion of community-based services (Gibson, 1992). Most countries consider their institutional rates for the elderly to be higher than necessary, and have tried to limit growth by shifting resources to community-based services. Community-based services are promoted to prevent or delay costly institutionalization, to respect the wish of most older people to remain at home for as long as possible and to reduce burdens on family care-givers (Jamieson, 1991; Monk and Cox, 1991).

The availability of family support is a key factor in both social and health policy strategies. Families, and particularly female relatives, assume much of the responsibility for the care of older people in the community (see also Chapters 3 and 4). Many caregivers are themselves elderly: in the UK 25% of caregivers are older people who often provide more demanding personal care and physical help services than that given by younger caregivers (Wenger, 1990).

Recognition of the resulting stress, isolation, fatigue, susceptibility to illness, financial demands, and jeopardy to employment prospects and other family responsibilities, has led to the call for services designed to relieve this burden. Family support services include tax subsidies and housing allowances, financial assistance to caregivers, respite care, and adult day care (Chappell, 1992) (see Section F). Many policies, though, are still based on the assumption that women will not be employed and so will be available to provide the needed care, an assumption that is no longer true for many women.

Although community-based services have expanded rapidly in Canada, Australia and the UK, they are not fully meeting demand. Many suffer from lack of coordination between health and social services, uneven distribution between rural and urban areas, and a general failure to help people learn what help is available and to what they are entitled. One way of meeting this challenge may be the creation of geriatric assessment teams, that is, multidisciplinary teams that provide case management for the elderly individual, to ensure a coordinated and vigorous response from available services that will enable most people to remain in their homes (Otis, 1992) (Section F).

Policy-makers in this area have long been concerned about the extent to which community-based services should supplant family care, adding considerably to public costs. Community services, however, supplement rather than supplant family care. The introduction of services has not affected the willingness of families to provide care, nor has it increased the use of public services. In the Canadian province of Manitoba, for example, 80% of the elderly receiving formal home care services also receive care from informal sources, usually family members; this rate is the same as before the introduction of universally available home care benefits (Chappell, 1992).

Social Policy Development on Income Support and Housing for Older People

Income Support

In the area of income security, policy in Canada, Australia and the UK involves a tangle of uncoordinated programmes that rely on both direct transfers of tax revenues, contributory plans and tax credits. The cost of these programmes, which is borne by younger people who are still working and paying tax, will become an increasing burden on a decreasing number of people. In addition, existing programmes fail to provide an adequate level of retirement income to those who, for whatever reason, did not earn enough during their working lives to qualify for benefits, while it continues to provide support to those elderly whose personal income is greater than the national average.

The principal source of income for people over 65 is public pensions, which supplies more than half of the cash income received by the elderly, with private pensions and investments making up most of the rest. The basic old-age security pension is a flat rate universal benefit funded by general revenues (see Chapter 2), but each country has an array of income supplements, spousal allowances, and veterans' and military pensions that may add to this. Some old-age security provisions and guaranteed income supplements are income-tested, but not tied to past earnings or other contributions. Canada, Australia and the UK also have programmes for benefits for people with special disability needs, for example assistive device and drug allowances, attendant care supplements, laundry for incontinent persons, and lump sum payments for disability-related equipment needs. A substantial number of people who are entitled to these benefits do not claim them (Victor, 1987; McDonald and Wanner, 1990).

In all three countries, public pensions and income supports are indexed to inflation, while private sector pensions are not. Public sector pension plans, for those who worked in the public sector, constitute a major source of retirement funding. The very old, women, and the disabled are the least likely to have any savings or occupational pensions. Women, with roughly a third of the level of pension coverage of men, have proportionally lower income levels than men, and rely more heavily on non-contributory income security plans than do men. This income gap has been closing in recent years with the introduction of spousal and widow benefit plans and changes in the laws of marriage and divorce that give divorced women access to their ex-spouses' public and private pensions (Gee and Kimball, 1987).

The tax structures in these three countries take age into account in ways that are advantageous to older people, through age and partial pension—income tax credits. These are not, however, universal sources of income since they only benefit those who would otherwise pay tax, which does not include everyone over the age of 65.

Housing (see also Chapter 24)

Housing policy has shifted in all three countries from providing specialist accommodation to enhancing the ability of the elderly to live independently within the community. In both Australia and Canada more than three-quarters of those over 65 own their own home, nearly all without mortgages, because of the favourable housing markets of the 1950s and 1960s and policies that made home ownership more feasible (Kendig, 1990). In the UK, home ownership among the elderly is much lower, roughly 50% in 1988, but may grow because of recent policies encouraging home ownership. Older people tend to own older homes in need of repairs, better heating and plumbing and the like (Walker, 1990).

Policies to meet the desire of most older homeowners to stay in their homes include schemes that defer taxes until the home is sold, loan programmes for major repairs and programmes providing funds for disability-related retrofitting and equipment. In Australia and Ontario, Canada, subsidies are provided to build 'granny-flats' — prefabricated units built onto an existing house which allow families to care for their elderly relatives while maintaining privacy. These are less common in the UK, although building societies do offer home improvement mortgages to older people, and pensioners can qualify to receive supplementary pension benefits to cover the costs of adaptations, and regular maintenance and insurance on their homes.

Affordable and adequate housing is especially difficult for older people who have never owned their own homes. In Australia, however, public housing was redirected in 1969 to consider the needs of older people, and by 1986 people over 60 accounted for a quarter of all households in public housing. Similar efforts have been made in Canada, while the UK, with its traditionally much lower home-ownership rate, has moved to put controls over rent increases to protect the elderly (Victor, 1987).

A range of residential homes or nursing homes are available in all three countries, housing about 5% of the elderly population (Chapter 2 and Section F). These are subsidized by the government for those unable to pay, except in Australia which opted to drop the income test. Much of this accommodation is provided by local or municipal authorities as well as voluntary organizations and housing cooperatives. In Australia and Canada there is a large private retirement home industry which has built communities exclusively for those who can afford it. In the UK the tendency has been to build sheltered accommodations for the elderly, which are small residences (up to 30 beds) with a warden, in existing communities or rural areas. These provide accommodation on the social model of care, whereas in Canada and Australia, nursing homes tend still to use the medical model of care (Johnson, 1990).

Because of perceived problems with the quality of care in residential and nursing homes, financial incentives to build specialty accommodation which would allow older people to continue living in the community were favoured in the 1980s. The belief that care provided in the home was less expensive than institutional care fits well with the political ideology of reducing the role of the public sector. However, despite a number of policies that promote community care, financial incentives for the commercial provision of institutional care in Australia and the UK have contributed to strong growth in this area in recent years (Jamieson, 1992).

Implementation of Health and Social Policies

In all three countries, national insurance covers the bulk of health care services for the whole population. In Canada and Australia, federal and provincial or state governments share the cost of services, although actual service provision is a state or provincial responsibility. Reimbursement to physicians in these two countries is on a fee-for-service basis, which provides few incentives to promote health or to provide the most appropriate services to people with chronic and disabling conditions.

In the UK, general practitioners receive most of their income through capitation payments, which encourage health promotion and illness prevention. It has been recognized for years that acute hospitals are not well equipped for the needs of older people with chronic, multiple and disabling conditions, and there is a recent trend for services for older people to be established in hospitals to provide integrated medical, nursing and allied care. Geriatric hospitals are reorienting to provide more acute and rehabilitative services, rather than indefinite long-term care. As well, day hospitals are becoming more common. The inpatient care of the acute and geriatric hospitals should be closely linked with community services, but coordination is proving difficult (Ham, 1992).

In Australia, health policies for older people were fundamentally revised in the 1980s; Canada's policies are now in the process of revision. These revisions place greater emphasis on health promotion and illness prevention. The Australian Better Health Commission of 1986 included specialized programmes to improve the level of knowledge about ageing in the community and to counteract stereotypes, as well as to improve lifestyle behaviour amongst older people and facilitate self-care and independence. The current federal goal in Australia seeks to decrease growth of institutional care by placing a limit on the number of institutional places available, promoting screening for eligibility for entry to nursing homes, and developing a broader range of community services (Healey, 1990). Similar objectives, for similar reasons, have been defined for community care programmes in the UK and Canada.

In the UK, the Griffiths Report of 1988 tried to deal with the fragmentation of services between health and social services by recommending that local authorities be responsible for all community care services, and develop these in consultation with the health authorities. Home help, for both older people and others with special needs, has shifted its emphasis from domiciliary services to that of providing more elements of personal care, especially for older, frailer clients. Nursing services, however, still fall mostly under local health authorities and arrangements for coordination with social services are not always effective (Lawson et al., 1991).

Community service structures differ in each state in Australia and each province in Canada, but service outputs are similar because of federal funding and requirements. In the UK there are wide variations between regions in the amounts and types of community services. Overall, resources for community services remain relatively sparse compared to resources for institutional care.

Conclusion

Although future trends are always difficult to predict, we seem to be witnessing in social policy for older people a fundamental change from age-based to needs-based servicing, from universal to targeted programming, and from institutional to home-centred service provision. The vast majority of older people are healthy and independent, but the rising numbers of the very old may mean that the need for care will increase in the future. On the other hand, future elderly may be even healthier than the current generation. It is clear in any case, that social policy for older people will always be a source of concern and debate throughout the world.

References

Andrews, G, Carr, S (1990) Health Care for the aged. In Kendig, H, McCallum, J (eds) *Grey Policy: Australian Policies for an Ageing Society*, pp. 110–126. Sydney: Allen, Unwin.

Armitage, A (1988) *Social Welfare in Canada: Ideals, Realities and Future Paths*, 294 pp. Toronto: McClelland, Stewart.

Banting, KG (1987) *The Welfare State and Canadian Federalism*, 263 pp. Kingston: McGill-Queen's University Press.

Chappell, NL (1992) *Social Support and Aging*, 104 pp. Toronto: Butterworth.

Driedger, L, Chappell, NL (1987) *Aging and Ethnicity: Toward an Interface*, 131 pp. Toronto: Butterworth.

Gee, EM, Kimball, MM (1987) *Women and Aging*, 142 pp. Toronto: Butterworth.

Gibson, MJ (1992) Public health and social policy. In Kendig, H, Hashimoto A, Coppard, LC (eds) *Family Support for the Elderly: The International Experience*, pp. 88–114. Oxford: Oxford University Press.

Ham, C (1992) *Health Policy in Britain: the Politics and Organisation of the National Health Service*, 286 pp. London: Macmillan.

Healey, J (1990) Community services: long-term care at home? In Kendig, H, McCallum, J (eds) *Grey Policy: Australian Policies for an Ageing Society*, pp. 127–149. Sydney: Allen, Unwin.

Jamieson, A (1991) Trends in home care policies. In Jamieson, A (ed.) *Home Care for Older People in Europe: A Comparison of Policies and Practices*, pp. 273–295. Oxford: Oxford University Press.

Jamieson, A (1992) Home care in old age: a lost cause? *Journal of Health Politics, Policy and Law* 17: 878–898.

Johnson, M (1990) Dependency and interdependency. In Bond, J, Coleman, P (eds) *Ageing in Society*, pp. 209–228. London: Sage.

Kendig, H (1990) Ageing and housing policies. In Kendig, H, McCallum, J (eds) *Grey Policy: Australian Policies for an Ageing Society*, pp. 92–109. Sydney: Allen, Unwin.

Lawson, R, Davies, B, Bebbington, A (1991) The home help service in England and Wales. In Jamieson, A (ed.) *Home Care for Older People in Europe: A Comparison of Policies and Practices*, pp. 63–98. Oxford: Oxford University Press.

McDaniel, SA (1986) *Canada's Aging Population*, 136 pp. Toronto: Butterworth.

McDonald, PL, Wanner, RA (1990) *Retirement in Canada*, 172 pp. Toronto: Butterworth.

Monk, A, Cox, C (1991) *Home Care for the Elderly: An International Perspective*, 171 pp. New York: Auburn House.

Otis, N (1992) *Identifying Care Alternatives for Older People: The Victorian Regional Geriatric Assessment Program*. No. 13, Lincoln Papers in Gerontology, La Trobe University, Melbourne, Australia.

Victor, C (1987) *Old Age in Modern Society: A Textbook of Social Gerontology*, 338 pp. London: Croom Helm.

Walker, A (1990) Poverty and inequality in old age. In Bond, J, Coleman, P (eds) *Ageing in Society*, pp. 229–249. London: Sage.

Wenger, GC (1990) Elderly carers: The need for appropriate interventions. *Ageing and Society* 10: 197–219.

Wray, LA, Torres-Gil, F (1992) Availability of rehabilitation services for elders: A study of critical policy and financing issues. In Ansello, EF, Eustis, NN (eds) *Aging and Disabilities: Seeking Common Ground*, pp. 55–67. New York: Baywood Publishing.

B

The Ageing Process

SECTION EDITOR: ANTHONY A VANDERVOORT

6

Biological and Physiological Changes

ANTHONY A VANDERVOORT

Some Theories of Ageing
•
Ageing Changes in the Motor System
•
Loss of Functional Cells from the Motor System
•
Sensory Function
•
Peripheral Neuromuscular System
•
Ageing and Muscle Strength
•
Changes in Protective Reflexes and Balance Control
•
Capacity for Adaptation in Older People
•
Cardiorespiratory Function
•
Cardiovascular Changes
•
Respiratory System Changes
•
Summary

Normal biological ageing causes a reduction in the body's reserve capacity. This effect can be observed in all body systems – muscular, skeletal, neural, circulatory, pulmonary, endocrine, immune. However, the rate and extent of decline vary widely among tissues and functions (Table 1), and between individuals. For example, maximum heart rate decreases steadily across the entire lifespan, while maximum muscle strength is well maintained in adults until the sixth decade. The declines which are observed at the system level are ultimately a reflection of either a loss of cells with ageing or a reduction in the capacity of a group of cells to carry out their specialized function.

Table I

Examples of variation in effects of age on physiological function

Variable	Effect
Maximum heart rate	Declines across entire age span
Blood count	No effect of age
Vital capacity	Declines from young adult age
Joint flexibility	Declines from young age
Muscle strength	Declines after middle age
Self-selected gait speed	Declines after middle age
Simple reaction time	Little effect of age
Choice reaction time	Slower in older people
Visual acuity	Decline begins in middle age
Hearing ability	Reduced in older people
Vestibular function	Reduced in older people
Stomach acidity	Reduced in older people
Renal function	Reduced in older people
Immune response	Reduced in older people
Reproductive hormones	Reduced after middle age

Note: These selected effects of ageing reflect the average response of healthy populations. The considerable variability that exists among individuals tends to increase in samples of older people. Gender also influences the timing and magnitude of some ageing effects.

Some Theories of Ageing

Loss of some physiological function is inevitable for all people as they grow older, even with an optimum lifestyle. Scientists have long been fascinated with the study of mechanisms underlying the ageing process. Why do cells in the sensorimotor cortex and basal ganglia of the brain deteriorate with ageing? Why is muscle atrophy observed in older men and women who have maintained a lifestyle of vigorous exercise? What causes the stiffening of connective tissue and the loss of bone mass in healthy, active older people? Many theories of ageing have been proposed and the prominence of each has waxed and waned, as new experimental evidence has appeared (Cristifalo, 1990).

One of the more prominent theories is the idea that there might be a critical group of cells whose deterioration initiates a chain reaction of effects throughout the body. Considerable attention has been devoted to the neuroendocrine system in general, and to the hypothalamus in particular, because of its key role in pacing adrenal glucocorticoid function and many aspects of body homeostasis. Certainly, the effects of some changes in hormonal control are profound, such as reduction of oestrogens/female menopause and the decline in growth hormone/loss of muscle mass in males.

Two general conceptual approaches merit consideration: first, that ageing is a genetically programmed event in a normal sequence from development to death; and second, that ageing occurs due to the gradual breakdown of cellular function. That senescence might possibly be programmed by the genetic regulation of a cell's DNA code has been elegantly demonstrated in fibroblast cells.

Whether the postmitotic nerve and muscle cells have a similar 'built-in' senescence is also of much interest to biologists, especially with respect to the search for genetic mechanisms that might somehow initiate the process. It is possible that there are specific genes which programme decline in function, or that over time the normally precise regulation of protein synthesis becomes eroded to the point that errors occur at various points in the process (e.g. the DNA code, transcription, mitochondrial response to the messenger RNA). The latter 'error theory' has led to many proposals for causative agents such as random mistakes that are not detected and repaired, radiation damage to the cells, crosslinking of molecules and the impact of free radicals on cell function. The latter proposal involves the concept that one of the byproducts of aerobic metabolism, a highly charged ion called a free radical, is destructive. While the cell has a limited protective system to handle these ions, accumulative damage may eventually lead to cellular dysfunction.

Ageing Changes in the Motor System

Age-related reductions in reserve capacity of the motor system result from a loss of properly functioning cells from the body over time. The nervous system, the muscles it controls, and the connective tissue and bones which transmit torques for movement all consist of specialized cells. Over time some of these cells either degenerate completely or change in structure. As the numbers of human nerve and muscle cells are thought to become fixed in a postmitotic state before or shortly after birth, their decline in later life is representative of important principles of the ageing process: it is intrinsic, progressive, deleterious and irreversible. Fries and Crapo (1981) noted, however, that normal ageing is often confounded with the effects of a sedentary lifestyle. Decreases in sensory function, motor control, strength and even metabolic capacity stem from the gradual reduction in number and function of excitable cells (see Chapters 7, 9 and 22).

Loss of Functional Cells from the Motor System

In one sense, the remarkable longevity of a human neuron or muscle fibre must be admired. Some people will live for over a century, and some of their cells will have been generating action potentials and manufacturing a wide array of proteins throughout that time. However, other excitable cells which were present at maturation will have disappeared, leaving a reduced reserve. This loss of neurons has been demonstrated throughout the nervous system, although there are regional variations in the extent to which this occurs (Brody and Vijayashanker, 1977). The existence of neuronal loss may be subtle and generally well-compensated for in even the oldest individuals. Excessive localized degeneration and cell loss is found in clinical conditions such as Parkinsonism (basal ganglia), senile dementia of Alzheimer's type (neocortex and hippocampus), or Friedreich's ataxia (cerebellum), but these are not part of the normal ageing process. It should also be noted that cells may still be present on anatomical observation, yet be dysfunctional because of biochemical changes.

Nerve cells communicate via neurotransmitters and hence it has been of considerable interest to investigate the effect of ageing on them (Magnoni *et al.,* 1991). Such research is complicated because of the complex nature of signalling — synthesis, release, diffusion, reception, postreceptor action and degradation of a given neurotransmitter — and the ever-growing variety of neurotransmitter chemicals found in the nervous system (acetylcholine, dopamine, norepinephrine, serotonin, gamma-aminobutryic acid (GABA) and many peptides including endorphins). However, with ubiquitous neurotransmitters such as acetylcholine and dopamine differences between young and aged nervous systems have been noted for each aspect of signalling. Finally, nerve cells also show a loss of dendritic and synaptic connections in aged nervous systems, along with microscopic changes such as accumulation of lipofuscin and neurofibrillary triangles. However, the remarkable redundancy of the nervous system also becomes apparent when it is realized that despite these changes mental function of most aged people remains adequate for an independent lifestyle (see Chapter 8).

Sensory Function

A decline in function of the body's various sensory systems is observed with ageing (Katzman and Terry, 1983). One of the most prevalent changes is the loss of visual acuity, leading to the need for reading glasses in middle-age. Other visual changes relevant to movement include decreased spatial discrimination, restriction in upward gaze and reduced ability to track objects.

Another well-known sign of ageing is hearing loss, which usually appears later in life than visual changes. Both the acoustic apparatus and related nerve pathways appear to undergo functional decline, which may produce communication pro-

blems in older people. As well, morphological changes appear in the vestibular organs, which contribute to decline in the ability to detect orientation in space. The olfactory system and taste receptors are also affected and the losses in these senses may lead to reduced appetite and poor nutritional status.

Of particular interest to physiotherapists is function of the somatosensory system in older people. Anatomical studies have demonstrated changes in the number and structure of specialized nerve ending receptors in the skin such as Meissner's and Pacinian corpuscles (Katzman and Terry, 1983). Older groups have been shown to be less sensitive to vibration, touch-pressure, cutaneous pain and temperature, especially in laboratory studies with precise quantitative methods. An important point to remember is that ageing produces variable differences in sensory function at different locations (see Chapter 8).

The nerves of older people show a small (about 10% or less) decline in maximal nerve conduction velocity (Hakansson *et al.,* 1991; Doherty *et al.,* 1993). Owing to the accuracy of electrophysiological measurement techniques and small variation between individuals, these differences are statistically significant, yet they appear to be of less importance to function. Older persons who have a pronounced slowing of nerve conduction velocity need further investigation for pathology (e.g. nerve entrapment or vascular insufficiency).

Physiotherapists should not assume that their own perception of a stimulus matches that of an older patient. A recent study on pain perception in groups of young and older women examined the effect of a 10 minute ice application to the forearm. The older women reported minimal discomfort from the procedure, while that reported by the younger women was significantly greater (Hakansson *et al.,* 1991). A similar difference between age groups was also observed with respect to discomfort felt during electrical stimuli of a nerve conduction velocity test.

These results on reaction to localized cooling should not be confused with age-related reductions in ability to tolerate and adapt to cold and hot ambient temperatures in the environment. Factors such as deterioration in hypothalamic control of body homeostasis, in combination with altered autonomic nervous system function and temperature sensation, lead to reduced ability to regulate body temperature. Hence extra precaution should be taken during situations such as strenuous exercise or hot/humid climates.

Peripheral Neuromuscular System

The central nervous system puts movement plans into action by activating motor units (MUs), each consisting of a single motoneuron and its family of innervated muscle cells. Considerable flexibility is built into the peripheral motor pathways due to the variability in contractile properties between these MUs. Using the electrophysiological technique of motor unit (MU) estimation, a striking decline in the number of excitable MUs present in skeletal muscles has been demonstrated – beginning in the seventh decade (McComas, 1977; Doherty et al., 1993). The functional implications of this loss of muscle mass are widespread and hence the atrophy is of much interest from both a biological and a rehabilitation perspective (see Chapters 7, 9 and 22).

Ageing Muscle

Modern radiological techniques allow accurate measurements of muscle cross-sectional areas in healthy people of different ages. The thigh muscles show significant reductions (25–35%) in size for older adults versus young, yet muscles of the upper limb do not atrophy to the same extent (Lexell, 1993). This regional difference suggests that the leg muscles studied were demonstrating a form of disuse atrophy (i.e. older adults had stopped exercising them as much). While this is an attractive hypothesis when trying to promote increased weight-bearing activity, there are also other factors gerontologists are studying such as changes in trophic supply from motoneurons and systemic levels of circulating hormones. Simple anthropometric measurements may be misleading in estimating muscle mass in older groups, as the overall shape and exterior girth of older peoples' limbs can appear to be unchanged if fat and connective tissue have replaced the disappearing muscle.

Among a number of skeletal muscles investigated, the vastus lateralis head of the quadriceps group has received particular attention from gerontologists (Lexell, 1993; Porter and Vandervoort, 1995). In one study of cadavers, the total number of muscle fibres observed decreased substantially with increasing age, such that an 80-year-old had about 50% fewer fibres than a young adult. There was also evidence of fibre atrophy, but this was specific to the Type II fast-twitch fibres and not observed in the Type I slow-twitch fibres. It is not known why the Type II fibres would be more susceptible to age-related deterioration, yet one encouraging finding is that those that are still remaining appear to be capable of hypertrophy during a weight-lifting programme.

The preferential atrophy of Type II fibres, and some evidence of fibre type grouping as well, have been interpreted as evidence of an ongoing denervation and reinnervation process that may favour the preservation of Type I fibres in older muscles. It is also postulated that some of the Type I motoneurons actually enlarge their own motor unit territory by capturing neighbouring fibres 'orphaned' by their deteriorating original axon. In support of this theory, the decline in the number of functional motor units is coupled with the appearance of some very large EMG potentials in the profile of an older muscle (McComas, 1977; Doherty et al., 1993).

Connective Tissue

Connective tissue is present throughout the body and the effects of ageing on it are readily apparent. The loss of elasticity in connective tissue causes the wrinkled appearance of the skin in older people. Connective tissues in other structures are also affected, ranging from the lungs to the muscles and joints.

Physiotherapists are often concerned with the changes in connective tissue that create stiffness in older people. The altered feel of joints and limitations to range of motion can be traced to the changes taking place in collagen and elastin components of their tissue structures. The network arrangement of collagen fibres normally provides useful structural support, yet with ageing they form excessive cross-linkages that reduce extensibility. There is also a loss of elastin, which not only forms a supporting structure for tissues it surrounds, but also has the important ability of returning to its original state after being stretched.

Thus the connective tissue within muscles and tendons plays a key role in maintaining the structural integrity of the contractile elements while transmitting their tension production to the attached bones. Structural proteins around the muscle sarcomeres such as titin and nebulin help to keep the actin and myosin filaments located at near optimal positions for generating maximum tension. However, this precise structural integrity of muscle can be disturbed by factors such as prolonged periods of immobilization or disuse — the resulting contracture can dramatically restrict

Table 2
Changes in muscle cells with ageing

Physiological function	Morphological or biochemical change
Reduced strength	Reduction in number of fibres Type II fibre atrophy Irregularities in sarcomere structure
Slowed contraction	Alteration in myosin ATPase enzymes Changes in sarcoplasmic reticulum function Type II fibre atrophy
Decreased excitability	Changes in sarcolemmal ionic pumps Dehydration and low potassium levels
Increased stiffness	Increased connective tissue within fibres
Reduced O_2 metabolism	Fewer mitochondria in sarcolemma Decreased aerobic enzymatic capacity Increased vascular resistance

torque generation and movements. Cartilage tends to become thinner and less well lubricated as the production of hyaluronic acid decreases in later life. This tissue is also reliant on movement because the cycle of compression and release forces (produced by alternate contraction and relaxation of active muscles) presses fluid and associated nutrients throughout the joint cavity (Walker, 1991).

Ageing and Muscle Strength

Although minor decreases in the strength of maximum voluntary contractions (MVC) of muscle begin to appear in middle age, important reduction does not become apparent until after the age of about 60 (Figure 1). During isometric tests, healthy people in their seventh and eighth decades score on average about 20–40% less on MVC tests than young adults, and the very old show even greater (50% or more) reductions. Males and females appear to show similar patterns of age-related deterioration (Doherty et al., 1993). Sedentary populations may also show greater loss in the lower limb musculature than upper.

Strength of concentric muscle actions (in which the muscle is allowed to shorten) is lower in older people than in young adults; at higher velocities of movement the age-related deficit is quite marked. However, the amount of strength deficit with age is consistently less for the eccentric type of muscle action (lengthening) than during either isometric or concentric muscle activity, and in some situations there may be no difference at all (Porter and Vandervoort, 1995). Thus, there is somewhat of a paradox created in which the changes with ageing that reduce strength when muscle shortens may actually enhance its perfor-

Figure 1 The relationship between maximum voluntary isometric muscle strength and age in healthy adults. The curvilinear pattern has been derived from a review of the literature, including the author's own research. Note that the decline with age does not become apparent until the sixth decade.

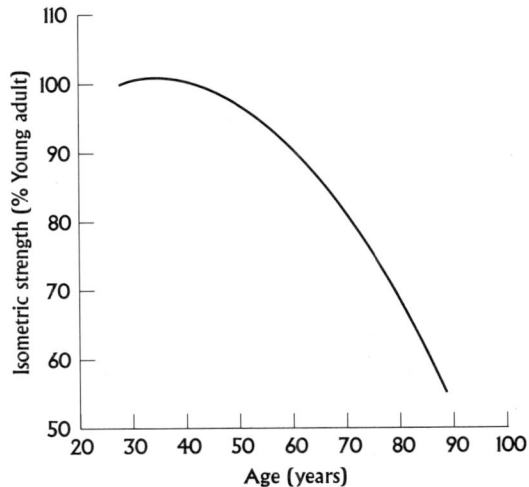

mance during eccentric loading. Although the explanation as to why muscles of older people have this relative advantage when lengthening against resistance remains to be fully clarified, it is a phenomenon worth noting. Perhaps their fatigue resistance for a given task would be improved if it could be done during eccentric loading rather than concentric (i.e. the muscle would be able to work at a lower relative intensity of maximum capacity).

Age differences in MVC strength may reflect either a reduced (atrophied) amount of muscle, or a reduction in muscle excitation via the descending motor pathways. The fullness of the motor drive was assessed by Vandervoort and McComas (1986) using a twitch interpolation technique – a brief percutaneous electrical shock was applied to the motor nerve during a well-practised maximal voluntary contraction of the ankle plantarflexors and dorsiflexors. Healthy elderly people, ranging in age from 60 to 100 years, were usually found to be able to activate their ankle muscles maximally in this simple isometric task; the superimposed twitch stimulus added little or nothing to their volitional force. Furthermore, older people have demonstrated quite reproducible isometric strength values in reliability studies, which provides additional evidence that they are highly motivated to achieve maximum strength scores. Thus, the primary mechanism to explain the age-related declines in strength must be a decreased excitable muscle mass. Indeed, there is good agreement between measures of strength loss and muscle atrophy in gerontology studies (Porter and Vandervoort, 1995). However, as this interpolated twitch described above was only applied to a simple, isometric, single-joint task, it is still quite possible that a lack of central nervous system coordination can be an important limiting factor during dynamic strength manoeuvres involving many muscle groups (Sale, 1988).

Muscles of older people contract and relax more slowly than in young adults. This slowing may stem from the reduced proportional contribution of Type II fibres to the twitch contraction, together with an age-related change in the muscle's calcium regulatory mechanisms. Slowing of a muscle contractile response confers an adaptation of greater efficiency for the excitable membranes of the associated motoneurons and their muscle fibres; the more slowly a muscle contracts, the lower is the frequency of nerve impulses required to attain a given muscle tension or reach tetanic fusion. This benefit for the central nervous system, along with the fact that Type I fibres take up more of the total muscle mass, may explain why even sedentary older people still demonstrate adequate fatigue resistance in their muscles. Indeed, healthy and fit older people could potentially experience less metabolic stress during a submaximal exercise bout than sedentary young adults, because their muscles have undergone a natural adaptation towards tonic activity (see also Chapters 9, 12 and 22).

Changes in Protective Reflexes and Balance Control

Slowing of contraction also has a disadvantage because it gives older muscle a reduced capacity for rapid production of force in protective reflexes (i.e. when ballistic, phasic reactions are required). This slowing combines with other changes in the neuromuscular system to magnify the functional deficit. For example, if an older person steps on an obstacle the kinaesthetic and pain sensations are less intense and nerve impulses slower to travel around the reflex loop to the muscle. After the signal arrives at the muscle, the actual generation of restorative torque is also slower and may not be in time to prevent a loss of balance. Also, the muscle response must act against increased passive resistance of the connective tissue structures of the antagonistic muscles, a factor which hinders rapid stretch and therefore rotation of aged joints, particularly in older women. Figure 2 shows how these two factors of reduced strength and increased stiffness combine to decrease the active range of motion values in older people (Vandervoort *et al.*, 1992) (see Chapter 22).

There is clear evidence of deterioration throughout the postural control system in association with the ageing process (Chapters 7 and 9). Although at some points these degenerative changes may seem to be small and insignificant, the summation of deficits will increase the risk of

Figure 2 A comparison of age effects on strength of the ankle dorsiflexor muscles, passive resistance against dorsiflexion, and active range of motion (ROM) in the dorsiflexion direction. The sample consisted of healthy men and women grouped in 5 year spans from 55 to 85. The weakened state of the very old females, plus increased passive resistance, limits active ROM. (From Vandervoort et al., 1992.)

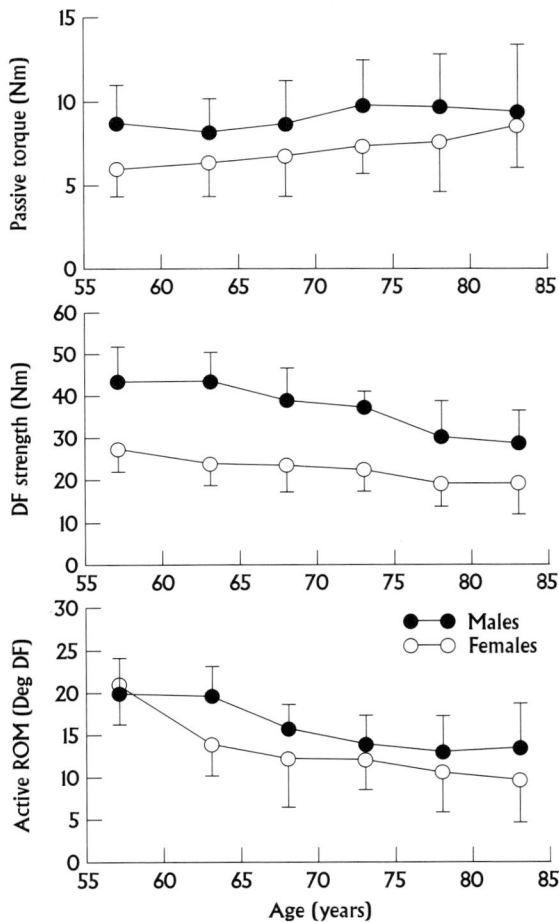

cal changes such as delay in the detection of imbalance and disorganization of central processing they put the older individual at increased risk (Patla, 1995).

Capacity for Adaptation in Older People

A key principle upon which physiotherapy with older people is based is that their tissues and organ systems still retain a capacity to adapt to a therapeutic stimulus. The adaptive response will vary widely depending on factors such as the initial level of the function and the intensity of the stimulus. Due to effects of ageing, older people may not respond in the same manner as young adults to interventions and care must be taken to individualize their physiotherapy programmes (Pickles, 1989). Few empirical studies of the effects of specific remedial exercise and modalities on older patients exist at present (see Chapter 12), and the physiotherapist will often need to rely upon clinical judgement and extrapolation of findings from clinical studies of young adults.

Recently, there has been a growing interest in the adaptive capacity of the ageing neuromuscular system (Marks, 1992). Can muscle cells that have survived into old age still respond to an 'overload' stimulus with hypertrophy? (See Chapter 12.) Can descending motor pathways adapt to increased demands and allow older adults to relearn the skill of coordinating a strong voluntary movement? (See Chapter 9.) Mounting evidence now supports the belief that cellular adaptation in both the muscular and nervous systems is possible at all ages. Until recently, for example, it was considered that strength increases in older people following a weight-

incorrect or inefficient response and a subsequent loss of coordination, particularly when attempting a taxing functional activity (e.g. going down stairs while carrying a load, moving sideways quickly to avoid a collision). Slower postural reflexes alone will not always be the cause of a fall, but combined with other biologi-

Figure 3   How multifactorial influences of ageing can impair mobility. The four key systems identified are all highly susceptible to the effects of inactivity. Thus, an older person who begins to withdraw from regular activity begins a spiral of increasing susceptibility to mobility problems.

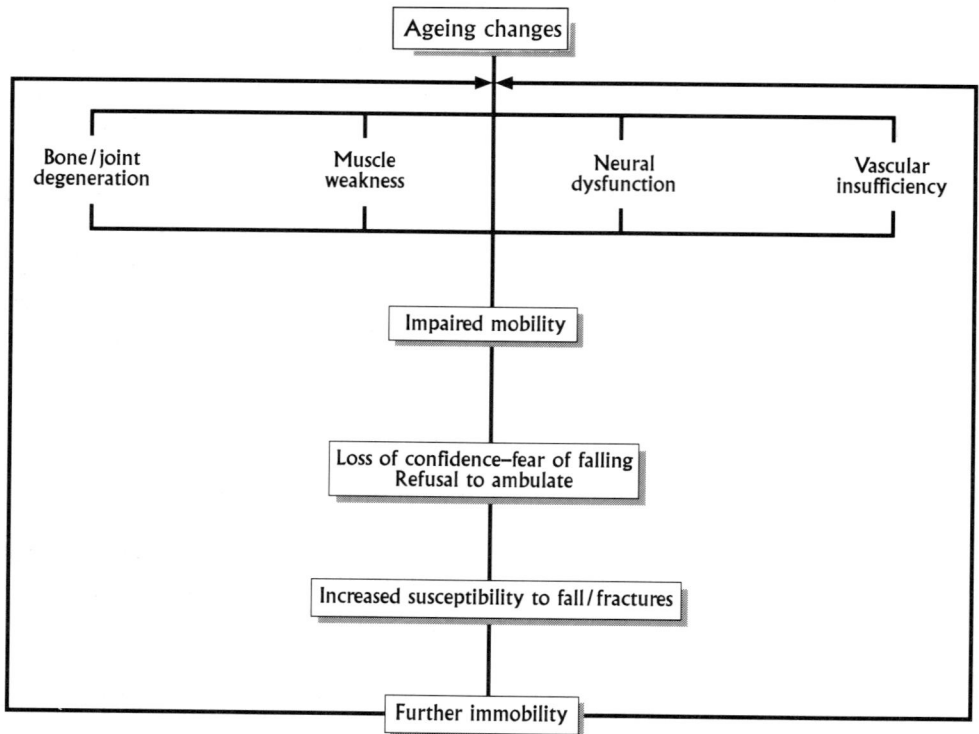

lifting programme resulted solely from increased neural drive, but significant hypertrophy of muscle cells has recently been demonstrated during such programmes (Porter and Vandervoort, 1995). This finding confirms that the cellular regulation of contractile proteins can still be stimulated to increase the production of myosin, actin and other muscle constituents. At least some of the deleterious age-related change in body composition is reversible, given the appropriate biological stimulus. It is useful to remember too that seemingly small changes in activity can make an impact on strength and function, especially in very old people who start from quite low baseline levels (Connelly and Vandervoort, 1995). (See Chapter 12.)

Cardiorespiratory Function

Many studies over the years have demonstrated an age-related decline in cardiorespiratory function, as exemplified by the body's maximum capacity to utilize oxygen (VO_2max) for metabolism (Wilmore and Costill, 1994). VO_2max can be expressed in absolute terms of total amount of O_2 consumed per minute (i.e. millilitres per minute) or relative to some expression of body mass, usually total weight in kg (i.e. ml per kg per min). When calculated with respect to total body weight, a rather striking difference is found between males and females. Sedentary males stay fairly constant in VO_2max until maturity (45 ml/kg/min) and then experience a decline of approximately 1% per year. Females, however, begin to decline in terms of relative VO_2max immediately after puberty because of their increased proportion of body fat; after this they have lower average values than males.

The primary cause of both the difference between genders and the age-related decline in aerobic capacity is the same: an increase of body fat relative to amount of metabolically active lean tissue present. This reduces the endurance of older people for weight-bearing activity. While other changes do take place in the cardiovascular and respiratory systems, the capacity for exercise in the healthy older person is primarily linked to the aerobic fitness of the skeletal muscle. In other words, the heart and lungs appear to remain capable of delivering an adequate supply of oxygenated blood to the working muscle for the normal daily activities of healthy older people (Paterson, 1992). It takes exercise at extreme levels of performance (e.g. Master athletes) or stress testing to expose the limitations of reserve capacity of the ageing cardiorespiratory system.

A recent large-scale study helps to illuminate the important effects of age-related changes in physical activity level and body composition on aerobic capacity (Jackson et al., 1995). VO_2max relative to body weight was measured in 1499 men ranging in age from 25 to 70 years. While average body weight did not differ across ages, average percentage of fat increased from 16.5 to 22.9% and the fat-free weight (which is mainly muscle) declined by 4.5 kg. Hence, both absolute and

relative VO_2max showed decreases with advancing age, but the yearly decline of approximately 0.5 ml/kg/min in the relative VO_2max was more pronounced. In fact, the effectiveness of a healthy lifestyle was simulated in a statistical model: if people were to reduce the usual age-related trends and actually lower their body fat and increase their activity level while growing older, they could minimize the normal loss of aerobic capacity by half. The remarkable benefits of fitness programmes for improving or maintaining the endurance of older people have also been demonstrated in numerous studies of acute exercise programmes and chronically trained Master athletes (Paterson, 1992) (see Chapter 12).

Cardiovascular Changes

One of our most potent symbols of being alive is the beating heart. Much attention has been paid to how various aspects of circulatory function change with ageing (Wilmore and Costill, 1994). These changes result in a decrease of reserve capacity in cardiovascular function that will affect exercise tolerance. The basal metabolic rate (BMR) of the 'resting' body has a VO_2 of approximately 3.5 ml/kg/min (in fact many tissues are still active, including the heart and lungs and excitable cells such as in the nervous system). The heart meets this demand by pumping about 5 litres of blood per minute as its cardiac output (CO), which in turn is determined by the rate (HR) and stroke volume (SV) per beat (e.g. 80 bpm × 60 ml per beat). Ageing actually makes this job easier because BMR declines throughout the lifespan, most rapidly during development and then gradually during the adult years, as a result of the loss of metabolically active tissue (lean body mass), together with a reduction in the actual rate of energy consumption by subcellular activities such as Na^+/K^+ pumps.

Exercise places dramatically increased demands on the working muscles for fuel and oxygen. The heart responds by increasing its output some 4–5 times. The primary mechanism used by the young adult to meet this demand is to increase heart rate, up to an average maximum of at least 200 bpm. However, the older heart loses this reserve at a rate of about 1 beat per year, starting from early childhood. Hence, a frequently used rule of thumb to estimate maximal HR in people is to calculate it as 220 bpm minus the age in years. There is considerable variability among individuals, however. The mechanism for this change appears to be changes in the amount and conductance of the cardiac pacing system (SA node and bundle of His), as well as decreased sensitivity to catecholamine stimulation. Second, to increase output the heart can enhance its stroke volume, but this capacity also appears to decrease somewhat in sedentary older people. The main mechanism for the ageing effect on SV appears to be due to stiffening of the heart wall, which in turn limits the capacity for its muscle fibres to be stretched during filling and take advantage of better length–tension mechanics (known as the Frank–Starling mechanism).

Most of the increase in cardiac output during exercise is channelled through the muscle vascular bed, due to the increased driving force of a raised blood pressure and an autoregulated opening of muscle microcirculation. With ageing, the arterial walls become stiffer and the peripheral vascular resistance (against muscle blood flow) is increased. This increased resistance is reflected in the rises in blood pressure with ageing. Fortunately, the muscle does have another option, which is to increase its extraction of O_2 from whatever blood flow it gets. This extraction is referred to as the arterial–venous O_2 difference, and can be readily increased with appropriate exercise training. A major benefit of this adaptation is that a more efficient, trained muscle will require less blood flow for a given VO_2, thereby reducing the heart's workload for any given submaximal exercise intensity.

Respiratory System Changes

Common clinical measures of pulmonary function show age-related decrements. Variables related to the ability to move air out of the lungs, such as vital capacity and forced expiratory volume in 1 s, show linear declines with age (Wilmore and Costill, 1994). As total lung capacity is not normally reduced, more of the lung capacity in older adults is taken up with a residual volume of air – amounting to 30% or more – that is not exchanged on a given breath. The primary mechanism of age-related loss is attributed to the increased stiffening of elastic tissues in both the lungs and chest wall, thereby reducing the effectiveness of their passive recoil after being stretched.

As it is of vital importance that the blood receive a fresh supply of oxygen and releases its carbon dioxide in the lungs, the pulmonary system actually has a large reserve. This reserve is somewhat diminished in old age, but is still usually adequate to keep an older person's arterial blood saturated with oxygen at rest and during moderate exertion (this is in the absence of notable pathology anywhere along the chain, e.g. absence of asthma, emphysema, heart failure or haemoglobin disorders). An untrained older person may be limited to a maximum of 60–80 litres of ventilation per minute, almost half that of a young adult. Fortunately, the many elements of pulmonary function, involving aspects of ventilation, diffusion and perfusion, appear to show less deterioration in older people who have stayed physically active (Johnson et al., 1994).

Summary

The ageing process is intrinsic, progressive, deleterious and irreversible. The biological basis of ageing remains a topic of great interest and likely reflects the complex interaction between a genetically controlled internal clock and gradual deterioration of cell function over time. The motor system is particularly susceptible to the ageing process because its nerve and muscle cells are postmitotic and thus irreplaceable. Many interrelated physiological changes with ageing can be linked to detrimental alterations of body composition towards increased fat and less muscle and bone mass. Coinciding with the ongoing ageing process can be the detrimental effects of a sedentary lifestyle of some older people, which also initiates reduction in reserve capacity. However, the capacity for physiological adaptation to increased activity patterns remains into very old age. There is a strong, positive relationship between amount of reserve capacity available for doing a physical task and the ability to delay fatigue. Even a small gain of physiological function may translate into functional improvement and greater independence for older people.

References

Brody, H, Vijayashanker, N (1977) Anatomical changes in the nervous system. In Finch, C, Hayflick, L (eds) The Handbook of the Biology of Aging. New York: Van Nostrand Reinhold.

Connelly, DM, Vandervoort, AA (1995) Low resistance training increases knee extension strength in very old females. Physiotherapy Canada 47: 15–23.

Cristifalo, VJ (1990) Overview of biological mechanism of ageing. Annual Review of Gerontology and Geriatrics 10: 1–22.

Doherty, TJ, Vandervoort, AA, Brown, WF (1993) Effects of ageing on the motor unit: a brief review. Canadian Journal of Applied Physiology 18: 331–358.

Fries, JF, Crapo, L (1981) Vitality and Aging. San Francisco: WH Freeman.

Hakansson, DM, Vandervoort, AA, Kramer, JF (1991) Effect of cold therapy on nerve conduction in young and elderly women. Physiotherapy Canada 43 (2): Suppl.

Jackson, AS, Beard, EF, Wier, LT et al. (1995) Changes in aerobic power of men, ages 25–70 yr. Medicine and Science in Sports and Exercise 27: 113–120.

Johnson, BD, Badr, MS, Dempsey, JA (1994) Impact of the ageing pulmonary system on the response to exercise. Clinics in Chest Medicine 15: 229–246.

Katzman, R, Terry, R (1983) The Neurology of Aging. Philadelphia: FA Davis.

Lexell J (1993) Ageing and human muscle: observations from Sweden. Canadian Journal of Applied Physiology 18: 2–18.

McComas, AJ (1977) Neuromuscular Function and Disorders. London: Butterworths.

Magnoni, MS, Govoni, S, Battaini, F et al. (1991) The ageing brain: protein phosphorylation as a target of changes in neuronal function. Life Sciences 48: 373–385.

Marks, R (1992) The effect of ageing and strength training on skeletal muscle. Australian Journal of Physiotherapy 38: 9–19.

Paterson, DH (1992) Effects of ageing on the cardiorespiratory system. Canadian Journal of Sport Sciences 17: 171–177.

Patla, AE (1995) A framework for understanding mobility problems in the elderly. In: Craik RL, Oatis CA (eds) Gait Analysis: Theory and Application. St Louis: Mosby.

Pickles, B (1989) Biological aspects of ageing. In: Jackson, OL (ed.) Physical Therapy of the Geriatric Patient, 2nd edn. New York: Churchill Livingstone.

Porter, MM, Vandervoort, AA (1995) High intensity strength training for the older adult – a review. Topics in Geriatric Rehabilitation 10: 61–74.

Sale, DG (1988) Neural adaptation to resistance training. Medicine and Science in Sports and Exercise 20: S135–145.

Vandervoort, AA, McComas, AJ (1986) Contractile changes in opposing muscles of the human ankle joint with ageing. Journal of Applied Physiology 61: 361–367.

Vandervoort, AA, Chesworth, BM, Cunningham, DA *et al.* (1992) Age and sex effects on mobility of the human ankle. *Journals of Gerontology: Medical Sciences* **47**: M17–21.

Walker, J (1991) Connective tissue plasticity: issues in histological and light microscopy studies of exercise and ageing in articular cartilage. *Journal of Orthopaedic and Sports Physical Therapy* **14**: 189–197.

Wilmore, JH, Costill, DL (1994) *Physiology of Sport and Exercise.* Champaign, Il: Human Kinetics.

7

Changes in Posture and Gait

SANDRA J OLNEY, ELSIE G CULHAM

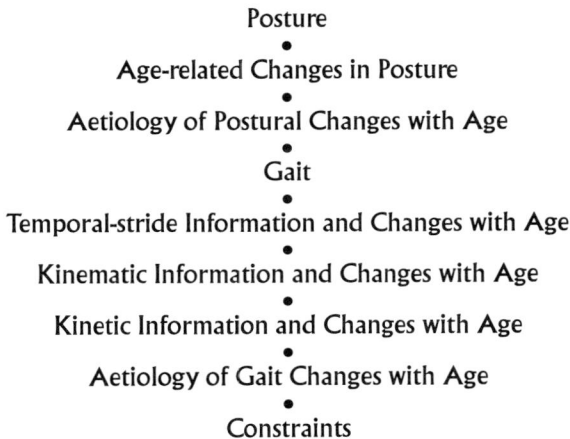

Posture
•
Age-related Changes in Posture
•
Aetiology of Postural Changes with Age
•
Gait
•
Temporal-stride Information and Changes with Age
•
Kinematic Information and Changes with Age
•
Kinetic Information and Changes with Age
•
Aetiology of Gait Changes with Age
•
Constraints

Posture

Static posture is defined by the arrangement of the body segments relative to each other. Optimal postural alignment is one which requires minimal energy to maintain and produces minimal stress on joints. In the standing position, optimal posture in the sagittal plane is most commonly described as one in which a plumb line dropped from the ear lobe will fall through the shoulder joint, midway through the trunk, through the greater trochanter, slightly anterior to a midline through the knee and slightly anterior to the lateral malleolus. The pelvis and hip are in a neutral position, the knee joint is extended and the ankle joint is in neutral dorsi/plantarflex-

ion (Figure 1). Abnormalities in alignment of one component of the skeleton will result in compensatory changes in adjacent regions.

Abnormalities in postural alignment and compensatory changes in adjacent regions will influence the manner in which a person moves. Walking is arguably the most thoroughly studied of all human motor activities. Early cinematographic records and hand calculations using data from innovative force or pressure devices have provided a wealth of fundamental information. Modern sensors and powerful computers have made it possible to collect and manipulate large volumes of data that have revealed some of the complexities of this fundamental human function and the effects of ageing.

Figure 1   Normal adult posture.

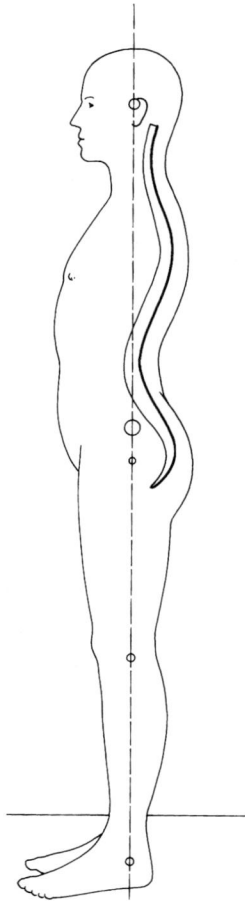

Age-related Changes in Posture

Alteration in the erect standing posture is one of several changes which occur in the musculoskeletal system as a consequence of ageing (see Chapter 6). Age-related changes occur primarily in the sagittal plane and include an increase in kyphotic curvature of the thoracic spine (Milne and Lauder, 1974; O'Gorman and Jull, 1987), a decrease in lumbar lordosis (Milne and Lauder, 1974), an increase in knee flexion angle (Brocklehurst et al., 1982), a more posterior hip position and anterior lean of the trunk above the hips (Woodhull-McNeal, 1992). These changes tend to begin above the age of 40 years and together contribute to the reduction in height and the stooped posture typically described in older people.

Despite the consistency with which the above changes are reported in the literature a 'typical posture' cannot be defined due to the marked variability in standing posture in older individuals. The postural changes are not inevitable and they do not necessarily occur together. While some changes may be attributed to primary causes, others are more likely the result of compensatory mechanisms which function to maintain an upright position.

Postural Types

Identification of postural subtypes may facilitate understanding the postural deviations and the interaction of the various abnormalities which occur. Postural types or subgroups have been described for both healthy and osteoporotic older individuals (Milne and Lauder, 1974; Itoi, 1991; Culham and Peat, 1994). Abnormalities in posture can be divided into two basic types, both of which involve an increase in curvature of the spine in the sagittal plane. One type of posture may be labelled thoracic kyphosis and the second a thoracolumbar kyphosis (Figure 2).

Spinal deformity often develops insidiously and objective measures of posture are needed to monitor change over time and to determine the effectiveness of treatment. Objective measures of spinal posture in the sagittal plane can be obtained using inexpensive, non-invasive clinical instru-

Figure 2 Changes in posture with age. (a) Type one posture – thoracic kyphosis; (b) type two posture – thoracolumbar kyphosis.

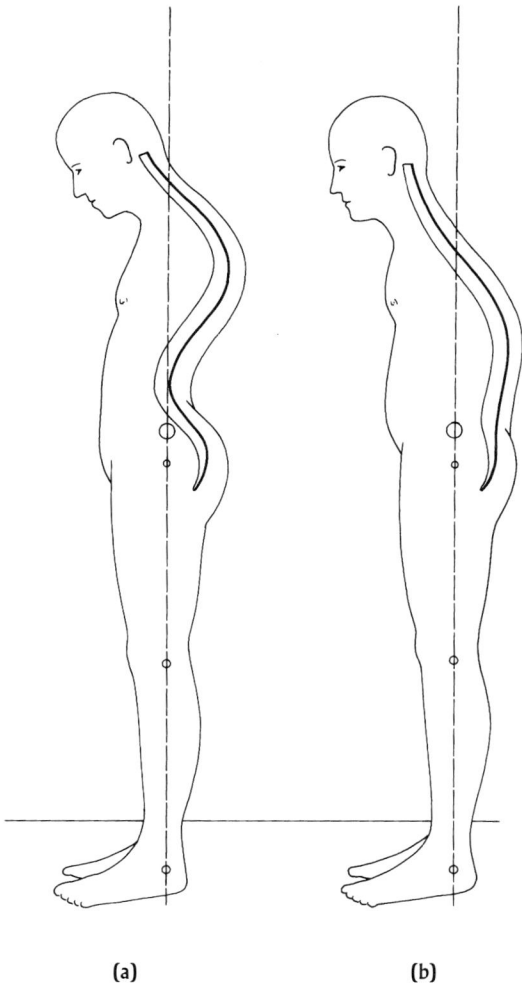

(a)   (b)

ments. Loss of height occurs with the development of spinal deformity and provides an objective measure of change that the patient can monitor independently. Spinal curves can be measured clinically using a flexicurve or an inclinometer. The flexicurve consists of a strip of lead covered by plastic which can be bent in one plane only. It retains the shape into which it is bent and can be used to copy any curved surface. The flexicurve is applied over the spinous processes from the seventh cervical vertebra to the sacrum and the location of spinous processes of interest are marked on the flexicurve. The curve is subsequently traced on paper and the spinal curvature calculated mathematically. An inclinometer consists of a protractor containing a freely swinging pointer suspended from its centre. Two attached feet which project from the base of the protractor are positioned along the spine. The gravity-dependent pointer records the angle of inclination of the spinal segment relative to the vertical. Slope or inclination of the upper and lower thoracic spine, upper lumbar spine and sacrum can be obtained by this method and thoracic and lumbar curvature calculated from these measures (Figure 3).

THORACIC KYPHOSIS

This is the most common postural abnormality which occurs with age and is defined by an increase in kyphotic curvature of the thoracic spine, with the apex of the kyphotic curvature located in the mid thoracic region. The increased thoracic curve is associated with maintenance of, or an increase in, the lumbar lordosis. Itoi (1991) called this type of posture a 'round back' or 'hollow round back', depending on whether the lumbar curve was normal or increased.

Itoi (1991) considered that the kyphotic curvature was the primary deformity in the women studied, and that the increase in lumbar lordosis in the hollow round back deformity was a compensatory mechanism developed to maintain a balanced spine. If sufficient compensation is provided by the lumbar lordosis no alteration in the hip and knee angles is required. If the curves are balanced this postural abnormality will also not necessarily result in a forward trunk lean described in the elderly population.

Figure 3 Spinal slopes in the sagittal plane as measured using an inclinometer.

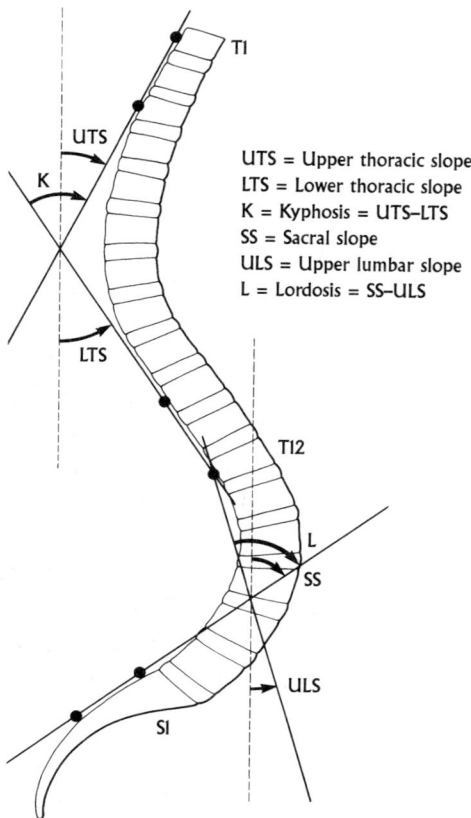

UTS = Upper thoracic slope
LTS = Lower thoracic slope
K = Kyphosis = UTS–LTS
SS = Sacral slope
ULS = Upper lumbar slope
L = Lordosis = SS–ULS

measured caudally from the first thoracic verte-brae, is increased relative to the vertical in subjects with this posture resulting in a forward head position (Culham and Peat, 1994). The forward tilt of the scapula in the sagittal plane is also increased compared to that found in subjects of the same age with no postural abnormality, but not to the same extent as the upper thoracic spine. The prominent dorsal ribs may prevent the scapula from tilting forward to the same degree as the upper thorax. The increasing dis-crepancy in inclination between the upper thoracic spine and scapula, as kyphosis increases, may result in a gradual lengthening of structures having attachment to the cervical spine and scapula, for example the levator scapula and rhomboid muscles and the suprascapular nerve, causing stretching and potential irritation of these structures.

THORACOLUMBAR KYPHOSIS

In people with this type of posture the apex of the kyphotic curvature is in the lower thoracic, thora-columbar or lumbar region, which results in either a thoracolumbar kyphosis or a total kyphotic curvature of the spine. In either case, there is a loss of the normal lumbar lordotic curvature. This postural type combines the 'lower acute kyphosis' and 'whole kyphosis' subgroups described by Itoi (1991) for osteoporotic women. In subjects with a thoracolumbar or total kyphotic curvature, com-pensation for the kyphotic curvature cannot occur in the lumbar region. Osteoporotic women with these types of posture were found to have a decreased forward tilt of the sacrum, increased posterior pelvic tilt, and an increased knee flexion angle in standing. Itoi (1991) postu-lated that the initial compensation for this type of kyphotic curvature was one of posterior sacral and pelvic tilt. The posterior pelvic tilt first results

When the apex of the curvature is in the thoracic region the ribs become prominent dorsally and the antero-posterior diameter of the thorax is increased. Culham and Peat (1994) reported that subjects with this type of posture had a significant increase in the protraction angle of the scapula and the angle between the scapular spine and the clavicle in the transverse plane compared to sub-jects without postural deformity in the same age range. It was thought that these changes were necessary to accommodate the increased antero-posterior diameter of the thorax.

The slope of the upper thoracic spine, as

in extension of the hip, but once maximal hip extension has been achieved, the femoral inclination angle increases and the knees flex (Itoi, 1991). Brocklehurst et al. (1982) reported a greater knee angle in standing in elderly subjects compared to younger subjects which was unrelated to degenerative changes in the knee joint. It appears likely that the knee joint angle increases when the kyphotic curvature in the lower spine cannot be compensated for at higher levels.

The thoracic spine curvature is not increased in this postural type, nor is there any increase in the antero-posterior diameter of the thorax. The trunk is inclined forward above the apex of the curve, resulting in an increase in the inclination of the upper thoracic spine and a forward head position, as observed in thoracic kyphosis. The forward trunk lean, or more anterior position of the centre of gravity of the trunk, reported by Woodhull-McNeal (1992), is more likely to occur in individuals with this type of spinal posture.

Culham and Peat (1994) measured shoulder complex position in subjects with a thoracolumbar kyphosis, and found that the inclination of the upper thoracic spine was significantly increased in this group when compared to women without spinal deformity, although the increase in the forward angulation of the scapula in the two groups was the same. There was no increase in the scapular protraction angle or the angle between the scapular spine and clavicle in the transverse plane as observed in the group with a thoracic kyphosis. With the spinal curvature at a lower level there is no increase in the antero-posterior diameter of the thorax and no need for compensatory alterations in the position of shoulder complex structures.

Aetiology of Postural Changes with Age

Spinal Fractures Secondary to Osteoporosis

Spinal osteoporosis, leading to fractures of the vertebral bodies, is the principal cause of kyphosis in ageing men and women (Milne and Lauder, 1976; O'Gorman and Jull, 1987). Osteoporosis is defined as a reduction in bone mass which increases susceptibility to fracture. Vertebral fractures due to osteoporosis involve the lower six thoracic and all the lumbar vertebrae. The upper thoracic and cervical vertebrae are rarely involved. Fractures show a consistent predilection for two sites, in the mid thoracic (T 7/8) and the thoracolumbar junction. Fractures cause anterior compression and wedging of vertebral bodies typically resulting in an acute increase in kyphosis, with the apex of the curve at the level of the fractures.

Milne and Lauder (1976) studied the relationship between the degree of kyphosis and shape of the vertebral bodies. Wedge deformity of the vertebral bodies was measured from radiographs of 486 men and women between 62 and 90 years of age. The length of a curved line drawn along the anterior and posterior aspects of the vertebral bodies from the upper border of T7 to the lower border of T12 was measured. The posterior measurement was expressed as a percentage of the anterior measure and this value was taken as the index of wedging. Kyphosis was measured in the same subjects using a surveyor's flexicurve. The degree of vertebral wedging and kyphosis both increased with age in men and women. Wedging explained 42% and 48% of the variation in kyphosis in men and women, respectively. While kyphosis was greater in women, the degree of wedging was not significantly different, indicating that factors other than vertebral fracture contribute to kyphosis in women. Similarly, in a study of 87 women with spinal osteoporosis, De Smet *et al.* (1988) reported that the number of anterior wedge fractures correlated significantly with the degree of kyphosis. However, many women with no fractures also had an accentuated curve leading the authors to conclude that non-skeletal factors also contribute to kyphosis.

Decrease in Physical Activity

A decrease in level of physical activity with age is also thought to contribute to increasing sagittal plane curvature of the vertebral column (Chapter 6). Decreasing levels of physical activity with age may result in a decrease in bone mass and increased incidence of vertebral fracture. Physical activity is known to positively influence bone mass achieved at skeletal maturity and to prevent bone loss later in life (see also Chapter 12). Astronauts exposed to weightless conditions and patients confined to bed have reversible bone loss from both the axial and appendicular skeleton. Athletes have significantly greater bone mass than people who do not exercise. The bones with the greatest increase in mass are those subjected to the greatest weight-bearing stresses during performance of the sport or exercise. Finally, it has been demonstrated that involutional bone loss in women can be decreased or reversed by exercise.

In addition, physical activity is necessary for maintenance of muscle strength and health of supporting connective tissues of the spine. Loss of tone and strength in these structures, particularly the back extensor muscles, will result in a decreased ability to counteract the anteriorly directed gravitational forces which tend to increase spinal flexion. Kyphosis angle has been reported to be significantly greater in subjects with 'average' versus 'above average' fitness levels in healthy postmenopausal women (Chow and Harrison, 1987).

Flexion Forces

The line of gravity falls anterior to the thoracic vertebrae, passes through the twelfth thoracic and first lumbar vertebrae and descends anterior to the second sacral vertebrae. Weight-bearing forces are therefore exerted on the anterior portion of the thoracic vertebral bodies and intervertebral discs; additional flexion forces will tend to further accentuate the thoracic curvature.

Factors such as muscle weakness, poor self-image, emotional or psychosocial stress and mimicking the habits of parents may all result in habitual poor posture, in which a person tends to slump forward, and gradually cause an exaggeration of kyphotic curvature. Chow and Harrison (1987) found that subjects with greater degrees of kyphosis tended to have 'poor posture' since childhood.

Occupations which involve repetitive or sustained forward flexion of the spine may also cause an increase in thoracic curvature. Service workers and farmers have a greater curvature than teachers or office workers. Dependent breasts in women may also be a factor.

Gait

Knowledge about gait can be classified into three types: temporal-stride, kinematic and kinetic information. The first two of these provide only descriptive information, while kinetic information may also provide insights into the probable causes of observed gait characteristics.

Temporal-stride Information

Temporal-stride measures are descriptive, and include stride length, cadence, speed of walking, the durations of stance and swing phases of each side and the phases of double support. The events are diagrammatically represented in Figure 4. The speed of walking, generally measured over several strides, is the average length of the stride divided by the average duration of the stride. The timing information given by the stride duration is more frequently expressed as step cadence, or the number of steps taken per minute when both right and left steps are included. The relationships between speed, stride length and cadence is:

$$\text{Speed (m/s)} = \frac{\text{stride length (m)} \times \text{step cadence (per minute)}}{120}$$

A decrease in either stride length or cadence will result in decreased speed.

Temporal-stride Changes with Age

The speed an individual chooses for daily ambulation is the most fundamental measure of gait performance. Self-selected walking speed has usually been reported to decrease with age (Chapters 6 and 9). The rate of decline in speed that has been reported by various authors reflects the differences in the populations studied as well as the methods used. Most studies have reported the decline to age 60 to be in the range of 1% to 2% per decade (Bendall et al., 1989), with rates of decline in the later decades ranging from 7% per decade (Bendall et al., 1989) to 16% per decade for men in one study (Himann et al., 1988). The reduction in walking speed has been largely

Figure 4   The major temporal events in the normal gait cycle.

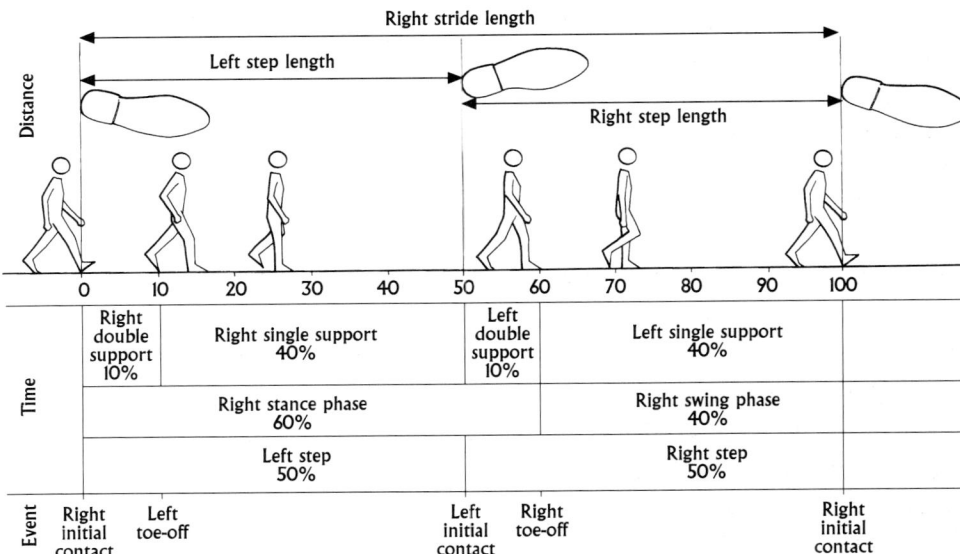

87

attributed to reduction in stride length rather than cadence. Although some authors have reported a reduced walking cadence in some older people (Murray et al., 1969; Gillis et al., 1986), those studying healthy and fit older persons have not found differences (Elble et al., 1991; Winter, 1991). In comparing older subjects with young subjects walking at the same speed, the older persons take shorter steps at a greater frequency to achieve the same speed. Although age-related decreases in walking speed are due largely to reductions in stride length, increases in speed by an older person are accomplished by the same relative increases in both stride length and cadence as those of a younger person (Ferrandez et al., 1990). These observations indicate that intentional modulations of velocity do not change with age.

The major temporal events in the gait cycle are shown in Figure 4. The proportions of the gait cycle spent in the stance phase is higher in older adults than in the young. Although normally occupying about 60% of the gait cycle, stance phase increases of up to 5% have been reported. Similar increases in double support time also occur with age. These changes are attributable to differences in self-selected speeds of walking, and are similar to the proportions found in young subjects walking at slow speeds (Ferrandez et al., 1990).

Kinematic Information

Kinematic information is also descriptive, and includes the positions of joint centres and the centres of mass of limb segments, as well as joint angles and their angular velocities and accelerations. One method of obtaining this information is video-based (Figure 5), in which a videotape is taken of the walking subject who has been suitably prepared with reflective markers placed on appropriate body landmarks; data are often automatically digitized and computer processing permits calculation of desired variables. A second method uses markers consisting of infrared diodes placed on the body parts, and special cameras which identify their location. Although the latter method is somewhat more cumbersome for the subject, it provides smaller marker error. The most commonly used kinematic data are the

Table 1

Mean Values of Temporal-Distance Measures Reported for Various Subject Ages

Source	Speed (m/s)	Stride length (m)	Cadence (steps/min)
Winter (1991)			
Mean age 24.6, N=2	1.43	1.55	111
Mean age 68.0, N=15	1.28	1.39	110
Murray (1969)			
Age 20–25, N=8	1.50	1.54	114
Age 81–87, N=8	1.18	1.26	109
Ferrandez et al. (1990)			
Age 60–69, N=28	1.00	1.09	106
Age 80–92, N=12	0.60	0.71	100

Figure 5   Subject taking part in collection of data for gait analysis.

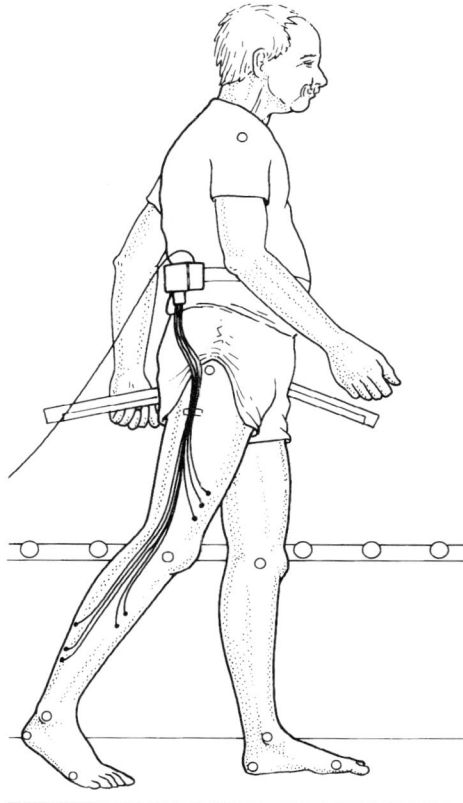

profiles of these variables obtained from repeated gait cycles.

Kinematic Changes with Age

Kinematic profiles of older people show small variations from those of young subjects. In all cases, however, the variability of these profiles has been reported to be reduced in older people. The ankle shows diminished range of motion, largely a result of a reduced plantarflexion excursion during push-off (Murray et al., 1969; Winter, 1991). While young adults extend their knee nearly fully at the end of swing, older persons complete the swing phase with the knee in several degrees

of flexion (Murray et al., 1969; Winter, 1991). Maximum extension and flexion of the knee as well as the dynamic range of knee movement have been reported to be reduced with age (Elble et al., 1991). Although there is one report of an increase in hip joint range over the stride (Winter, 1991), other authors have reported a decrease (Murray et al., 1969) or a trend towards a decrease, particularly in extension (Elble et al., 1991).

The results from studies of foot clearance are inconsistent. Some authors have reported the clearance to be greater in persons over 65 years (Murray et al., 1969), while others have reported values similar to those of younger adults (Winter et al., 1990; Elble et al., 1991). Heel contact velocity in the horizontal direction has been reported to be significantly increased in the elderly despite walking at slower speeds (Winter, 1991). This velocity rapidly decreases to zero upon weight bearing, as a result of friction force between the heel and the floor. If the friction is reduced (see Chapter 26), for example on polished floors, the potential for slipping becomes greater.

The head provides a stable platform for the visual system during gait. The differences between the accelerations of the head and the pelvis while walking have been compared in the young and old, as the reduction in acceleration between the pelvis and head represent the effectiveness of a damping effect by the trunk. Although pelvic accelerations are lower in older people (Winter, 1991), the head accelerations are significantly higher.

Kinetic Information

Kinetic information includes knowledge about the variables that are the causes of the kinematic patterns seen, and therefore is capable of providing explanatory as well as descriptive information. These variables include forces, moments of force and joint powers. The most common method of analysis uses inverse dynamics with a link segment model. In this method the forces from the floor on the most distal segment, the foot, are measured, as well as the mass of the foot segment, its position and motion. This information permits calculation of the net joint moment and the forces that must have been present at the ankle in order that the motion could occur. Having solved the problem at the ankle, the analysis proceeds to the lower leg segment in the same manner, then to the thigh and trunk.

Joint moments in the plane of progression can be

used to express support and balance. The support moment is the sum of the hip extensor, knee extensor and ankle plantarflexor moments across stance phase. It is remarkably consistent despite variations in the contributions from the hip, knee and ankle. In fact, the moment required at the hip to balance the large mass of the head, arms and trunk essentially determines its shape and amplitude, and the moment of the knee shows a 'trade-off' with it. The degree to which they trade off can be expressed as covariance, and used as an index of balance (Winter, 1991).

The net muscle power across a joint can be calculated as the product of the net moment of the muscles about a joint and the net angular velocity, so that the value of the power at any instant is sensitive to both the strength of the muscle contraction and the speed of the movement. Energy for walking is generated by concentric contractions and absorbed by eccentric muscle activity. The greatest contributions to the work of walking are made by the ankle plantarflexors at push-off and the hip flexors commencing simultaneously but continuing into early swing phase (pull-off). Minor contributions are made by the hip extensors in early stance phase.

Kinetic Changes with Age

Because only two sets of kinetic data have been reported for older people (Olney et al., 1989; Winter, 1991), their generalizability is not known. The moment of force profiles of the young and older people were similar with one exception: the plantarflexor moment during push-off was reduced in older persons with a consequent reduction in power generation (Figure 6; see Chapter 26). The net positive work performed

Figure 6   Mean power profiles of young subjects walking at natural speed (1.44 m/s dotted line) compared with the elderly walking at natural speed (1.09 m/s, solid line), slow speed (0.64, dash-dot line) and very slow speeds (0.40 m/s, dashed line). Note decrease in push-off power of ankle plantarflexors (A2) and increase in absorption by knee extensors (K3).

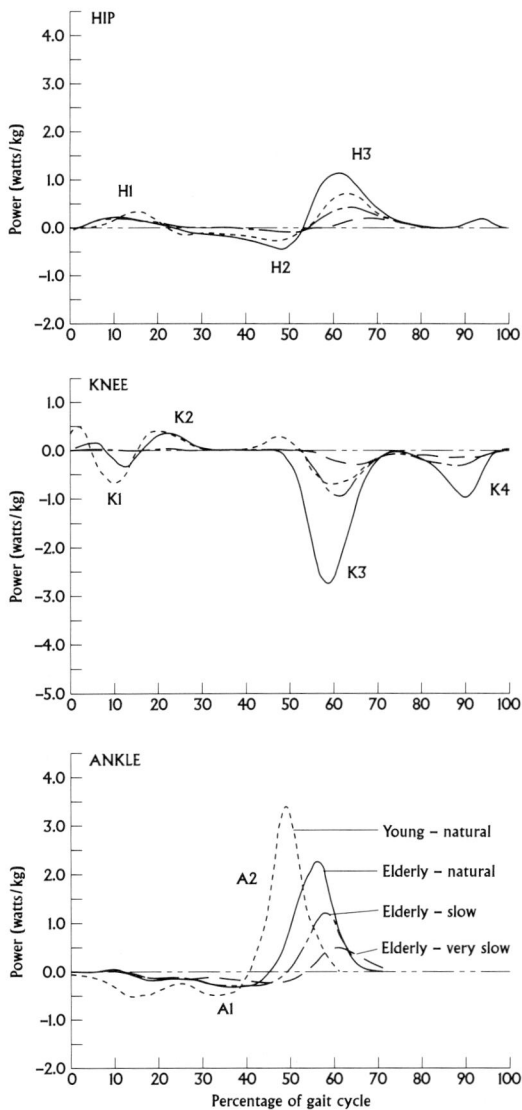

during push-off was further diminished in older persons by the larger amount of absorption by the knee extensors during the late stance phase. Winter (1991) has also reported a reduction in the absorption by the knee flexors in older persons in late swing, just prior to heel contact; this is thought to reduce deceleration of the swinging leg, resulting in higher horizontal heel contact velocities. A kinetic change with age related to balance was the degree of trade-off between the moment profiles of the hip and knee. A lower index of balance was found for the older subjects.

Aetiology of Gait Changes with Age

The temporal and stride, kinematic, and kinetic changes in the gait with ageing can be grouped into two categories: those consistent with subtle physiological changes in the sensorimotor system (Chapter 6) and those that are consistent with motor adaptations that promote safer walking (Chapter 9).

Differences Consistent with Subtle Physiological Changes

It is not possible to separate with any degree of certainty the changes in gait resulting from the direct effects of physiological decline from those that are functional adaptations to this decline. However, when an altered characteristic of the gait cannot be construed as providing any adaptive or compensatory function, it would be reasonable to attribute it to deterioration of the sensorimotor system.

The horizontal heel velocity at heel contact falls in this category. Despite lower overall gait velocities, it has been reported to be significantly higher in older people (Winter, 1991). As the person makes contact with the floor, the horizontal friction force of the floor rapidly causes the velocity to reduce to zero. The higher horizontal velocity requires a higher friction force to oppose the tendency to slip and, on slippery floors or icy surfaces, the excessive horizontal heel velocity would increase the risk of a slip-induced fall (see also Section F). Older people also demonstrate reduced mechanical power absorption at the knee before heel contact and later and lower electromyographic activity of the hamstrings. As the absorption by the hamstrings is needed to reduce the velocity of the swinging limb, the reduction in absorption cannot be construed as being functional to the gait. The placement of the heel on the floor at a near zero horizontal and vertical velocity is a complex task requiring precise motor control and feedback. Its decline, consistent with the reduction in hamstring muscle activity and reduced energy absorption, may be due to either deterioration of the quality of the feedback or the motor control processes.

Similarly, the higher horizontal head acceleration found in older subjects is dysfunctional to the purpose of providing a consistent visual platform. This may indicate a deterioration in the trunk balance control system, attributable to deterioration in the sensorimotor system, or may indicate that the vestibular system has reduced gain, that is, it may require more acceleration input to monitor the accelerations experienced by the head for use in the control of gait and posture. In the latter case, the increased acceleration is a functional adaptation.

The decrease in the degree of trade-off between the moment profiles of the hip and knee, the index of balance, cannot be considered to be a functional change, and is likely attributable to degradation in the sensorimotor system.

The intrasubject and intersubject variability of kinematic, kinetic and electromyographic profiles of older persons have been consistently reported to be less than those of younger subjects (Winter et al., 1990). In other words, they are more stereotyped in their motions; they show less stride-to-stride variation than younger subjects as well as being more like each other in performance. They may have lost some of their neural plasticity, or their ability to perform the activity with the wide range of variations that are characteristic of younger subjects.

Differences Consistent with Motor Adaptations

A number of changes in gait are best explained as functional adaptations. Some gait characteristics promote stability. Walking is a very unstable activity; during single stance phase the centre of mass lies entirely outside the base of support, passing near the medial border of the foot. It is reasonable that older subjects may unconsciously choose to walk in a manner that increases the proportion of stance time and double support time and, therefore, their stability. The increase in absorption at the termination of stance is likely a biomechanical byproduct of this functional modification. At the same time, a vigorous push-off at the termination of double stance would have the potential to increase destabilization, and may account for a reduction in vigour in older subjects. In addition, as the risk of slipping is increased in older subjects by a higher horizontal approach velocity, the force vector at the time of heel contact is more vertically aligned, and less likely to result in a slip if the step length is decreased. Further, by bending the knee slightly, the foot reaches a position of stability more quickly (see also Chapter 9).

Constraints

Age itself is a poor explanation for change, as it begs the questions as to the physical or environmental conditions (constraints) that may interact to display the changes. Although our understanding of the specific constraints, their roles, their influence and their mutability is rudimentary, a few deserve special mention. We may consider the degree to which these constraints are likely to be responsible for the changes in timing, kinematics and kinetics that are identified above, consider the degree to which these changes are mutable, and in this way speculate on their potential for remediation.

Normal gait depends upon free passive joint mobility, appropriate force-generating capabilities of muscle action, and sufficient levels of work capability or fitness. Joint mobility is known to decrease with age, though none of the declines approach the limits needed for gait (James and Parker, 1989). It is unlikely that joint range is an important constraint under normal circumstances. The force levels generated by most major muscle groups during level gait is also far below their maxima. The one exception is the ankle plantarflexor group, which produces a very high level of muscle contraction with each step. In fact, calf strength has been a significant predictor of natural walking speed (Bendall et al., 1989). Strength may thus be an important constraint (Chapter 6), and its decline partially responsible for the reduced walking speed. As

large strength gains even in the very old have been reported from exercise programmes (Fiatarone et al., 1990), the possibility of increasing gait speed exists. It has been suggested that the general fitness level is an important constraint in gait (Cunningham et al., 1986); training programmes directed at increasing fitness have resulted in increases in self-selected walking speed in men 60–65 years of age. Results of this sort suggest some potential for fitness type of training in gait remediation (Chapter 12).

Normal gait also requires sufficient sensory input from the visual, vestibular and proprioceptive systems. Ageing is known to be associated with some decline in each of these systems, but little is known about the potential for reversal of these.

Further knowledge about the specific constraints, their influence, and the mutability of the constraints on gait would all improve our understanding of their relationships to ageing and the possibilities for their remediation.

References

Bendall, MJ, Bassey, EJ, Pearson, MB (1989) Factors affecting walking speed of elderly people. *Age and Ageing* 18: 327–332.

Brocklehurst, JC, Robertson, D, James-Groom, P (1982) Skeletal deformities in the elderly and their effect on postural sway. *Journal of the American Geriatrics Society* 30: 534–538.

Chow, RK, Harrison, JE (1987) Relationship of kyphosis to physical fitness and bone mass in post-menopausal women. *American Journal of Physical Medicine* 66: 219–227.

Culham, E, Peat, M (1994) Spinal and shoulder complex posture. II: thoracic alignment and shoulder complex position in normal and osteoporotic women. *Clinical Rehabilitation* 8: 27–35.

Cunningham, DA, Rechnitzer, PA, Donner, AP (1986) Exercise training and the speed of self-selected walking pace in men at retirement. *Canadian Journal on Aging* 5: 19–26.

De Smet, AA, Robinson, RG, Johnson, BE, Lukert, B (1988) Spinal compression fractures in osteoporotic women: Patterns and relationship to hyperkyphosis. *Radiology* 166: 497–500.

Elble, RJ, Thomas, SS, Higgins, G, Colliver, J (1991) Stride-dependent changes in gait of older people. *Journal of Neurology* 238: 1–5.

Ferrandez, AM, Pailhous, J, Durup, M (1990) Slowness in elderly gait. *Experimental Aging Research* 16: 79–89.

Fiatarone, MA, Marks, EC, Ryan, ND, Meredith, CN, Lipsitz, LA. Evans, WJ (1990) High-intensity strength training in nonagenarians. *Journal of the American Medical Association* 263: 3029–3034.

Gillis, B, Gilroy, K, Lawley, H, Mott, Wall, J (1986) Slow walking speeds in healthy young and elderly females. *Physiotherapy Canada* 38: 350–352.

Himann, JE, Cunningham, DA, Rechnitzer, A, Paterson, DH (1988) Age-related changes in speed of walking. *Medicine and Science in Sports and Exercise* 20: 161–166.

Itoi, E (1991) Roentgenographic analysis of posture in spinal osteoporotics. *Spine* 16: 750–756.

James, B, Parker, AW (1989) Active and passive mobility of lower limb joints in elderly men and women. *American Journal of Physical Medicine and Rehabilitation* 68: 162–167.

Milne, JS, Lauder, IJ (1974) Age effects in kyphosis and lordosis in adults. *Annals of Human Biology* 1: 327–337.

Milne, JS, Lauder, IJ (1976) The relationship of kyphosis to the shape of vertebral bodies. *Annals of Human Biology* 3: 173–179.

Murray, MP, Kory, RC, Clarkson, BH (1969) Walking patterns in healthy old men. *Journal of Gerontology* 24: 169–178.

O'Gorman, H, Jull, G (1987) Thoracic kyphosis and mobility: The effect of age. *Physiotherapy Practice* 3: 154–162.

Olney, SJ, Grondin, RC, McBride, ID (1989) Energy and power considerations in slow walking. *Abstracts of the XII International Congress of Biomechanics, Los Angeles*, p. 117.

Winter, DA (1991) *The Biomechanics and Motor Control of Human Gait: Normal, Elderly and Pathological*, 143 pp. Waterloo: University of Waterloo Press.

Winter, DA, Patla, AE, Frank, JS, Walt, SE (1990) Biomechanical walking pattern changes in the fit and healthy elderly. *Physical Therapy* 70: 340–347.

Woodhull-McNeal, AP (1992) Changes in posture and balance with age. *Aging – Clinical and Experimental Research* 4: 219–225.

8

Cognition and Learning

LESLEY A BAINBRIDGE

Introduction
•
Cognition in Later Life
•
Factors Affecting Cognition and Learning in Later Life and Implications for Practice
•
Strategies for Facilitating Improved Cognition and Learning in Older Adults with Organic Brain
Dysfunction
•
Conclusion

Introduction

Physiotherapists are educators. Whether teaching as part of a formal patient education programme, participating in public education forums, or interacting with patients on an individual level, physiotherapists constantly engage in the process of education. Educating older adults requires an understanding of the processes of cognition (or 'knowing' in the broadest sense of the word including information, sensation and perception) and learning in the context of later life so that appropriate and rewarding educational experiences and treatment interventions with older people can be planned, implemented and evaluated (see also Chapters 9, 10 and 12).

The myths surrounding ageing perpetuate many of the barriers to learning for the older adult. 'You can't teach an old dog new tricks' is a commonly held misperception by older adults themselves (Chapter 3). Ryan (1992), for example, has suggested that age-based memory stereotypes can interfere with performance of the older adult because of societal or individual beliefs based on myth. Many of these myths will change with future cohort groups now entering the realm of the older adult. Battersby (1985) stresses that we learn to be old, using parents and grandparents as role models. As these role models change through better and more accessible education and a commitment to a healthier lifestyle, so may the patterns of ageing.

Several general observations about older people are often overlooked. First, each older person is an individual. Older persons do not comprise one homogeneous group with respect to cognition or to learning (Chapter 4). In most experimental tests, the differences between younger and older subjects is quite small, yet the individual differences among the older subjects is large (Perlmutter and Hall, 1985). Fry (1992, p. 304) suggested that 'the profiles of intellectual potential and consequence in old age continue to be varied and dynamic, and the range of individual differences is enormous'. Even where cognitive decline is clearly related to pathological changes, as in a patient with Alzheimer's disease, '. . . each person loses different abilities at different times and each responds differently to interventions' (Danner et al., 1993). A recognition of the individual nature of older adults, exaggerated as it is by the rich and varied tapestry of life experiences (Simpson, 1992), will help physiotherapists to ensure effective interventions. It will also support the current focus on client-centred or client-driven care by acknowledging the older adult's individual goals.

Second, indicators of cognitive decline do not necessarily appear suddenly in later life. Experiences such as persistent repetitions of thought processes, a decreased ability to hold and manipulate several ideas at one time, and a perceived shrinking of vocabulary, can occur as random, isolated incidents at any time of life. As these occasional, often annoying experiences become progressively more common and frequent in later life normal cognition is found to be altered (Perlmutter and Hall, 1985). This general observation will help to demystify the changes in cognition and learning that are normally associated with ageing.

Third, context is a critical consideration when exploring cognition in later life. Research methods put cognitive experiments in the laboratory setting, thus depriving the older adult of a familiar context. The extent to which this affects the research results is not yet clear but Schaie (1990) claimed that competent behaviour by individuals in their 80s and 90s can be expected in familiar surroundings and circumstances. Salthouse (1990) has also observed that cognitive functioning tested in older adults differed significantly in the laboratory setting from that found in the context of regular occupational and daily activities. This general observation has implications for physiotherapists as they plan and implement treatment interventions and educational experiences (Chapters 10, 12 and 13).

This chapter will explore cognition and learning in the older adult. It will describe cognitive changes in later life and will relate these changes to learning and to the role of the physiotherapist. The discussion will focus mainly upon memory and intellectual ability as two of the key features associated with cognition and learning. Although the chapter is not intended to cover pathological conditions that affect cognition and learning, a brief review of some strategies for compensating for organic brain dysfunction in older people will be provided. Implications for physiotherapy practice will be covered and barriers to education for older adults will be explored so that the physiotherapist can consider strategies for minimizing obstacles (Chapters 3, 4 and 10).

Cognition in Later Life

Cognition comprises several components such as memory, communication, language and writing ability, motor skills, learning, problem solving and intellectual ability (Fry, 1992; Danner et al.,

1993). This section will discuss cognition in the contexts of memory and intelligence. Implications of the effects of the ageing process on memory and intelligence for the practice of physiotherapy will be discussed.

Memory

Memory ability has a major influence on learning for older adults (Fry, 1992). According to Perlmutter and Hall (1985, p. 207), it '. . . has to do with the retention and retrieval of information or skill that has been learned' and it comprises some of the most exclusively individual characteristics of all people, but most especially older persons. Gose and Levi (1985) describe how memory serves to define our individuality:

- It is the basis of all knowledge we have about ourselves and the world.
- It registers, stores, and makes available information about countless things we have experienced in life, from childhood to a moment ago.
- It records our emotions and feelings.
- It is used in the performance of all the skills we have, from riding a bicycle, knitting, and driving a car, to speaking our own or a foreign language.
- It records our sensory experiences and makes it possible to recognize something we have seen before, or can see in the mind's eye; something we have heard before, or can hear in our minds; or to recognize an odour, a taste, a touch.

To understand the changes in memory that are considered part of the ageing process, it is important to understand the underlying concepts of memory. Until recently memory was recognized as having three stages: sensory, short-term or primary, and long-term or secondary (Perlmutter and Hall, 1985) but in recent years the term

'working memory' has been introduced by Baddley (1986, 1992). Memory serves three functions for the manipulation of information: registration, retention, and retrieval or recall (Fry, 1992). The following section will describe the stages and components of memory, how they interact, and how they are influenced by the ageing process. Implications for physiotherapy practice will be introduced.

SENSORY MEMORY

Sensory memory forms the shallowest component of memory. It processes environmental information for brief periods of time after which it must be processed at a deeper level if it is to be retained. Examples of sensory memory include sights, sounds, fragrances, tastes, etc. (Perlmutter and Hall, 1985). This phase is not deemed to be a primary consideration in the ageing process.

SHORT-TERM OR PRIMARY MEMORY

Short-term memory stores information long enough to undertake immediate action such as dialing a telephone number once it has been read from the telephone book. It is in short-term memory that information is sorted and, when appropriate, encoded or recorded for use at a later date. This process of storing information requires organization and individuals will use their own organizational strategies to assist them in eventual retrieval (Perlmutter and Hall, 1985).

Age related changes have been demonstrated in short-term memory. Fry (1992) suggests that short-term memory decreases if manipulation of the material is required or if the individual is required to pay attention to more than one task at a time. Short-time memory processes tend to slow with age and although there is no reduction in the amount of storage room for information, it takes longer to access it (Perlmutter and Hall, 1985).

LONG-TERM OR SECONDARY MEMORY

Long-term memory is considered to have unlimited storage room, containing all the information we have gleaned through experience and knowledge acquisition. Problems with retrieval suggest that the true depths of long-term memory can never be tapped consciously, but the information still resides in the storage area. This stage of memory has two components: episodic and semantic. Episodic memories are 'the conscious recollection of personally experienced events' (Baddley, 1989, p. 42) and 'include everything that happens to us, so that each memory is linked with a time and a place' (Perlmutter and Hall, 1985, p. 219). Examples include recalling a party, a sporting event, a dinner menu or a special birthday. Semantic memories include knowledge of the world (Baddley) and 'are organized factual knowledge' (Perlmutter and Hall, p. 219). Examples include remembering the number of provinces in Canada, the capital cities of Australia, the names of the British monarchy, or the number of inches in a foot. Information that requires longer storage than that available in short-term memory is encoded in long-term memory where it is held until needed at which time it is transferred back to short-term memory for conscious manipulation.

Semantic memories tend to remain intact during ageing but episodic memories show signs of vulnerability. Retention of information in storage does not appear to be affected by age but retrieval of the information does appear to be impaired. This may be due to difficulty with encoding the information and with transferring it to long-term memory and accessing it again (Perlmutter and Hall, 1985).

WORKING MEMORY

Baddley (1986, 1992) has suggested replacing the concept of short-term memory with working memory. This term 'refers to a brain system that provides temporary storage and manipulation of the information necessary for such complex cognitive tasks as language comprehension, learning and reasoning' (1992, p. 556). Although short-term memory was initially conceptualized as a single unit of memory, Baddley and his colleagues have suggested that the concept of working memory captures the storage and processing functions through three subcomponents: the central executive or 'attention-controlling' system and two 'slave systems', the visuospatial sketch pad (visual images) and the phonological loop (storage and rehearsal of speech-based information). The central executive's primary function is that of coordinating the resources within the two slave systems. When this coordination function is disrupted, cognitive dysfunction results. Working memory is particularly vulnerable to the effects of ageing due to the complex nature of simultaneous storage and manipulation of information (Craik et al., 1989; Hutch and Dixon, 1990; Salthouse, 1990). Hutch and Dixon (1990, p. 261) also suggest that 'if ageing is associated with diminished working memory capacity, then a substantial portion of the observed age differences in performance may be related to a reduction in this resource'.

The concept of working memory, appears to provide a useful framework for studies of adult cognition. Working memory has provided a rich source of laboratory findings related to memory and has enhanced the study of psychometrics in recent years. There are, however, some practical applications. The ability to comprehend complex material is contingent upon a functional working memory, yet simple material can still be managed with a dysfunctional working memory (Baddley, 1992). Baddley (1986) suggests that registering of information in older persons remains intact but that the ability to use the information to change behaviour declines. The speed of processing information and the ability to register new information and to process it simultaneously both slow with ageing. These observations correlate closely to the factors affecting cognition in a later section of the chapter.

THE PROCESS OF MEMORY

Gose and Levi (1985) use three 'Rs' to identify the three phases of memory: registering, retaining and retrieving. The ability to register new information in memory depends upon attitude or a belief and self-confidence in the ability to remember; the reasons behind remembering or the importance of the information; the attention paid to remembering or the use of all senses to aid in registering; and organizing of individual ways in which people highlight new information in memory for easier retrieval.

Retaining information is connected to memory and can take place in both short-term or long-term memory. Short-term retention is used for information which is either quickly forgotten or which is being sent on to long-term memory. Organizational strategies such as repetition or grouping can assist the transfer to long-term memory. Long-term memory is the expansive filing system used to store the clues or links with previous information so that, through association, retrieval becomes easier. General knowledge and personal experience form the two parts of long-term memory (Gose and Levi, 1985).

Retrieval of information takes place through recall or through recognition. Recall means searching memory for information and reproducing it whereas recognition means associating new information with something already in memory. Recall needs the help of all senses to act as prompts to the information being sought. Recognition is easier than recall but also relies heavily on all senses (Gose and Levi, 1985).

Some aspects of memory in older adults are particularly important for the physiotherapist to consider when working with older learners. Older persons may believe that they cannot remember, they may perceive some information as irrelevant and therefore not important to remember, they may be distracted and thereby decrease their attention to the new information being presented, they may have difficulty concentrating or summarizing information into clues, or they may have difficulty linking new information to that which already exists (Gose and Levi, 1985). Loss of memory is not a significant feature of normal ageing. The pace at which information is registered or retrieved may slow down, but most older adults can still remember well. As discussed earlier, memory is an intensely individual process, so generalizing the effects of age on memory is difficult. There are, however, strategies that can assist memory in older adults. Perlmutter and Hall (1985) suggest the following:

- organizing material by category
- identifying verbal aids to memory e.g. making words out of the first letters of each item
- creating a vivid image of items
- developing a plan for rehearsing material
- frequent repetition of material

Intellectual Ability and Ageing

Woodruff-Pak (1988) discusses the concepts of fluid and crystallized intelligence. Fluid intelli-

Table 1
The Effects of Ageing on Memory

Stages of memory	Key characteristics	Effects of ageing
Sensory memory	Shallowest component Brief processing of information Examples include sights, sounds, fragrances	Minimal changes due to ageing
Short-term (primary) memory	Short time frame Small capacity ($\leqslant 7$ items) Sorting and encoding stage Example includes storing a telephone number long enough to dial and then, if necessary, encoding it for future use	Capacity decreases if manipulation of material required or if attention must be paid to more than one task at a time Increase in processing and retrieval time
Long-term (secondary) memory	Unlimited storage room Contains information gleaned from experience and knowledge acquisition over the lifespan Consists of two types of memories: episodic and semantic Examples include (1) episodic: memories of a party or a sporting event and 2) semantic: factual memories such as capital cities and provinces' names	Semantic memories remain intact Episodic memories are vulnerable, although more to retrieval than retention
Working memory	Replaces the concept of short-term memory Refers to a system for temporary storage and manipulation of information rather than a unitary phase of memory	Susceptible to the effects of ageing due to the complexity of simultaneous storage and manipulation

gence represents the biological basis of intelligence or 'the fluidity of the mind' (p. 324). It is also described as a relatively formless type of intelligence that is independent of experience or education and as the 'ability to perceive complex relations and to engage in short-term memory. [It] also involves the ability for concept formation, reasoning, and abstraction' (Fry, 1992, p. 309). Examples include rote memory, inductive reasoning, and memory span (Woodruff-Pak, 1988; Fry, 1992).

Crystallized intelligence 'is learned information' (Woodruff-Pak, 1988, p. 324). It is also described by Fry (1992, p. 309) as 'a function of experience and knowledge of the intellectual and cultural heritage of society'. Fry suggests that crystallized intelligence is affected by education and experience and provides examples that include general information, vocabulary and numerical and practical reasoning. Fry also introduces the concept of practical intelligence, described as 'the pragmatics of applying intellectual skills to every day activities' (1992, p. 309). This type of intelligence is

Table 2
The Effects of Ageing on Intelligence

Types of intelligence	Key characteristics	Effects of ageing
Fluid intelligence	Biological basis Relatively formless Independent of experience or education Relates to complex relations and the ability to engage in short-term memory Examples include rote memory, memory span and inductive reasoning	Declines with age
Crystallized intelligence	Learned information A function of experience and knowledge Examples include general information and vocabulary	Remains relatively stable across the lifespan
Practical intelligence	Application of intellectual skills to everyday life Related to crystallized intelligence	Remains relatively stable over the lifespan

related to crystallized intelligence and favours the perspective that experience and individual motivation affect the cognitive ability to address the needs of everyday life.

These concepts of intelligence are important to consider in relation to the ageing process. Fluid intelligence appears to decline as a part of ageing yet crystallized and practical intelligence remain fairly stable across the lifespan (Fry, 1992), and are therefore the areas of most promising focus for educational interventions and activities. Fry suggests that fluid intelligence can be improved through appropriate learning experiences and that gains in the areas of performance accuracy and problem solving have been noted.

The Older Adult Learner

Learning, as mentioned earlier, is difficult to separate from cognition. Memory and intellec-tual ability have been discussed as key elements of cognition and therefore this section will address some general comments about the older adult.

Learning is most often defined as the process of acquiring knowledge, skills and abilities (Chapter 9). Baddley (1989) suggests that there are two types of learning, procedural and declarative. Procedural learning 'comprises the acquisition of skills e.g. learning to type', while declarative learning is 'the acquisition of new knowledge or experience e.g. remembering to go to a typing class' (p. 42) and is a conscious recollection of the past. The integration of these two types of learning creates what Baddley calls good learning, defined as a systematic encoding of incoming material, integrating and relating it to what is already known (p. 55). As various aspects of cognition are affected in later life, it is important to understand that these can affect learning for older individuals.

Battersby (1985) calls for a much more definitive meaning for education in later life. He encourages those pursuits that enable the older person to gain control over some aspects of their lives. For example, the relative importance of learning to play bridge and learning how to manage retirement funds must be determined with the client, so that learning priorities can be established. Education and learning in the context of later life can be defined in many ways. Physiotherapists will need to explore their own conceptualization of education in later life in their clinical practice.

Fry (1992) reinforces the need to consider individual differences in older persons while bearing in mind the general areas in which ageing appears to affect performance. He suggests that 'the formulation of appropriate educational strategies and therapeutic interventions consistent with the learning potential of individual persons' is critical in approaching learning in the older adult (p. 308) (see Chapters 9, 10 and 12). Schaie (1974, p. 805) suggests that the literature supports the concept 'that people can and do function at a high [intellectual] level throughout life, and thus can be expected to continue the educational process into very old age'. He argues that the development of specific programmes to 'reverse the cultural and technological obsolescence of the aged' would go a long way to improving the learning experiences of older adults and to integrating older persons more fully into society (see Chapters 3 and 5).

Adaptation to the effects of ageing is, in reality, a learning experience for the older adult. Changes in sensory, physical and cognitive systems in the extreme can seriously hamper performance but for most of the ageing population substitution and compensation become the normal learning experience as the way to keep functional in daily life and most people do it well (see Chapters 2 and 22).

Factors Affecting Cognition and Learning in Later Life and Implications for Practice

Consideration of the factors affecting cognition in later life can provide a valuable array of tools for the physiotherapist when approaching interventions with an older client. Three types of factors influence cognition and learning in the older adult – population factors, environmental factors and activity or task factors – and these present conditions that facilitate learning and those that create barriers (see also Chapter 9).

Population Factors

Older adults often expect that their memory will fail them or expect to fail at other cognitive tasks (Perlmutter and Hall, 1985; Schaie, 1990; Fry, 1992). These expectations are born of stereotypical images of ageing and are also related to cohort effects. They may also cause an older adult to stop trying, yet if cognitive skills are not used, they will decline. Fear or expectation of failure can be addressed through emphasis on ability and recognition of effort in a safe, non-judgemental environment. Showing respect for past achievements and setting achievable goals may also help (Simpson, 1992) (Chapter 3).

Cohort differences can influence cognitive changes (Schaie, 1974; Perlmutter and Hall, 1985). The level of education is important; the more education an individual has received, the more likely it is that cognitive decline can be minimized. Consideration of the educational background of clients may provide clues useful in maximizing the learning process. Many older adults growing up half a century ago received little formal education and it is probable that it is a long time since they participated in educational activities. This may affect their memory and learning skills.

Depression can also affect cognitive performance and should be considered as a potential factor in cognitive performance and learning ability when working with older adults (Perlmutter and Hall, 1985).

Health status affects mental performance (Simpson, 1992). The existence of health problems appears to adversely affect performance of older adults on intelligence tests. Healthy older adults may be likely to learn more easily than those in poor health, but one cannot generalize on this point (Chapter 2).

Physical condition can influence the older adult's intellectual performance (Perlmutter and Hall, 1985). Regular exercise and physical conditioning can improve speed and performance on simple cognitive tasks (Chapter 6).

Environmental Factors

Context may influence the ability of older individuals to perform cognitively to their maximum level (Perlmutter and Hall, 1985). If skills are taken out of the context of every day life, performance may suffer. Physiotherapists should consider performance in an institutionalized setting, such as a hospital outpatient department, in relation to performance in the home or other familiar surroundings (Chapters 5 and 24).

Anxiety negatively affects cognition in older adults (Perlmutter and Hall, 1985). Fear of failure or an overanxious need to succeed can seriously hamper performance. Providing genuine reinforcement in a safe environment can help to overcome the adverse effects of anxiety. The use of a friendly, pleasant voice and maintaining a warm affect will help to dispel anxiety (Simpson, 1992). Key characteristics of an environment conducive to learning for older adults include active listening, exploration of fears, seating that encourages conversation and constructive feedback that provides building blocks for learning. Creating a learning environment that does not focus on youth-oriented programming, marks, degrees and fixed schedules but creates flexibility and emphasizes ability, will go a long way to decreasing anxiety.

Past experiences and familiarity with subject matter will affect learning and memory in older adults (Perlmutter and Hall, 1985). Information is stored and used in the context of every day life. Forcing older clients to process information in a void will minimize the learning experience. Consideration of the importance of familiarity with the content and context of material will enhance the older adult's ability to learn and/or remember. Changing the learning situation, geographically, as well as practically, can be a vital step in getting the most from physiotherapy intervention.

Geographical factors can influence access to learning opportunities. These are often some of the most difficult to overcome, as they may involve public policy and funding availability. Many older people do not drive and the supply of volunteer drivers is limited. Public transport may not be available, particularly in rural communities. Transportation for persons with disabilities can be creatively addressed in some communities and the organization of educational opportunities in settings such as community centres or church halls may help to address the problem of geography (see Section F).

Activity or Task Factors

The speed of learning and memory processing is another critical consideration when dealing with older adults (Perlmutter and Hall, 1985; Simpson, 1992; Fry, 1992; Danner et al., 1993). Older persons take more time to learn and more time to produce the answer. If they are feeling rushed or fatigued performance will be hampered; ensuring the older client has a rest before physiotherapy intervention may help to reduce the effects of fatigue (Simpson, 1992). Individual pacing therefore becomes a key to ensuring the most effective learning experience for the older adult (see Chapter 9).

Motivation affects learning and cognition (Perlmutter and Hall, 1985; Simpson, 1992) — if there is no reason to learn or remember information, why bother? Ensuring that the learning experience is meaningful to the older client will, again, ensure the best intervention outcomes from the client's perspective.

The complexity of information can also affect cognitive performance in older adults (Fry, 1992). Cognitive tasks should be kept simple enough to be managed yet complex enough to prevent boredom. It may be helpful to focus on manageable components of larger issues or broader goals. Gradual progression from simple to complex concepts and procedures also facilitates learning by older adults.

Distractibility, or inability to focus on a learning task, can detract from an older person's cognitive performance (Perlmutter and Hall, 1985). The relevance of new information is critical (Fry, 1992); irrelevant information can get in the way by causing an irritating distraction. Careful selec-

tion and presentation of clearly relevant material will help to focus the older adult's attention on the task at hand.

Interference can affect learning in older adults (Perlmutter and Hall, 1985; Fry, 1992). Proactive interference refers to old material getting in the way of new material. For example, it is more difficult for older people to form new word associations using formerly common association: black / white and high / low are more difficult to learn when realigned as black / high and white / low. Retroactive interference refers to new material interfering with old material. Thus, attempting to learn a new list can make remembering an old list more difficult. Recall and recognition can both suffer from interference. New material should be presented in ways that capitalize upon relevant old material, while allowing irrelevant material to be lost.

Performing two tasks at once can seriously compromise the older adult's ability to perform well (Simpson, 1992). Communication should be phrased in simple terms and all unnecessary words should be dropped. Group work almost always involves concentrating on more than one thing at a time and, therefore, keeping group size small (6 to 8) may help to accommodate the effects of group work.

Visual input is profitable to old and young people alike. This effect does not decline in later years and so provides an excellent strategy for working with older adults (Fry, 1992; Danner et al., 1993). As with any material, the visual images, or pictures, must be meaningful to best assist in cognitive performance. The use of visual imagery also provides flexibility in the learning experience and adds to the range of approaches for facilitating learning.

Strategies for Facilitating Improved Cognition and Learning in Older Adults with Organic Brain Dysfunction

Physiotherapists engaged in education of older adults need to be able to recognize signs of confusion or disorientation that may be interfering with the learning process and to provide appropriate intervention and consultation. Strategies which may be useful in addressing learning in older adults with organic cognitive impairment have been summarized by Danner *et al.*, (1993):

- Where language and writing ability are compromised:

(a) speak slowly using simple sentences
(b) use the same word for the same object each time
(c) give time for a response and if none, repeat the communication in the same way
(d) look at the client to gain his or her attention before speaking
(e) use one-step commands
(f) use non-verbal clues to trigger memory
(g) ask the client to repeat an answer if it is not understandable (see Chapter 10).

- Where memory is compromised:

(a) use sensory channels (touch, smell, taste, hearing)
(b) assist the client to start the activity
(c) use visual clues, e.g. a picture of a toilet over the bathroom door
(d) use sequencing by placing objects in the order in which they will be used

- Where learning is compromised:

(a) use repetition

(b) use statements, not questions
(c) limit decision making e.g. give a choice between two items, not a whole range of items

Conclusion

This chapter has focused on cognition and learning in the older adult. Physiotherapists should recognize that the unique characteristics of older persons require special consideration when planning, implementing or evaluating educational programmes or approaches with, not for, the older adult population. Myths that continue to surround the ability or desire of older adults to learn must be strongly contested.

References

Baddley, A (1986) *Working Memory,* 289 pp. Oxford: Clarendon Press.

Baddley, A (1989) The psychology of remembering and forgetting. In Butler, T (ed.) *Memory, History, Culture and the Mind,* pp. 33-60. Oxford, New York: Blackwell.

Baddley, A (1992) Working memory. *Science* **255**: 556–559.

Battersby, D (1985) Education in later life: what does it mean? *Convergence* **18**: 75–79.

Craik, FI, Morris, RG, Glick, ML (1989) Adult age differences in working memory. In Vallar, G, Shallice T (eds) *Neuropsychological Impairments of Short-term Memory.* New York: Cambridge University Press.

Danner, C, Beck, C, Heacock, P, Modlin, T (1993) Cognitively impaired elders: using research findings to improve nursing care. *Journal of Gerontological Nuarsing* **19**: 5–11.

Fry, PS (1992) A consideration of cognitive factors in the learning and education of older adults. *International Review of Education* **38**: 303–325.

Gose, KB, Levi, GH (1985) *Dealing With Memory Changes as You Grow Older.* Vancouver: Typeworks.

Hutch, DF, Dixon, RA (1990) Learning and memory in ageing. In Birren, JE, Schaie, KW (eds) *Handbook of the Psychology of Aging,* pp. 258–271. San Diego, London, Sydney: Academic Press Inc.

Perlmutter, M, Hall, E (1985) *Adult Development and Aging,* pp. 206–266. New York, Chichester: John Wiley & Sons.

Ryan, EB (1992) Beliefs about memory changes across the adult life span. *Journal of Gerontology: Psychological Sciences* **47**: 41–46.

Salthouse, TA (1990) Cognitive competence and expertise in ageing. In

Birren, JE, Schaie, KW (eds) *Handbook of the Psychology of Aging*, pp. 310–320. San Diego, London, Sydney: Academic Press Inc.

Schaie, KW (1990) Intellectual development in adulthood. In Birren, JE, Schaie, KW (eds) *Handbook of the Psychology of Aging*, pp. 291–305. San Diego, London, Sydney: Academic Press Inc.

Simpson, J (1992) Growing older: changes in mental performance. In French S (ed.) *Physiotherapy A Psychosocial Approach*, pp. 273–285. London: Butterworth-Heinemann.

Woodruff-Pak, D (1988) *Psychology and Aging*, pp. 286–341. Englewood Cliffs, NJ, Sydney, London: Prentice-Hall Inc.

9

Motor Learning Concepts Applied to Rehabilitation

LAURIE R SWANSON, JULIE A SANFORD

Introduction
•
Age-related Changes in Cognition and Motor Performance
•
Motor Learning
•
Factors that Affect Motor Learning
•
Summary

Introduction

Knowledge about the effect of age on skills and behaviours is crucial for the maintenance and development of functional abilities of older adults. An understanding of the effects of age on the ability to perform and learn motor skills will enable the physiotherapist to help older adults to maximize their participation in a variety of recreational and work-related skills, as well as developing adaptive skills in response to physical limitations (see Chapters 6, 7 and 8).

Motor learning is the study of how motor skills are acquired. The purpose of this chapter is to present concepts from the field of motor learning that are relevant to rehabilitation of older adults. The first section reviews briefly what is known about the age-associated changes in cognition and motor performance in normal older adults. The next section examines general concepts in motor learning that are necessary to understand the process involved in learning a new skill involving movement. In the following section specific concepts in motor learning are presented that can be used to guide therapeutic interventions.

Age-related Changes in Cognition and Motor Performance

Ageing and Cognition

A common finding is that cognitive functioning declines with increasing age (Salthouse, 1991). Some of the cognitive functions found to be affected by ageing include encoding input, selectively attending to appropriate stimuli, searching and retrieving from long-term memory, and using working memory to integrate information and formulate an action (Kausler, 1994). In particular, Salthouse (1990) has concluded that some of the age-related changes in cognitive functioning can be attributed to reductions in the capabilities of working memory. These capabilities include simultaneous storage and processing of information. Changes in the various mechanisms involved in cognitive skills ultimately can affect the ability to learn, remember, and solve problems (see Chapter 8).

Ageing and Motor Performance

In addition to changes in cognition, there are age-related changes in how older adults perform previously learned skills (which is the area of motor control). Generally, older adults are slower in both preparing and executing movements. In particular, they respond differently to variables that influence movement planning, and they tend to show differences in the kinematics of movement when compared to younger adults. Older adults also tend to use different cognitive strategies during the planning and execution of movements (Kausler, 1994). For example, they tend to trade off speed for accuracy. Given the changes in motor performance that occur with age and the associated changes in performance

strategies, these findings have implications for how older adults learn motor skills. More specifically, older adults may utilize learning variables differently than young adults (see Chapter 7).

Influence of Age-related Changes on Motor Learning

Unfortunately, there are only a few studies that directly address the influence of age on the variables thought to enhance motor learning (Kausler, 1994). Some of the important variables that influence learning in younger adults include information feedback, practice schedules, and pre-practice training. Preliminary work indicates that normal older adults use these variables in a similar way as younger adults (Swanson and Lee, 1992; Carnahan et al., 1993). Until further research is completed, the overriding assumption is that these same concepts can be incorporated into therapeutic interventions with older adults. Future work will clarify the extent of the generalizability of these motor learning concepts to both normal and disabled older adults.

Motor Learning

Definition of Motor Learning

Motor learning is a set of processes associated with practice or experience leading to relatively permanent changes in the capability of responding (Schmidt, 1988). More simply, motor learning addresses how practice conditions contribute to the acquisition of skilled movements.

Motor learning is one area of study in the overall field of motor behaviour, which is the study of principles of human skilled movements. Motor control is another area involving neural, physical and behavioural organization of movement. As this term is often used interchangeably with motor learning, some confusion may be created in the literature. Finally, motor development is the study of age-related changes in motor control and learning across the lifespan.

Historical Perspectives on Motor Learning

The research field of motor learning is multidisciplinary and has been investigated by physiologists, psychologists, and kinesiologists. More recently, physiotherapists and occupational therapists have become involved in this field in relation to the application of the motor learning principles to therapeutic interventions. Depending on their training, the scientists who study this field work along a wide continuum, investigating the neural basis of learning at one end and the behavioural features of human motor performance at the other. Behavioural research investigates variables that influence the acquisition of skilled movement.

Stages of Motor Learning

Most theories suggest that motor learning involves a progression through different performance stages (Gentile, 1972). These stages are characterized by a progression from performance that is under cognitive control and which relies heavily on verbal mediation and attention to a performance stage that is much more automatically regulated. The purpose of rehabilitation is to learn adaptive skills or to re-learn previously functional motor skills. In both situations new motor learning is the goal, and the assumption is that there is a close theoretical parallel between the stages of learning a new motor skill and the stages of learning during rehabilitation.

The Role of Practice

Practice is considered fundamental to motor learning. One description of the role of practice is called the Power Law of Practice (Fitts and Posner, 1967). It describes the performance change in a motor skill during acquisition. The Power Law states that improvement in performance is the greatest during the initial practice stages. With increasing practice one sees a diminishing return in terms of the amount of improvement. That is, improvement in performance increases at a slower rate as the person becomes more skilled. However, while performance improvements slow down, they do not stop altogether.

Much of the motor learning research that addresses changes with advancing age has been directed at the effects of ageing on practice gains. These studies indicate that older adults benefit from practice and that this benefit indicates that the older adult can improve the cognitive operations that mediate performance. But generally, their performance does not reach the same level as that of young adults (Light, 1990). Although older adults can improve performance with practice, these studies provide little insight into the effects of age on the learning process.

Performance Gains: Temporary or Permanent?

A key issue in motor learning research is the distinction between performance and learning. Learning is a process of change and cannot be observed directly. Rather, learning must be inferred from performance. Historically, learning has been inferred from two types of performance scores. The most traditional method is to examine the change in performance over practice (Schmidt, 1988). The problem with such a method is that temporary changes in performance during practice do not necessarily reflect the more permanent nature of performance change required by definitions of learning. In fact, there are some variables that affect temporary performance changes during practice that have quite different effects when permanent changes are assessed.

The more appropriate assessments of learning involve retention tests, which are evaluations of performance of the motor skill after a period of no practice. Retention tests provide an indication of the relative permanence of the performance change, after all temporary influences on performance have subsided (e.g. fatigue). Changes gained within a physiotherapy treatment session may reflect a combination of temporary performance change and learning. In order to assess learning, performance needs to be assessed at a later time (e.g. at the beginning of the next therapy session).

Factors that Affect Motor Learning

Before discussing the specific factors that affect motor learning two caveats need to be considered. First, the majority of research in motor learning has been conducted on young adults and there may be limits to the application of the findings to older persons. However, the preliminary research on older adults indicates that generally, although the older adults do not achieve the same level of performance as younger adults, older adults do use the learning variables in a similar way to younger adults (Chapter 8). Sec-

ond, the vast majority of research on motor learning in normal adults has focused on the early stage of learning. Individuals who are participating in rehabilitation programmes are in the early stage of learning and as a result, the findings from this research are relevant to rehabilitation. The important factors considered in the early stage are those which impact on the cognitive processing of the learner (Chapter 8). Three variables that have a direct impact on performance improvements in this stage are feedback, practice schedules, and prepractice training. Given that the focus of rehabilitation is on new learning, these factors will also influence the efficiency of learning during the therapeutic interventions. The examination of each factor will include: an explanation of the concept; traditional view in therapy; research evidence; and guidelines for implementation.

Augmented Feedback

Feedback is a broad term referring to information about the achievement of a movement goal (Schmidt, 1988; Magill, 1993). Feedback is considered to be 'augmented' if it is provided by an external source and is supplemental to the information derived from sources such as proprioceptive, touch and visual receptors.

Augmented feedback is usually classified as either knowledge of results (KR) or knowledge of performance (KP). KR is defined as verbal, post movement information about the outcome of the action in terms of the environmental goal, such as the time taken for a client to stand from a sitting position. KP is also augmented feedback, but different in that it is related specifically to the nature of the movement pattern produced, such as the straightness of the elbow or the distribution of weight transferred in the sit to stand.

Most of the research that has been conducted on

the effectiveness of KR and KP has been designed to investigate the impact of various manipulations on motor learning (Schmidt, 1988; Magill, 1993). This research is relevant to physiotherapy interventions, in which the provision of feedback is fundamental. An overall goal of therapy is to enable the client to learn the skill by developing self-assessment and self-correction skills. The way the therapist provides feedback can either assist or be detrimental to the client's attempt to acquire this skill.

The research investigations involve the scheduling of when and how KR and KP are provided to the learner, and include the following specific manipulations: frequency, summaries, bandwidth, and timing techniques. As most of the research has been conducted using KR, the remainder of the chapter will be restricted to these data.

FREQUENCY OF KR

Augmented feedback that is provided after only a small proportion of the total number of practice repetitions made by the learner will be more beneficial for learning than when it is provided after each individual practice attempt.

Currently, the general wisdom in therapy is to provide feedback to the performer as often as possible. This view is based on the traditional theory that the amount of feedback is directly proportional to the amount of learning — the more feedback, the better.

The proportion of motor attempts that are followed by feedback, relative to the total number of attempts (termed 'relative frequency'), is an important variable in learning. However, research shows that less frequent feedback (e.g. 50% relative frequency) is as beneficial or better for learning than feedback after every repetition

of the task (Vander Linden et al., 1993). Reduced feedback is especially effective if given relatively frequently early in practice, then gradually reduced in frequency (termed 'faded' feedback frequency) as the performer achieves more competency at the skill (Wulf and Schmidt, 1989; Winstein and Schmidt, 1990).

The results of this research suggest that the physiotherapist should: give feedback relatively frequently to maintain motivation, but not on every repetition, or learners may become too dependent on the feedback; use frequent feedback only until the learner achieves the basic movement pattern; and give feedback often in early practice, gradually withdrawing it as performance proficiency improves.

SUMMARY KR

Feedback that is provided as a summary about a number of repeated attempts is more effective than feedback provided after each individual attempt. This principle is not often applied by physiotherapists, who have believed that providing immediate feedback is more beneficial in rehabilitation settings. Feedback after every trial does improve the performance, but not the retention or the learning of a skill. When measures of learning were assessed after a period of time, people who received summary feedback were better at remembering the skill (Carnahan et al., 1993). Schmidt (1991) suggests that the optimal summary length will be related to the complexity of the task: relatively short summaries are more effective for complex tasks (which contain large amounts of information to remember), while relatively long summaries are more appropriate for simple tasks (which have low information loads).

It is suggested that physiotherapists use summary feedback by having the learner repeat the task three or four times and then providing feed-back — by either reviewing each repetition or summarizing the information from the individual repetitions, increasing the number of repetitions included in the summary if the task is very simple and decreasing the number in the summary if the task is very complex.

BANDWIDTH FEEDBACK

Feedback is given if the performance falls outside a predetermined bandwidth of acceptability. No feedback is given if the error is small and falls within the acceptable bandwidth. When no feed-back is provided the learner understands that the attempt was successful.

Traditionally, when teaching new motor skills physiotherapists allow for a margin of error before feedback about the error is provided; as learning progresses, this margin of tolerance is reduced.

Studies on bandwidth feedback effects have usually been conducted by manipulating the size of the tolerance limits about the movement goal (such as the accuracy demands of the goal). Results have shown that learning was facilitated when the provision of feedback was based on a 10% bandwidth of correctness, as compared to 5% and 0% bandwidths (Winstein, 1991). Studies also suggest that while reducing the bandwidth tolerance will improve performance, learning may be degraded if the bandwidth becomes too small (Lee et al., 1994). This is similar to the concept described earlier that too frequent KR is detri-mental to learning.

Physiotherapists are advised, therefore, to use a bandwidth for acceptable error when deciding whether or not to provide feedback. The toler-ance limits for setting the bandwidth are reduced as competency improves. Be careful not to use too stringent a bandwidth.

TIMING OF KR

Ultimately, the learner must learn to self-assess performance using the feedback that is always available (i.e. intrinisic feedback). Augmented feedback that is provided too soon after the completion of an attempt will prevent the learner from assessing his or her own intrinsic feedback, and is detrimental to learning. Learning is enhanced by delaying feedback, and using that delay period to encourage the learner to evaluate their own performance. During this delay period, the learner has time to think about the feedback before making the next attempt. This approach contrasts sharply with the traditional physiother-apy belief that providing feedback about perfor-mance as soon as possible after the attempt is the best way to facilitate learning.

Studies have shown that providing feedback immediately after an attempt has been completed will enhance the acquisition of a motor skill. However, the quality of performance deterio-rates when performance is later required on a retention test where augmented feedback is no longer provided. In contrast, delaying feedback is more beneficial to learning, especially if the per-former is encouraged to evaluate performance during this delay period (Swinnen et al., 1990).

Physiotherapists are advised to delay giving feed-back at the completion of the task rather than providing instantaneous feedback, and to encou-rage learners to evaluate their own performance. After providing feedback, the learner should be allowed some time to think about and understand how to change performance before starting the next repetition.

Practice Schedules

The practice schedule defines how components within a task should be learned and how the practice of multiple tasks should be organized. Practice schedule variables include part versus whole practice of a task, variability of practice, and blocked versus random practice of different tasks. In younger adults manipulations of practice schedules that actively engage the learner in the cognitive processes are more beneficial for learning than schedules that require less active participation. Future research will clarify the extent to which older adults can gain a similar benefit from these practice schedules.

PART VERSUS WHOLE PRACTICE

When learning a skill, should the whole skill be practised or should components of the skill be practised separately? Guidelines suggest that part or whole practice depends entirely on the type of skill being practised.

Physiotherapists generally believe that part practice of a complex skill will be beneficial for the learner. For example in sit to stand, practising leaning forwards before lower limb extension may facilitate execution of the whole skill. Once the components are learned, the parts of the skill should be integrated and the whole skill should be practised. This principle is applied to the teaching of all motor skills.

The research on part versus whole practice suggests that the best way to practise depends on the type of task — discrete, serial or continuous (Magill, 1993). Discrete tasks have a clear beginning and end, and are relatively short in duration. The movement decision is made before the movement starts (e.g. turning on a light switch). Serial tasks are a series of discrete task strung together as a whole (e.g. making soup from a can). Con-

tinuous tasks have an arbitrary beginning and end; they are of long duration and decisions or corrections are made throughout the movement (e.g. walking or driving).

The research further suggests that if the skill is naturally separated into discrete subcomponents which represent the same action as the required skill (i.e. a serial task such as making a cup of coffee), then part practice can be beneficial to learning the whole skill. However, if the parts do not represent the same action as required by the whole skill (i.e. with discrete tasks such as tying a shoelace, or with continuous tasks such as walking) then whole practice is better (Magill, 1993). It is important, therefore, for physiotherapists to analyse the nature of the skill (i.e. serial, discrete or continuous) to be learned before deciding whether or not to practise its component parts.

VARIABILITY IN PRACTICE

Providing a wide range of practice variations throughout the learning process allows the learner to become more adaptable to new performance situations. To date many physiotherapists have believed that when learning or relearning a particular type of motor skill (such as sitting to standing), practice should concentrate on a single variation or version of the task (such as using the same chair for all attempts), and that this task should be mastered before other variations of the task are attempted (e.g. using chairs of different heights).

Research has shown, however, that although practice which is restricted to repeating exactly the same version of a task does facilitate the learning of that task, performance on related tasks is not facilitated. In contrast, practice on a range of task variations does facilitate performance when a new variation of the task is encountered (Schmidt, 1988).

It is suggested that as the client learns a particular task (e.g. arising from a sitting position), the practice should vary along some dimension such as different heights of chairs, different types of chairs (arm versus no arm chairs) and different seating surfaces (soft versus hard). The variability of practice experience should be constructed to span the range of variations experienced in everyday life.

BLOCKED VERSUS RANDOM PRACTICE

Blocked practice applies when the client is trying to learn more than one different type of task such as rolling, sitting up from lying, getting up from a bed, and drinking from a glass. In a blocked schedule, all of the practice of one task is completed before the next task is practised. A random practice schedule is one in which the different tasks are interspersed in the practice session. The important concept here is that when learning more than one skill, practising all of the skills in a random schedule is detrimental to performance, yet facilitates learning. In contrast, blocked practice is beneficial for performance, but detrimental to learning.

Physiotherapists have traditionally considered that when more than one motor skill is practised in a therapy session, learning is facilitated by concentrated effort on one task at a time. However, many research studies, using a wide variety of tasks (mostly discrete), have shown that although random practice is detrimental to performance (relative to blocked practice), it enhances learning (Magill and Hall, 1990). Different practice schedules appear to affect cognitive functioning in different ways. Blocked practice enables the learner to perform skills more automatically and more quickly, perhaps due to processing the requirements of the skill at a more superficial level, whereas random practice forces greater cognitive analysis of the similarities and differences between skills being practised. Recent research also suggests that several repetitions of a task within a random schedule may be a good compromise in order to avoid too much performance decrement, while maintaining the benefits of purely random practice (Al-Ameer and Toole, 1993).

It is suggested that when learning of more than one task is involved, practising the tasks in a random schedule is preferable to a blocked schedule. If the tasks are difficult, two or three repetitions should be used before switching to a new task. It should be understood that although random practice causes decrements in immediate performance, better learning will eventually result.

Prepractice Training

There are a variety of practice techniques that enhance motor performance and learning but do not involve actual movement. These practice techniques can be effective both prior to actual physical practice or when interspersed between periods of physical practice. These techniques include mental practice and observational learning.

MENTAL PRACTICE

Mental practice is the cognitive rehearsal of a physical skill in the absence of overt physical practice. Mental practice of a skill involves asking clients to spend a period of time thinking about themselves performing that skill. This type of practice enhances the performance of motor skills, especially when combined with physical practice.

Mental practice has not been used in traditional physiotheraphy. Several studies show that mental practice is beneficial for new motor learning as well as preparing to perform a skill (Magill, 1993). Much of the work in this area has been directed to enhancing performance in athletes; to date only one study has reported the benefits of mental practice in the learning of new motor skills in rehabilitation (Linden et al., 1989).

Techniques used for mental practice should involve a preperformance review where the learner focuses attention on the behaviour required to complete the movement pattern. After the performance, further mental rehearsal should be undertaken to allow the learner to 'replay' the skill and consider which aspects of the movement produced the results of his or her performance.

OBSERVATIONAL LEARNING

Providing a demonstration (modelling) of a motor skill can give a considerable amount of information quickly, and in a way that is sometimes difficult to achieve with verbal instructions. A method that combines demonstration with physical practice and feedback demonstrations optimizes learning.

Physiotherapists have always demonstrated skills as an intuitive method of instruction. Considerable research supports this view that modelling provides concise visual information about a motor skill that facilitates learning (McCullagh, 1993). The evidence also indicates that learning is enhanced if the individual demonstrating the skill (the model) is also trying to learn the skill. In addition to watching the model, the learner needs to receive the feedback that the model is using to learn the skill. Physiotherapists are therefore encouraged to use demonstrations to supplement verbal instructions. Periods of practice should be alternated with demonstrations and information provided about the relevant aspects of the performance by the model during the demonstration.

Summary

This chapter has presented some of the principles of motor learning that can be applied to rehabilitation of older adults. It has focused on specific variables within information feedback, practice schedules, and prepractice training that are particularly relevant to the learning involved in rehabilitation, although there are many other areas in the field of motor learning. It is important to remember that these principles have been developed mainly from research on younger adults. As research continues on motor learning in older adults, the applicability of the principles will be more firmly established. In the meantime these principles are intended as guidelines for therapeutic interventions with both younger and older adults (see also Chapter 12).

Acknowledgements

The authors would like to thank Tim Lee for his helpful comments on an earlier draft of this chapter. Preparation of this work was funded in part by a grant from the Ontario Ministry of Health awarded to the co-authors.

References

Al-Ameer, AA, Toole, T (1993) Combination of blocked and random practice orders: Benefits to acquisition and retention. Journal of Human Movement Studies 25: 177–191.

Carnahan, H, Vandervoort, AA, Swanson, LR (1993) The influence of aging on motor learning. In Stelmach, GE, Homberg, V (eds) Sensorimotor Impairments in the Elderly, pp. 41–56. Dordrecht: Kluwer.

Fitts, PM, Posner, MI (1967) Human Performance. Belmont, CA: Brooks Cole.

Gentile, AM (1972) A working model of skill acquisition with application to teaching. Quest 17: 1–23.

Kausler, DH (1994) Learning and Memory in Normal Aging. San Diego: Academic Press.

Lee, TD, Maraj, BKV, Swanson, LR (1995) Effect of adaptive bandwidth knowledge of results on motor learning. Unpublished

Light, KE (1990) Information processing for motor performance in aging adults. *Physical Therapy* **70**: 820–826.

Linden, CA, Uhley, JE, Smith, D, Bush, MA (1989) The effect of mental practice on walking balance in an elderly population. *Occupational Therapy Journal of Research* **9**: 155–169.

McCullagh, P (1993) Modeling: Learning, developmental, and social psychological considerations. In Singer, RN, Murphey, M, Tennant, LK (eds) *Handbook of Research on Sport Psychology*, pp. 106–126. New York: Macmillan.

Magill, RA (1993) *Motor Learning: Concepts and Applications*, 4th edn. Dubuque, IA: Brown.

Magill, RA, Hall, KG (1990) A review of the contextual interference effect in motor skill acquisition. *Human Movement Science* **9** :241–289.

Salthouse, TA (1990) Working memory as a processing resource in cognitive aging. *Developmental Review* **10**: 101–124.

Salthouse, TA (1991) *Theoretical Perspectives on Cognitive Aging*. Hillsdale: Erlbaum.

Schmidt, RA (1988) *Motor Control and Learning: A Behavioural Emphasis*, 2nd edn. Champaign, IL: Human Kinetics.

Schmidt, RA (1991) Frequent augmented feedback can degrade learning: Evidence and interpretations. In Requin, J, Stelmach, GE (eds) *Tutorials in Motor Neuroscience*, pp. 59–75. Dordrecht: Kluwer.

Swanson, LR, Lee, TD (1992) The effects of aging and schedules of knowledge of results on motor learning. *Journal of Gerontology: Psychological Sciences* **47**: 406–411.

Swinnen, SP, Schmidt, RA, Nicholson, DE, Shapiro, DC (1990) Information feedback for skill acquisition: Instantaneous knowledge of results degrades learning. *Journal of Experimental Psychology: Learning, Memory and Cognition* **16**: 706–716.

Vander Linden, DW, Cauraugh, JH, Greene, TA (1993) The effect of frequency of kinetic feedback on learning an isometric force production task in nondisabled subjects. *Physical Therapy* **73**: 79–87.

Winstein, CJ (1991) Designing practice for motor learning: Clinical implications. In Lister, MJ (ed) *Contemporary Management of Motor Control Problems: Proceedings of the II STEP Conference*, pp. 65–76. Alexandria: Foundation for Physical Therapy.

Winstein, CJ, Schmidt, RA (1990) Reduced frequency of knowledge of results enhances motor skill learning. *Journal of Experimental Psychology: Learning, Memory and Cognition* **16**: 677–691.

Wulf, G, Schmidt, RA (1989) The learning of generalized motor programs: Reducing the relative frequency of knowledge of results enhances memory. *Journal of Experimental Psychology: Learning, Memory and Cognition* **15**: 748–757.

C

Working with Older People

SECTION EDITOR: ANTHONY A VANDERVOORT

10

Effective Communication

JB ORANGE, ELLEN B RYAN

Nomenclature
•
Communication Between Health Care Providers and Older Clients
•
Normal Age-related Changes in Speech, Voice, Hearing, Language and Communication
•
Speech and Voice, Hearing, Language and Communication Disorders in Older Adults
•
Communication Strategies with Older Adults
•
Summary

There is little question that communication is critical to humans. Nearly all tasks in which humans participate invariably involve communication. Communication serves to establish and develop physical, social and emotional links between one another. Communication also provides a means by which individuals can participate in their health care such as describing symptoms and following spoken, written, or gestured instructions. For adults 65 years of age or over, communication is of paramount importance because it empowers them. Decisions about the course of their lives or the nature of their physical and mental health care are dependent on them possessing effective communication skills. Moreover, health care providers' use of appropriate interaction strategies, as well as supportive com-

municative environments, promotes independent decision-making. However, the communicative disorders suffered by older adults, inappropriate communication by care providers, and communication-impaired environments can isolate older adults, foster dependency and insecurity, lower self-esteem, and reduce their chances of optimizing their health.

In the USA, it is estimated that communication problems occur in over 30% of adults 65 years of age or over (Campbell Brown, 1990). Prevalence rates of communicative disorders among older adults in Canada, the UK, Australia, New Zealand and other developed nations vary greatly depending on the nature of the problem (i.e. hearing versus speech versus language disorders) and the place of residence (i.e. home versus institution), but a similar overall rate is thought to apply. As the proportion of adults 65 years of age or over in developed countries continues to grow, comparable increases in the proportion of older adults with communication impairments are expected in the coming decades. The link that exists between the importance of communication to older adults and the high prevalence rate of communicative disorders among this cohort shows clearly that care providers, and in particular health care providers such as physiotherapists, must be prepared to address the communicative needs of this expanding segment of the population. Moreover, evidence of stereotyped-based, inappropriate communication directed towards older clients by care providers makes communication education an essential component of their training (see also Chapters 4 and 8).

The purpose of this chapter is to present a brief overview of the age-related changes in communication and some common communication difficulties experienced by older adults, and to discuss communication strategies that physiotherapists might find useful in their daily therapeutic interactions. Important terms are defined to establish clear distinctions among communication disorders. Two models outlining the communicative predicament of older adults and the communication enhancement approach for health care providers are summarized to help establish a framework for the effective communication techniques. Examples of strategies are provided to illustrate the need for clinicians to problem solve as they select individually tailored supportive techniques suited to the heterogeneous communication and cognitive skills of older adults (Chapter 8).

Nomenclature

Communicating effectively with older adults requires that care providers know the difference between various types of speech, hearing, language, voice and communicative disorders. The following terms are presented which highlight important distinctions.

'Speech' is often referred to as the sounds that people say. Speech can be divided into production and perception domains. Speech production involves the activity of making and modifying sounds, while speech perception (i.e. hearing) includes receiving, discriminating, and processing spoken sounds. Speech production consists of the complex coordination of dynamic neuromuscular movements necessary for respiration, phonation (i.e. vocal fold vibration), resonance (i.e. movement of velum — soft palate), articulation, and prosody (i.e. duration of sounds, rate and volume of speaking, pitch changes, syllable stress, etc.). It is estimated that humans produce 12–14 sounds per second during normal speech which require between 120 000 and 140 000 neural events! When one considers that adult speaking rates range between 150 and 180 words per minute and that each English word has on average six sounds, that adds up to millions of neural events per minute just to make sounds! Speech perception, or hearing, is a complex series of acoustic and cognitive processes involved in receiving and interpreting speech sounds. Hearing, like speech production, is often underestimated in its importance until it becomes impaired.

'Language' is a system of shared, culturally bound, symbols that represent ideas, as well as a set of rules that control how symbols are displayed. Grammar, vocabulary and word order (i.e. syntax) are three primary elements of language. The ability to use language in sophisticated and complex ways is a key defining characteristic of humans. For example, humans speak sounds, write letters, and use sign languages or gestures in which combinations of symbols represent meaningful words and complex relationships of ideas.

The term 'voice' refers to the production of a sound signal (i.e. vocal tone) through the vibration of the vocal folds in the larynx. The vocal tone is modified by musculoskeletal structures such as the pharynx, soft palate, oral and nasal cavities, teeth, tongue, lips and jaw to give clarity to speech sounds (Chapter 4).

The final term, 'communication', refers to the exchange of ideas through spoken, written, signed, touch, smell or non-verbal means (e.g. gestures, facial expressions, body posture). Communication involves speech, hearing, voice, language and cognitive (i.e. attention, perception, memory, judgement) processes. Communication is used to establish and develop relationships and effect control over one's life. Communicating is particularly important for older adults who may be at risk of being isolated from others as a result of a various pathologies (e.g. stroke, neurodegenerative diseases such as Parkinson's disease), and changes in social roles (e.g. retirement) or mental and marital status (e.g. dementia and widowhood) (see also Chapters 3 and 5).

Communication Between Health Care Providers and Older Clients

Whereas there are age-related and disease-related changes that affect communication for some older adults, it is important to keep in mind the influences that health care providers exert on interactions with their clients. Health care providers who act as the primary communication partner of older adults control in many ways the amount, content, structure and context of communicative interactions. Just as older adults may need support more than ever for effective communication, health care providers can often undermine attempts by constraining opportunities or even modifying older adults' communication to suit stereotyped expectations (Chapters 3 and 11). The Communication Predicament of Ageing presented in Figure 1 depicts the manner in which the communication of care providers can sometimes reduce the chances for communication success with older adults (Coupland et al., 1991; Ryan et al., 1995). The model suggests that communication partners often modify their talk to older adults based on false assumptions and stereotyped expectations of how older adults communicate. The over-accommodated communication by partners helps to elicit age-biased communication from older adults and reinforces dependence, incompetence and poor self-esteem. The model, therefore, takes into consideration the dyadic and reciprocal influences fundamental to the concept of communication.

Field studies of social interactions between care providers and older adult care receivers in North America, Europe and Australia support several conclusions (Shadden, 1988; Coupland et al., 1991; Baltes et al., 1994). Formal care providers of chronic care, both in institutions and in the home, regularly provide social reinforcement that shape dependent behaviours and usually ignore care receivers' self-care activities. This pattern of reinforcement establishes reliance upon the care provider and leads to reduced self-care skills and decreased self-esteem. Over-

Figure 1   The communication predicament of ageing.

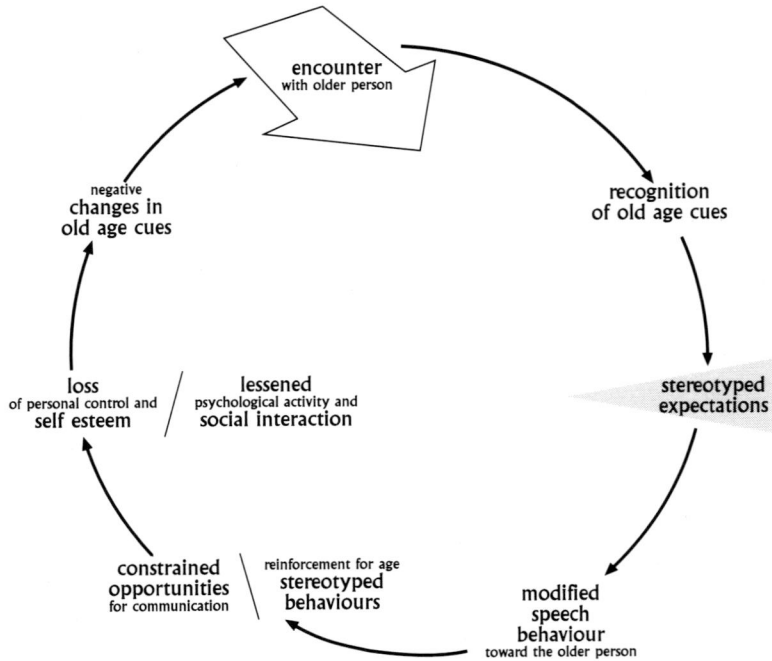

helping, rather than encouraging continued use of existing independent behaviours, takes less time but is dangerous to the overall functioning of older adults (Chapters 11 and 22). Studies have shown that dependence-inducing behaviours occur even in reactivation units that have the explicit goal of enhancing independence.

Despite the clear mission statements of facilities and compassionate care providers, talk with institutional residents, especially those with cognitive impairment (see Chapter 8), occurs mainly in the context of staff tasks and a narrow interpretation of health care. Even in the context of activities of daily living such as bathing and dressing, health care providers often miss opportunities for human-to-human connection. It would appear that the agenda of care providers is viewed as a higher priority than the advancing of social inter-

actions. This is particularly unfortunate for interactions with cognitively impaired older adults where health care providers, who ignore residual skills, may be placing their patients at further risk of isolation and stigmatization.

Baby talk, patronizing communication, and infantalizing behviours occur often in institutions, to some extent in home care, and even among families. Although often well-intentioned, communicating with older adults in baby talk and other patronizing ways conveys a fundamental lack of respect. Use of baby talk to older adults residing in institutions (i.e. high pitch and exaggerated intonation pattern accompanied by simplified grammar and vocabulary) has been found to be linked much more to the care provider than to characteristics of the resident receiving this talk. Sometimes older adults seeking community-based services are patronized through behaviours such as non-listening, offering little opportunity for decision-making, pats on the head, exaggerated praise for everyday activities, overly superficial conversation, slow but loud talk, and a focus on topics related to the past (see Chapter 11).

These findings raise questions about the optimal ways health care providers can and should communicate with the older adults for whom they provide care. There are no simple rules for talking with older adults; nor is there a 'cookbook-recipe' outlining the sequential steps one should follow. Some older adults suffer from various combinations of communication, cognitive, medical, neurosensory and mobility problems for which accommodations need to be made; some do not suffer any chronic problems. Some expect us to talk with special deference because of their age; others seek a friendly relationship before accepting care. For example, care providers are faced with the dilemma of addressing a new client either by their last name (e.g. Mrs. Jones) or by their first name (e.g. Mary). The challenge to clinicians to modify communications to the individual needs and preferences of older adults is termed the Communication Predicament of Caregivers. The following sections highlight the heterogeneity of speech, voice, hearing, language and communicative skills and disorders of older adults and reinforce the need for health care providers of all professions to accommodate their communication on an individual basis.

Normal Age-related Changes in Speech, Voice, Hearing, Language and Communication

Several recent excellent texts are devoted entirely to discussing the changes in speech (see also Chapter 8), voice, hearing, language and communication related to normal ageing processes. The reader is referred to books by Bayles and Kaszniak (1987), Chapey (1994), Clarke (1993), Lubinski (1991), Maxim and Bryan (1994), Ripich (1991), Shadden (1988) and Willmot (1991) that provide clear, detailed, and thorough presentations and from which the following overview is drawn.

Speech and Voice

Speech production involves respiration, phonation, resonance, articulation and prosody. Voicing consists primarily of phonation, but the other subsystems of speech are involved in sound modulation. Age-related changes across speech and voice subsystems include reduced strength, rate, duration, range and speed of motion. For respiration, this means increased rigidity of the chest wall and associated musculoskeletal structures that drive speech production. The decreased compliance, however, has only a minor influence during normal speech and voicing tasks. Reduced loudness, fewer syllables per breath group (i.e. amount spoken on one breath of air), and longer inter- and intra-sentence pauses may be apparent in the speech of older adults.

Calcification, thinning, and stiffening of laryngeal cartilages, atrophy of laryngeal muscles, as well as deterioration of mucous secreting glands, create a less dynamic voicing system. These age-related biological and physiological changes may result in perceived lower pitch in older females and increased pitch in males, reduced pitch control and range, harsh or breathy voice quality, and shorter maximum voicing time.

Atrophy of velar muscles (i.e. soft palate) occurs in conjunction with progressive declines in muscle control and elasticity of pharyngeal muscles. The combination of these changes results in small increases in perceived hypernasality.

The minor changes in articulation associated with ageing are based on several factors. Alterations in the bony composition of the mandible and maxilla distort the tempromandibular joint, and restrict normal movements affecting clarity, accuracy and speed of sound production. Decreased strength of the muscles of the tongue, lips and face, loss of teeth, fewer oral secretions, and diminished touch and pressure sensitivity in the oral cavity lead to perceptions of slow rate of articulation, imprecise consonants and reduced clarity. Some characteristic speech and voice features of older adults include slow speech rate, harsh or hoarse voice quality, lower volume, hypernasality, slow articulation and imprecise consonants.

Hearing

Hearing impairment in older adults, commonly referred to as presbycusis, is one of their most prevalent chronic conditions. The prevalence of hearing problems among Canadians between 65 and 74 years of age is over 13%, for those 75 to 84 years of age over 22%, and for those 85 years of age and over nearly 50% (Statistics Canada, 1992). The numbers are even higher for older adults who reside in residential and chronic care facilities. Similar rates of hearing impairment have also been reported among older adults in other developed countries.

Age-related structural changes in the outer and

middle ear include losses of resilience, elasticity and flexibility of the pinna (i.e. outer ear), ear canal, tympanic membrane (i.e. ear drum), middle ear bones (i.e. ossicles) and the Eustachian tube, which connects the middle ear to the nasopharynx. These age-related changes, in concert with atrophy of the muscles that support the three middle ear bones, lead to poor conductive hearing levels. Degeneration of hair cells and supporting cells, and reductions in the vascular supply to the inner ear (i.e. cochlea) contribute to sensoryneural based hearing impairment. Subtle changes in the central auditory system include losses of neurons in subcortical auditory pathways and structures, and in cortical regions responsible for sound perception and interpretation (i.e. superior temporal gyrus).

The overall effect of the age-related changes in hearing is that high-frequency tones (e.g. women's voices), especially those above 2000 Hz, are more severely affected than low tones. Tinnitus, or 'ringing-in-the-ears', sometimes co-occurs with presbycusis. Hearing losses in both ears occur more frequently in men than in women.

Language

Language skills change with ageing. However, reports on the exact nature of these changes varies considerably between studies. This is hardly surprising as language is a complex mental system that is interdependent on other cognitive processes — most notably attention, perception and memory processes (Chapter 9).

Subtle problems such as naming people, objects, and pictures (i.e. anomia) may emerge with ageing and are thought to be related to slower access to and retrieval of items in mental vocabularies. Recent evidence suggests that the size of the vocabulary of older adults can increase with age, although the active spoken and written vocabularies used every day may gradually decline. Older adults store new information with less elaboration, imagery and organization than do younger people, which may contribute to their naming problems. However, the relationships among word storing strategies, mental associations of word meanings, and word recall and retrieval processes in older adults remain unclear (see Chapter 9).

One of the major issues in age-related changes in language among older adults is their reduced ability to understand spoken and written material beyond single sentences (e.g. instructions, stories and conversations). While it is agreed, generally, that there are no age-related effects for recognizing single words and understanding word meanings, age effects in comprehension have been observed for complex grammatical material and structures containing words that occur infrequently in a person's vocabulary. These age-related difficulties in listening and reading comprehension may reflect a combination of problems in motor systems and cognitive and language processes.

The spoken language of older adults does not usually contain errors in grammar or word order but may be long and elaborate in detail. There is conflicting evidence over whether older adults versus younger adults produce less grammatically complex sentences. Any changes that do exist, however, exert little impact on effective everyday language use.

Communication

Studies of age-related changes in communication among older adults have addressed the social uses of language in a variety of contexts. Only a small minority of older adults are loquacious, thus debunking the myth that *all* older adults are overly talkative. The evidence concerning verbosity indicates that some older adults may tend to generate multi-word verbal and written responses containing indefinite terms (e.g. this, someone, thing), errors of referencing, and reduced syntactic complexity. Moreover, some may digress from the main topic of conversation, giving the impression of increased talkativeness. However, analysis of the conversations of older adults has shown their resourcefulness and flexibility in adapting to communication partners, topics of conversation, and contextual influences. Older adults demonstrate robust skills in maintaining conversation, and logically and sequentially shifting the topic of conversation when appropriate, which may help to minimize problems in interactions. Further stories told by older adults versus younger adults receive more favourable ratings for interest and clarity.

A key point in age-related changes in communication is that older adults adapt their communication goals as part of successful ageing — adapting goals to fit changing skills, limitations, and resources. Hence, they may make trade-offs, such as using simpler grammar when telling complex, interesting stories (Kemper, 1992), relying more on written lists and instructions than on their own memory, or restricting their friendship network to a few close friends, without bothering to make new acquaintances.

Speech and Voice, Hearing, Language and Communication Disorders in Older Adults

Age-related disorders of speech and voice, hearing, language and communication have been the focus of intense research over the past two decades. One of the difficulties faced by researchers and clinicians alike has been distinguishing age-related from non-age-related changes – that is, determining whether or not the older adult suffers from a clinical disorder. The wide range of performance of older adults contributes to this difficulty. Decisions as to whether the changes constitute a disorder should only be made on the basis of a comprehensive and thorough understanding of lifespan development and the range of individual variability.

Speech and Voice

The most frequent impairment in speech production among older adults is dysarthria – a motor speech disorder in which there are impairments in the muscle systems that control respiration, phonation, resonance, and articulation.

The profile of speech features associated with dysarthria varies depending on the aetiology (e.g. progressive or non-progressive, focal or diffuse neural pathology), site of damage (e.g. peripheral and/or central nervous systems), the severity of the disease, age of person, presence of co-occurring medical or psychiatric problems, medications being taken, and primary spoken language, among others. For example, an individual with moderate-to-severe hypokinetic dysarthria associated with Parkinson's disease and an individual with moderate-severe amyotrophic lateral sclerosis (ALS) may both exhibit moderately unintelligible spontaneous speech, but for different reasons. The individual with Parkinson's disease is most likely to display monotone, short, rapid rushes of speech that contain inappropriate silences. Conversely, the individual with ALS is most likely to exhibit hypernasality, a slow rate of speaking, harsh voice quality, and short phrases. Strategies to improve their intelligibility will vary because of the differences which underlie their poor speech production.

Another speech disorder that occurs in older adults, often co-occurring with the language disorder aphasia, is apraxia of speech. Rare in its pure form, apraxia of speech is a disturbance in the capacity to programme mentally the motor sequences required for the production of sounds. The speech of an older adult with apraxia of speech will contain inconsistent speaking errors, unlike the consistent speech problems observed in individuals with dysarthria.

Voice impairments in older adults frequently result from laryngeal cancers that occur secondary to smoking (Doyle, 1994). Surgical resection of all or part of the larynx and its supporting musculoskeletal tissues (i.e. laryngectomy) results in loss of the voice. After this surgery, some patients can be taught to use the upper portion of their oesophagus to produce 'oesophageal speech'. Others unable to master this technique may benefit from the insertion of a voice prosthesis containing a vibrating reed which produces 'vocal' tones that can be modulated to approximate speech sounds. Still others elect to use an electro-larynx that mechanically generates 'vocal' tones via an electrically vibrating device.

Hearing

As noted previously, presbycusis is the term that describes the biological ageing of the auditory system and the hearing losses observed in older adults that occurs as a result of cumulative intrinsic and extrinsic factors (Salomon, 1991). Intrinsic factors include changes in the vascular supply to the inner ear, genetic predisposition, and inner ear sensory cell and nerve degeneration. Extrinsic factors include a poor dietary profile, acute or chronic noise exposure, and use of ototoxic drugs such as those used in the treatment of various forms of cancer. Prolonged over-exposure to loud noises accounts for the largest portion of hearing impairments in older adults, especially among males. The classic profile of hearing impairment typical of presbycusis is a progressive, binaural, symmetrical sensorineural hearing loss of high frequency sounds above 2000 Hz that emerges late in adulthood.

The most frequent complaints of hearing-impaired older adults are problems with hearing acuity and discrimination, particularly in noisy environments (e.g. restaurants) or locations with poor acoustics (e.g. large auditoriums, halls, or places of worship). Another common complaint is tinnitus, or 'ringing-in-the-ears', which often results from changes in the vascular supply to the inner ear or from taking salicylates (i.e. aspirin) (Willmot, 1991).

Language

By far the most prevalent form of language disorder in older adults is aphasia. Aphasia is a disorder of language that results from focal neurological damage, most often a cerebral vascular accident (CVA, i.e. a stroke), to the language dominant cerebral hemisphere, which is almost always the left. Cognitive impairment, if it does occur in individuals with aphasia, is usually minimal and limited to complex mental processes such as memory, organization/planning, or problem-solving. The type of stroke, severity, and the site of lesion in the language dominant hemisphere all influence the nature of the language problems. There are two major types of aphasia — non-fluent and fluent aphasia.

Individuals suffering a CVA to the anterior portions of the language dominant hemisphere will most likely exhibit non-fluent or anterior aphasia, of which Broca's aphasia is the most typical. The language profile of an individual with non-fluent aphasia includes limited, often grammatically incorrect, spoken output that is termed 'telegraphic' because of the high proportion of nouns and verbs and the few connector words such as prepositions, articles (e.g. the, a), and pronouns. Word-finding difficulties may be apparent. Listening and reading comprehension are less impaired and are definite strengths. Repetition of words and sentences is mildly to moderately impaired. Apraxia of speech may co-exist with the language problems.

Individuals suffering a localized CVA to the posterior portion of the language dominant hemisphere will most likely display fluent or posterior aphasia, of which Wernicke's aphasia is the most typical form. The language profile of an individual with fluent aphasia includes copious spoken output that sometimes contains nonsense words (i.e. neologisms), or words related to the intended words by sound (e.g. 'bat' for 'pat') or meaning (e.g. 'hat' for 'scarf'). Anomia, or word-finding difficulties, may be quite severe. Listening and reading comprehension are frequently severely impaired, as is repetition of words and sentences.

Communication

The most frequent form of communicative disorder in older adults that a health care provider is likely to encounter is associated with the syndrome of dementia. Dementia is an acquired, progressive, degenerative impairment that affects the mental activities associated with memory, communication and language, personality, visuoperceptual skills, and cognition (i.e. abstraction and judgement) (Cummings and Benson, 1992). The prevalence of dementia in the older adult populations of developed countries is expected to reach shocking proportions during the first three decades of the twenty-first century, unless there are major medical breakthroughs in prevention and treatment.

Communication and language problems, based in part on deteriorations in memory, occur in over 85% of individuals with Alzheimer's disease (Cummings and Benson, 1992). The communication and language profiles of an individual with Alzheimer's disease vary with the clinical stage of their illness (i.e. early-mild, middle-moderate, late-severe). Subtle naming problems appear in the early stage along with subtle changes in the social appropriateness of words and sentences. Listening and reading comprehension are generally intact, except for complex language structures. Problems may occur in following multi-partner conversations. As the disease progresses to the middle clinical stage, anomia becomes more pronounced, spoken output lacks substantive words (i.e. nouns, adjectives, adverbs, verbs), and individuals experience greater difficulty participating in conversations. Communication becomes a significant challenge during this stage, both for the individual with Alzheimer's disease and for their care providers. By the late clinical stage, verbal output may be limited to periodic nonsense words, islands of fluent and coherent single words, and repetitions or partial repetitions of themselves or what others say to them. Listening and reading comprehension are severely impaired.

Communication Strategies with Older Adults

In contrast to the Communication Predicament of Ageing described earlier, Ryan *et al.* (1995) have developed a model that promotes a comprehensive approach to communication with older adults. Based on communication accommodation theory (Coupland *et al.*, 1991) and a health promotion perspective, the Communication Enhancement Model outlined in Figure 2 takes into consideration the roles of both the care provider and the older adult as well as the environmental influences within which interactions occur. The framework of the model incorporates three determinants of communication (i.e. accommodated communication based on individual needs, individualized assessment and supportive environments) that care providers can target to establish effective communication with older adults. Baltes *et al.* (1994) demonstrated the potential for reversing the communication predicament in an institutional context with systematic staff training.

While the Communication Predicament Model discussed earlier suggests that the modified speech behaviours of care providers are based on recognition of old age cues (e.g. age, physical features such as white hair or stooped posture, or institutional setting) and stereotyped expectations of performance, the Communication Enhancement Model promotes modifications of communication and assessment protocols on an individual basis; modifications that are free of preconceived negative views of performance. In view of the variations in the communicative performance of older adults, the concepts of individualized accommodated communication and individualized assessment are particularly rele-

Figure 2   Communication enhancement model.

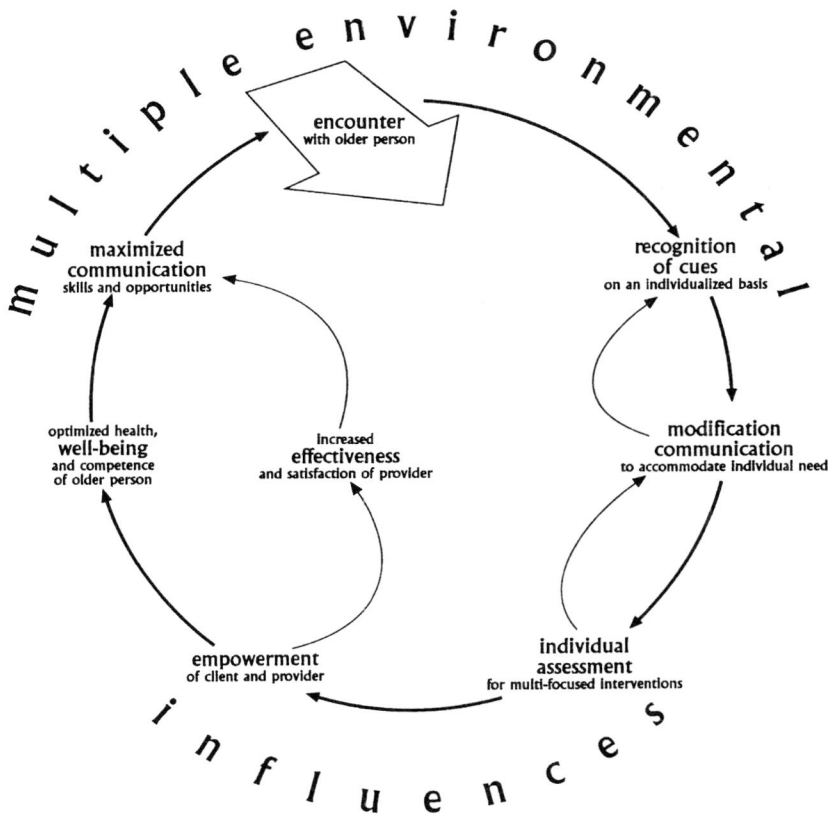

Figure 2   Communication enhancement model.

vant for health care providers such as physiotherapists. Further, the impact of multiple physical and psychosocial environments on individualized communication is especially important for caregivers who provide care to older adults in long-term and chronic care facilities where environments may restrict rather than support communication. Therefore, care providers who operate within the framework of these three determinants of communication enhancement will provide opportunities for older adults to develop greater control over decision-making through empowerment, to optimize their sense of well-being, and to maximize communicative effectiveness. Interaction strategies used by care providers that are based on the model are more

likely to suit the speech, voice, hearing, language, or communication changes and disorders unique to each older adult.

The following sections and accompanying tables contain examples of interaction strategies that operate within the framework of the Communication Enhancement Model and target the communication changes and disorders observed in older adults. Before discussing them, however, a few caveats are warranted. First, the heterogeneity of speech, voice, hearing, language, and communication skills of older adults require that health care providers respond to needs on an individual basis. Clinicians must be prepared to accept that strategies which work well for one person's difficulty may not work for the same problem exhibited by another. A useful strategy common to all interactions with older adults, regardless of the nature of their communicative disorder, is patience. Second, the strategies outlined below are not meant to be either prescriptive or exhaustive. There is no 'cookbook-recipe' method to strategy selection or use. Third, and most important, care providers must be prepared to use their clinical problem-solving skills to select and develop suitable approaches. The examples outlined in the accompanying tables should be considered starting points in the process of developing and using communication enhancement strategies.

One of the key themes in this chapter is that human communication is a complex process with multiple mediating factors. The Communication Predicament of Ageing and the Communication Enhancement Model identify clearly important influences on communication with older adults. Establishing appropriate and individualized accommodated communication with older adults requires flexibility, adaptability, and critical thinking.

Table 1

Strategies for Helping Older Adults with Speech and Voice Disorders

Dysarthria

- Ask person to slow-down or speed-up speaking rate depending on profile of impairment
- Finger tapping on table-top, lap, or leg may slow articulation and increase intelligibility
- Syllable-by-syllable, word-by-word, or over-exaggerated speaking may aid clarity and reduce bursts of speech
- Remind person to take full breaths before speaking
- Use questions that signal clearly what you DID or DID NOT understand, e.g. 'Do you mean _____?', 'I don't know what _____ means?', 'Speak slower / faster / louder', 'Say the last two words again (slower / faster / louder), please. I didn't quite get them.'
- Ask person to say or to repeat the key words
- Do not pretend to understand — acknowledge that you did not understand the message and provide specific feedback about the nature of your misunderstanding
- Use your full and undivided attention when listening
- If after repeated attempts to understand, ask person to use alternate / augmentative communication (e.g. gesture, write, picture or language boards, computer-synthesized voice system) — be familiar with her / his system
- If alternative / augmentative communication options fail, acknowledge continued problems and suggest that you return to the topic or conversation in few minutes after a rest or time-out period
- Minimize background distracting visual, auditory, olfactory and tactile 'noise' to highlight spoken messages (e.g. turn off television or radio, turn away from visually distracting windows or hallways, move out of areas with a lot of other people who are talking, leave areas that smell bad)
- Move to their level (i.e. crouching), especially if older adult is in a wheelchair — get close to person after asking permission, and especially if unable to speak loudly

Laryngectomy

- Use your full and undivided attention when listening
- Ask questions that signal clearly what you DID or DID NOT understand; do not pretend to understand
- Ask person to write out word(s) that are problematic
- Minimize background distracting visual, auditory, olfactory and tactile 'noise' to highlight spoken messages
- Get close to person after asking permission
- Minimize your shock reaction to the possible unusual vocal quality of an electro-larynx or oesophageal speech

Strategies for Speech- and Voice-impaired Older Adults

Strategies for interacting with older adults suffering from speech and voice disorders are outlined in Table 1. The suggestions are directed primarily toward the care provider who should provide unambiguous feedback and act as a facilitator. Interactions with alaryngeal speakers can be intimidating, especially if they are using oesophageal speech or an electro-larynx. Speech and voice clarity may be severely compromised in older adults using either of these methods of voice production.

Strategies for Hearing-impaired Older Adults

There are several key supportive strategies that care providers should consider when interacting with hearing impaired older adults and trouble shooting the problems of hearing aids (see Table 2). It is important to note that not all older adults suffer from hearing problems. For those who do,

Table 2
Strategies for Helping Older Adults with Hearing Problems

Hearing Aid Related

- Trouble shooting to make sure hearing aid is functional:
  'O' setting is OFF; 'M' setting is microphone = ON; 'T' setting is for interfacing with telephones; 'NSF' setting is Noise Suppression for use in locations with a lot of background noise
- Hearing aid battery should be placed properly in the aid; a battery lasts approximately 3–4 weeks of everyday use (i.e. 12–16 hours)
- Ensure earmoulds (i.e. piece that fits in ear) and tubing (in 'behind-the-ear' and body aids) are free of obstructions (e.g. wax or twists) and seated properly in the ear and on the aid
- A whistling or high-pitched sound indicates one or more of the following:
  earmould is not seated properly
  volume control set at near maximum volume
  hole in earmould tubing
  aid is working when hand or object is cupped over aid
- Although many older adults are hearing impaired, do not assume your partner is until it is confirmed
- Do not speak on behalf of a hearing-impaired older adult; translating or clarifying information, when called upon, is more supportive of their independent communication
- Minimize background distracting visual, auditory, olfactory and tactile 'noise' to highlight spoken messages (e.g. turn off television or radio, turn away from visually distracting windows or hallways, move out of areas with a lot of other people who are talking, or places that are offensive in their odour or are too cold or too warm)
- Face the person at their eye level when speaking to them; do not speak to them from a great distance
- Get the person's attention before speaking by calling their name or lightly touching distally on limbs – do not call or speak to them from another room
- Make sure your face is free from distracting movements (e.g. eating, chewing food, smoking) and is clearly illuminated to aid with speech-reading
- Speaking to a hearing-impaired person over the phone is more difficult because of poor sound transmission as well as lack of facial, gestural and non-verbal cues
- Speak slowly and at a slightly louder than normal volume; shouting distorts sounds and draws unnecessary attention to hearing problems
- Explicitly introduce new topics in a conversation (e.g. 'Let's now talk about your recent trip to _____. Tell me about what you did on the trip to _____.')

though, their hearing difficulties are not often linked with cognitive disturbances; care providers should not assume that hearing difficulties are linked with declines in mental abilities. The care providers' manner of interaction (e.g. use of attention getting signals, rate of speaking, supportive physical and psychosocial environments) should always suggest that the older adult is cognitively capable of functioning as a competent communicator. Care providers may also need to dispel the unfounded fears of hearing-impaired older adults who feel that their hearing problems may be related to the onset of dementia. Strategies based on the framework of the three components of the Communication Enhancement Model, like those outlined in Table 2, help avoid misunderstanding, embarrassment, frustration and anxiety.

Misconceptions continue to persist concerning the extent to which hearing aids can 'correct' hearing problems. Hearing aids are sophisticated electrical devices designed to amplify sounds; nearly every type amplifies *all* sounds. The non-selective amplification of all sounds by hearing aids (except for some recent models fitted with noise-suppression circuitry) creates many difficulties for hearing-impaired older adults who frequently suffer speech discrimination problems in addition to declines in hearing acuity. Many (but not all) hearing-impaired older adults benefit from a hearing aid. Using a hearing aid appropriately and becoming accustomed to wearing one can be challenging, as it demands a great deal of intense attention by the user. Ironically, while hearing aids are intended to support communication and facilitate interactions, some older adults avoid using them because of the difficulties encountered in acclimatizing to the amplification of all sounds and because of the fear of being stigmatized.

Strategies for Older Adults with Aphasia

Table 3 contains information on strategies to improve communication environments, while Table 4 deals with strategies to help older adults with aphasia. The strategies in Table 3 also have broader application to non-aphasic older adults. Changing features in the physical and psychosocial environments by minimizing the influences of a communication-impaired environment (Lubinski, 1981) increases opportunities for interaction, costs very little, can be minimally intrusive, and can be a common sense way of improving communication between care providers and older adults.

Communication with older adults suffering from aphasia can be particularly frustrating for all participants, especially if health care providers do not understand or appreciate the nature of the language problems or the extent of retained abilities. Individuals with aphasia experience language-based difficulties in speaking, writing, listening and reading comprehension, as well as difficulty in the use and comprehension of non-verbal behaviours (e.g. facial expressions and gestures). Cognitive impairment, unlike that observed in dementia, is minimal and is limited primarily to central and higher order cognitive processes such as memory and problem-solving. The language difficulties of older adults with aphasia do not render them incapable of making their needs known or of making informed decisions. Consequently, health care providers must avoid talking about their client in front of them as if they are not there, and should not assume that the lack of communication signals indicates a lack of mental capability. The strategies outlined in Table 4 emphasize approaches that optimize inde-

Table 3

Strategies for Improving Communication Environments

Communication-impaired Environment (Lubinski, 1981)

- Settings that contain few opportunities for successful and meaningful communication
- Minimize influences of communication-impaired environment:
  be sensitive to the value of communication; promote this perception among colleagues and others
  eliminate rules which restrict quantity and quality of communication
  provide acceptable communication partners
  offer reasons to talk
  support privacy for communicating
  increase accessibility to other adults and supportive physical and psychosocial environments
  offer multisensory stimulation where appropriate
  help develop self-worth of older adults

Physical Environment

- Identify optimum number of conversation partners that facilitate interactions; consider those who are unfamiliar with the older adult
- Keep lighting optimal and make sure background noise is minimal
- Avoid competing messages such as blaring noise from the television, radio, or street
- Keep smells acceptable and temperature comfortable
- Arrangement, mobility, accessibility, comfort and composition of furniture can facilitate interactions, e.g. round tables invite, facilitate and help maintain interaction
- Accessible and private locations support personal, private-intimate conversations

Psychosocial Environment

- Gather relevant biographical information about new client beforehand to optimize conversational topic selection and to identify shared interests
- Include talk on a wide range of topics
- Always view person as potential communicator, praise all communicative attempts regardless of their level of success and type of disorder; ignoring person's communicative attempts may signal overall rejection
- Encourage family involvement in communication, where appropriate
- Do not talk about the person in front of her/him

Internal Environment

- Consider person's personality, work experiences, and relationship with family members
- Consider person's previous and present social roles
- Be aware that being tired will make communication more difficult and less rewarding

Adapted from Lubinski (1981)

pendence and control of communication for older adults with aphasia.

Strategies for Older Adults with Dementia

Communication with older adults who suffer not only from communication and language pro-blems, but also from immediate and recent memory impairments, changes in personality, visuospatial difficulties and impairments in judgement, poses significant and unique challenges to health care providers. These are the problems faced by family caregivers on a daily, moment-to-moment basis. Caregivers need to adjust speech, language and non-verbal features, take

Table 4

Strategies for Helping Older Adults with Aphasia

- Enquire about the type of aphasia, the levels of impairment, and retained abilities from speech-language pathologist or consulting physician(s); this helps focus individualized accommodated communication

Anomia: Word-finding Difficulties

- Provide longer periods of time for response(s)
- Provide the target word if requested or if person becomes anxious or frustrated
- Suggest time-out's following unsuccessful attempts (two to three tries); acknowledge that both of you are experiencing difficulty and tell person that you will come back later or will return to that topic in a few minutes; remember to get back!
- Provide sound, synonym, or sentence completion clues if you think you know word
- Ask person to spell, write out, gesture, or use synonym for the target word(s)

Other Speaking Problems

- Limited or unintelligible verbal output does not mean mental incompetence; do not assume cognitive impairment because of speaking problems
- Focus on communication of meaning and message rather than on correct word use; do not correct person if she/he uses wrong words or has poor grammar
- Repeat back what you think the person said to let her/him know what you have (mis)understood
- Learn the capabilities or limitations of person's augmentative/alternate communication devices (e.g. computer-based communication systems, synthesized voice communication devices, paper printer systems, word/alphabet boards)
- Encourage all attempts at communication, even through the use of singing or recitation of stereotyped phrases

Listening Comprehension Problems

- Get person's attention first by calling name or gently touching distally on limbs
- Ask one question or pose one idea at a time
- Ask Yes/No questions rather than open-ended questions (e.g. 'What did you do over the weekend?')
- Use forced choice question format (e.g. 'Do you want to start with the arm exercises or with the wax bath?')
- Use familiar vocabulary in short, grammatically simple sentences
- Use gestures, facial expressions, pictures, written information, music, or videos to augment what you say to her/him; avoid too much redundant information as that may overwhelm person
- Rephrase using synonyms rather than adding new information

into consideration memory limitations and premorbid and current personality status, as well as consider the emotional components and conversational strategies necessary to optimize effective communication. It is unreasonable to expect that caregivers will take into consideration all at once all of these areas that impact on communication. A more reasonable expectation, however, is that they should make accommodations in one domain at a time, observing the impact of the adjustment, and using critical thinking skills to determine why the accommodation did or did not work. The complexity of the cognitive, communicative, and behavioural disturbances exhibited by individuals with dementia requires caregivers to consider a comprehensive approach to appropriately accommodated communication (Orange *et al.*, 1995). The suggestions presented in Table 5 are intended to provide a starting point for the development and use of some effective options.

Table 5
Strategies for Helping Older Adults with Dementia of the Alzheimer's Type

Language

- Limit use of pronouns (e.g. he, she, they, this, that, everyone); use proper nouns instead
- Use direct statements (e.g. 'Lift your right leg') and minimize technical terms and jargon
- Limit colloquialisms because the person may interpret terms literally, such as 'Hop up onto the exercise table'
- Use Yes/No questions or modify questions to provide a choice, e.g. 'Do you mean stiffness *here* [pause] or stiffness *here?* (while pointing to or touching specific locations); minimize use of open-ended questions (e.g. 'Where is your stiffness?') — they provide too many choices

Conversation

- Never argue the logic of a point, e.g. 'You don't need to go to work. You retired 10 years ago.'
- Explain what you are doing as you are doing it, e.g. aspects of your physical examination or therapy
- When the person repeats sentences/ideas to a point that bothers you, distract by changing the topic or by using familiar music or videos
- Learn and use the person's background and personal history to make conversation meaningful and relevant
- Link topics — a new topic should be related to the old one; or state clearly that you are changing the topic
- Use signals that specify exactly what you misunderstood, e.g. 'I don't understand what — means?'
- If you are unable to get the person to understand, acknowledge the problem and change the topic

Memory

- Act as the person's memory trigger; do not assume that the person will search her/his own memory
- Minimize effects of poor memory on communication:
  follow routines
  give instructions in small steps; one at a time
  give ample time for the person to respond

Speech

- Use pauses between words or sentences to group important information
- Stress syllables and words to highlight information, e.g. 'Did you do your arm exercises *this morning* [pause] or *this afternoon?*'
- Speak clearly, slowly, and calmly; your speech should not be hurried or abrupt and your language not harsh

Body and Other Non-verbal Language

- Use calm facial expressions, body movements and posture; becoming angry or over-excited may alarm and confuse
- Move close and to the person's physical level, e.g. crouching for those who are wheelchair bound; minimize distractions and focus the person's attention
- Get person's attention first before talking, e.g. call out name or touch on hand to (re)gain attention and to reassure; do not touch until your presence is known

Emotions

- You do not always have to speak to communicate
- Respond to the person's *message,* not her/his *words*
- Acknowledge the emotions of person (isolation, fear and loneliness), e.g. 'I understand you feel frustrated. I would feel frustrated too if . . .'
- An empathetic tone and response will signal that you understand the person's feelings of loneliness, anxiety, and helplessness

Continued over

Table 5 (Continued)
Strategies for Helping Older Adults with Dementia of the Alzheimer's Type

Perceptions and Attitudes

- Do not use 'secondary baby talk' (i.e. exaggerated pitch, shrill tone, and loud voice) and terms of endearment (i.e. 'Sweetie', 'Dearie'), nick or pet-names, and non-verbal behaviours that may suggest incompetence, dependency, or lack of respect
- Avoid making statements in front of persons that you do not want them to know
- Work through your own views of older adults with cognitive impairment, recognizing that feelings of resentment, anger, or disgust will show through your body language and speech and will have a harmful impact on the care you provide

Adapted from Orange *et al.* (1994)

Table 6
When To Refer Older Adults to Speech–Language Pathologists and Audiologists

Speech, Voice, Language, Communication

- Sudden or gradual onset of unexplained slurred or unintelligible speech
- Sudden or gradual development of harsh, hoarse, or breathy voice quality
- Unexplained weakening of voice as day progresses
- Unexplained sudden or gradual onset of hypernasality
- Sudden or gradual onset of listening or reading comprehension problems
- Sudden or gradual onset of problems with word order, grammar, or accurate use of words – spoken output does not seem to make sense
- More than just 'normal age-related' problems are apparent, such as:
  word-finding difficulties
  memory problems
  withdrawal from social interactions

Hearing

- Older adult complains that people speak too softly or that they mumble
- Older adult asks repeatedly for people to speak louder or to repeat what they said
- Older adult complains of hearing constant ringing in ears
- Others complain that older adult's television, radio, or recorded music is too loud
- Others or older adult complains that background noise makes it difficult to hear

Adapted from Clark (1993).

Summary

Age-related changes in speech, voice, hearing, language and communication have been the focus of intense attention by researchers over the past 15 years. Much important information has been gathered on the biological, phychosocial and cognitive-related influences on communication with older adults. Recent findings have shown the importance of communication as a valuable clinical tool for health care providers as well as promoting interdisciplinary collaboration in developing communication strategies targeted to the individual needs of older adults (see Table 6 for suggestions about referrals to speech–language pathologists). Most importantly, however, we have come to recognize the significance of effective communication with and by older adults to help establish and maintain their optimal levels of emotional and physical well-being. It is clear that approaches which signal a positive enabling attitude are likely to enhance communication and to support independent decision-making among older adults.

References

Baltes, MM, Neumann, E-M, Zank, S (1994) Maintenance and rehabilitation of independence in old age: An intervention program for staff. *Psychology and Aging* 9: 179–188.

Bayles, K, Kaszniak, A (1987) *Communication and Cognition: Normal Aging and Dementia.* San Diego: College-Hill Press / Little, Brown.

Campbell Brown, S (1990) The prevalence of communicative disorders in the aging population. *Proceedings of the Research Symposium on Communication Sciences and Disorders and Aging,* pp. 14–25. Rockville, Maryland.

Chapey, R (1994) *Language Intervention Strategies in Adult Aphasia,* 3rd edn. Baltimore: Williams & Wilkins.

Clarke, L (1993) *Communication Disorders of the Older Adult: A Practical Handbook for Health Care Professionals.* New York: Hunter / Mount Sinai Geriatric Education Center.

Coupland, H, Coupland, J, Giles, H (1991) *Language, Society and the Elderly.* Oxford: Basil Blackwell.

Cummings, JL, Benson, DF (1992) *Dementia: A Clinical Approach,* 2nd edn. Boston: Butterworth-Heinemann.

Doyle, P (1994) *Foundations of Voice and Speech Rehabilitation Following Laryngeal Cancer.* San Diego: Singular Publishing Group.

Kemper, S (1992) Language and aging. In Salthouse, TA, Craik, FIM (eds) *The Handbook of Aging and Cognition,* pp. 213–270. Hillsdale, NJ: Lawrence Erlbaum Associates.

Lubinski, R (1981) Environmental language intervention. In Chapey, R (ed) *Language Intervention Strategies in Adult Aphasia,* pp. 223–245. Baltimore: Williams & Wilkins.

Lubinski, R (1991) *Dementia and Communication.* Philadelphia: Mosby.

Maxim J, Bryan K (1994) *Language of the Elderly: A Clinical Perspective.* San Diego: Singular Publishing.

Orange, JB, Molloy, DW, Lever, JA *et al.* (1994) Alzheimer's disease: physician-patient communication. *Canadian Family Physician* 40: 1160–1168..

Orange, JB, Ryan, EB, Meredith, SD, MacLean, M (1995) Application of the Communication Enhancement Model for longterm care residents with Alzheimer's disease. *Topics in Language Disorders* 15 (2): 20–35.

Ripich, D (1991) *Handbook of Geriatric Communication Disorders.* Austin: PRO-ED Inc.

Ryan, EB, Meredith, SD, MacLean, MJ, Orange, JB (1995). Changing the way we talk with elders: Promoting health using the Communication Enhancement Model. *International Journal of Aging and Human Development* 41 (2): 87–105.

Salomon, G (ed.) (1991) Hearing in the aged. *Acta Oto-Laryngologica* (Suppl.) 476: 7–285.

Shadden, B (1988) *Communication Behavior and Aging: A Sourcebook for Clinicians.* Baltimore: Williams & Wilkins.

Statistics Canada (1992) *Canadians with Impaired Hearing* (Special Topic Series from the Health and Activity Limitation Survey, No 82–615, Vol. 5). Ottawa: Statistics Canada.

Willmot, JF (1991) *Aging and the Auditory System: Anatomy, Physiology, and Psychoaccoustics.* San Diego: Singular Publishing.

11

Applications of Perceived Control and Learned Helplessness

LEAH E WEINBERG

It has been suggested that having personal or internal control and therefore predictability, over events in one's life is essential to well-being, adaptation to life conditions and survival (Rodin *et al.*, 1985). Both enhanced and diminished opportunities for personal control are reported to have significant effects on the emotional, cognitive and physical well-being of older people (Rodin and Langer, 1977). Challenges to the older adult's sense of perceived control are likely to arise from the multiple chronic health conditions and social or environmental losses that accompany ageing.

The construct of control and some of the concepts related to perceptions of control, such as learned helplessness, have become dominant areas of research related to older people. Learned helplessness is hypothesized to result from exposure to uncontrollable events (Seligman, 1975). The individual 'learns' that their responses are independent of outcomes, and expects that all outcomes are beyond personal control. Learned helplessness is characterized by adverse effects on cognition, affect, motivation, and may result in loss of self-esteem (Seligman, 1975; Abramson et al., 1980). How and why this sense of control may be influenced by, or influences, the ageing process is not clear. Moreover, how control orientation (i.e. mastery or helplessness) affects cognitions, affect, motivation, and behaviour in older people is not well understood.

Conflicting results have been reported regarding stability or change in control beliefs over time, the specificity or generality of control beliefs over situations, the benefits or adverse consequences of internal or external control (Rotter, 1966), and the correlates or determinants of control in older people (Rodin et al., 1985; Lachman, 1986). Although some of the control-related concepts discussed below have not been firmly established, they provide a useful framework for understanding control-relevant influences in working with older people. The remainder of this chapter explores the concepts, measures and applications of control and learned helplessness in working with older people.

Locus of Control

Locus of control (LOC) (Rotter, 1966) refers to perceptions about internal or external locus of control over reinforcements. Internal locus of control orientation is described as the generalized expectancy that outcomes (or reinforcements) are the result of the effectiveness of one's own efforts, behaviour, or relatively enduring characteristics. External locus of control orientation refers to the generalized expectancy that outcomes (reinforcements) are randomly determined by unpredictable forces such as chance, luck or fate, or as the result of the actions of powerful other people (non-random forces).

LOC in older people has been measured using Rotter's (1966) internal–external (I–E) locus of control scale. This scale measures the extent to which people believe they exercise personal control over their lives (considered to be internal control), or the extent to which they believe events or outcomes are determined by luck, chance, fate, or powerful other people (considered to be external control). The scale is a uni-dimensional construct with internal and external (I–E) control orientation represented as opposite ends of a continuum. Individuals have been referred to as 'internals' or 'externals', indicating the strength and direction of their control orientation along the continuum.

Maintaining a strong sense of internal control has been associated with better physical and mental health and well-being among institutionalized older people, especially when opportunities to maintain control have been sustained (Rodin and Langer, 1977). Distinctions have been made between perceived control and actual or behavioural control. Perceived control is generally defined as the perception or expectation that outcomes are possible and contingent on the individual's decisions, choices, and actions, regardless of the objective level of control or actual behavioural control undertaken. Older people's perception of personal control may be as important to health and well-being as overt behavioural responses (Rodin et al., 1985).

However, the exact relationships between control and ageing are still to be determined. It is not clear if general or global I–E control beliefs (as measured by Rotter's scale) stay the same, increase, or decrease with advancing age. Some clarification of control beliefs has been reported using multidimensional and domain specific measures of control.

Multidimensional Measures of Control

Multidimensional measures of control differentiate the multiple sources of control such as self, chance and other people into separate dimensions. In contrast to Rotter's unidimensional I–E control scale, multidimensional scales have been developed which measure general control beliefs in three subscales, internal control, external control-chance, and external control-powerful others (Levenson, 1974, cited in Lachman, 1986). These multidimensional scales measure control beliefs which may influence people in a global way across all behavioural domains, or limited to a specific domain of behaviour, such as health (Wallston and Wallston, 1981).

Multidimensional and domain-specific measures may be more salient for measuring control beliefs in older people. Older people may be particularly sensitive to increases in external sources of control in their lives by chance (e.g. accidents) or powerful other people (e.g. health care givers). It is suggested that older people recognize the influence and importance of external sources of control such as chance and powerful others, while at the same time being able to preserve their sense of internal control (Lachman, 1986).

Thus, expectancies about control among older people may show particular age-related changes in specific dimensions, and in specific domains such as health or intellectual functioning (Lachman, 1986) (see Chapter 8). General measures of control may conceal important age changes in control beliefs, which multidimensional and domain-specific measures may reveal.

Health Locus of Control

Considerable attention has been directed towards the relationship between ageing, control and health (Rodin et al., 1985). Health locus of control refers to generalized expectancies about whether one's health is controlled by one's own behaviour or by external forces. It is not clear to what extent older people believe they control their health outcomes, desire or want to take responsibility for personal (interal) control over their health, or believe that health professionals control, or are responsible for their health outcomes.

The Multidimensional Health Locus of Control (MHLC) scale (Wallston and Wallston, 1981) assesses the extent to which someone believes that health outcomes are the result of internal (personal) factors, or that health/illness is determined by external-chance factors (luck, fate), or external-powerful others (e.g. doctors, nurses, physiotherapists). The use of this scale with older people has demonstrated that, compared to younger adults, older people were more externally oriented in their health beliefs, and were particularly likely to believe that powerful other people have great control over their health (Lachman, 1986). Conceivably, increasing exposure to health professionals may increase external control beliefs over health in older people.

In additon to general health locus of control beliefs, scales relevant to specific conditions (e.g. osteoporosis, arthritis, breast self-examination) have been developed. These scales may be more useful in understanding older adults' health-related beliefs, health behaviours and health outcomes, including psychosocial adjustment to chronic illness (Affleck *et al.*, 1987b). For example, examination of the older person's perceptions of control, predictability, or helplessness in arthritis can assist health practitioners to understand the degree to which older clients cope or are overwhelmed by their disease or disability. In addition, these scales may indicate the extent to which older people want personal control or health care provider control over the course of their disease or the symptoms, and the degree of active participation individuals want to take in their own health care. By using this information in conjunction with clinical findings, physiotherapists may be able to respond more appropriately to the individual perceived needs of older people in rehabilitation programmes.

Primary and Secondary Control

Perceived primary control is defined as an individual's attempt to gain control by bringing the environment into line with his or her wishes. Perceived secondary control refers to control obtained when the individual brings him or herself into line with environmental forces (Rothbaum *et al.*, 1982). Secondary control may be a way for older individuals to maintain perceptions of control in a low control environment, for example in a hospital or nursing home. Patient behaviour such as anger or reactance may be attempts to maintain primary control. Passivity, withdrawal, helplessness, or being the 'good patient', may be manifestations of secondary control (Taylor, 1979). These theoretical constructs may explain some of the behaviours older people display in health care settings, especially when there are constraints on an individual's attempts to maintain perceived control.

Learned Helplessness

The notion of control is also related to the condition of 'learned helplessness', which is believed to result from exposure to uncontrollable events (Seligman, 1975). This condition is thought to result from 'learning' that outcomes are uncontrollable, expecting that future outcomes will be uncontrollable, and believing that any response is futile because, regardless of the effort expended, the outcome will remain the same. Proponents of this theory assert that learned helplessness leads to cognitive, motivational and emotional deficits (Abramson *et al.*, 1980).

Cognitive deficits are described as the inability to identify contingencies between responses and outcomes when they do exist, so that reduced or ineffective efforts are made to develop new responses or coping behaviours. Motivational deficits are characterized by reduced efforts to engage in voluntary responses or activities, while emotional deficits may include depressed affect and reduced self-esteem (Abramson *et al.*, 1980). Learned helplessness is a term often used to describe or explain the passive, dependent, depression-like behaviour of older people who are residents in long-term care institutions (Solomon, 1982; Rodin *et al.*, 1985). Interventions to overcome learned helplessness in older people usually involve methods designed to enhance the individual's sense of perceived personal control (Rodin and Langer, 1977; Rodin *et al.*, 1985).

Control, Learned Helplessness and Attributions

Feelings of control, and a sense of personal mastery or helplessness are thought to be influenced by the causal attributions (causes or explanations) a person makes about events or outcomes. For example, Abramson *et al.* (1980) have theorized that people develop causal attributions about their feelings of helplessness along three dimensions: locus (internal versus external); globality (general versus specific); and stability (stable versus changeable).

The locus dimension describes the internal/external locus of causality (internal-causal factors located within the individual, external-causal factors located in the environment). Globality indicates whether the cause is generalized across many situations, or is specific to one situation. The stability dimension determines if the cause is unstable or enduring. Weiner (1986) argues that controllability (i.e. the cause is subject to volitional or personal control or is not controllable) is another important dimension. Helplessness is hypothesized to result when a cause is attributed to internal, stable, uncontrollable, and/or global factors.

Weiner (1986) suggests that people routinely seek causal explanations for outcomes and events in their lives, particularly those which are unexpected, negative or important. He states that the underlying properties or dimensions of causal attributions determine or guide a person's subsequent cognitive, affective and motivational reactions and behaviour. The locus dimension (i.e. attributing the cause to factors within the individual or within the external environment) will be strongly associated with particular affective or emotional changes such as increases or decreases in pride, self-esteem and self-efficacy. Further, the stability dimension would be associated with expectations of success of control and mastery for an unstable cause, or failure and helplessness when the cause is stable. Emotions connected to the stability dimension would range between feelings of hopefulness and hopelessness. The controllability dimension, which indicates whether or not the cause can be influenced by the person, is related to emotions such as shame, guilt or anger.

Thus, how older people perceive and interpret their personal abilities and their social environment, in various situations, will determine feelings of personal control and mastery, or conversely, feelings of lack of control and helplessness. The success or failure of older persons in rehabilitation programmes may be influenced by the attributions they make about the cause of their disabilities and handicaps and their expectations about being able to influence or control them.

Applications of Control, Learned Helplessness and Attributions

A fall represents an unexpected, negative and important event for the older person. How older people perceive, interpret and explain the cause of a fall may influence the efforts and activities undertaken to prevent future falls. The older person may search for causal attributions; was the fall due to their own limitations such as arthritis or visual or balance problems (internal factors), or due to the surroundings such as a slippery pavement (external factors)? Are these causes stable and enduring, or can one expect to change or influence the cause? Are the causes subject to (personal) control, or are they perceived to be uncontrollable? Further, are they global, affecting a wide variety of situations, or related to specific conditions?

Causal ascription to internal, stable, uncontrollable reasons (e.g. diminished vision or arthritis) may lead to feelings of helplessness in preventing future falls, reduced motivation to take any protective actions, and depression about not being able to prevent falls or injury. In contrast, causal ascription to internal, unstable and controllable reasons such as decreased strength which is subject to remedial interventions such as strengthening exercises (Chapters 6 and 12), may lead to expectancies of future increased strength, motivation to participate in a strength training programme, and a mastery control orientation about prevention of future falls (Chapter 7).

Furthermore, attributions may play an important role in evaluating feelings of personal control or helplessness in relation to psychosocial adaptation and health behaviours in chronic diseases (Affleck et al., 1987a). For instance, causal attributions by rheumatoid arthritis patients about the causes of their illness, disease remission or exacerbations may be associated with feelings of mastery or helplessness either over the disease itself, over the symptoms (Affleck et al., 1987b), or with the extent of functional difficulties or disease severity (Affleck et al., 1987a). Patients who more actively search for the cause of their illness report greater functional difficulties and greater helplessness. Preoccupation with attributions about the causes of a chronic illness such as rheumatoid arthritis may derive from an inability to exercise effective control or predictability over the disease or its symptoms.

Attribution of symptom exacerbation and remission to personal behaviours would suggest that these events are amenable to personal control. Thus, behaviours such as increased rest,

pacing of activities, the use of thermal agents, and exercise may be perceived as effective ways to gain control over symptoms. Control over remissions may be less predictable and less subject to personal control, but subject to more control by external factors such as doctors and changes in medications (Affleck et al., 1987a).

Factors Contributing to Loss of Control and Learned Helplessness

Opportunities for older people to exercise personal control may be limited by both biological (internal) and environmental (external) factors. The range of outcomes that are attainable or controllable by older people may be influenced by internal factors such as poor health status, multiple chronic health conditions and declining physical abilities (Rodin et al., 1985) (see Chapters 6 and 22). Environmental challenges to the older person's sense of control may arise from losses that accompany older age such as loss of roles, loss of spouse, loss of identity through retirement, or loss of home (Rodin et al., 1985).

At the same time as the older person is experiencing diminished (internal) control over outcomes, control by external forces (i.e. chance, luck or powerful other people) may be increasing. For example, a fall by an older person may be considered a random event caused by chance or bad luck. In addition, the influence of (powerful) health care professionals may escalate when older people require more interaction with the health care system (see Chapter 5). This is particularly evident in institutional environments which require individuals to relinquish control over many aspects of their daily activities, and to have their lives controlled by doctors, nurses and physiotherapists (Taylor, 1979). Finally, the negative stereotypes of ageing, including those held by health care professionals and the elderly themselves, may further contribute to feelings of incompetence, lowered self-esteem, and expectancies of diminished control over desired and valued outcomes (Solomon, 1982; Rodin *et al.*, 1985).

Solomon (1982) has argued that the social antecedents of learned helplessness and the creation of dependency in older persons in the health care setting are related to negative stereotyping of the elderly by health care providers, unequal interpersonal exchanges, and behaviours typically associated with sick and healer roles. By considering older people as frail, dependent, mentally and physically incompetent, caregivers indicate their low expecations about the level of physical and mental behaviour the older person is capable of achieving (Chapter 3). These negative expectations become incorporated into the social climate of health care institutions, they contribute to restrictions of choice and autonomy of older people, and they effectively reduce the older person's control over outcomes or reinforcements. Thus within health care environments, helpless, dependent behaviour in older people is too often expected, sanctioned, and reinforced (Baltes and Reisenzein, 1986).

Furthermore, negative labels such as non-compliant and unmotivated are often applied to older people when they do not conform to the expectations of care providers. For example, rehabilitation of older persons may progress in small increments and require a longer time than the physiotherapist expects. Older people become vulnerable to external cues regarding their personal mastery and competence. This may result in feelings of incompetence and low self-esteem in the older person, implying that the older person has made an internal, stable, uncontrollable attribution about his/her own abilities.

Negative stereotypes and negative expectations of the elderly may interfere with their true potential to achieve successful outcomes in rehabilitation programmes (Chapters 3 and 4). The physiotherapist may view an older person as having a low priority in a busy clinical practice and have low goal expectations for rehabilitation. A reduction in the opportunities for older persons to participate in active therapy programmes may diminish their true rehabilitation potential (Chapters 9, 12 and 13), contributing further to dependency and helplessness. Current research on the positive effects of strength training even in very old, debilitated individuals may help to dispel these negative stereotypes and promote higher expectations about the potential for rehabilitation and independence in older people.

Institutionalized Older People

The most seminal studies of control and ageing are the field studies involving control-enhancing interventions with older people living in institutions (Rodin and Langer, 1977). These studies strongly suggest that feelings of decreased control are associated with negative mental and physical health outcomes in older people. On the other hand, provision of sustained opportunities to increase and exercise control has been reported to be associated with positive outcomes on health and well-being among institutionalized older people (Rodin and Langer, 1977).

The prevalent stereotype of institutionalized older persons is that of passive, withdrawn, dependent individuals who exhibit learned helplessness, and who are expected to decline functionally in both physical and psychological abilities. This is due in part to one of the prevailing criteria for admission into a long-term care institution, namely, an objective measure of incompetence for self-care or independent living which serves to reinforce the negative view of the resident held by staff (Chapter 3). Baltes and Reisenzein (1986) reported that staff behaviour in nursing homes supported dependent behaviours of residents, while efforts of residents at independent behaviours were discouraged. They called this a 'dependency-support script', indicating that this was the dominant interaction pattern of residents and caregivers.

A similar, but less consistent pattern of behaviours was found between older persons living at home in the community and their informal (i.e. family members) and formal caregivers (i.e. home care nurses) (Baltes et al., 1994). One could interpret these findings as indicative of caregivers attempting to fulfil the caregiver role, that is, to 'take care' of the older person, and to 'take control' over decisions regarding the older person. Such behaviours by both formal and informal caregivers induce dependency and helpless behaviours in older people.

Since the dependent, helpless behaviours of older nursing home residents do not necessarily reflect a need for assistance, educational intervention programmes for staff may be necessary to retrain staff in how to maintain and rehabilitate independent behaviour in these older people. For example, an intervention consisting of a training and education programme for nursing home staff which included communication skills, facts about ageing and the role of the social environment in the development of dependency, discussions about helping styles and models, and basic behavioural principles in the management of desirable and undesirable behaviours was undertaken by Baltes et al. (1994). This resulted in a significant

increase in independence-supportive and control-enhancing behaviours on the part of staff, and more self-reliant behaviour on the part of residents when they interacted with staff.

The series of studies reported by Baltes et al. (1994) illustrates the importance of the social environment (Chapter 5) and the attitudes (Chapter 3), expectations, and actions of health care professionals (Secton F) in the creation of dependency, helplessness and incompetence in older people. These studies emphasized that dependency and/or helplessness do not have to be the norm for older residents in long-term care institutions, or older persons living in the community.

An example of dependency-inducing behaviours on the part of nursing home staff is the inappropriate use of wheelchairs by ambulatory nursing home residents (see Chapter 25). Nursing homes represent an environment in which wheelchair use is often the norm, regardless of the need for such assistance. Staff often require residents to use a wheelchair for convenience and expediency. New residents may take their cues from the staff that they are slow in ambulating from place to place, or that they are at risk for falls, and therefore they need to use a wheelchair. Residents who want to be 'good patients' may comply with staff expectations that 'slow' residents will use a wheelchair (Taylor, 1979). These residents may also be demonstrating secondary control by bringing themselves into alignment with environmental forces by using a wheelchair (Rothbaum et al., 1982).

Loss of ambulation in elderly nursing home residents may be directly related to these environmental cues. The more a person uses a wheelchair instead of walking, the more debilitated they become, and the more assistance they require, thus inducing feelings of loss of control, incompetence and helplessness. The physiotherapist may be able to facilitate feelings of control in these residents by setting up an exercise and ambulation programme with individual residents, and monitoring the frequency, distance, and endurance of residents' ambulatory efforts over a period of time. However, staff education and support is essential to the success of such control-enhancing programmes (Rodin and Langer, 1977; Baltes *et al.*, 1994).

Summary

The construct of control, and the related concepts of mastery, helplessness and causal attributions provide some insight into how personal control may be influenced by the ageing process, and how control may be experienced by older people. The attributions older people make about health-related events and outcomes may influence their expectations, motivation, and behaviour in rehabilitation programmes. In the course of their work with older persons, physiotherapists may discover the attributions older people make about their health problems, and alter maladaptive interpretations. This process is known as attributional retraining (Weiner, 1986), and is designed to enhance feelings of control and mastery over outcomes and facilitate subsequent expectations and motivated behaviour.

People differ in the extent to which they desire personal control, particularly in the health domain. A high level of personal control is usually considered to be beneficial to health and well-being. However, in some instances, trying to maintain personal control in uncontrollable situations, or when a high level of internal control is beyond the coping ability of the individual (Rodin *et al.*, 1985), the stress induced may lead to negative health consequences.

Clearly, it is important for older people to have opportunities to exercise personal control over desired and valued outcomes. However, there is also a need to balance the forces of internal and external control in meeting the needs of older people. The rehabilitation potential of older individuals may be influenced by both their own control-relevant beliefs and those of the physiotherapist. Providing older people with options congruent with their control perceptions may not always be possible. There may be a difference between the older person's preferred expectancies or perceptions of control and actual capability of control. In addition, underestimating the true potential of the older person may undermine efforts by the older individual to exercise control and achieve successful outcomes in rehabilitation settings. It is the physiotherapist's responsibility to ensure that the optimal balance of control forces is incorporated into rehabilitation and health promotion programmes designed to help older people.

References

Abramson, LY, Garber, J, Seligman, MEP (1980) Learned helplessness in humans: An attributional analysis. In Garber, J, Seligman, MEP (eds) *Human Helplessness* pp. 3–34. New York: Academic Press.

Affleck, G, Pfeiffer, C, Tennen, H, Fifield, J (1987a) Attributional processes in rheumatoid arthritis. *Arthritis and Rheumatism* 30: 927–931.

Affleck, G, Tennen, H, Pfeifer, C, Fifield, J (1987b) Appraisals of control and predictability in adapting to a chronic disease. *Journal of Personality and Social Psychology* 53: 273–279.

Baltes, MM, Reisenzein, R (1986) The social world in long-term care institutions: Psychological control toward dependency. In Baltes, MM, Baltes, PB (eds) *The Psychology of Control and Aging*, pp. 315–343. Hillsdale, NJ: Erlbaum.

Baltes, MM, Neumann, E, Zank, S (1994) Maintenance and rehabilitation of independence in old age: An intervention program for staff. *Psychology and Aging* 9: 179–188.

Lachman, ME (1986) Locus of control in aging research: A case for multidimensional and domain-specific assessment. *Journal of Psychology and Aging* 1: 34–40.

Rodin, J, Langer, EJ (1977) Long-term effects of a control-relevant intervention with the institutionalized aged. *Journal of Personality and Social Psychology* 35: 897–902.

Rodin, J, Timko, C, Harris, S (1985) The construct of control: Biologicaly and psychosocial correlates. *Annual Review of Gerontology and Geriatrics* 5: 3–55.

Rothbaum, F, Weisz, JR, Snyder, SS (1982) Changing the world and changing the self: A two-process model of perceived control. *Journal of Personality and Social Psychology* 42: 5–37.

Rotter, JB (1966) Generalized expectancies for Internal versus External control of reinforcement. *Psychological Monographs: General and Applied* **80** (1, Whole No. 609).

Seligman, MEP (1975) *Helplessness*. San Francisco: WH Freeman.

Solomon, K (1982) Social antecedents of learned helplessness in the health care setting. *The Gerontologist* **22**: 282–287.

Taylor, SE (1979) Hospital patient behaviour: Reactance, helplessness, or control? *Journal of Social Issues* **35**: 156–184.

Wallston, KA, Wallston, BS (1981) Health locus of control scales. In Lefcourt HM (ed.) *Research With The Locus of Control Construct* Volume 1 *Assessment Methods*, pp. 189–243. New York: Academic Press.

Weiner, B (1986) *An Attributional Theory of Achievement Motivation and Emotion*. New York: Springer-Verlag.

12

Exercise and Activity Programmes

SCOTT G THOMAS

Introduction
•
Assessment of Needs, Abilities and Progress
•
Goal-directed Exercise and Activity
•
Benefits of Exercise and Methods of Prescribing
•
Considerations in Exercise Programming for the Older Adult
•
Summary

Introduction

Exercise and physical activity can help to overcome a particular disability (Chapter 22), increase the capacity to function, or simply provide pleasure. Physical activity can benefit people of all ages, but is especially critical to the health of older adults. A sample of the effects of regular exercise is shown in Figure 1 using the Movement Continuum Model of Physical Therapy (Cott *et al.*, 1995). Publications about exercise and ageing provide important information about possible benefit of regular physical activity; physiotherapists help older adults turn these possible benefits into actual results.

Older adults experience physical activity in forms as diverse as digging in the garden and ballroom dancing. They have equally diverse reasons for participating, or not participating, in a given activity. Physiotherapists work to identify and implement exercises and activities that will meet the physical, social and psychological needs of their older clients.

A comprehensive understanding of the benefits that derive from specific types and levels of physical activity is essential. Shuffle board has undeniable social benefits; however, its effect on cardiorespiratory health is negligible. Home calisthenics may be useful for increasing flexibility and muscular endurance, but they have no effect on building a social support network. Knowledge regarding the relationship between

Figure 1   Possible benefits of exercise for older adults across the movement continuum. [Adapted with permission from *Physiotherapy Canada*.]

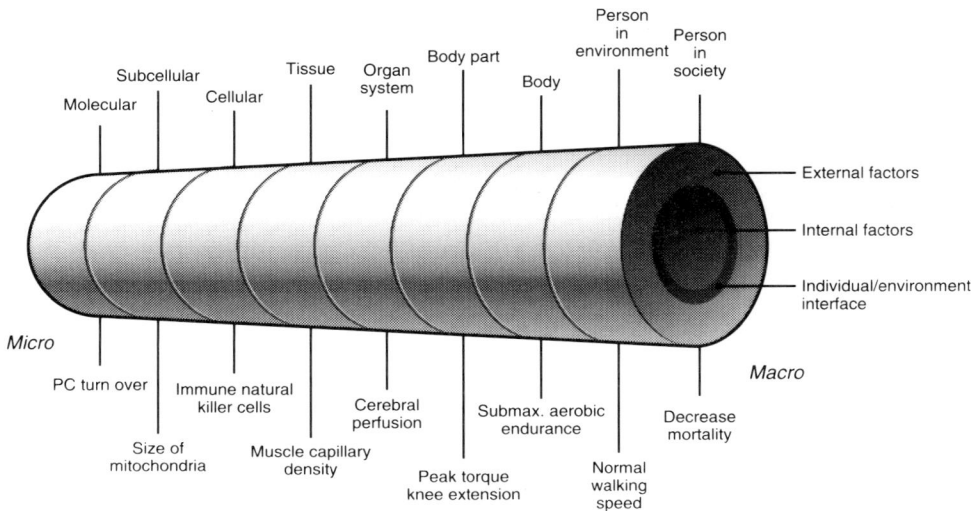

specific exercises and specific benefits will help the healthy older client in making an informed decision about a suitable programme.

Knowing which type and intensity of physical activity can provide a desired benefit is half the battle; assisting the older adult in adopting and maintaining participation in the appropriate activity is the other half. Knowing what is best is no guarantee of doing what is best. Participation in physical activity may be divided into adoption and maintenance phases. Continued participation depends on other factors including perceived health, behavioural skills, spouse support, perceived available time and access to facilities. People are more likely to drop out if they are depressed or anxious, if the programme is too expensive or monotonous, and if the exercise leadership is uninspiring (Dishman, 1988). Healthy older adults have many possible sources of information and assistance in becoming more physically active. Governments in many nations use advertising to deliver the public health message that physical activity is beneficial

(Chapter 5). Recreation specialists have developed programmes for older people, and other health professionals promote exercise and may mount exercise programmes. Physiotherapists provide expertise concerning how movement affects older people who span the continuum from health to severe disability.

Assessment of Needs, Abilities and Progress

Goal Development

In working with older people, assessment of what they want out of the process is especially crucial. The broad goals of physical activity participation are improved physical, psychological and social functioning, but the formulation of a physical activity programme or exercise prescription requires identification of more specific goals. The rehabilitation of specific deficits should be placed in the context of what activities the older client would like to perform (Chapter 9).

Surveys of older adults suggest that they participate in physical activity for much the same reasons as younger people. The primary reason for participating is to feel better (93%), while the percentage of people citing doctor's advice as an important reason increases from 35% for 10- to 24-year-olds to 55% among those over 65 (Canada Fitness Survey, 1982). Probing for more specific information will help in setting realistic and relevant goals. Does the client believe that exercise will allow them to resume playing tennis, enjoy a walking tour, play with their grandchildren, or take care of themselves at home?

A physical activity history can identify activities that the older adult has previously enjoyed. Information regarding current physical activity habits is especially valuable. Those who are currently inactive should start slowly, but have the most potential for improvement; those who are currently active may quickly achieve the prescribed exercise level, but will show less marked improvement. Several extensive physical activity questionnaires are available but those which are tailored for the older population are preferable (Washburn et al., 1990; Voorips et al., 1991).

Many of the barriers to participation in physical activities are the same as for younger adults; lack of social and family support, lack of time, pressure of work and family commitments, and inconvenient exercise locations (Canada Fitness Survey, 1982). Fear of injury or re-injury is a common concern that limits participation of older people. Therefore, exercise programmes for the older adult must minimize the risk of injury through selection of appropriate exercise modes and intensities. The existence of chronic illnesses may also constrain participation in physical activity, either through incapacity or through fear. The physiotherapist needs to be clear what hesitations an older client may have that may prevent their adopting and maintaining a physical activity habit.

Screening

Most older people are apparently healthy, independent and can enjoyably participate in physical activity. Yet chronic disease becomes more prevalent with age, and the safety of older adults in exercise programmes becomes an increasing concern. If a physical limitation exists, identification of the type and degree of impairment and disability will allow a programme to be developed which is specific to the older client's needs and abilities. The screening process should detect changes in any of the systems listed in Table 1. Some of this information may be available from a medical or health history, but much will need to be gathered by the physiotherapist. The inital step in the screening process is to identify possible problems; the second step is to confirm the problem's existence; the final step is to ascertain the severity of the problem. The tools listed in Table 1 can be used to identify possible problems. The screening process is tailored to the population, the tools at hand and the total respondent burden.

In general, screening should be a process to determine what type of exercise is appropriate under specific conditions, not of eliminating the possibility of exercising. The screening process should identify conditions that might change the risk/benefit ratio of exercise participation for the client. The dangers of exercise for the older adult are often less than the dangers of inactivity. However, recommendations regarding specific contraindications to aerobic exercise participation do exist (Van Camp and Boyer, 1989).

Few of the screening tools which are available are

Table 1

Screening for Physical Activity

System	Example of deficit	Example of a tool to detect
Cardiorespiratory	Orthostatic hypotension	PAR Q
	Previous myocardial infarction	PAR Q
	Risk factors	Interview
Musculoskeletal	Osteoporosis	
Neural	Balance deficit	One leg support time
	Sensory loss (hearing)	Interview
Metabolic	Non-insulin dependent diabetes mellitus	Medical history
	Hypothyroidism	Medical history
Integrated function	Unable to perform some physical activities of daily living	Barthel
	Decreased mobility	Timed up-and-go

specifically for the older adult. The PAR Q (Physical Activity Readiness Questionnaire) is very useful for many populations (American College of Sports Medicine, 1993) including older people, but was originally developed for use with adults aged 20 to 65. Geriatric Functional Assessment tools are age specific but, unfortunately, few are suitable for locating where on the broad spectrum of normality a person's physical function falls.

Assessment

Piscopo (1985) has listed several specific reasons for using a fitness test:

- to determine base-line data for initial exercise prescriptive programming,
- to determine the physical fitness status at various points in the programme,
- to motivate the participant — help create interest in programme activities,
- to analyse needs, strength, and weaknesses of specific fitness parameters,

- to assess the attainability of desired programme objectives,
- to determine the value of exercise types and procedure's avowed purposes,
- to assist the participant to assess his or her level of performance,
- to provide clues for the programme director to evaluate programme content and effectiveness

Information from such an assessment will help to determine an appropriate starting point for the programme, what progress is being made, and if the ultimate goal has been attained (Cole *et al.,* 1994). Feedback from an assessment can increase the participant's self-efficacy and, as Piscopo's list indicates, may provide motivation for continued activity.

An exercise assessment may be a final step in the screening process. Cardiovascular, metabolic, neural or musculoskeletal deficits may not manifest themselves when the subject is at rest or during normal activities of daily living. The stress produced during an exercise assessment may reveal impairments that would limit the level of participation or change the requirement for monitoring or supervision. The client may report angina, or electrocardiographic monitoring may reveal ST segment depression at a specific heart rate during an exercise stress test. Further cardiovascular investigation might indicate that it is safe for the client to exercise as long as intensity is kept below the anginal threshold.

All participants should have some form of assessment, be it simple or complex. A knowledge of the client's health status, treatment goals, and the measurement properties of the tools will help guide the choice of an appropriate test battery. In general, simple measures require complex interpretation, and sophisticated measures can be simply interpreted. The measures which address various dimensions (Table 2) vary in quality, level of sophistication and difficulty in administration. Tests that relate as closely as possible to the activities which the older adult wants to perform should be selected. Thus, use a walking test for clients who plan on a walking programme, and an upper extremity muscular endurance test for those who plan to exercise by paddling a boat.

BODY COMPOSITION

A decrease in muscle mass and an increase in body fat mass can impair the functional capacity of the older adult even if total body mass remains relatively constant. Excess body fat, particularly excess body fat on the trunk, is associated with increased risk of morbidity and mortality. Body composition can be assessed in older people using a variety of methods (Table 3). Body mass index has been used extensively for population studies, but is less useful for assessing an individual. High values (> 30) indicate further assessment is required. Sophisticated imaging techniques are not widely available and their use for routine assessments is not justified. Body density measures using hydrostatic weighing are not appropriate for older adults. Estimation of lean body mass and fat body mass from body density is less precise in older adults.

Skinfold and girth measures are useful to determine the changes in the body composition of an older adult. Training-induced decreases in body fat and increases in muscle mass can be detected by an experienced appraiser using the measures indicated in Table 3. However, the ability to esti-

Table 2
Physical Capacity Dimensions to Measure

Level	Simple/general	Intermediate	Complex/specific
Body composition	Body mass index	Subcutaneous fat thickness (skinfolds)	Body density, imaging methods
Aerobic	Walk tests	Submaximal heart rate response	Measured maximal oxygen uptake
Flexibility	Sit-and-reach	Goniometer	Electro-goniometer
Muscular strength	1 repetition maximum	Isometric strain gauge	Isokinetic dynamometer
Muscular endurance	Number of repetitions to failure	Time to failure with isometric hold	Decrease in work output during repeated dynamic exercise
Motor function	Timed up-and-go	Functional reach	

Table 3
Body Composition Measurement Methods

Raw measures		Calculated values		Body composition indicator
Body size	Height	Body mass index		Indicator for further testing
	Weight	$BMI = \dfrac{Body\ Mass\ (kg)}{Height^2\ (m^2)}$		
Skinfold thickness	Tricep	Sum of		Overall body adiposity
	Bicep	skinfolds (SOS)		
	Medial Calf			
	Subscap		Sum of trunk	Trunk adiposity
	Suprailiac		skinfolds (SOTS)	
Girths	Waist	Waist:hip		Trunk adiposity
	Hip	ratio WHR $= \dfrac{Waist\ (cm)}{Hip\ (cm)}$		

mate accurately the percentage of body fat with those methods is limited by age-related changes in skin and in the proportion of fat stored subcutaneously rather than around the internal organs. Skinfold thickness measures are more sensitive to change in adiposity than is a measure of body mass alone. Many older clients are concerned about their appearance and feedback about progress in changing body composition will be welcomed and may act as an incentive for continuing participation in their physical activity programme.

AEROBIC ASSESSMENT

Aerobic fitness is determined by the capacity of the cardiorespiratory system to deliver oxygen to and remove carbon dioxide from the tissues, and the capacity of the active muscle to use oxygen (Chapter 6). Aerobic metabolism generates the vast majority of energy used by the body. Even sleeping is an aerobic activity! Assessment of the capacity to generate energy aerobically provides information about the ability to participate in normal activities, and the size of the physiological reserve capacity for participating in enjoyable physical activity.

Wasserman *et al.* (1994) provide a useful review of aerobic exercise testing and interpretation in a variety of clinical populations. Monitoring during submaximal testing of a healthy older person should include observations, pulse rate and rating of perceived exertion (Borg, 1986). If possible, blood pressure should be monitored, and electrocardiogram (single lead or more) and oxygen saturation tests performed. If cardiovascular risk factors such as a family history of heart disease, history of smoking or elevated blood lipid levels are present, careful monitoring becomes critical.

ASSUMPTIONS AND AGE

Aerobic fitness declines with age by approximately 10% per decade. Since VO_2max is typically between 10 and 40 ml/kg/min (3–10 METs) in the older population, a low starting level (1.5–2 METs) and small increments (1–2 METs) between test levels are recommended. Interpretation of test results can be difficult, since assumptions that are justified for the young, healthy adult may not hold for older persons. For example, the assumption that maximal heart rate can be predicted from the subject's age is tenuous at best in older people. This uncertainty also makes it less accurate to use the Astrand prediction of VO_2max from submaximal test data.

Many older people take medications which can alter the response to exercise (American College of Sports Medicine, 1993). Variations in medication and dosage between test occasions can lead to the false impression that cardiorespiratory fitness has changed. Physiotherapists should consider and consult about whether the test should be completed when the client is on or off medication.

Aerobic fitness may be quantified by measuring or estimating the maximum rate at which oxygen can be consumed (VO_2max). A direct measure of VO_2max is recognized as the 'best' measure of aerobic fitness, since it is reliable and has high face and predictive validity. However, the costs are high in terms of equipment, time, client effort and discomfort. Submaximal measures of aerobic fitness typically measure the physiological strain associated with a known rate of work. Physiological strain is most often assessed using heart rate. Many medications (beta-blockers, antidepressants) alter the heart rate response to exercise; the use of other strain indicators, such as perceived exertion, may be preferred for older adults who are on medication. The higher the heart rate for a given work load, the lower the aerobic fitness. Performance tests, such as the 6 or 12 minute walk, or the mile and a half walk / run, may be submaximal or maximal depending on the effort of the participant.

PERFORMANCE TESTS

Performance tests are seldom useful as measures of aerobic fitness in older people because the test result may be strongly influenced by factors such as pacing, learning, encouragement, or orthopaedic limitations, rather than depending on the capacity of the cardiorespiratory system. Cunningham et al. (1982) found that aerobic power accounted for only 15% of the variance in client selected walking speed. The self-paced walk test does have the advantage of being submaximal and client-paced. Other performance tests may pose an unacceptably high risk if the participant can not be closely monitored while making a maximal or near maximal effort. While performance tests are very useful as summary measures of functional ability, they do not provide information on what limits the client's function to that level.

SUBMAXIMAL TESTS

Submaximal tests have the advantage of requiring less expense and expertise, while producing less client discomfort than maximal tests. The results from submaximal tests may be interpolated and reported as the rate of work at a given heart rate (e.g. Physical Work Capacity, in watts at heart rate of 120, PWC_{120}) or heart rate at a given oxygen uptake (Heart Rate at $VO_2 = 1.5$ l/min, $HR_{1.5}$). These values (PWC_{120} or $HR_{1.5}$) are useful in quantifying the aerobic fitness of an older adult; they are less useful in comparing aerobic fitness between older adults. For a 60-year-old a heart rate of 120 bpm probably represents 75% of their maximum; for an 80-year-old it represents 85% of maximum. Thus the same PWC_{120} corresponds to different relative intensities.

Estimation of VO_2max from submaximal test results assumes a maximal heart rate, and a known oxygen uptake for the test work rate. The standard deviation for predicted maximal heart rate is approximately 12 beats per minute. In the young adult that represents approximately a 6% (12/200) range. In the older adult it corresponds to a larger error (8%, 12/150). Efficiency (work rate/energy consumption) and thus the oxygen cost of a given work rate may change with ageing. The accuracy of VO_2max estimation is limited by the use of equations developed from a younger population sample. The advantage of estimated VO_2max values is that they can be readily compared with age-specific norms. This allows an older client to be informed, for example, that he or she is above average, or in the top 20% of their age group.

MAXIMAL TESTS

VO_2max has been directly measured on thousands of older adults. The risks of maximal testing are higher than for submaximal testing. The maximal value provides a physiological reference point from which the intensity of exercise can be gauged. Performing a maximal test in a controlled environment reassures an older adult that they are capable of exercising vigorously.

Figure 2 illustrates the oxygen cost and work rate parameters for three commonly used test protocols which may be suitable for testing apparently healthy older people. The first two protocols may be used to conduct a submaximal test if they are halted at a submaximal heart rate, or continued to a symptom or effort-limited maximum to assess maximal aerobic capacity. Older inactive adults take longer to reach a steady oxygen uptake, ventilation and heart rate in response to exercise. Consequently they should exercise for more time at each stage of a submaximal test.

At approximately 50–70% of VO_2max ventilation increases rapidly and blood lactate concentration rises. The point at which this occurs has been labelled the Ventilation Threshold (V_ET), Lactate Threshold (LacT), or Anaerobic Threshold (AnT). The threshold is used as a submaximal marker of aerobic fitness since it increases with

training, and relates to the ability to perform aerobic tasks of relatively high intensity. Measurement of the threshold requires sophisiticated equipment and data processing but provides a submaximal, objective indicator of aerobic fitness.

The choice of a maximal or submaximal test procedure will depend on the facilities available, the health of the client, and the type of programme in which they may participate. The level of exertion (heart rate or RPE) reached during testing should be greater than that achieved during training. If possible, a maximal test with measured gas exchange should be used. If that approach is not available, a submaximal test with the result reported as PWC_{120} or $HR_{1.5}$ is the next best choice. The chosen test modality (cycle, treadmill, step, arm ergometer) should correspond as closely as possible with the older client's planned activity.

FLEXIBILITY

A decrease in flexibility is a hallmark of ageing. Flexibility is more dependent on physical activity pattern than age or gender. Flexibility in shoulder adduction is significantly higher for independent older persons compared to those who are institutionalized (Cunningham et al., 1993). MacDougall et al. (1991) have reviewed the methods and normative values for flexibility measurement and training in young adults and athletes, but there have been no systematic explorations of flexibility in the older adult.

Flexibility is joint-specific and primarily determined by the muscle–tendon complex. It is affected by temperature, and therefore the values measured will depend on room temperature and previous activity (warm up). Indirect measures such as the Wells and Dillon 'sit and reach test' are based on measurement of linear

Figure 2   Aerobic fitness testing protocols.

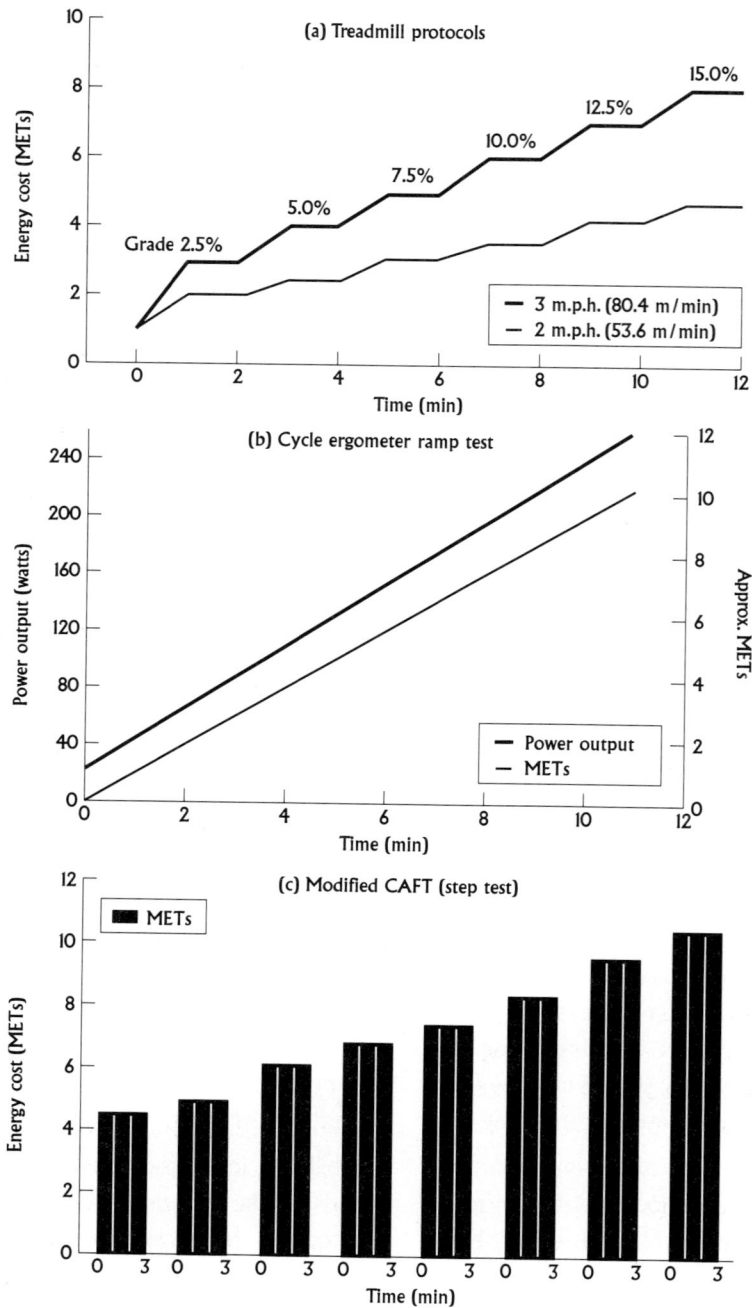

(a) Treadmill protocols

(b) Cycle ergometer ramp test

(c) Modified CAFT (step test)

distance between body segments or from an object. They are influenced by body dimensions (long arms and short legs are an advantage for the sit and reach) and involve movement at several joints. They are useful as rough summary measures, but provide little information about exactly where the limited range of motion exists.

Direct measurements of angular displacement, which are more readily compared between people, can be made with goniometers and flexometers. The goniometer is readily available and familiar to physiotherapists but must be used with a standardized test protocol (MacDougall et al., 1991). Reliability is more easily achieved with the Leighton flexometer, which is suitable for simple movements, although it may not be appropriate for back range of motion.

MUSCULAR STRENGTH (SEE CHAPTER 6)

There is growing recognition of the importance of strength in maintaining an independent, active lifestyle. Measurement of strength in the older adult presents many of the same challenges as encountered with younger clients. Physiotherapists must select from isometric, isotonic and isokinetic movements, concentric and eccentric contractions, and choose between isolating a particular muscle group and testing a functional movement which involves several muscles. The total number of measures used should be limited to protect the client from the effects of fatigue. Risk of injury may be reduced if the muscle temperature is increased by exercise before testing.

Specific strength tests which mimic the movements used in training will demonstrate larger gains than more general tests. The maximum change will be observed when the older adult tests and trains with the same device. Strength measures during functional activities will be most useful in demonstrating the impact of training on the client's life.

As with aerobic testing, the measures available vary in sophistication and specificity. Low reliability for strength of Grade 3 and above renders manual muscle testing useful only with the weakest of older adults. Isometric strength can be reliably measured using a portable device such as a modified sphygmomanometer (Cole et al., 1994), a cable tensiometer, or a hand grip dynamometer. Grip strength is important to function and normative values are available. Grip strength is a rough indicator of overall strength and several studies have associated increased risk of falling with weak grip strength (Simpson, 1993). Training-induced change in strength can be readily identified if isometric testing and training are performed at the same joint angles. The importance of such change for daily life or typical physical activities may be limited, however.

Isokinetic test devices are becoming more widely available and may be useful in quantifying age- or training-related change in the force–velocity curve. Due to a combination of fast twitch fibre loss, increased stiffness, and neural control changes, velocity of movement is slower in older people. As a result, the older adult may not reach a high test velocity on an isokinetic device. The maximum velocities at which they can produce force will differ between joints and between individuals.

Isotonic tests of one repetition maximum (1–RM) are more safely performed with equipment such as the 'Universal' gym than with the more widely available free weights. Bench press and leg press tests involve the action of several muscle groups and provide an overall measure of upper and lower extremity strength.

MUSCULAR ENDURANCE

Tests of muscular endurance evaluate the ability to continue exerting large forces over a 30–150 second period. Muscular endurance is dependent on both the size of the muscle and on the ability to supply energy anaerobically. Muscle mass declines with age, stores of high-energy compounds are smaller and anaerobic enzyme activity is reduced. Muscle endurance is important in many activities such as gripping a suitcase handle or carrying a load.

Muscular endurance is quantified in isometric, isotonic or isokinetic activities. Isometric endurance may be measured as time to failure while exerting a large (e.g. 80% relative to 1 RM) force. Isotonic endurance is quantified as number of repetitions to failure, and isokinetic as the decrease in force exerted over a specific number of repetitions (usually 15–30) (MacDougall *et al.*, 1991). Muscular endurance shows less decline with ageing than strength.

In the past, concerns about the effects of resistance exercise on blood pressure decreased the frequency of strength assessment and strength training for the older adult. However, several recent studies have conclusively proved that resistance training is safe and efficacious for the healthy and frail older adult (Govindasamy and Paterson, 1994; Porter and Vandervoort, 1995).

Goal-directed Exercise and Activity

There is general agreement that exercise is good for the older adult. Some of the numerous benefits which derive from participation in regular physical activity were summarized in Figure 1; others include:

- improved mood, decreased anxiety, increased vigour (Chapter 19),
- improved cognition (Chapter 8),
- increased aerobic fitness, increased cardiorespiratory endurance,
- improved blood lipid profile,
- increased flexibility and range of motion,
- increased bone density (Chapter 16),
- increased muscle strength and endurance (Chapter 6),
- increased muscle mass and decreased fat mass.

However, there is little public recognition that specific benefits are associated with specific exercise programmes. The older adult may be interested in process-related goals such as 'having a good time', or in outcome-related goals such as 'improving my figure'. After goals have been identified with an older client and their current physical abilities assessed, the physiotherapist should next identify which exercise programme will allow the achievement of these goals.

Exercise prescription is based on a few important principles — overload, specificity and reversibility. The overload principle states that for a physiological adaptation to result a greater than usual stress must be applied. This is a critical principle in assessing the worth of sweeping recommendations such as, 'people over 65 should walk three blocks every day'. This distance may represent an appropriate stimulus for an older adult who walks one block per day, but would cause detraining in the Master athlete who already runs 5 kilometres per day. The second training principle is specificity. Physiological adaptations are specific to the energy system, the muscle groups, and in many cases the movement pattern used as the training stimulus. The third principle, reversibility, is a source of hope and despair: existing physical capacity is lost through inactivity, as well as regained from exercise and activity programmes.

The exercise stimulus is conveniently described using the FITT acronym: F, frequency sessions per week; I, intensity of an exercise session; T, time or duration of an exercise session; and T, type of exercise describe the exercise stimulus at a given point in the programme. A final descriptor, progression, specifies how the exercise stimulus will be changed over time.

Exercise recommendations for the older adult must consider the narrowed range of appropriate exercise stimuli. As Figure 3 indicates, young adults can adapt to a wide range of exercise dosages; due to age-related physiological declines and deconditioning, the older adult will have positive adaptations to a smaller range of exercise intensities. Too large a stimulus may result in injury, overtraining or simply in the participant refusing to continue participating, while too small a stimulus may fail to produce any training effect.

Benefits of Exercise and Methods of Prescribing

Social and Psychological Benefits

Anecdotal evidence and common experience maintains that exercise improves an older adult's self-esteem, confidence, social network and well-being. Hard scientific evidence of these benefits has proven somewhat more difficult to collect (Gitlin *et al.*, 1992).

There is evidence that acute and chronic exercise reduce depression and anxiety in younger and older adults (Emery *et al*, 1991). The effect is more pronounced in those who are initially depressed or anxious. In young adults acute exercise increases positive effect (vigour, confidence), but the affective benefits in older adults are less clear.

There is little information regarding how the affective results may vary when any of the components of the FITT prescription are changed. The setting and programme characteristics are important in producing social benefits for older adults. Obviously, calisthenics in their own homes are unlikely to produce the social benefits of group participation in a neighbourhood walk followed by tea and cakes. Physiotherapists should be aware that opportunities for social interaction and fun strongly influence an older person's continued participation in the activity programme, as well as their social and psychological health.

Aerobic Fitness

Regular participation in aerobic exercise programmes produces significant change in the cardiorespiratory function of older adults. Increases in aerobic fitness measures such as VO_2max, PWC_{170}, $HR_{1.5}$, V_ET have all been reported as well as increases in maximum ventilation, blood volume, maximum cardiac output, muscle capillary density, and muscle aerobic enzyme activity (Govindasamy and Paterson, 1994). Improvements in the ability to use oxygen through increased capillarization or increased muscle enzyme activity are more pronounced than changes in the ability to deliver oxygen through improved cardiac function.

Aerobic exercise by older adults also produces decreased vascular resistance, increased high density lipo-proteins, and decreased blood lipid concentrations. It also helps to maintain or increase bone density, improves glucose tolerance, decreases fat stores and increases lean body mass; these changes counteract the expected changes with ageing. Exercise advocates have pointed out that exercise benefits can be the

Figure 3   Theoretical relationship between stimulus intensity and adaptive response in healthy young and old and frail people.

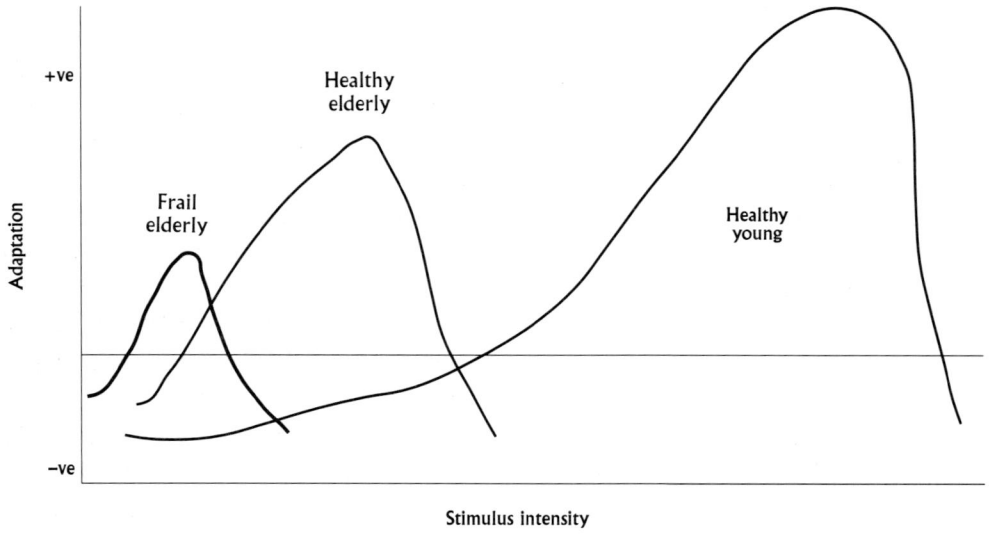

Figure 4   Effect of aerobic training intensity on change in VO_2max in older adults.

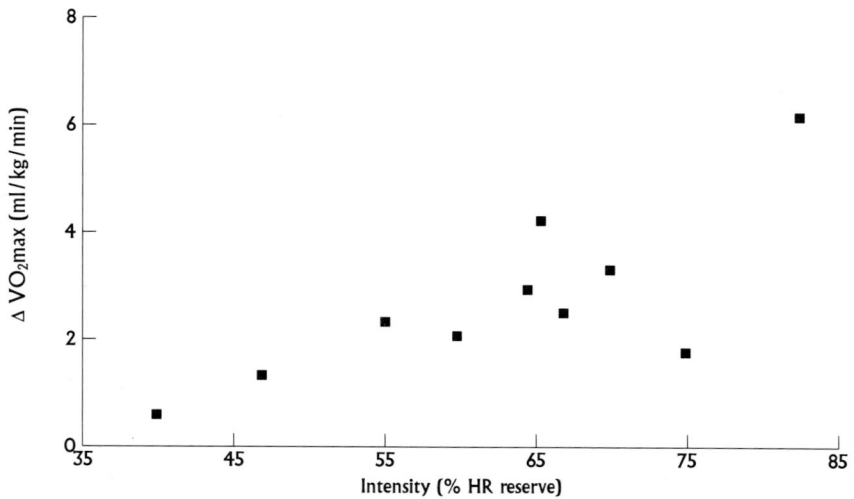

equivalent of decreasing physiological or functional age by five to 20 years.

The relation between the size of exercise stimuli and the size of the training effects has been examined. In general, higher training intensities produce larger response (Figure 4).

The average change in VO_2max in aerobic training studies of older adults is between 5 and 25%. The larger percentage increases are observed when the pre-training VO_2max is low and the training intensity is high. Increases in submaximal aerobic exercise endurance capacity can be dramatic. For example, before training older men were able to exercise on the treadmill for just 7 min while after completing 9 weeks of endurance training they were able to exercise at the same level for 21 min (Govindasamy and Paterson, 1994). The change in ability to exercise at submaximal levels has a great impact on functional capacity. Aerobic training reduces the older adult's heart rate, ventilation, and rating of their exertion level. The reduced disruption of homeostatis and reduced sense of effort permit the older adult to participate in more activities for a longer period of time.

The FITT approach can be used as a guide for prescribing aerobic exercise for the older adult. Table 4 indicates that there is a range of values for each component of the prescription. The client's current physical capacity and goals will guide the physiotherapist's choices within the designated ranges; frequency, intensity and time are often manipulated jointly to achieve specific goals. High-frequency, moderate-intensity, long-duration exercise programmes are ideal for promoting fat loss. On the other hand the largest gains in maximum oxygen uptake may be achieved with high-frequency, high-intensity, short-duration prescriptions. Improvements in blood lipid profile require a moderate to high programme. Previously sedentary older adults should start with a low intensity (50% of VO_2max) moderate frequency (3–4 week), short duration (10–15 min) programme. Duration should be increased before intensity. Changes in intensity and duration should not increase the total volume of exercise by more than 10% every week. Changes in connective tissue develop more slowly than aerobic fitness capacity, so keen participants may have to be advised to progress slowly to avoid injury.

Since the intenstiy of aerobic exercise is often set

Table 4
Aerobic Training Prescription (FITT approach)

Variable	Range	Low end	High end
Frequency	3–6 times per week	Start of programme Time constrained	Late in programme Very limited physical capacity
Intensity	60–80% HRmax 50–85% VO_2max	Start of programme Limited capacity Fat loss goal	Late in programme Performance goals
Time	15–60 min per session	Start of programme	Fat loss goal Intensity low
Type	Large muscle groups, rhythmic	Aquabics Walking	Aerobics Jogging

relative to maximum heart rate or maximum oxygen uptake, maximal testing is used to provide those values for calculating an appropriate training intensity. As previously discussed, maximum heart rate can be roughly estimated from age, and maximum oxygen uptake can be roughly predicted from the response to submaximal exercise. Alternative methods of setting exercise intensity include using ratings of perceived exertion and the anaerobic threshold.

Training intensity typically is set at 11 to 13 on the original Borg scale (scale range 6 to 20) or 4 to 6 on the revised version (scale range 0 to 10). Older adults, even more than other age groups, should receive careful instruction and practice with the scale before using it to regulate their exercise intensity. Lack of recent exercise experience may have decreased their ability to 'listen' to their body's messages about the suitablity of exercise intensity. It is very useful to have the older adult rate the exertion for each level of a maximal test so that they can later anchor their perceptions relative to the maximum. Monitoring a combination of heart rate and perceived exertion may be the best method of carefully regulating exercise intensity.

Flexibility

Decreases in range of motion can limit function, impede participation in physical activities and increase the probability of injury (Chapter 22). Increases in range of motion can be achieved with a modest investment of effort and time by most older adults. Flexibility is a labile component of physical capacity and frequent exercise (5–7 days per week) is recommended. Specific recommendations regarding length of hold (minimum of 10 s) and intensity of the sensation of stretch (just short of pain) have been made, but there is little research evidence on which to base specific

recommendations such as a 10 s versus 30 s hold. Several types of movement and stretching (ballistic, static, PNF) may improve flexibility, but generally slow stretching and holding the stretched positions for some time are most appropriate for developing flexibility in the older adult, while keeping the risk of injury to a minimum. Flexibility may be improved and maintained through participation in activities such as Tai Chi, which are pursued for their own sake. Specific exercises have been recommended to increase flexibility (Shephard and Thomas, 1989; Makrides and Campagna, 1992) and programmes of movement such as that originated by Feldenkrais have been promoted.

Muscular Strength and Endurance

Recent research has dispelled many myths about strength and muscular endurance training of older people (Govindasamy and Paterson 1994; Porter and Vandervoort, 1995). Injuries are often associated with previous orthopaedic problems and therefore a careful history may help in avoiding problems. Older adults can safely participate in resistance training and can significantly increase their muscle strength (ability to exert force), muscular endurance (ability to continue exerting large forces), and muscle mass. From studies with healthy older adults and with frail older adults, it is known that muscle strength is an important determinant of function – a determinant which can be modified through exercise. To exert large forces, fast twitch muscle fibres, which decrease in number and size with age, must be recruited. Resistance exercise may be the best way of maintaining the viability of fast twitch motor units in the older adult. Substantial increases in both strength and muscular endurance are observed with training of older adults. Low initial strength levels have been increased by 174%, and even in highly active older women strength was increased through resistance training by 5–65% (Porter and Vandervoort, 1995).

Muscular strength and muscular endurance are distinct components of physical capacity. However, in prescribing resistance exercise, specificity and progression are common considerations.

Training-induced changes in muscle strength and endurance are specific to position and velocity. In prescribing and monitoring training progress it is important to remember that training effects are largest for the type of resistance exercise used in training. For example, gains from isometric training of elbow flexion at 90° will be small outside the range of 80–100°. Isotonic exercise with free weights or a machine is usually more readily available than isokinetic training. Free weights are more readily available than machines, but require more skill to use safely. Transfer of the effects of strength training to activities of daily living has been demonstrated. Eccentric strength is perserved better than concentric strength with ageing, but little information is available regarding the effect of eccentric training in the older adult. In the young adult eccentric training poses a greater risk of muscle tissue damage, but if carefully prescribed can strengthen connective tissue.

Progression is a key factor in providing effective resistance training. Because gains in muscular strength and endurance are large, and may be rapid, the prescription must be revised frequently (every 1–2 weeks) on the basis of repeated testing. The initial gains, which may be due to learning and ill-defined neural factors, are very encouraging for the older participant, and feedback from testing will help motivate continued participation.

There is a wide range of frequencies and intensities and types of resistance training which may be employed to increase strength and/or muscular endurance. Frequency can, and should, be less with resistance training (two to three sessions per week) than with aerobic training (three to five sessions per week). It should be emphasized to over-eager clients that the strength gains occur following the training sessions, not during the session itself. Intensity is set relative to the maximum weight which can be lifted once (1RM), or as the maximum weight which can be lifted for a given number of repetitions (reps). Since the frequency of injury increases markedly with 1RM training relative to exercise at more moderate intensities, it is not advisable to use 1RM training with older people.

The FITT approach must be stretched somewhat to describe the time spent in a resistance training session. The amount of time spent in the programme will vary with the number of muscle groups exercised and the number of sets which are completed in a session. To minimize muscle soreness beginners should start with one set and progress to three sets per session over 4–6 weeks.

Strength Training

A variety of programmes have proved effective for increasing the strength of older adults. Table 5 indicates that, as with other age groups, the initial 2–3 weeks of a strength training programme should involve a low volume and low intensity of exercise.

Muscle hypertrophy does occur with strength training of the older person but is much more modest (10–20%) than the large changes in strength. Older women whose socialization may make them fear development of bulging muscles can be reassured that the combination of gender and age ensures that only an Olympian effort will produce marked hypertrophy.

Table 5
Strength Training Prescription (FITT approach)

Variable	Range	Low end	High end
Frequency	2–3 times per week	• Start of programme • Time constrained	• Late in programme
Intensity	60–75% 1RM, 10–15 repetitions 75–90% 1RM, 3–6 repetitions	• Muscle endurance • Start of programme	• Late in programme • Muscle strength
Time	1 set 3 sets	• Start of programme	• Fat loss goal • Intensity low
Type	Isometric Isotonic Isokinetic	• Calisthenics • Household objects	• Weight machines • Free weights

Muscular Endurance

The intensity for developing muscular endurance is less than for increasing muscular strength. The total training time will be greater because a larger number of repetitions (10 to 15) will be performed in each exercise set. Training frequency is the same as for development of muscular strength (two to three times per week).

Other instructions which are common to programmes emphasizing development of muscle strength or endurance are: balance muscle groups (agonist, antagonist); use the full range of motion; use large muscle groups first; keep breathing; and use a spotter.

Both muscular strength and muscular endurance are desirable for the older adult and many people will have limited time and energy to devote to resistance training. For those people a middle training intensity of 75–80% of 1RM and six to ten repetitons in each of three sets may be ideal. Increases in muscular strength will improve muscular endurance in activities where a fixed force is exerted or weight lifted. Improvements in mus-

cular endurance result in little change in muscular strength.

Body Composition

In middle age body mass increases or remains constant as muscle mass is lost and fat accumulates as a result of reduced participation in physical activity and changes in the hormonal milieu (decreased growth hormone and steriod hormone levels). In later life, body mass declines as muscle mass loss is augmented by loss of fat mass, body water and bone mineral content. Decreased muscle mass, bone mineral content and increased fat mass result. None of the changes are desirable and many turn to exercise as a method of halting or reversing the changes. Resistance exercise is showing promise as means of replacing lost muscle mass and maintaining or increasing bone mineral content. The energy expenditure required for aerobic exercise can decrease adiposity and help maintain lean body mass in the face of reduced caloric intake.

Energy expenditure during aerobic exercise is proportional to the volume of work completed. Moderate intensity exercise, performed frequently with a large muscle mass, for long periods of time is ideal for maximizing energy expenditure. Unfortunately, few older people are willing to devote large amounts of their time to prolonged exercising. As the duration of a session is decreased exercise intensity could be increased to hold the total caloric expenditure constant. Use of this strategy is limited by the older adult's aerobic capacity. The optimum solution differs according to the older client's preferences, but in general a 45-min session at approximately 60% of VO_2max, three or more times per week, in combination with moderate caloric restriction (deficit of 500 calories per day) will produce more noticeable fat loss. Caloric restriction alone is not recommended because lean body mass (muscle and water) losses occur. Body mass loss should not exceed 1 kg per week.

Maintenance of lean body mass is important to physical capacity and function. Research findings are accumulating which suggest that resistance exercise may be effective in both increasing muscle mass and decreasing adiposity. Energy expenditure during resistance exercise is not substantial but the increased muscle mass which results from intense training requires increased energy expenditure to maintain. As a result total energy expenditure is increased and adiposity may be reduced. The older adult can increase muscle cross-sectional area by 10–20% through resistance training. The resistance training must be intense (greater than 70% 1RM) and programme participation prolonged (greater than 3 months) enough to cause significant muscle hypertrophy. The minimum intensity of resistance exercise which is effective in slowing age-associated decline in muscle mass probably varies with somatotype and hormonal milieu.

Several studies have demonstrated higher bone density in physically active older adults compared to their sedentary peers. Longitudinal studies have demonstrated slower loss or increases of bone mineral content with aerobic or resistance exercise. The effect is confined to the bones which are stressed during the exercise and is lost following termination of participation. Weight-bearing physical activities such as walking and jogging are more effective than weight-supported activities such as swimming (Snow-Harter and Marcus, 1991). The intensity of either resistance or aerobic exercise must be carefully monitored in the presence of decreased bone density. The ideal approach is to start exercising early in adulthood, increase peak bone density and continue exercising throughout life to preserve bone density.

Considerations in Exercise Programming for the Older Adult

There are several considerations in establishing exercise programmes which are common to all ages and others which are particular to older adults (American College of Sports Medicine, 1993). Changes in sensory acuity, in tolerance to environmental stressors, differences in activity preferences, and increased health risks must all be considered if programmes are to be successful.

Home programmes have proved successful with older adults only when accompanied by frequent (weekly or biweekly telephone contact) (Barry and Eathorne, 1992). The importance of social contact to the older adult suggests that group programmes are more likely to provide a stimulus for continued participation. As well, the increased requirement for monitoring responses to exercise suggests that a supervised programme will be safer and more effective.

Successful programmes have a low probability of injury, regularly assess the response to training and provide appropriate feedback. Programme leaders must be enthusiastic and should be realistic role models. Peer leadership should be developed and encouraged whenever possible. The participants should set goals for themselves and, if appropriate, complete a self-contract. The support of significant others (family, friends, spouse) is critical to continued participation. Finally, group participation, variety and fun should be part of the programme. Music is often an important part of group programmes (Barry and Eathorne, 1992).

This chapter has emphasized the importance of prescribing exercise which will allow the older participant to achieve specific goals. However, if the goal is primarily 'joie de vivre' then the detailed prescription approach may not be appropriate. The physiotherapist's role may simply be to identify what activities are available and possible. Some healthy older adults are capable of participating in activities from 5-week canoe trips to gymnastic competitions; they provide an important role model of what may be possible. Respect for the diversity of interests and physical abilities of older adults requires that an individual approach be used whenever possible.

Decreases in thermoregulatory ability make regulation of the environment for exercise more important. If the exercise environment cannot be controlled, participation should be limited in hot weather; early morning or late evening are the best times to avoid the heat (Shephard and Thomas, 1989). Hyperthermia is more likely in the older adult, who should be encouraged to drink fluid before (approximately 500 ml) and during water breaks (150 ml every 15 min) which are part of the programme. Drinking only when thirsty will result in dehydration.

Cold injuries may occur in winter, if care is not taken, because of impaired temperature perception or wetting of protective clothing. Dressing in layers and removing and replacing layers as body temperature changes will help prevent hypothermia. Poor skin circulation increases the risk of frostbite and blister formation so frequent inspection of exposed skin is recommended during outdoor winter activities.

The following case study is a single example of how to apply some of the concepts which have been considered in this chapter. It is not meant to form the basis of a 'cookbook' approach but to illustrate how the information can be employed practically in a specific case.

Case Study

Mrs Smythe was widowed five years ago at the age of 64 but has a strong social support network with her family (sisters and three children) and friends. She is a member of the neighbourhood community centre but lives independently in her own single-storey house.

Mrs Smythe had been healthy and physically active (walking, gardening) until recently. She fell ill with influenza 6 weeks ago and has made a very slow recovery. She spent most of 2 weeks in bed, and needed her family to help with the meals and housework. She feels depressed about her reduced energy and is concerned about her ability to return to her previous activities and independence in living. She would like to increase her physical capacity at least to the point where she can handle her previous activities comfortably and also develop some reserve capacity.

Preliminary screening reveals no personal

or family history of cardiovascular disease and no positive response to the PAR Q. Mrs Smythe's blood pressure (132/84) and pulse rate (72) are within normal limits. Her posture is good and she has not had a fracture since the age of 8 when a fall from a tree resulted in a broken arm. Her balance was adequate to stand on one foot for 55 s with eyes open and 40 s with eyes closed. Yet when she stood up from a chair she appeared unsteady.

She used glasses to complete the physical activity questionnaire but was able to read a notice about an exercise class, which was posted on a bulletin board, without them. She responded to all spoken questions. The report from her family physician suggests that she has an unusually good health history with no metabolic disease, and no hospitalizations other than for childbirth. She used over-the-counter 'cold remedies' during her illness, but had not thought the flu serious enough to inform her physician. She has not yet returned to performing all household tasks. Her timed get-up-and-go test was completed in 28 s.

Her screening tests suggest that she can safely participate in a general conditioning programme. Her recent sedentary lifestyle suggests that she is very deconditioned and can expect substantial gains from participating in exercise. Her physical activity history indicates that she is interested in walking, and she has also expressed an interest in strengthening her upper body. Her slow performance on the get-up-and-go test and her unsteadiness on rising suggest that her recent illness may have left her with some postural hypotension.

As a result of her expressed desires to improve her overall physical capacity, energy level and strength her baseline assessment included aerobic capacity, muscular strength and endurance test components. Body composition was assessed using just height (155 cm) and weight (62 kg) to calculate BMI (24). Aerobic testing included an incremental treadmill test to volitional fatigue, after she had been familiarized with the Borg scale for rating perceived exertion. During the test an electrocardiogram was used to assess heart rate and watch for ECG abnormalities. Maximum oxygen uptake was estimated from the maximal work level achieved by applying the ACSM equations to the maximal grade (12%) and speed (110 m/min) which Mrs Smythe achieved. Mrs Smythe reported that she stopped due to overall fatigue and just before stopping she rated her exertion as a 19 (very, very hard). Her heart rate at the end of the test was 150 beats per minute and her ECG showed no abnormality.

Her test results indicated her aerobic fitness is average (24 ml/kg/min, 6.8 METs) for her age and gender. Given her recent inactivity and previous moderate activities this result suggested that she may be genetically well endowed for aerobic activity. Mrs Smythe was surprised and pleased by these test results.

The sit-and-reach test results tests suggest that Mrs Smythe should make flexibility exercises part of her routine. She will spend 10 – 15 min following the main portion of her programme performing a selection of stretching movements as part of a 'warm-up' routine.

Mrs Smythe's hand grip strength was symmetrical (right and left both 7 kg) but slightly below average. Measurement of strength with the modified sphygmomanometer suggested some weakness of the knee extensors (15 kg, predicted 19), elbow flexors (12 kg predicted 17 kg) and dorsiflexors (13 kg, predicted 15). Bench press was below average reported values (20 kg). These results indicated that Mrs Smythe would benefit from a strengthening programme. Details of a suggested training programme for Mrs Smythe are given in Table 6.

Table 6
Suggested Training Programme for Mrs Smythe

Week	Setting	Activity	Intensity	Time
1	Physiotherapy clinic	Instruction Aerobic (days 1, 3, 5) and Strength (days 2, 4)	Walk-treadmill @ 60% HRmax=90 bpm Grip, bench @ 60% 1RM Arm raise	15 min 2 sets, 5 reps 5 reps/side
2	Physiotherapy clinic, individual	Aerobic Strength	Walk-treadmill @ HR 90 bpm Grip, bench Arm raise	20 min 2 sets, 10 reps 5 reps/side
3	Physiotherapy clinic, individual	Aerobic Strength	Walk-treadmill @ HR 105 bpm Grip, bench, arm curl @ 65% 1RM Arm raise	20 min 2 sets, 10 reps 10 reps/side
4	Physiotherapy clinic, individual	Aerobic Strength Retest strength	Walk-treadmill @ HR 105 bpm Grip, bench, arm curls @ 65% 1RM Arm raise 1 kg	25 min 3 sets, 10 reps 10 reps/side
5	Physiotherapy clinic, group	Aerobic Strength	Walk-corridor @ HR 105 bpm Grip, bench, arm curl Arm raise 1 kg	25 min 3 sets, 10 reps 10 reps/side
6	Physiotherapy clinic, group	Aerobic Strength Retest strength and Aerobic (submax)	Walk-corridor @ HR 105 bpm Grip, bench, arm curls @ 70% 1RM Arm raise 1 kg	30 min 3 sets, 5 reps 10 reps/side
7	Community-based programme	Aerobic Strength	Walk-track @ HR 105 bpm Grip, bench, arm curls Arm raise 1 kg	30 min 3 sets, 10 reps 10 reps/side

Table 6 (Continued)
Suggested Training Programme for Mrs Smythe

Week	Setting	Activity	Intensity	Time
8	Community-based programme	Aerobic Strength	Walk-track @ HR 110 bpm Grip, bench, arm curls Arm raise 1.5 kg	30 min 3 sets, 10 reps 10 reps/side
9 and beyond	Community-based programme	Aerobic Strength Retest aerobic and strength Reassess goals	Vary activities; consider mall walking, Volksmarches Vary routine; consider circuit training	30 min

Summary

Physiotherapists can play a vital role in promoting the health of older people through providing physical activity recommendations and exercise prescriptions (see also Chapter 13). Physical frailty occurs when the older person can no longer adapt to any physical stresses. The range of safe and effective intensities declines with inactivity. A health promotion approach which increases physical capacity also enhances the older adult's ability to respond positively to exercise. Increasing physical activity and physical fitness before impairments are clinically evident is more effective than trying to ameliorate health problems that have reduced the client's capacity to respond. The benefits associated with exercise will improve client's health so that he or she is better able to cope with acute health challenges, such as illness or injury.

The physiotherapists who work with older clients have a unique opportunity to develop individualized exercise programmes that are based on the client's goals and abilities. This specificity increases the probability that a change to a more physically active lifestyle wil be sustained. As experts in movement and movement impairments, physiotherapists are the best possible resource for the older adult.

References

American College of Sports Medicine (1993) *ACSM's Resource Manual for Guidelines for Exercise Testing and Prescription.* Malvern, Lea & Febiger.

Barry, HC, Eathorne, SW (1992) Exercise and aging: Issues for the practitioner. *Medical Clinics of North America* **78**: 350–376.

Borg, GAV (1986) *The Perception of Exertion in Physical Work.* London, MacMillan.

Canada Fitness Survey (1982) *Fitness and Aging.* Ottawa: Fitness Canada.

Cole, B, Finch, E, Gowland, C, Mayo, N (1994) *Physical Rehabilitation Outcome Measures.* Toronto: Canadian Physiotherapy Association.

Cott, C, Finch, E, Gasner, D et al. (1995) The movement continuum theory of Physical Therapy. *Physiotherapy Canada* **47**: 87–95.

Cunningham, D, Rechnitzer, P, Pearce, M, Donner, A (1982) Determinants of self-selected walking pace across ages 19 to 66. *Journal of Gerontology* **37**: 560–564.

Cunningham, DA, Paterson, DH, Himann, JE Rechnitzer, PA (1993) Determinants of independence in the elderly. *Canadian Journal of Applied Physiology* **18**: 243–254.

Dishman, RK (1988) *Exercise Adherence: Its Impact on Public Health.* Champaign: Human Kinetics.

Emery, CF, Burker, EJ Blumenthal, JA (1991) Psychological and physiological effects of exercise among older adults. *Annual Review of Gerontology and Geriatrics* **4**: 218–238.

Gitlin, LN, Powell-Lawton, M, Windsor-Landsberg, LA et al. (1992) In search of psychological benefits: Exercise in healthy older adults. *Journal of Aging and Health* **4**: 174–192.

Govindasamy, D, Paterson, DH (1994) *Physical Activity and the Older Adult: A Knowledge Base for Managing Exercise Programs.* Champaign: Stipes Publishing Company.

MacDougall, JD, Wenger, HA, Green, HJ (1991) *Physiological Testing of the High-performance Athlete*. Champaign: Human Kinetics.

Makrides, L, Campagna, P (1992) *Elderfit: A Guide to Exercise for Seniors*. Halifax: Dalhousie University.

Porter, MM, Vandervoort, AA (1995) High intensity strength training for the older adult. *Topics in Geriatric Rehabilitation* 10: 61–74.

Piscopo, J (1985). *Fitness and Aging*. New York: John Wiley & Sons, Inc.

Shephard, RJ, Thomas, SG (1989) *Fit After Fifty*. North Vancouver: Self-Counsel Press.

Simpson, J (1993) Elderly people at risk of falling: The role of muscle weakness. *Physiotherapy* 79: 831–835.

Snow-Harter, C, Marcus, R (1991) Exercise, bone mineral density, and osteoporosis. *Exercise Sport Science Reviews* 19: 351–388.

Van Camp, SP, Boyer, JL (1989) Exercise guidelines for the elderly. *The Physician and Sports Medicine* 17: 83–88.

Voorips, LE, Rvelli, ACJ, Dongelmans, PCA *et al.* (1991). A physical activity questionnaire for the elderly. *Medicine and Science in Sports and Exercise* 23: 974–979.

Washburn, RA, Jette, AM, Janney, CA (1990) Using age-neutral physical activity questionnaires in research with the elderly. *Journal of Aging and Health* 2: 341–356.

Wasserman, K, Hansen, JE, Sue, DY *et al.* (1994) *Principles of Exercise Testing and Interpretation*. Philadelphia: Lea & Febiger.

13

Health Promotion Programmes

ELIZABETH C HENLEY, ROBYN L TWIBLE, LINDA KREMER

Introduction

Promoting health is every health care professional's responsibility and health promotion within the practice of gerontology offers the physiotherapist an exciting challenge. Health promotion should be considered in *all* actions, activities and interventions performed by physiotherapists. Promoting health with their clients must become a way of life. This means that physiotherapists should promote health when interacting with a client on a one-to-one basis; organize or assist in the organization of health promotion activities with their client groups; and work with the relevant community to help them identify community health needs and assist them in developing strategies to promote health. Additionally physiotherapists must become active and involved in the development of health policies, and act as advocates for promoting health even if only at a local level. Some physiotherapists must take on this responsibility at state / provincial and national levels.

Background to Health Promotion

To be able to undertake health promotion activities with older clients it is necessary to have a clear definition of health promotion and of the various models that can be utilized. It is also necessary to understand the philosophical issues that underpin health promotion and the relevant theories and strategies that are required to design, implement and evaluate any health promotion activitiy for the older population.

Definitions of Health Promotion and Models

Since the 1980s there has been much debate over the term health promotion and its relationship to allied and similar terms such as public health, prevention, health education and wellness. In 1986 the World Health Organization (WHO) organized an International Conference on Health Promotion in Ottawa, Canada, the outcome of which was the development and dissemination of the Ottawa Charter for Health Promotion (Figure 1). The Ottawa Charter identified prerequisites for health – peace, shelter, education, food, income, a stable ecosystem, sustainable resources, social justice and equity. This document has provided the foundation on which most nations have established their own health promotion policies and programmes.

WHO Definition of Health Promotion

The definition of health promotion contained in the Ottawa Charter provides an umbrella definition which encompasses all of the above health promotion terms and more importantly identifies a generic philosophy which underpins any action aimed at promoting health. Health promotion is the process of enabling people to increase control over, and to improve, their health (Chapter 1). To reach a state of complete physical, mental and social well-being, an individual or group must be able to identify and to realize aspirations, to satisfy needs, and to change or cope with the environment. Health is, therefore, seen as a resource for everyday life, not the objective of living. Health is a positive concept emphasizing social and personal resources, as well as physical capacities. Therefore, health promotion is not just the responsibility of the health sector, but goes beyond healthy lifestyles to well-being. The Ottawa Charter for Health Promotion has five major components: building healthy public policy; creating supportive environments; strengthening community action; developing personal skills; and reorienting health services (see also Chapter 5).

Health Promotion Models

The literature abounds with many classifications of the types of health promotion models or strategies (Wilcock, 1990; Ewles and Simnett, 1992). These include: health education; preventative health; healthy public policies; community development; organizational development; envir-

Figure 1   The Ottawa Charter for health promotion.

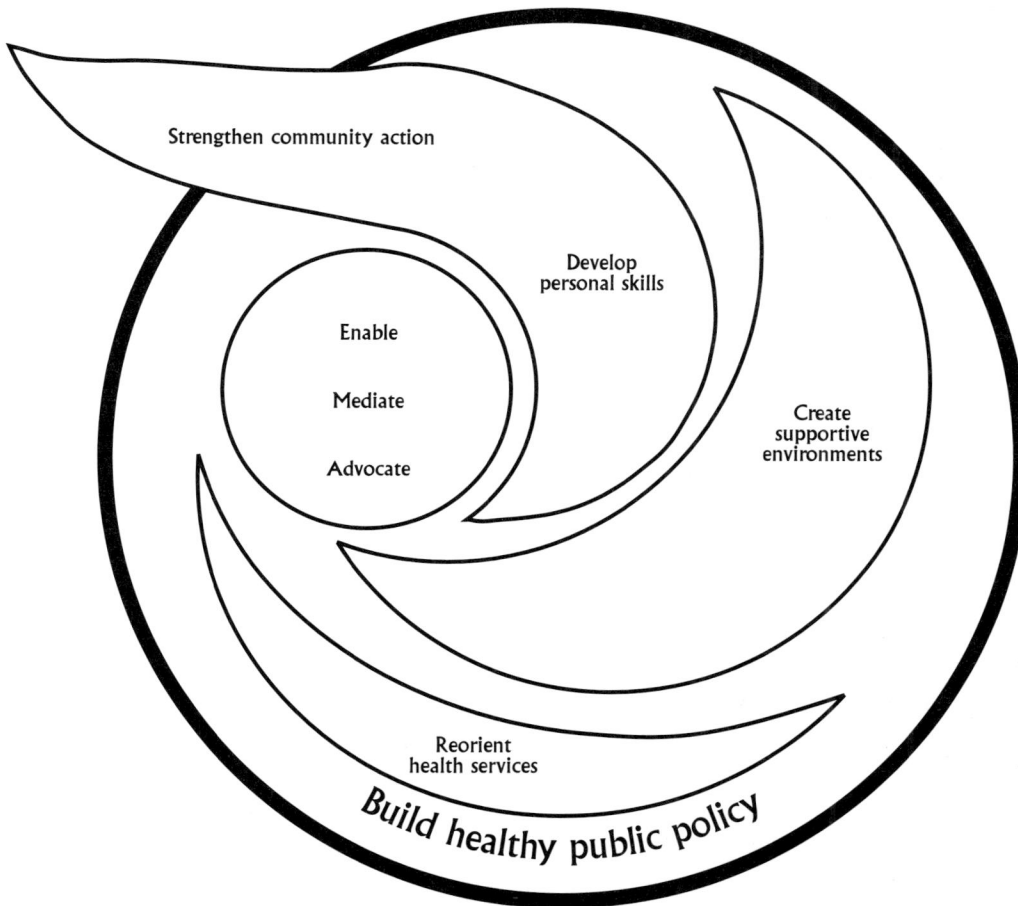

onmental health measures; social equity; regulatory activities; wellness; and ecology.

Health Education (Primary, Secondary and Tertiary)

Health education is the promotion of specifically planned educational opportunities for people to learn about health and as a result make voluntary changes to their behaviour to enable them to choose a more healthy lifestyle. Health education

by physiotherapists can take place on a one-to-one basis; in small groups; through mass media campaigns; or via a health fair.

Primary health education aims to prevent ill health and therefore is directed towards healthy people. It includes programmes designed by physiotherapists on topics such as back care, keeping fit and active, and safety in the home and community. Secondary health education focuses on informing clients about their personal health in an effort to improve their health, or prevent their condition from deteriorating. Such programmes would include cardiac and respiratory rehabilitation programmes, osteoporosis exercise programmes and incontinence workshops. Tertiary health education is directed towards educating clients and their carers about how to maximize their potential for healthy living, when there is no medical intervention that can improve their health status; for example, stroke programmes.

Preventative Health

Preventative health is also often referred to as public health. It involves strategies aimed at preventing ill health to the public at large (see Chapters 2, 5 and 12). Some examples of the types of activities offered as preventative health include: immunization programmes, mass screening programmes, occupational health and safety, protection services, clean water supply and waste disposal/sanitary systems. Physiotherapists might undertake falls prevention programmes or fitness assessments for older people (Chapter 12) or work with town planners to provide safe environments.

Healthy Public Policies

Public policy is thought to have the single most important influence on the health of older people (Cumming and Scanlon, 1994). It involves developing and implementing public policies that promote health in all aspects of the community's life. The development of these policies is a combined effort between government departments, non-government agencies, health professionals and the general public (Chapter 5). Physiotherapists may take an active interest and lobby agencies regarding policies such as anti-smoking legisla-

tion, transportation, access issues and building code regulations.

Community Development

Community development in this context is a strategy which relies on community participation to promote individual and group responsibility for the health and welfare of their community. It is one of the cornerstones of both the Ottawa Charter and the WHO Alma Ata Declaraton on Primary Health Care. Opportunities are provided for the community to identify its own health needs and take actions to address them. This could result in the establishment of self-help groups, development of new services or enhancement of existing facilities and services. For example, physiotherapists might become involved with community members to help them identify their own needs, e.g. in the establishment of a self-help group for stroke clients.

Organizational Development

In this approach, organizations develop policies and take actions that promote the health of their staff and customers, by ensuring healthy food choices in the canteen, providing a smoke-free environment, installing non-slip floor coverings, producing 'healthier' products, and using biodegradable packaging. For example, physiotherapists might consult with manufacturers and suppliers of mobility equipment and exercise equipment to provide advice and suggestions for improved designs of particular products.

Environmental Health Measures

The focus of this approach is to make the physical environment, whether at home, at work or in the community, conducive to optimal health, through basic public health measures such as provision of clean water and uncontaminated food, as well as additional measures to control pollution and eliminate hazards that may cause accidents. Physiotherapists should ensure that the physical environment of their own facility promotes optimal health by eliminating hazards, having good lighting, using large reader-friendly print in their handouts, and providing appropriate furniture.

Social Equity

This aspect of health promotion focuses on the advancement of social and economic changes that increase the individual's and community's knowledge, motivation, resources and opportunities for health (Chapter 5). This process is often initiated by action groups or individuals within the community, who then seek support from other groups and individuals in the community to bring about the changes. It involves lobbying of politicians, governments and other organizations or groups, and includes increasing community awareness on specific issues by the use of mass media campaigns. This type of intervention usually seeks to address issues such as adequate income, equal access and other inequalities that are the prerequisites for health. Physiotherapists may become involved in and support the community action groups.

Regulatory Activities

This approach refers to the political and educational activities directed at politicians, policy-makers and planners, which are aimed at lobbying and implementing legislative changes and voluntary codes of practice which directly or indirectly promote better health in the community. Such activities could include the improved labelling of foods, controlled advertising of alcohol, or increased taxation on cigarettes. Physiothera-

pists could provide advice and/or lobby relevant agencies about issues that promote or impede health of the community, with special emphasis on fitness and mobility. Activity could also involve such issues as compulsory labelling of mobility equipment to ensure safe usage.

Wellness

The 'wellness' approach promotes and fosters attitudes and actions that lead to optimal health and life satisfaction. It is a holistic philosophy which seeks to obtain a balance of body, self, environment and culture and is seen by some as the ultimate position on the illness/health promotion continuum. Physiotherapists should act as role models by maintaining their own healthy lifestyle, as well as promoting this philosophy among community groups.

Ecology

This approach could be seen as the global equivalent of the wellness model. It seeks to obtain harmony between all living organisms, their environment, habits and modes of life. Inherent in its approach is sustainability of resources and the development of world-wide policies and actions to health and well-being for all.

Health Policy and Health Promotion

At the time of the release of the Ottawa Charter, another Canadian document was produced *Achieving Health for All*, which provided a framework for health promotion (Figure 2). Three challenges were identified: reducing inequities in health; increasing the prevention effort; and enhancing people's capacity to cope. Three

Figure 2   A framework for health promotion, Government of Canada 1986.

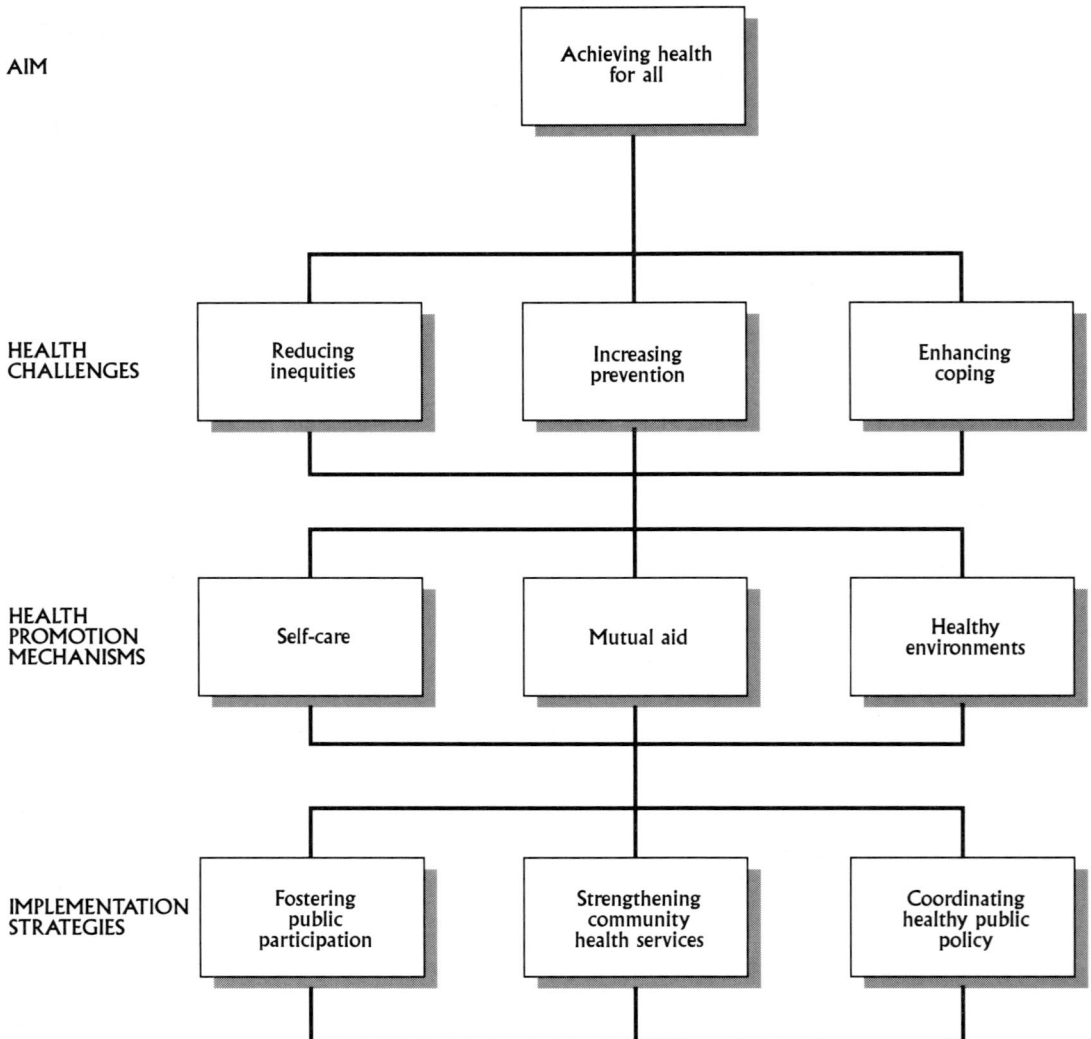

mechanisms were proposed by which these challenges might be met: self-care; mutual aid; and healthy environments. Three strategies suggested to implement these mechanisms were: public participation; strengthening community health; and coordinating healthy public policy. Rehabilitation professionals were challenged to develop new avenues of practice and service

delivery to meet the developing needs of the community.

In 1988 the Australian Federal government published a report, *Health for all Australians*, which was put forward as part of Australia's commitment to the WHO 'Health for All by the Year 2000' programme. This report dealt with ways in which the health system might better address health improvement and take more seriously its responsibilities in prevention and health promotion. One of the specific target populations identified by the report was older people. In response to this report, various state governments developed health policies and programmes specifically directed towards older people. One such initiative was the Report of the Healthy Older People Project (1989) which outlined a health promotion policy for older people in New South Wales. Subsequent to establishment of these government policies, many programmes have been instigated, such as the NSW North Coast Fall Prevention Project, the Medication Education Project in Sydney, the Stroke Risk Education Programme and the Older People Enjoying Life Project (Cumming and Scanlon, 1994).

Health and Behaviour

Factors that involve the individual or community and their willingness to become involved in health promotion initiatives, to be empowered to change their behaviour as a result of these involvements, are vital to the success of health promotion initiatives.

Motivation, Health and Behaviour Change

One of the misconceptions of society is that the acquisition of knowledge about poor health practices and the preferred healthy alternative is sufficient motivation for people to change their behaviour. Motivation is dynamic, not static, and may reflect the stage an individual (or community) has achieved in adopting and developing a new behaviour (Egger et al., 1990). Motivating

positive health behaviour is complex and draws upon many of the models of motivation and individual behaviour change; for example, the cognitive dissonance model, Maslow's hierarchy of needs, the health belief model, social learning theory, protective motivation theory and the theory of reasoned action (Chapter 8). Cummings et al. (1980) identified the following six factors common to all models of motivation and behaviour change:

1. Accessibility to health care.
2. Evaluation of health care.
3. Perceptions of symptoms and threat of disease.
4. Social network characteristics.
5. Knowledge of disease.
6. Demographic characteristics.

The above factors can be translated into a model for planning health programmes, which encompasses the following characteristics:

1. A change in behaviour is considered desirable in order to avoid injury and disease.
2. Change is based on rational use of information.
3. The change has the support of a person's peer group.
4. Change can be accomplished by specific activities.
5. Barriers to change can be overcome.

The change is applicable to the specific demographics of a group, e.g. age, ethnicity, socio-economic status.

(adapted from Egger et al., 1990)

Empowerment

Katz (1984) defines empowerment as access to and control over resources (Chapter 11). It is inherent in one of the five global health promotion components outlined in the Ottawa Charter, that of *strengthening community action.* Empowerment for health promotion provides a base from which individuals and the community can address social inequalities. The resolution of such inequalities will have a positive impact on the health of individuals and the community. In practical terms, it means that the target population for any health promotion activity must be actively involved in the health promotion process right from the beginning. Hawe *et al.* (1990 p. 21) state 'even in relation to national health goals,...there is a view that communities must gather data and view their own situation and translate goals into something achievable on the local level for there to be an impetus for action'. Breslow (1992) concurs with this statement based on a study of the health promotion needs of an inner-city population. To be effective programmes need to be developed by the people they are intended to serve (Chapter 5). The Australian Better Health Commission (1986) also stressed the need to encourage active community participation in developing an awareness of healthy living. In health promotion, community participation depends on individuals becoming aware of, interested in, motivated towards and having access to, programme development and implementation.

Philosophical Issues

Values and Beliefs Related to Health

Twible (1992) pointed out that older people's awareness of links between their habits and diseases or conditions may be limited. It is important, therefore, to establish what knowledge base exists prior to programme planning (Heckler, 1985). Specifically, health promotion pro-

grammes for older people start with consultation with the client group and must begin with needs assessment to identify risk factors and specific health issues and concerns pertinent to this community group (Lanning and Fliesser, 1986; McCormick, 1986).

Current Issues in Health Promotion for Older People

Health for All Australians (1988) identified a range of current issues in health promotion of relevance to the older population, in particular:

- Importance of maintaining independence including social and financial factors,
- Prevention of accidents and injury,
- Self-management of chronic diseases,
- Reduced manual and mental dexterity,
- Physical isolation due to design of public transport systems and access to facilities,
- Negative perceptions and stereotyping of older people with consequent personal difficulties,
- Incontinence,
- Sensory losses,
- Mental health problems,
- Loneliness.

Chronic Conditions Leading to Disability

The Report of the Healthy Older People (HOP) Project (1989) suggested a number of chronic conditions which tend to become disabling, often because of the ensuing mobility problems. Each of these may react with other conditions and compound the disabling effects. Prevention of disabilities arising from these conditions has become the focus of many health promotion programmes. The major chronic conditions identified through the HOP project research were:

- Arthritis,
- Incontinence,
- Cardiovascular disease,
- Osteoporosis leading to fractures,
- Foot problems,
- Sight problems,
- Hearing problems,
- Dementia and related disorders.

Special Features of Health Promotion Programmes for Older People

There are unique issues to be considered when developing programmes for older people (Cummings and Scanlon, 1994). Older people are not a homogeneous group and programmes should reflect this diversity. Factors that need consideration include:

1. *Age diversity of older people* The age range for older people can be from 60s to over 100 years. The youngest of these will have different demands and requirements than the oldest group.
2. *Focus of programme* The focus should be on wellness and quality of life, to reduce morbidity and mortality, and prolong life. Health promotion programmes must often concentrate on prevention of disability rather than prevention of disease and address such issues as loneliness, social support and life satisfaction, as well as addressing physical needs.
3. *Personal skills and self-confidence* Programmes should aim to improve personal skills and self-confidence to allow participants to articulate their concerns; create an environment where the individual's comments are valued and provide appropriate feedback as an indication that their opinions are taken seriously.
4. *Assertiveness* Older people must be given the opportunity to differentiate between assertive (positive) behaviour and aggressive behaviour.
5. *Logistical considerations* Consider aspects such as the venue and its lighting, noise and distraction levels, access to the building and toilet facilities, as well as public transport and parking facilities.
6. *Gender* In Australia, 58% of those aged 65 years or more and 71% of those aged 86 years or more are women (Rowland, 1991) (Chapter 2). Therefore women will be the target of most health promotion programmes and their special needs must be taken into account. It is often necessary to introduce ways to enable them to be involved separately from their male counterparts.
7. *Ethnic Background* Today, industrialized countries will have older people from many different ethnic backgrounds. Materials used in health promotion programmes in these countries will need to be adapted (in content, context and semantics) for use with a diversity of ethnic groups, taking into account their different attitudes, beliefs and behaviours about health issues. The concept and importance of independence, for example, may have an entirely different meaning in the UK and in Vietnam.
8. *Health of carers* Many older people are looked after by family members or by a spouse. These caregivers are also an appropriate target group for health promotion programmes (separate from their involvement in programmes related to those for whom they provide care).
9. *Health promotion in nursing homes* A large

percentage of old-old people live in an institutional setting. Health promotion programmes can be directed to improving their quality of life in this environment (see also Chapters 2 and 3).

10. *Cognitive impairment* Cognitive impairment is unusual in people less than 75 years old. Any strategies must direct special attention to the issue of cognitive impairment (Chapter 8) which is more common in the 75+ age group.

11. *Loss of study participants because of death* This may become a problem in programmes involving the old-old, because of the increased mortality rate with age.

The Health Promotion Process

The phases in the health promotion process include acceptance, needs assessment, analysis of the data to determine the problem areas, planning the programme, implementation and evaluation (Hawe *et al.*, 1990).

Acceptance

The first phase in the health promotion process is acceptance by the physiotherapist that there is a need for a health promotion programme, followed by a decision to do something about it. It includes a decision to be proactive, rather than waiting for others to take action. The 'target group' for intervention may be individuals, a small group or a community population.

Needs Assessment

A needs assessment is then made. Although the importance of needs assessment prior to health promotion planning is now widely recognized,

earlier programmes were frequently instituted without consumer consultation.

Bradshaw (1972) described four different types of need, each being identified by a different method:

1. *Normative need:* What expert opinion defines as need, e.g. serum cholesterol levels above 5.6 mmol/l require intervention (Chapter 12)

2. *Expressed need:* What you can infer about health needs of a community by observation of use of services

3. *Comparative need:* Examining the services provided in one area to one population and using this as a basis to determine the sort of services needed in another area with a similar population

4. *Felt need:* What people in the community say they want or what they think are the problems that need addressing.

Attention to all four types of need increases the chance of constructing a comprehensive view of the community's problems. These needs should then be prioritized. The needs assessment provides the team with a broad picture of the health problems in the community and then helps the team make decisions about the sort of health interventions that should be planned and mounted. Needs assessment should be viewed as part of the intervention process itself and can be the beginning of active community interest and involvement to ensure continued interest and impetus for action (Hawe *et al.*, 1990; Breslow, 1992). Facilitating community participation in health promotion is also one of the cornerstones of the Ottawa Charter (1987). The most successful and sustainable programmes are those that focus on priorities that meet the perceived needs of the community.

There are five steps in the needs assessment phase

which focus on data collection and gathering a range of opinions to identify the priority problem:

1. *Data collection via the consultation process.* Get a feeling for the types of issues that may be perceived as being important and the breadth and depth of their concerns, by talking to a large cross-section of people living and working in the community (or related to the target group), e.g. residents, health agencies, community organizations, local doctors, ethnic organizations. This step can be informal or may use more formal approaches such as structured interviews, questionnaires, or group data gathering techniques.
2. *Data collection via public records and statistics.* A great deal of data may be available from government sources and non-government organizations (or from hospital records, if the intention is to develop an in-house programme) which would be useful in health promotion planning. Results of any previous surveys or other research already done in that community should also be examined.
3. *Presentation of findings.* Invite all who have contributed to the project to view the progress thusfar, including community members. Present the information clearly and in a way that is likely to generate comments and analysis.
4. *Determining priorities.* The target group next determines priorities for action. One of the most useful methods of consensus decision making in community groups is the nominal group technique (NGT) where a structured process is used to rank problems (Delbecq and Van der Ven, 1971). This approach has been used successfully in a health promotion project for veterans and war widows in Australia (Twible, 1992).
5. *Identifying the health problem and document-*ing in a measurable, meaningful form. Identification and documentation of the health problem, its magnitude and the population at risk require careful attention. With respect to the 'fractured hip' population, for example, the problem statement may read that 'in Area X the incidence of hip fractures resulting from falls in older people, aged 65-75 years, has increased by 6% in the past 2 years'. By stating the problem in such a way the team has described a baseline from which to measure the degree of success in reducing the problem.

Analysis of the Data to Determine the Problem Areas

The focus of this phase is to develop a detailed profile of the target group, what exactly is happening with this health problem, who is experiencing the health problem and why. Careful attention to this part of planning the programme will help the team to avoid mistakes commonly made by other programmes. This process includes:

1. *Literature review.*
2. *A description of the target group.*
3. *Exploration of the health problem.* The target group should be consulted to determine how they perceive the problem, its causes, consequences and impacts on the individual, family and community, and what the best strategies to deal with the problem might be. Open-ended questions are a very useful way of uncovering beliefs and attitudes that will need to be addressed during the implementation phase. Group methods such as focus group technique and NGT are recommended for this part of the process (Hawe *et al.* 1990).
4. *Analysis of causal factors.* These factors can be subdivided into three main categories: predis-

posing factors, e.g. knowledge, attitudes, beliefs about exercise; enabling factors, e.g. availability of programmes to take part in; and reinforcing factors, e.g. reduction in insurance premiums, mass media campaigns.

Planning the Programme

Planning the programme involves establishing goals, objectives, subobjectives and strategy objectives (see also Chapter 12 and Section F). Goals are what the team ultimately wants to achieve by running the programme; they must be stated specifically, relating the place, person or target group, and time framework for the changes. Objectives describe the specific changes the team wants to bring about in the target group and subobjectives describe what has to happen before an objective can be achieved. Strategy objectives describe what is done in the programme to achieve the objectives, e.g. running media campaigns or holding workshops (Hawe *et al.*, 1990).

Selection of strategies and activities for the programme is largely dependent on the team's philosophy in health promotion and the setting in which the programme is to be carried out. With older people, the most effective style of learning relies heavily on highly interactive sessions with individuals or small groups, although well-organized mass media campaigns are also effective.

Teaching materials to be developed may include handouts, flyers, special equipment and audiovisual material. Pilot trials of these materials will ensure that they will be acceptable and meet the needs of the target group.

Training sessions for staff in the use of these materials are desirable to ensure that all personnel have a good understanding of the project and their own roles in it.

Implementation

Developing a programme manual is a useful way of listing and describing procedures for implementation and administration of the programme. Documentation of decisions made about changes and a regular updating of programme protocols are essential. A detailed budget needs to be drafted.

Evaluation

The final phase in the health promotion process is evaluation. It is often the one step which receives the least attention and consequently is poorly done. Performing an evaluation allows the team to judge the value of its programme to the target group. Evaluation must be planned before the programme is started, so that the right type and amount of data are collected. In many health promotion programmes the lack of preliminary planning of the evaluation process has resulted in difficulty in assessing whether or not the health promotion activity has been successful (Cumming and Scanlon, 1994).

Evaluation methods fall under two broad categories: qualitative methods, which seek to interpret the meaning of the programme for the people involved; and quantitative methods, which involve measuring variables of interest and changes occurring as a result of the programme, using standardized measures. Qualitative methods are particularly useful in projects with older people as they provide for a detailed examination of problems in a social setting and can be used to find out why a programme did or did not succeed (Cummings and Scanlon, 1994). Quantitative methods are particularly powerful tools in establishing needs, developing baseline profiles and measuring changes in health status outcomes. This approach enables statistical analysis of the data, and increases the generalizability of conclusions.

Evaluation or evaluative research can be subdivided into three sections: process evaluation, which measures the activities of the programme and how well it was delivered; impact evaluation, which measures the immediate effect of the programme; and outcome evaluation, which measures subsequent or long-term effects of the programme.

Four main elements are assessed during the process evaluation: whether the programme reaches the target group; whether the participants are satisfied with the programme; whether all activities of the programme are being implemented; and whether the materials and components of the programme are of good quality (Hawe *et al.*, 1990). As a general rule, new programmes rely more on qualitative methods in the early stages of the evaluation process, while more established programmes use more quantitative analysis to measure the magnitudes of changes that are produced.

Learning Styles and Media

Geragogy

The term geragogy was proposed by Johns (1988) and is used to describe the process involved in stimulating and helping older people learn. It deals with the unique instructional considerations that relate to teaching older people who are frail, disabled and in need of assistance (Chapters 2 and 22). Older people who do not fall into this category should have learning experiences that are appropriate for any adult, i.e. andragogy. The following discussions relate to considerations applicable to both groups of older people.

A Quality Learning Experience for Older People

Creating a positive learning environment (physical and psychosocial) is instrumental to successful learning (Chapter 8). The physiotherapist acts as a facilitator, motivator and guide in the learning process rather than a giver of information. The following, based on a review of the literature, are features that must be considered when designing learning experiences for older people:

- Consult with participants (re content, priorities, learning activities, time and location, etc.) prior to planning any learning experience.
- Ensure that participants' basic needs are met so that they can attend to the learning experience.
- Clearly show that what is being learned is relevant and beneficial to the learner's life and how it contributes to society as a whole. Ensure the content is well organized, meaningful, relevant and based on a clear focus.
- Focus on and emphasize learning that provides learners with knowledge, skills and resources that maintain or improve their independence.
- Learning activities should be, where possible, experiential in nature and based on the interests of the target population.
- Use learning experiences that draw upon the learner's varied lifespan experiences and provoke curiosity.
- Explain to the learners that emphasis will be given to thinking, reasoning, problem-solving and understanding the relevance and relationship of what they are learning to their everyday life.
- Offer a range of learning experiences related to the given topic / idea / concept being learned.

Give clear uncluttered examples that are relevant to the target population.

- Structure the learning activities so that there are opportunities for the learners to proceed at their own rates. Ideas should be limited, have a clear focus and avoid many rapidly changing stimuli. Allow sufficient time for the participants to process information.
- New information is acquired when a strong central focus is presented and distractions are kept to the minimum.
- Ideas / issues / information should be reinforced a number of times in different contextual settings — especially when a new concept is being introduced.
- Use highly organized material designed to assist in the retention of key ideas.
- Use a recognition type of test or familiar everyday activities to aid recall of information rather than pure recall. Timed tests are not suitable for older people.
- To ensure maximal participation provide a multimedia approach, a range of learning experiences and a variety of perspectives and personnel to present information, especially their peers as well as actual participants.
- Facilitate the learning process by providing encouragement, guidance and reinforcement. Help the participants to minimize their weaknesses and use their assets. In this way, they will achieve success and devlop or maintain self-confidence and self-esteem (Chapter 11).
- Create an atmosphere which encourages interaction, warmth and friendship as well as developing a spirit of camaraderie and a common goal for the group.
- Encourage and provide opportunities to extend and explore areas of interest either inside or outside the learning situation.
- Regularly review and summarize what has been learned. Ideally focus on three to five main points.
- Continually ask for feedback and undertake some form of evaluation.

Media

A combination of print, audio and visual materials may need to be developed to:

- promote the programme
- reinforce what has already been learned
- provide future reference
- be an integral part of the learning experience.

Print Material

The most effective print materials:

- Use dark print on light backgrounds. Black on white is best.
- Use a plain, clear typeface of at least 14-point size.
- Use white space to break up paragraphs.
- Use clear, straightforward language.
- Avoid colour combinations with low contrast, such as blue with green, or pink or yellow on white.
- Avoid script or ornamental print.
- Avoid using all capital letters, even in titles; words in uppercase and lowercase combinations are easier to read.
- Avoid narrow margins.
  (adapted from ParticipACTION, Canada, 1992)

Audio Material

Hearing loss is one of the most common physiological changes in ageing. It is important, therefore, that the physiotherapist is well positioned and projects their voice sufficiently so that all the audience can see and hear. Background noise should be minimized and the participants asked if the volume is too high or low, so that any necessary adjustments can be made. It may be necessary to use a microphone.

Visual Material

Older people are a heterogeneous group. Pictures that stereotype older people as being all alike should be avoided, as should images of frailty. Pictures should show healthy older people in all aspects of life, including minority groups. Positive images that demonstrate independence should be presented of those with mobility limitations. Members of the group should be asked what type of media they prefer. Blurry or wavy images should be avoided as they are distracting to those whose visual acuity is diminished.

Language

Is the leaflet easy to understand? The answer to this question deals with the issue of readability; texts with words of one or two syllables are more easily understood and require a lower level of comprehension than polysyllabic words. If material is hard to read the message may be missed. The language used should be directed at the individual person and be written in a way that is convincing. Is there anything offensive or irritating in the leaflet or material? Older people are particularly sensitive about use of offensive or irritating language. Material that refers to chronological age should be avoided. It should be ensured that materials translated from one language to another are culturally sensitive and do not conflict with cultural norms. Older people prefer clear, practical articles of about 500

words, for example, that provide how-to tips and clarify health issues. In addition to content, information on availability of services and programmes should be included (ParticipACTION, 1992).

Conclusion

More attention to health-promoting behaviours and activities is required as people get older. Older people are a more diverse group than any other age group due to varied lifetime experiences and environmental influences, as well as showing great variation in their levels of health and activity. They have developed a resilience in dealing with set-backs in order to maintain their ability to function as individuals within a community. Physiotherapists have the background knowledge and expertise to work with this population, to improve their ability to make informed choices regarding health behaviours, to access health/community resources, and to advocate for changes in health services or environmental design/planning. Health promotion is not a separate and distinct service. It is a value, an attitude, a process and an approach which should be part of every physiotherapist's regimen. It involves individuals, communities and institutions working together to encourage independence and enhance the quality of life of older people as they enjoy their later years in life.

References

Better Health Commission (1986) *Looking for Better Health.* Canberra: Australian Government Printing Service.

Bradshaw, J (1972) The concept of social need. *New Society* March: 640-643.

Breslow (1992) Empowerment, not outreach: Serving the health promotion needs of the inner city. *American Journal of Health Promotion* 7: 7-9.

Cumming, R and Scanlon, K (1994) *Health Promotion and Older People: A Guide to Evaluation.* Sydney: NSW Health Department.

Cummings, KM, Becker, MH, Maile, MC (1980). Bringing the models together: An empirical approach to combining variables used to explain health actions. *Journal of Behavioural Medicine* 3: 123-145.

Delbecq, AL, Van der Ven, AH (1971) A group process model for problem identification and programme planning. *Journal of Applied Behavioural Science* 7: 466-492.

Egger, G, Spark, R, Lawson, J (1990) *Health Promotion Strategies and Methods.* Sydney: McGraw-Hill.

Ewles, L, Simnett, I (1992) *Promoting Health: A Practical Guide,* 2nd edn. London: Scutari Press.

Hawe, P, Degeling, D, Hall, J (1990) *Evaluating Health Promotion: A Health Worker's Guide.* Sydney: MacLennan & Petty.

Health for All Australians (1988) Canberra: Australian Government Printing Service.

Healthy Older People (1989) Sydney: NSW Department of Health.

Heckler, MM (1985) Health promotion for older Americans. *Public Health Reports* 100(2).

Johns, M (1988) *Geragogy: A Theory for Teaching the Elderly.* New York: Haworth Press.

Katz, R (1984) Empowerment and synergy: Expanding the community's healing resources. In *Studies in Empowerment.* New York: Hawthorne Press.

Lanning, NM, Fliesser, YL (1986) The rainbow to wellness. *The Canadian Nurse* 82: 23-26.

Larau, LS, Heumann, LF (1982) The inadequacy of needs assessments of the elderly. *The Gerontologist* 22: 324-333.

McCormick, B (1986) Getting a second chance: Wellness for seniors. *Hospitals* 20: 60-61.

Ottawa Charter for Health Promotion (1987) *Health Promotion* 1:447-460.

ParticipACTION (1992) *Live it Up! A Guide to Healthy Active Living in the Senior Years.* Toronto: ParticipACTION.

Rowland, DT (1991) *Ageing in Australia.* Melbourne: Longman Cheshire.

Twible, RL (1992) Consumer participation in planning health promotion programmes: A case study using the nominal group technique. *Australian Occupational Therapy Journal* 39: 13-18.

Wilcock, AA (1990) *Health Promotion and Occupational Therapy.* Melbourne: WFOT Congress.

D

Management of Impairments and Disabilities

SECTION EDITOR: JANET M SIMPSON

14

Goal Setting

CHERYL A COTT

Setting physiotherapy goals with older people who have complex problems can be very challenging. The purpose of this chapter is to outline the process whereby the physiotherapist sets treatment goals and evaluates outcomes with older people.

The goal setting process outlined here is based on the Movement Continuum Theory of Physical Therapy (Cott *et al.*, 1995), on the premise that movement is the central unifying concept of any physiotherapy approach. According to this theory, every person has a Preferred Movement Capability (PMC), which refers to the person's chosen movement ability, and a Current Movement Capability (CMC), which refers to the person's present movement ability. In usual circumstances, a person's PMC and CMC are the same; however, pathology and developmental factors can create a differential between the person's preferred level of movement and their current level of movement (a PMC/CMC differential). Physiotherapy is indicated when such a differential exists, or when there is the potential for this differential to develop (see Chapters 5, 6 and 8).

In order to set appropriate treatment goals, it is important for the physiotherapist: (a) to identify the older person's goals; (b) to determine the source(s) of the discrepancy between the person's CMC and PMC, through a detailed assessment; (c) to determine the modifiability of these sources; (d) to set appropriate physiotherapy

189

goals, and the necessary interventions to achieve those; and (e) to select appropriate outcome measures to evaluate attainment of these goals.

Identifying the Older Person's Goals

The first step is to determine the older person's reasons for seeking physiotherapy. What is the reason for the referral or consultation? What are the expectations of the older person for physical therapy? If the referral or consultation has been initiated by someone other than the older person, it will be important to know the goals of the referring source, and to determine whether these goals are meaningful to the older person.

The physiotherapist must take the time to interview older persons to ascertain the movement difficulties that they are experiencing and the level of function that they would prefer to have. Without this information, the physiotherapist will have difficulty establishing realistic and meaningful treatment goals. For example, PMC differs between older people depending on their functional requirements and the availability of support. Being able to walk 20 feet independently ten times a day may be sufficient mobility for a sedentary person who lives alone in a small apartment with full support services. However, this level of movement would be unsatisfactory for the person living in sheltered accommodation who had to walk to a communal dining room for meals. It is important, prior to setting treatment goals, to find out why the older person requires physiotherapy and what functional level they hope to achieve (Squires *et al.*, 1991).

It is not always possible for older people to articulate their goals clearly. They may have cognitive or communication impairments that limit their ability to formulate or communicate their wishes; they may not have a clear idea of what the potential is for changing their movment; they may feel dependent on the physiotherapist and be unable to take responsibility for helping to plan their treatment; or they simply may not wish to make these kinds of decisions. In these situations the physiotherapist may need to consider the goals of the family or caregivers, always remembering that the goals of the older person may differ from those of their families and caregivers. This does not negate the importance of family or caregiver goals, particularly in the instance of the older person with profound cognitive impairment when physiotherapy goals might be directed to improving or maintaining functional levels of the older person in order to ease the burden of caregiving.

Determining the Current Movement Capability and the Source(s) of the PMC/CMC Differential

The physiotherapist must next determine the factors that are limiting the older person's current movement ability and the potential modifiabiity of those factors. Determination of the current level of movement capability (CMC) is made using an objective physiotherapy assessment which identifies the internal and external factors that are constraining the CMC.

The traditional physiotherapy assessment includes evaluation of range of motion, muscle strength and endurance (Chapters 6, 7 and 12), sensation, posture and gait, exercise tolerance, and functional skills (Axtell and Schoneberger, 1990; Goldstein, 1991). If cardiopulmonary or neurological disease is present, assessment should be extended to include these systems. Particular emphasis is placed on the assessment of functional performance since impairments such as declines in range of motion or muscle strength do not necessarily translate into functional disability. For example, functional range of motion in hip flexion is approximately 110 degrees (Boone and Azer, 1979). Increases in hip range of motion beyond that point may have little effect on performance of functional activities.

In addition to considering physiological factors that might be affecting movement, it is also important to consider psychological factors such as the client's mood, cognitive status, and cultural and spiritual background (Chapters 8 and 9). Older people have a wealth of life experiences that produce a wide variety of coping styles and attitudes towards health and disabiity. Caution must be exercised before labelling an older person as 'unmotivated' or 'uncooperative'. Recent experiences such as the loss of a spouse or the fear of losing independence will influence an older person's enthusiasm or interest in moving, as will factors such as perceptual deficits or fear of falling.

Cognitive impairment is an important consideration with older people (Chapter 8). The incidence of cognitive impairment is disproportionately high in older people requiring physiotherapy. It may not be necessary or appropriate for the physiotherapist to formally assess mental status as this will routinely have been done by the physician and the information can be easily obtained from the medical or nursing records. Informally, the physiotherapist will want to know how the older person's cognitive abilities

such as his or her ability to follow and remember instructions to problem-solve and to learn motor skills are limiting the CMC.

The assessment process may need to accommodate for changes in the older person's ability to participate in a lengthy evaluation session. It may take a number of sessions to complete the assessment and it may also be necessary to choose assessment procedures that capture the most information with the least number of activities. For example, rather than evaluating range of motion and muscle strength at each joint in the lower extremities, it may be more energy and time efficient to check first how the older person is able to get up out of a chair three times in a row. This single assessment procedure will provide important information about functional range of motion, strength, exercise tolerance and balance that may be more relevant to identifying problems with functional mobility than the results of the more traditional range of motion and muscle strength assessment (Tinetti and Ginter, 1988). If this assessment procedure reveals specific areas of concern, a more detailed assessment of target areas is then warranted.

After establishing the older person's current movement capability, the next step is to develop hypotheses on possible reasons for the difference between the older person's preferred level of movement and his/her current movement ability. At this point, the physiotherapist must consider all of the factors that could be contributing to the PMC/CMC differential, in addition to internal physical and psychological factors, in the context of their social and physical environment.

Movement is context dependent and, particularly for older people, it is essential also to understand the individual's physical and social surroundings and the external environment that indirectly affects the individual (Holliday et al., 1992). Architectural and ergonomic factors in the environment such as lighting, floor surfaces, height of beds, chairs and toilets, and the presence of stairs can impede or enhance mobility. For example, the older person may want to be able to walk independently to meals, but the presence of stairs or the distance to the dining room may be the main factor limiting their preferred movement ability.

An older person's environment is not just made up of physical properties – of equal and interrelated importance are the social and emotional characteristics of that environment. Caregivers are critical to the social environment, for it is their interaction with the older person that fosters dependence or independence. Dependency behaviours may be encouraged, albeit inadvertently, by caregivers. Key to the social environment is caregiving that provides the older person with choices and fosters independence, a sense of control and autonomous functioning.

The physiotherapist will need to judge whether the client's social environment is impeding or supportive to their preferred movement ability. For example, when trying to regain independence in walking after a fall, an older person's physical status may be such that with practice, there is the potential for the return to independence, yet the policy of the institution is to use physical restraints with all individuals with a history of falls. In this instance, the person's social or caregiving environment may be the main factor limiting their current movement ability, rather than any physiological considerations.

Determining the Modifiabiity of the Sources of the PMC/CMC Differential

The focus of physiotherapy is to minimize the PMC/CMC differential by improving the CMC, either by modifying internal physical or psychological factors and/or by modifying the older person's physical or social environment. When setting goals for older persons, it is important for the physiotherapist to understand the modifiability of the sources of the PMC/CMC differential. This is complicated in older people by the interaction of normal age changes with the effects of disease and the environment, and the presence of co-morbidity.

The physiotherapist may identify a number of factors limiting the older person's CMC, and, given a finite amount of treatment time, will need to prioritize which factors to target. The physiotherapist should consider the extent to which each factor is limiting the older person's ability to function and the degree to which physiotherapy can modify each factor (O'Neil et al., 1992).

Each individual has a theoretical finite ability to move that can be biologically, psychologically and/or socially determined and that is affected by the process of ageing (Cott et al., 1995). For example, declines in maximal achievable heart rate with age will set limits on the effects of cardiac training in a 75-year-old person as compared to a 20-year-old person; depression or lack of interest in performing certain activities will limit how successful the older person is in performing those activities; and attitudes of caregivers may impede the older person's mobility. Levels of function and mobility prior to the current injury or illness are an important consideration for setting realistic goals; however, if the current episode was precipitated by a period of decreasing mobility and deconditioning, there may still be potential for increasing function to levels greater than those immediately preceding the current injury or illness.

Until recently there was little information on the influence of physiotherapy on modification of movement impairments and disabilities in older people (Chapter 22). However, recent studies have indicated that it is possible to improve both the strength and mobility of older people.

Modification of the older person's external environment to improve the CMC might involve the utilization of appropriate assistive technology or the education and training of caregivers. Modification of these external factors becomes particularly important when there is little chance of modifying the internal physical factors that are limiting movement.

For example, the older person may wish to be able to go to the toilet independently. He or she may have reached full potential in terms of modifying internal physical factors in that he or she is able to walk to the toilet independently with a walker, but it takes time and effort to do so. However, if that person also has urgency and frequency, it may be necessary to modify the physical environment by putting a commode at the bedside to facilitate function.

Setting Appropriate Physiotherapy Goals

Having established the older person's goals for treatment, the source(s) of the PMC/CMC differential and their potential for modification,

appropriate physiotherapy goals must next be clarified. These goals may be targeted at prevention of further increases in the PMC/CMC differential (prevention goals), at improvement of the CMC (intervention goals) and at adaption of the external environment (adaption goals).

When working with older people with complex problems, it is often necessary to incorporate all three types of goals into a comprehensive rehabilitation programme. For example, when working with an older person with a hemiplegia who is confined to a wheelchair, physiotherapy goals might be directed at: preventing secondary complications related to immobility such as contractures, pressure sores and deconditioning (prevention goals); ensuring that the person has achieved or is maintaining their maximum CMC in terms of their physical abilities (intervention goals); and ensuring that the physical and social environment are appropriately adapted to maximize movement potential through the prescription of assistive devices and the training of caregivers in appropriate transfer techniques (adaption goals).

The physiotherapy goals should be challenging but achievable, specific and measurable, and meaningful to the older person (Cott and Finch, 1991). Goals should not be so challenging that the older person feels discouraged about his or her ability to meet them. For example, the older person who has become deconditioned through inactivity may be discouraged at the thought of the amount of energy it will require to return to walking independently for long distances, no matter how much they may want to do so. It is usually helpful to break overall goals down into smaller steps, that give the client something to work towards, yet can be reasonably achieved in a short period of time. Successful achievement of early goals is key to ensuring the older client remains committed in continuing to pursue more difficult long-term goals. The first few goals could be to walk to the bathroom twice a day, gradually progressing to walking to meals daily. Particularly in the early stages, these goals should relate to functional activities that are important to the older person.

Goals must be specific and measurable, in order to determine whether they have been achieved.

Selecting Appropriate Functional Outcome Measures

Functional limitations are usually classified in terms of reduced physical, psychological, and social tasks and activities. All three need to be considered in an overall picture of functional capacity. Functional assessment is an attempt to evaluate the most important aspects of the behaviour, the objective and subjective worlds of the person through standardized methods that can be applied by people with a wide variety of backgrounds and training. Physiotherapists largely concentrate on physical function measures, but need always to keep in mind that many aspects of the other two components interact considerably with physical function.

There are a number of outcome measures available to physiotherapists that can be used to measure functional limitations such as balance (Berg et al., 1992), endurance (Cunningham et al., 1986), mobility (Podsiadlo and Richardson, 1991), and functional performance (Carr et al., 1985; Seaby and Torrance, 1989). An excellent resource for further information on these and other outcome measures is *Physical Rehabilitation Outcome Measures* (Cole et al., 1994), available through the Canadian Physiotherapy Association. A useful

companion guide is the *Standards for Administering Tests and Taking Measurements* from the Chartered Society of Physiotherapy.

The Functional Autonomy Measurement System (SMAF) (Hebert et al., 1988) attempts to address these limitations in functional measures by attempting to operationalize handicap by not only quantifying the person's performance on five sectors of functional activity, but also by estimating the available resources to compensate for any identified disability. For example, if an older person has a disability in that he or she needs assistance to transfer, and that asistance is available, then he or she would not be considered to have as great a handicap as a similar person who did not have that assistance available.

Developing and Implementing Treatment / Management Strategies

Once the goals and outcome measures have been established, the physiotherapist develops and implements appropriate physiotherapy strategies, targeted at the hypothesized sources of the PMC/CMC differential. Many of these strategies may be the same as those used for younger populations, but they may need to be modified to accommodate for age changes in physical and cognitive performance. O'Neil et al. (1992) identified two broad categories of therapeutic procedures specific to the frail elderly: general conditioning training, which includes activities addressed at improving internal physical factors or impairments; and functional activity training, which includes training in bed mobility, transfers, wheelchair operation, gait and activities of daily living (ADL). General conditioning training will precede or accompany functional activity training.

Evaluating Outcomes and Resetting Goals

After a period of time specified in the original assessment, physiotherapy goals should be re-evaluated and re-set, as appropriate (see also Chapter 12). At this point, the original hypotheses about the source(s) of the PMC/CMC differential are either substantiated or need to be re-addressed. If goals have been achieved or are in the process of being achieved, the original hypotheses are substantiated and treatment/management strategies should be halted or continued as appropriate. If goals have not been achieved, the original hypotheses should be reviewed, new goals developed and treatment/management strategies revised. If initial intervention goals have not been met after a suitable trial of physiotherapy, it may be necessary to re-evaluate the potential modifiability of internal physical factors, and possibly shift the focus of attention to modifying the environment (adaptation goals).

Conclusion

Setting physiotherapy goals for older people is challenging. Physiotherapists must have a broad base of knowledge about the effects of ageing, disease and the environment on older people's ability to move. They must develop an ability to problem-solve creatively, in order to address the complex issues that exist, particularly in frail, elderly people.

The goals that physiotherapists are most familiar with are intervention goals, which may not always be appropriate or feasible for many older people. Instead, the focus may need to be directed to prevention and adaptation goals, with which physiotherapists may be less comfortable or familiar. However, physiotherapists who work with older people enjoy the challenge of being creative and innovative and find personal satisfaction in contributing to the quality of life of their older clients, and in helping them to meet their goals.

References

Axtell, LA, Schoneberger, MB (1990) Physical therapy. In Kemp, B, Brummel-Smith, K, Ramsdell, JW (eds) *Geriatric Rehabilitation*, pp. 157-175. Boston: Little, Brown and Co.

Berg, KO, Wood-Dauphineee, SL, Williams, JI, Gayton, D (1989) Measuring balance in the elderly: preliminary development of an instrument. *Physiotherapy Canada* 41: 304–311.

Berg, KO, Wood-Dauphineee, SL, Williams, JI, Maki, BE (1992) Measuring balance in the elderly: validation of an instrument. *Canadian Journal of Public Health* 83: 7–11.

Boone, DC, Azer, SP (1979) Normal range of motion of joints in male subjects. *Journal of Bone and Joint Surgery* 61: 756.

Carr, JH, Shepherd, RB, Nordholm, L, Lynne, D (1985) Investigation of a new motor assessment scale for stroke patients. *Physical Therapy* 65: 175–178.

Cole, B, Finch, E, Gowland, C, Mayo, N (1994) *Physical Rehabilitation Outcome Measures*. CPA in cooperation with Health and Welfare Canada and the Canada Communications Group – Publishing, Supply & Services Canada.

Cott, C, Finch, E (1991) Goal-setting in physical therapy practice. *Physiotherapy Canada* 43(1): 19–22.

Cott, CA, Finch, E, Gasner, D. *et al.* (1995) The movement continuum theory of physical therapy. *Physiotherapy Canada* 47(2): 87–95.

Cunningham, DA, Technitzer, PA, Donner, AP (1986) Exercise training and the speed of self-selected walking pace in men at retirement. *Canadian Journal on Aging* 5: 19-25.

Goldstein, TS (1991) *Geriatric Orthopaedics: Rehabiliatative Management of Common Problems*. Gaithersburg, MD: Aspen Publishers Inc.

Hebert, R, Carrier, R, Bilodeau, A (1988) The functional autonomy measurement system (SMAF): Description and validation of an instrument for the measurement of handicaps. *Age and Ageing* 17: 293–302.

Holliday, PJ, Cott, CA, Torresin, WD (1992) Preventing accidental falls by the elderly. In Rothman, J and Levine, R (eds) *Prevention Practice: Strategies for Physical Therapy and Occupational Therapy*, pp. 234-257. Philadelphia: WB Saunders.

O'Neil, MG, Woodard, M, Soss, V *et al.* (1992) Physical therapy assessment and treatment protocol for nursing home residents. *Physical Therapy* 72: 596-604.

Podsiadlo, D, Richardson, S (1986) The timed 'up and go': A test of basic functional mobility for frail elderly persons. *Journal of the American Geriatrics Society* **39**: 142-148.

Seaby, L, Torrance, G (1989) Reliability of a physiotherapy functional assessment used in a rehabilitation setting. *Physiotherapy Canada* **41**: 264-271.

Squires, A, Rumgay, B, Perombelon, M (1991) Audit of contract goal setting by physiotherapists working with elderly patients. *Physiotherapy* **77**: 790-795.

Tinetti, ME, Ginter, SF (1988) Identifying mobility dysfunctions in elderly patients: Standard neuromuscular examination or direct assessment. *Journal of the American Medical Association* **259**: 1190-1193.

15

Postural Instability and Falling

JANET M SIMPSON

Definition of a Fall
•
Size of the Problem and Seriousness of the Consequences
•
Reasons for Falling
•
The Goals of Physiotherapy
•
Physiotherapy Assessment: Initial Considerations
•
Detailed Physiotherapy Assessment
•
Physiotherapy Management
•
Summary

Postural instability and falling not only pose a huge threat to elderly peoples' welfare and quality of life, but present physiotherapists with a major challenge. The likelihood of falling increases in old age, and so physiotherapists who specialize in rehabilitation of older people find that instability-related problems form a substantial part of their caseload. In fact, resolving non-specific balance problems may be considered a speciality of this area of clinical practice.

Definition of a Fall

Isaacs (1992, p. 67), defined instability as: 'impairment of the ability to correct displacement of the body during its movement through space'. Instability puts the person at risk of falling, but deciding what constitutes a fall, especially for research purposes, is not straightforward. Numerous definitions have been made, mostly taking account of at least three of the following factors:

1. that some part of the person comes to rest on the ground or some lower level i.e. below the waist,
2. that this event is unexpected and unintentional,
3. that the circumstances were not such that a normally fit person would have fallen, e.g. slipping on ice,
4. that the event cannot be explained as being the

result of a major intrinsic event, e.g. stroke, syncope, or heart attack.

Not all falls result in sudden, harsh contact with the floor or furniture. Some may follow a totter, with grasping at furniture or the wall on the way down to the floor. At other times a person may come to rest on the floor or on the ground in a slow but uncontrollable fashion. For example, a person may slide to the floor after falling asleep in a slippery chair.

Size of the Problem and Seriousness of the Consequences

A prospective community study in the USA revealed that 32% of participants, all over 75 years old, fell at least once during the one-year follow-up period, and 25% fell at least three times (Tinnetti et al., 1988). These figures confirm findings from previous studies in the UK, and New Zealand. Furthermore, the rate of falls increases to around 50% among people over 80 years old. The incidence is even higher among residents in institutions. One recent study in south east England showed that approximately 45% of people in geriatric medicine wards were at risk, varying from 14% to 100% depending on admission policy and whether the ward provided acute care or slow stream rehabilitation (Simpson and Mandelstam, 1995).

The UK Department of Health reported that in 1991 in England, falls were the major cause of death from accidents among people aged over 65 years. The US National Safety Council Report for 1988 had also identified falls as the leading cause of accidental death in people aged 65 years and over. Falls are also expensive for health services if they result in the person being admitted to hospital. Although the total number of fractures following falls is very high, only a small proportion (6–10% is the most often quoted range) result in serious injury, although 24% of the participants in a recent study were reported to have sustained serious injury (Tinetti et al., 1988).

Older people are often admitted to hospital after being found on the floor after a fall. Many spend over an hour there, some even days, before being found. 'The long lie', defined as 'a period of one hour or more lying on the floor after a fall' (Isaacs, 1992, p. 77) can have serious consequences: pressure sores, bronchopneumonia, dehydration, hypothermia, and delirium as well as emotional trauma.

A fear of falling is prevalent among older people. This fear is not confined to people who have fallen already; many who have not done so may suffer, whereas many fallers do not (Maki et al., 1991). Over 50% of the fallers in one survey said they were not afraid of falling, while 25% were so afraid that they had curtailed their activities (Tinetti et al., 1988). Such concerns may not only reduce the older person's quality of life, but also foster muscle weakness and postural instability, and thus exacerbate the risk of falling.

A fall can come as a great shock to someone who, although technically old, considers themselves as fairly fit and active for their age. They may experience considerable loss of self-confidence and may also restrict their activities. Usually, physicians are quick to identify reasons for this type of fall: heart problems, anaemia and acute illnesses, so physiotherapists may have little contact with this group.

Reasons for Falling

Recurrent, unexplained falling among old people, i.e. where no cause is immediately obvious, is no longer accepted as just a sign of old age, but as an indication that something is wrong and merits investigation. Falls in old age, especially among frail people, are commonly described as being multifactorial in origin, as few can be attributed to a single cause. The traditional medical model, in which a problem is related to a single disease or aetiology, is rarely applicable. The accumulated effects of multiple aetiologies which combine to affect postural skills and progressively reduce the person's threshold of stability, lead to the majority of falls. The risk of falling increases with the number of a person's disabilities (Tinetti *et al.*, 1986).

Three models of falls risk will be summarized: an epidemiologically based model (Tinetti and Speechley, 1989); a postural control model (Black *et al.*, 1993, p. 318); and the clinical model described by Studentski *et al.* (1994).

Epidemiological Model

The epidemiological approach emphasizes the multifactorial nature of most falls among older people and seeks to identify contributory factors. These include: chronic, predisposing intrinsic risk factors, situational factors, both intrinsic and extrinsic to the person, and the activity in which the person is engaged at the time of the fall.

Chronic predisposing risk factors are intrinsic characteristics of the older person that chronically impair stability, for example musculoskeletal or neurological disease and associated impairments. Sensory and mental impairments come into this category, as do the effects of medications. In contrast, short-term intrinsic risks encompass obvious reasons for falling such as syncope and stroke, but also other factors such as infections, fatigue and emotional stress.

Keeping one's balance demands attention. Some falls occur when the activity demands more attention than usual of an older person, such as walking on uneven or stony ground. Some activities that lead to falls may be classed as imprudent, like climbing a step-ladder to clean the top of a cupboard, but the majority of falls occur for no obvious reason during everyday activities in the home. In a study of fit community dwelling elders, 40% of falls occurred in the person's home during activities necessary for daily living and almost 30% could be attributed to inattention, whereas just over 30% occurred in connection with hazardous or imprudent activities (Reinsch *et al.*, 1992).

The risk factors that tend to receive most attention from the rehabilitation team are the extrinsic or environmental risk factors in the home such as poor lighting, slippery floors, loose rugs, as well as inappropriate spectacles, ill-fitting footwear, and thoughtlessly chosen clothing.

Postural Control Model

A postural control model of falling which is particularly useful to physiotherapists has been described by Black *et al.* (1993). This model emphasizes the potential mismatch between external threats to balance and the capacity of the person to resist them. The postural control model suggests two main reasons for falls:

1. When the postural system is unable to compensate for an external mechanical perturbation or external sensory perturbation. The mechanical perturbation may be externally

produced – being jostled, standing in a moving bus – or self-induced – walking, bending over, pushing a door. The latter are normally compensated for by anticipatory postural adjustments whereas it is not possible to compensate for unanticipated perturbing forces such as an uneven paving stone or other trips and slips. An external sensory perturbation can arise from the illusion of self-motion created when the next train moves, or by certain carpets which distort the proprioceptive information from the foot and ankle.

2. In response to an internal physiological perturbation that disrupts or shuts down operation of the control system itself. This can happen either by interference with perfusion of the postural centres of the brain or brainstem: transient ischaemic attacks, postural hypotension etc.; or by disruption of the operation of the sensorimotor systems producing dizziness or vertigo.

The authors point out that the largest proportion of falls experienced by older people are probably attributable to some form of mechanical perturbation that disturbs postural equilibrium. Whether or not an external perturbation will result in a fall is dependent on the effectiveness of the stabilizing reactions of the postural control system. Increased risk of falling in older people may arise from:

1. Greater likelihood of experiencing more frequent or more severe perturbations or both (e.g. from impaired motor control, disordered gait, cognitive or perceptual deficits that impair ability to identify and avoid environmental hazards).
2. Reduced ability to recover from perturbations that are easily withstood by healthy adults.

Clinical Model

Studentski et al. (1994) observed that fit older people and those who are bed-ridden rarely fall. From this they reasoned that the most important indicator of fall risk is difficulty with balance and mobility and that these problems are most likely among frail older people who are both mobile and unstable. Simpson (1993) reviewed prospective studies that identified muscle weakness as contributing to fall risk. However, Studentski and her associates suspect that poor postural competence, although a necessary risk factor for falling, is not a sufficient one and that the risk it poses may be modified by behavioural, social and environmental factors. They describe a clinical model of fall risk which encompasses four predefined domains:

1. *Mobility* – the person's ability to remain upright during a series of progressively more difficult mobility tasks.
2. *Environment* – the extent of threat or support provided by the dwelling.
3. *Attitude toward risk* – how the person resolves conflicts between independence and safety.
4. *Social support* – the degree to which a person feels he is receiving social support within his or her environment.

High versus low risk was determined by a simple mobility screen:

- *Low risk* – cannot sit independently for 60 s, cannot stand. Descends stairs step-over-step without using handrail. Descends stairs as above and also can tandem walk (tandem walk – at least five out of six heel to toe steps).
- *High Risk* – can sit, cannot stand. Walks but does not meet criteria for adequate ambulation (i.e. step length at least twice foot length, symmetric stride and the ability to follow a straight

path). Meets criteria for ambulation but cannot descend stairs.

Although there was some overlap between the two groups, recurrent falls occurred significantly more often in the high-risk than in the low-risk group. Most falls involved people who could stand but had abnormal gait.

The Goals of Physiotherapy

There are three aspects to physiotherapy in the management of older people at risk of becoming recurrent fallers or who are already in that category. The first, which dominates the literature, is prevention of further falls; the second is training clients to cope with further falls; and the third is restoring confidence and self-esteem.

Health promotion programmes are devised for not-yet-at-risk ageing people and many physiotherapists and health visitors are involved at this level. But in this chapter we are concerned with older people already deemed to be at risk, because they have any combination of a history of falling, poor postural control, or an admitted fear of falling. To reduce risk among this client group physiotherapists identify those factors, both intrinsic and extrinsic, contributing to the person's fall risk that are amenable to physiotherapy intervention, and then intervene accordingly. Dealing with an older client's lack of confidence in their own postural skills is also an important aspect of prevention.

Interventions to reduce the effects of further falls are directed at preventing unnecessary immobility and its consequences. Doing so may also impact on confidence. Furthermore intercurrent fallers, who may otherwise show little evidence of gait or postural abnormality, need help to regain their self-esteem. In summary, the aims of physiotherapy with older people who have fallen or are at risk of doing so are to:

1. improve their ability to withstand threats to their balance,
2. improve the safety of their environment,
3. prevent them suffering the consequences of a long lie on the floor,
4. restore their, and their carer's confidence in their ability to move about as safely and effectively as possible in their environment.

Physiotherapy Assessment: Initial Considerations

The purpose of assessment is to identify and record enough information to allow an effective physiotherapy treatment plan to be drawn up and, in due course, to be evaluated. In the busy clinical situation physiotherapists must be sharply focused. The factors related to the postural system being unable to compensate for an external mechanical perturbation are precisely the problems for which physiotherapists have the skills to intervene. To this end assessment must be focused on identifying postural-control-related disabilities and specific underlying impairments amenable to physiotherapy intervention.

If the client has not yet received a medical examination, physiotherapists may become aware of signs and symptons which may indicate a reason for falling which would be more appropriately dealt with by a physicaian — for example the client taking four or more prescribed drugs, especially sedatives, or who complains of dizziness on standing (Tinetti and Speechley, 1989; Black et al., 1993). It may also be necessary to bring other problems to the attention of other appropriate health care professionals.

This assessment establishes the older person's pre-intervention state, so that later comparison with the post-intervention state can indicate effectiveness of the treatment programme.

It is also important for the physiotherapist to determine the extent to which the client is able and willing to cooperate with an intervention programme and whether the carers will be willing to cooperate in the rehabilitation programme.

If fatigue is a factor, assessment may have to be spread over several sessions, particularly when the person is very old and frail.

Classification of Fallers

Fallers are classified as occasional fallers, intermittent fallers or recurrent fallers. Other older people may be defined as being at risk of falling.

- *Occasional faller.* The fall probably has an extrinsic, situational explanation. Gait and balance are normal, general health is good – may suffer from a blow to self-esteem.
- *Intermittent or intercurrent faller.* Subject to intermittent or one-off dysfunction, which may be caused by an acute illness or a transient disorder of the circulatory system. There may be a complete medical explanation and falling will stop once this has been remedied.
- *Recurrent faller.* According to Studentski *et al.* (1994) 'recurrent' means two or more falls in 6 months. General health is poor but there is no complete medical explanation for the falls.
- *At risk.* People who have not yet fallen but who appear to be at high risk according to the criteria delineated in the clinical model. General health may be poor. The physiotherapist or other health care professional may have observed them to be at risk.

Four categories of information should be sought:

1. *Intrinsic predisposing problems.* Chronic, intrinsic predisposing impairments underlying poor postural skills and associated disabilities that contributed to previous falls or might lead to further falls and that are amenable to rehabilitative intervention.
2. *Extrinsic situational problems.* Environmental hazards, extrinsic to the person, that contributed to previous falls and that might lead to further falls.
3. *Coping strategies.* Strategies the older person, and if appropriate, his/her carer, have in place for coping with a fall. What happened after the last fall?
4. *Psychological sequelae.* Psychological consequences of the fall that might lead to self-imposed restriction of activity.

If there is no clear environmental hazard associated with most of the falls, recurrent fallers can be suspected of hosting a variety of impairments that result in chronically poor postural control. Deconditioning and weakness in the anti-gravity muscles may be suspected, especially if repeated falls occur in circumstances in which it would be highly unlikely for a fit older person to fall. Indeed, this factor significantly differentiates between fallers and non-fallers in many surveys (Simpson, 1993).

Furthermore, recurrent fallers may have suffered one or more long lies, so particular attention needs to be paid to their own, and their carers', methods of coping with previous falls and to whether or not they have sound strategies in place for coping with future falls – as no doubt there will be more of these! Many recurrent fallers may express fear of falling and admit to have restricted their activities for this reason.

People for whom there is a clear medical explanation for their falls which has been successfully treated, may not be at risk of further falling. For example, insertion of a pacemaker may have corrected a cardiac arrhythmia, or the cause of anaemia may have been identified and treated. Other conditions associated with falls may remain unidentified and untreated, however; the physiotherapist should be alert to this possibility.

Detailed Physiotherapy Assessment

Measurement for pure research may be as complicated and expensive as there are funds to pay for it. In the clinical situation, however (which is nevertheless a research situation with a particular patient), measurement techniques must not only be valid and reliable, but must be quick and easy to use, easy to carry about, and preferably be cheap. At best they should require no more than a stop watch, a tape-measure or other portable instrument.

A key distinction during selection is whether the measure is to identify the presence or extent of a problem or to pick up a clinically significant change, i.e. to discriminate or to be responsive. An instrument is not always useful for both tasks.

Some of the measures mentioned in this section are described in the Canadian Physiotherapy Association's (CPA) compendium of the measures most frequently used in Canada (Cole et al., 1994). The grouping is by the levels of outcome of chronic disease. Sometimes it can be difficult to decide at which level a procedure measures, so no claims are made that the groups assigned are definitive. Nor should the measures listed to be regarded as a definitive selection; many more have been published. Physiotherapists specializing in rehabilitation of older people who work in the same service or the same geographical region should band together to decide which battery of measures is most useful to them.

Measurement of Handicap

Measurement at this level is not common in the clinical situation although highly recommended in research. The Philadelphia Morale Scale has been recommended for assessment at this level by the Royal College of Physicians of London and the British Geriatrics Society (Simpson and Forster, 1993). Interestingly, a score less than 10 out of 17 on this scale was a risk factor for falling among elderly people admitted to intermediate care facilities in New York state (Tinetti et al., 1986). However, it has yet to be shown that reducing the risk improves morale.

Environmental hazard assessment

This encompasses more than just the identification, by the client or by a professional, of hazards in a person's home such as loose rugs, slippery floors, broken steps; it means all hazards extrinsic to the client, including clothing and the behaviour of other people. Except for overwhelming balance threats, being pushed or even attacked by another person, many of these factors are minor and would not precipitate a fall in a fit older person. However, frail old people often lack the physiological reserves to cope with many minor balance threats, and it is thought that environmental factors contribute to most of their falls.

Unsafe footwear and unsuitable clothing can pose a threat to balance and should be assessed under this heading. Balance is an attention-demanding activity, so that elderly people with poor postural skills may need to concentrate very hard on keeping their balance, even during simple activities of daily living. If they become distracted by concern about the possibility of their trousers falling down, or by uncomfortable footwear, then the risk is considerably increased. Incontinence garments, in particular, can pose serious hazards. Pads inserted into loose fitting knickers or underpants, rather than being held in place with the correctly matching, well-fitting pants, may slide out of position and inhibit walking. Worse can happen to a woman wearing a skirt; the pad can drop to the floor and the natural reaction to stoop quickly to pick it up may possibly result in a fall. Not only can carelessly chosen incontinence garments be a risk factor for falling, but they are also a barrier to confident mobility.

House assessments, or home visits with the patient present, are often managed by a health visitor, occupational therapist or physiotherapist. Tideiksaar (1986) has produced a useful checklist for identifying hazards in a person's home.

Measurements of Disability

Risk of falling is a huge disability: the mobility screen is useful to identify people at risk (Studentski et al., 1994). The timed up-and-go (Cole et al., 1994) can also be used to pick out people with poor postural skills. The rating in degrees of 'normality' is not as helpful as doing so in degrees of 'safety', but this modification is still being tested. The timed element also makes the test responsive to change.

Tinetti (1986) also emphasizes observation of clients performing balance-related manoeuvres in order to identify performance deficits that will be targeted for retraining. Being at risk is related to inability to perform key functions safely: to walk, to manage steps, to stand and reach, to sit down and stand up, and to transfer, as well as to be able to withstand a mild perturbation. Postural ability during functional tasks may be either rated or timed. Tinetti (1986) gives rules for deciding whether or not each manoeuvre has been carried out normally.

Many of these manoeuvres can be timed although there may be lack of consensus of how long or how quick is most desirable. Stability has been related to gait speed, but time to walk a measured distance may be difficult to assess in a person's home if a walkway of sufficient length cannot be cleared. Allowing a turn introduces another element. Speed over 3 metres may be all there is space to assess or a functional distance (e.g. bed to toilet) may be most appropriate for that particular client. Walking devices may be used. The same normal footwear should be worn each time, and a decision has to be made between a standing or a walking start.

Another ability clearly necessary for safe function is the ability to stand without holding on to a support. The client should be allowed to hold on at first but then asked to let go when timing begins. This manoeuvre is included in several motor and function tests, but no consensus about time limits emerges. As with most of the timed tests, the final score should be the mean of three trials, to increase the reliability of the measure.

Measurements of Impairment

Once the client's balance-related disabilities have been identified the physiotherapist next seeks the underlying impairment. This may be muscle weakness, joint stiffness, pain, fear, or something else.

At this level there is no shortage of tests and instruments with which to collect baseline data. Physiotherapists should be able to identify clients who have psychological concerns related to their mobility. Two sets of information are needed: whether or not the person is afraid of falling (impairment) and second whether the person has restricted their activities through fear (disability).

Fear of falling has been defined as a lasting concern about falling. Questioning about fear will differ according to whether the interviewee is a recurrent faller, at risk, or has sustained a sudden onset of falling for medical reasons. Recurrent fallers are unlikely to be surprised at being posed a simple question, 'Are you afraid of falling?' and given the choice of responses 'Not at all', 'somewhat' 'very much' (Maki et al., 1991). Clients may find it helpful to be allowed to make their choice of response from an array of possible answers written clearly on cards.

A rather more indirect approach may be indicated for clients in the 'at risk' group and for intermittent fallers. A simple open-ended probe may be all that is necessary to elicit their reaction. Examples are:

'How did you feel after the fall',
'How do you feel about the falls'

If the client clearly has no problem this fact should be recorded (score = 'not at all') but the matter need not be pursued. On the other hand, if any degree of anxiety is manifest, some quantification is indicated, perhaps using Maki et al.'s question. Clients should be encouraged to voice their fears – at some length if necessary – as they may not have had the chance to do so previously. Particular attention should be paid to any information that may indicate a fruitful approach to restoring confidence.

Tinetti et al. (1994b) have operationalized 'fear of falling' in terms of self-efficacy. However the ten questions of the 'Falls Efficacy Scale' (FES) sound similar to self-assessed ADL items and clients may have difficulty differentiating one from the other. Among community-dwelling elders, FES scores were significantly related to levels of fear of falling and to self-reported functional ability. Many items touch on abilities beyond the capability of frail older people. The items on the scale may be useful for documenting responsiveness to interventions.

Clients in all groups who express fear should be questioned about any activities they avoid because of fear or that they are now nervous of performing. These activities will, with the client's agreement, be the focus of rehabilitation and set the goals of treatment.

Physiotherapy Management

Physiotherapy interventions are directed at preventing further falls, at preparing older people to cope with further falls, and at helping people regain confidence in their own postural skills. The emphasis varies between different clients.

It is not usual for occasional or intermittent fallers to be referred for physiotherapy, so many people with loss of confidence are left to cope with their problems as best they can. Recurrent fallers and those at risk, on the other hand, are usually treated during admission to acute care. Too often the solution to their instability problems has been to provide a walking aid and ensure that the person knows how to use it. Sometimes 'gait training' is merely following along behind a client who is walking unsteadily towards an ill-defined goal. Physiotherapists now appreciate that an active interventionist rehabilitative approach is needed.

Only a few intervention studies have been completed and most are of little help in choosing specific treatments for this group of clients. Interventions have been general rather than specific (Reinsch et al., 1992). However, a targeted, multiple-risk factor intervention, the Yale FICST study, which included physiotherapy, did have a statistically significant success in reducing falls during one year follow-up (Tinetti et al., 1994a). The community-dwelling participants were at least 70 years of age, independently ambulant (and so not particularly frail), and each showed at least one of eight falls-risk factors: two related to medication, evidence of hypotension and five mobility-related factors. The latter included any reduction in walking or transfer or balance ability, leg or arm muscle strength or range of motion. Koch et al. (1994) described the physiotherapy approach dealing with each of these specific problems. Besides the impact on falling, confidence in balance ability, as meased by the FES, improved more in the intervention group.

Increasing Postural Stability and Ability to Resist Balance Threat

At the end of the Yale study described above, two types of participants showed the greatest difference between intervention and controls in terms of specific risk reduction. These were people who had started with problems of balance or transfers and those who took four or more prescription medications.

The outcome of this investigation lends support to the hypothesis, also suggested by Studentski et al. (1994), that in order to reduce the risk of falling older people's postural skills need to be improved. This should be achieved by strengthening and increasing the endurance in the lower limb muscles, and through balance training.

Several prospective studies point to weakness in the lower limbs being more common among older people who have fallen than among those who have not; weak ankle dorsiflexors may be particularly critical (Simpson, 1993). Weak legs may precipitate falls, as when a person is unable to complete a transfer successfully, or unable to stand long enough without holding on to something to successfully manage clothing after using the toilet. Weakness may reduce the person's ability to resist falling once a perturbation has occurred.

The Yale group were clearly surprised that a greater effect for leg muscle strengthening exercises did not emerge in their study. They attributed this to the insensitivity of manual muscle testing and to the intensity and duration of the programme not having been great enough. Their surprise is understandable as it is known that even frail, very old people enjoy strenuous exercise and can improve quadriceps strength by using high-intensity, resisted exercise (Fiatrone and Williams, 1993) or low-intensity exercise (McMurdo and Rennie, 1994).

In the clinical situation, time for rehabilitation may be limited. Physiotherapists are advised to devise regimes concentrating on the movements and activities at which the client wishes to become more stable, and to do so by applying the exercise physiological principles of specificity and overload. A regime should be as intensive, in terms of repetitions per session and number of sessions per day, as the client can tolerate, and in hospital or institutions it can be supplemented by general fitness circuits using equipment such as a Kinetron, Westminster weight and pulley systems (Smith et al., 1995). Regimes devised for clients to follow in their own homes should follow the same principles (Koch et al., 1994). An obviously useful exercise is sit-to-stand; an increase in the speed to complete this manoeuvre reduces the risk of falling, probably by increasing muscle strength. Koch *et al.* (1994) described the scheme of progressive balance exercises used in the Yale study. Other schemes are to be found in the neurorehabilitation literature and evidence is emerging that balance exercises such as Tai Chi can reduce risk of falling. Frail older people should be helped to increase their ability to:

- Stand unsupported or with the minimum possible support, progressing to standing while doing up belts and buttons, reaching for objects on higher and higher shelves, picking up objects from chair-seats and from the floor. (Higher level clients can try standing with eyes closed, standing on foam of increasing thickness, even doing both.)
- Withstand perturbations by compensatory stepping in response to a gentle push on the sternum or laterally on the pelvis.
- Walk steadily (without support of another person) for the maximum distance needed in their own home (emphasize even step lengths). Training should begin with the shortest distance the client feels confident of tackling.
- Turn on the spot with fewer and fewer steps, about four to six maximum.
- Cope with steps of increasing height.

Increasing the Safety of Older People's Environment; Reducing Environmental Hazards

Common sense suggests that removing hazards in people's homes will reduce their risk of tripping. However, there is little hard evidence to support this assumption. Tinetti *et al.* (1988) found no independent association between falling and environmental hazards in the home, whereas Studentski *et al.* (1994) found that the environmental domain was a much weaker predictor of falling that either mobility factors or, interestingly, clients' tendency to avoid risk. Participants in a New Zealand community study most commonly fell over objects not identified as potential hazards by an occupational therapist. Over 1000 loose mats had been identified as potential hazards, but only five of them actually caused falls. The great majority of falls occurred over household objects (chair legs, foot rests, toilet seat frames) in uncluttered environments (Campbell *et al.*, 1990). These results do not mean that home hazard assessments are redundant, but rather that attention to these alone cannot be expected to prevent falling.

It is not always possible to predict what is going to cause the trip, and clients do not always comply with instructions for environmental changes. Poor lighting may be corrected easily but may not be welcomed by the client, who fears a rise in electricity costs. A person may like having a particular rug in a particular place, and resent a suggestion for change.

It will probably be of most value, as Reinsch *et al.* (1992) suggest, to add an increasingly cognitive focus to fall prevention, 'training older adults to be vigilant for environmental hazards in the house and in the community as well as teaching them to act preventively and to consider the risks they are taking'. Training can be interpreted as discussing with older people how they and their carers propose to maximize the safety of their home. Home visits should include practice with those activities most likely to lead to accidents and to find alternatives to those which cannot be carried out safely. A house-proud person may need to be reassured that visitors are not going to notice if the top of the cupboard has not been dusted! However, one home safety assessment and educa-

Figure 1.   The Sabine solution to dealing with a fall.

Martin Sabine, cofounder of a company producing simple but effective aids for patient movement, has developed the following solution for raising a person from the floor when no hoist is available. This enables one or two people to safely raise even a fairly dependent person from the floor onto a chair.

1. Assuming that the person is lying on his back, first check that it is medically safe to move him (if in doubt *don't*). If there are no contraindications, reassure him and make him comfortable whilst you collect the items you will require. These are two ordinary kitchen-type chairs, some cushions or thick books such as telephone directories. Place these in a handy position.

2. Turn him over onto his weaker side, so that his stronger arm is upper-most. Bend his hips to 90° and help him to place his top hand on the floor close to his body so that it can be used to assist on the next phase.

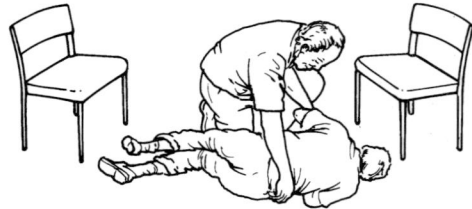

3. Kneel close to his body, level with the hips, and lean over to grasp the hip that is resting on the floor. Now ease him into an all-fours position, supporting his trunk with your legs and body.

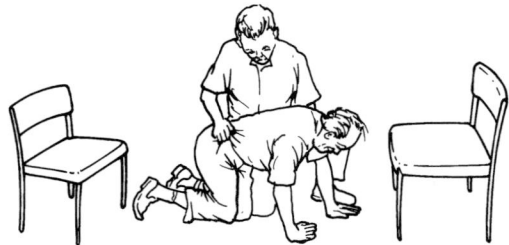

4. Help him to place his arms on the chair which you have previously placed close to his head. Carefully adjust his position to ensure that he is stable.

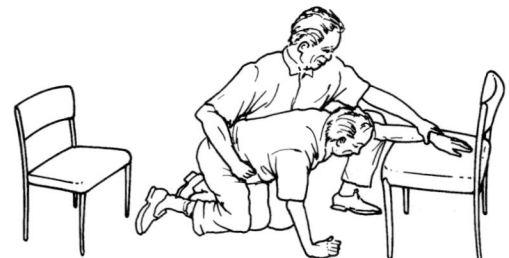

5. Using cushions or telephone directories, block the person's knees, one at a time, in order to raise the rear portion of his body about 15 cm (6 in) from the floor.

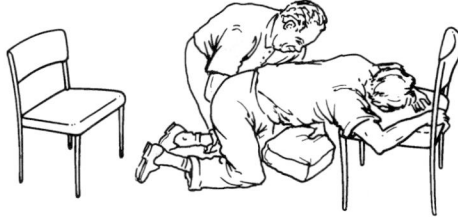

6. Having ensured that he is comfortable and safe, place the other chair behind him, tilting it, so that his bottom rests on the chair in an apparently seated position.

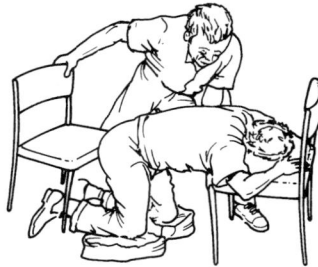

7. Supporting his trunk with one arm and stabilizing the chair with the other, ease him and the chair backwards until the chair is in a normal position and then adjust his posture if necessary.

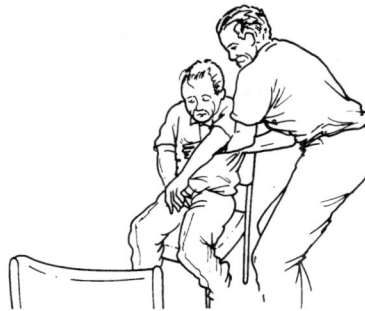

8. This technique can readily be adapted for two people.

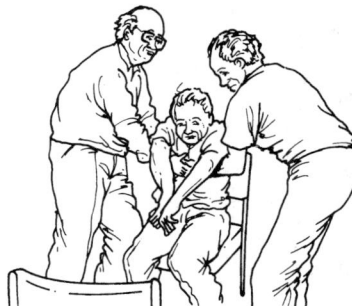

Note: Like all load movement techniques the method described above requires some skill, particularly in those who wish to teach it to others. You are advised to practise the manoeuvre using a light-weight model until you have achieved the necessary competence.

tional programme did not lead to the programme participants implementing any more safety precautions than the control group, both groups fell equally often (El-Faizy and Reinsch, 1994).

Coping with a Fall and Preventing a Long Lie and its Consequences

Commonly frail older people are unable to get up without assistance after a fall. Even those who can manage to get up with ease when at their best in the morning, may be unable to do so when tired later in the day.

Five people in the New Zealand study each had two falls after which they lay on the ground for more than 1 hour; one person lay for 12 hours, one for 7 hours. In this study people lay for 1 hour or more after 27 falls (Campbell *et al.*, 1990). Over a third of the older people questioned in a British study also claimed to have spent 1 hour or more on the floor after their last fall; more than one half of all fallers had had to wait for help to come (Simpson and Mandelstam, 1995). Since prolonged periods on the floor, especially if the person is unable to move, may lead to hypothermia, bronchopneumonia and pressure sores, as well as to the embarrassment of not being able to use the toilet and to pangs of hunger and thirst, physiotherapists are strongly urged to teach all their older clients how to get up from the floor without assistance from others.

This has not been a common procedure; only a small proportion of elders at risk appear to be willing and able to learn this skill (Simpson and Mandelstam, 1995). Many old people are reluctant to confront the problem of falling, denying that there is a risk, and over-estimating their own ability to get up from the floor. Carefully adapted teaching techniques requiring considerable skill and expert judgement are required of the phy-

siotherapist for success to be achieved (Reece and Simpson, 1996).

Nevertheless, people at risk of falling need to be helped to face up to the risk and be guided to work out strategies for coping when the next fall happens. Clients will have to be taught how to prevent hypothermia, pressure sores and bronchopneumonia and taught well enough for them to remember the advice in an emergency. Panic can set in at this time and previous lessons may be forgotten. Carers may need to be taught how to get an old person up from the floor without endangering themselves. The Sabine Method has been developed for this purpose (Figure 1). When the old person at risk lives alone and is unable to get up with ease a care-alarm may be the solution. However, just installing the system is not enough. An older person needs careful training in how and when to use the alarm. Although these recommendations seem to accord with common sense, evidence is awaited to show that teaching patients how to cope with a fall actually prevents the complications of a long lie.

Restoring Confidence in Balance Ability

Successful educational and intervention programmes should instill feelings of self-efficacy in older clients and restore confidence in their own ability to cope. In turn, fear of falling and the associated fear of not being able to get up should be reduced, and this may lead to greater confidence in walking and less risk of falling. Some evidence of improved confidence comes from the Yale intervention study in which the FES scores were significantly reduced among participants (Tinetti *et al.*, 1994).

A psycho-physiotherapeutic approach may be particularly useful when managing these problems. The person's assumptions of incompetence may be challenged by providing opportunities to practise balance tasks of increasing difficulty, i.e. by graded exposure to balance threat. The physiotherapist ensures that the chosen task is within the client's physical competence and once it has been performed successfully the client is encouraged to acknowledge their achievement and recognize their own competence.

Summary

Postural instability and falling are now recognized as disabilities meriting careful assessment and intervention by members of the multidisciplinary team rehabilitating older people. Physiotherapy is directed at intrinsic and extrinsic risk factors, in particular to improving ability to withstand balance-threats, to increasing safety of the environment, preventing the consequences of a 'long lie', and to restore confidence in functional balance ability. Tests, measures and checklists are available to assess degree of risk and the disabilities and underlying impairments associated with the risk of falling and guide decision-making in each of the four goal areas. Likewise, research findings are becoming available to guide the development of effective physiotherapy interventions in these areas. Guidelines for the rehabilitation management of this client group have been produced by the author in consultation with the Association of Chartered Physiotherapists with a Special Interest in Elderly People and with the Association of Chartered Physiotherapists in the Community (Simpson et al., 1998).

References

Black, SE, Maki, BE, Fernie, GR (1993) Aging, imbalance and falls. In Sharpe, JA and Barber, HO, *The Vestibular-Ocular Reflex and Vertigo*, pp. 317–335. New York: Raven Press.

Campbell, AJ, Borrie, MJ, Spears, GF et al. (1990) Circumstances and consequences of falls experienced by a community population 70 years and over during a prospective study. *Age and Ageing* 19: 136–141.

Cole, B, Finch, E, Gowland, C, Mayo, N (1993) *Physical Rehabilitation Outcome Measures*. Toronto: Canadian Physiotherapy Association.

El-Faizy, MJ, Reinsch, S (1994) Home safety intervention for prevention of falls. *Physical and Occupational Therapy in Geriatrics* 12: 33–49.

Fiatarone, MA, Evans, WJ (1993) The etiology and reversibility of muscle dysfunction in the aged. *Journal of Gerontology* 48 (Special Issue 77–83).

Isaacs, B (1992) *The Challenge of Geriatric Medicine*. Oxford: Oxford University Press.

Koch, M, Gottschalk, M, Baker, D et al. (1994) An impairment and disability assessment and treatment protocol for community-living elderly persons. *Physical Therapy* 74: 286–295.

Maki, BE, Holliday, PJ, Topper, AK (1991) Fear of falling and postural performance in the elderly. *Journal of Gerontology* 46: M123–131.

McMurdo, ME, Rennie, LM (1994) Improvements in quadriceps strength with regular seated exercise in the institutionalized elderly. *Archives of Physical Medicine and Rehabilitation* 75: 600–603.

Reece, A, Simpson, JM (1996) Teaching elderly people how to cope after a fall. *Physiotherapy* 82: 227–235.

Reinsch, S, MacRae, P, Lachenbruch, PA, Tobis, JS (1992) Why do healthy older adults fall? Behavioural and environmental risks. *Physical and Occupational Therapy in Geriatrics* 11: 1–15.

Simpson, JM (1993) Elderly people at risk of falling: The role of muscle weakness. *Physiotherapy* 79: 831–835.

Simpson, JM, Forster, A (1993) Assessing elderly people: should we all use the same scales? *Physiotherapy* 79: 836–838.

Simpson JM, Harrington R, Marsh N (1998) Managing falls among elderly people. *Physiotherapy* 84: 173–177.

Simpson, JM, Mandelstam, M (1995) Elderly people at risk of falling: do they want to be taught how to get up again? *Clinical Rehabilitation* 9: 65–69.

Smith, S, Simpson, JM, Hastie, IH (1995) Elderly people need more exercise: a functional exercise system. *Physiotherapy* 81: 605–610.

Studentski, S, Duncan, PW, Chandler, J et al. (1994) Predicting falls: the role of mobility and non-physical factors. *Journal of the American Geriatrics Society* 42: 297–302.

Tideiksaar (1986) Preventing falls: Home hazard checklists to help old people protect themselves. *Geriatrics* 41: 26–28.

Tinetti, ME (1986) Performance-oriented assessment of mobility problems in elderly patients. *Journal of the American Geriatrics Society* 34: 119–126.

Tinetti, ME, Speechley, M (1989) Prevention of falls among the elderly. *New England Journal of Medicine* 320: 1055–1059.

Tinetti, ME, Williams, TF, Mayewski, R (1986) Fall risk index for elderly patients based on number of chronic disabilities. *American Journal of Medicine* 80: 429–434.

Tinetti, ME, Speechley, MI, Ginter, SF (1988) Risk factors for falls among elderly persons living in the community. *New England Journal of Medicine* 319: 1701–1707.

Tinetti, ME, Baker, DI, McAvay, G *et al.* (1994a) A multifactorial intervention to reduce the risk of falling among elderly people living in the community. *New England Journal of Medicine* 331: 822–827. (See also letter on p. 872.)

Tinetti, ME, Mendes de Leon, CF, Doucette, JT, Baker, DI (1994b) Fear of falling and fall-related efficacy in relationship to functioning among community-living elders. *Journal of Gerontology* 49: M140–M147.

16

Osteoporosis and Osteoporotic Fractures

ELSIE G CULHAM

Pathophysiology
•
Classification and Aetiology
•
Diagnostic Tests
•
Prevention and Treatment
•
Summary

Osteoporosis is a clinical syndrome where bone mass is lower than that expected for an individual of a given age, race and gender resulting in bone weakness and a high risk of fracture. It is the most common metabolic bone disease in older people (Chapter 4) estimated to affect one in four women and one in ten men over the age of 50 years in North America. Osteoporosis is the major cause of fractures in older individuals and postmenopausal women leading to premature death, considerable disability, and enormous medical costs (Josse, 1989) (Chapter 15). The number of individuals sustaining osteoporotic fractures is expected to rise because of increased longevity and the rising geriatric population. Physiotherapists will play a key role in the development and implementation of programmes designed to prevent osteoporosis and the resulting fractures

as well as in the treatment of older adults with osteoporotic fractures. To provide optimal care, physiotherapists must understand the disease process, the consequences of skeletal fracture and the role of education and exercise in prevention and management of this syndrome. This chapter will provide information about the pathophysiology and aetiology of osteoporosis and outline preventative and treatment strategies with particular emphasis on physiotherapy.

Pathophysiology

The adult skeleton consists of approximately 80% cortical (compact) bone and 20% trabecular (cancellous, spongy) bone. Cortical bone, composed of layers or lamellae of bone organized around a nutrient (Haversian) canal, predominates in the shafts of the long bones of the appendicular or peripheral skeleton. Trabecular bone consists of vertical and horizontal plates of bone surrounded by a cortical shell. This type of bone is concentrated in the vertebrae, pelvis and ends of long bones (Riggs and Melton, 1986).

Bone is a dynamic tissue which undergoes constant remodelling throughout life. It is able to adapt to physical stresses placed upon it and is capable of repair in cases of trauma. The ability of bone to remodel over time is due to activity of the bone cells. During normal remodelling osteoclasts tunnel into cortical bone or into lacunae on the surface of trabecular bone resorbing bone by dissolving both mineral and osteoid. Osteoblasts simultaneously lay down new bone in the resorption cavities, creating a new structural unit of bone. In young bone, absorption/resorption are tightly coupled and bone mass is maintained (Simon, 1993). Bone remodelling occurs on the bone surfaces. Since trabecular bone has a greater surface to volume ratio than cortical bone, remodelling occurs to a greater extent. It has been estimated that the turnover rate of trabecular bone is 30% annually compared with a 10% annual turnover of cortical bone (Simon, 1993).

The loss of bone mass in osteoporosis may be due to either excess bone resorption or to a decrease in bone formation rate. In the first case, resorption may be greater than normal creating large tunnels due to osteoclast activity. Although osteoblasts may be functioning normally, insufficient osteoid is synthesized to fill the defect. In the second scenario, resorption is normal but bone formation is defective. Regardless of the mechanism, bone resorption always exceeds formation resulting in an overall decrease in bone mass. The remaining bone is morphologically and chemically normal.

Classification and Aetiology

Osteoporosis is classified as primary or secondary. Secondary osteoporosis occurs in cases where bone mass is reduced subsequent to pathological processes including endocrine disorders (hypogonadism, hyperparathyroidism, hyperthyroidism), nutrient-absorption deficiencies, bone marrow malignancy, prolonged use of drugs which influence bone metabolism such as corticosteroids, and renal failure (Josse, 1989). Primary osteoporosis refers to cases where the aetiology is unclear and has been divided into two types depending on the subject's age and sex. Type I (postmenopausal) osteoporosis occurs in women in the postmenopausal years (age 50–70 years) and is characterized by a period of accelerated loss, primarily of trabecular bone (Josse, 1989). This type of osteoporosis is often associated with a high rate of bone turnover in which resorption is increased and bone formation is inadequate to compensate. Vertebral fractures and Colles' fractures of the forearm are the most common fractures in this group. Type II (senile) osteoporosis occurs in both men and women over the age of 70 years. This type of osteoporosis is associated with slow and proportionate loss of trabecular and cortical bone due primarily to a decrease in bone formation. Hip fractures are more common in this population.

Several risk factors, associated with the development of primary osteoporosis, are outlined in Figure 1. These include the normal ageing process, gender, genetic predisposition, race, body mass and life style factors including activity level, inadequate calcium consumption and alcohol and tobacco use.

Figure 1   Conceptual model of aetiology of fractures related to primary osteoporosis.

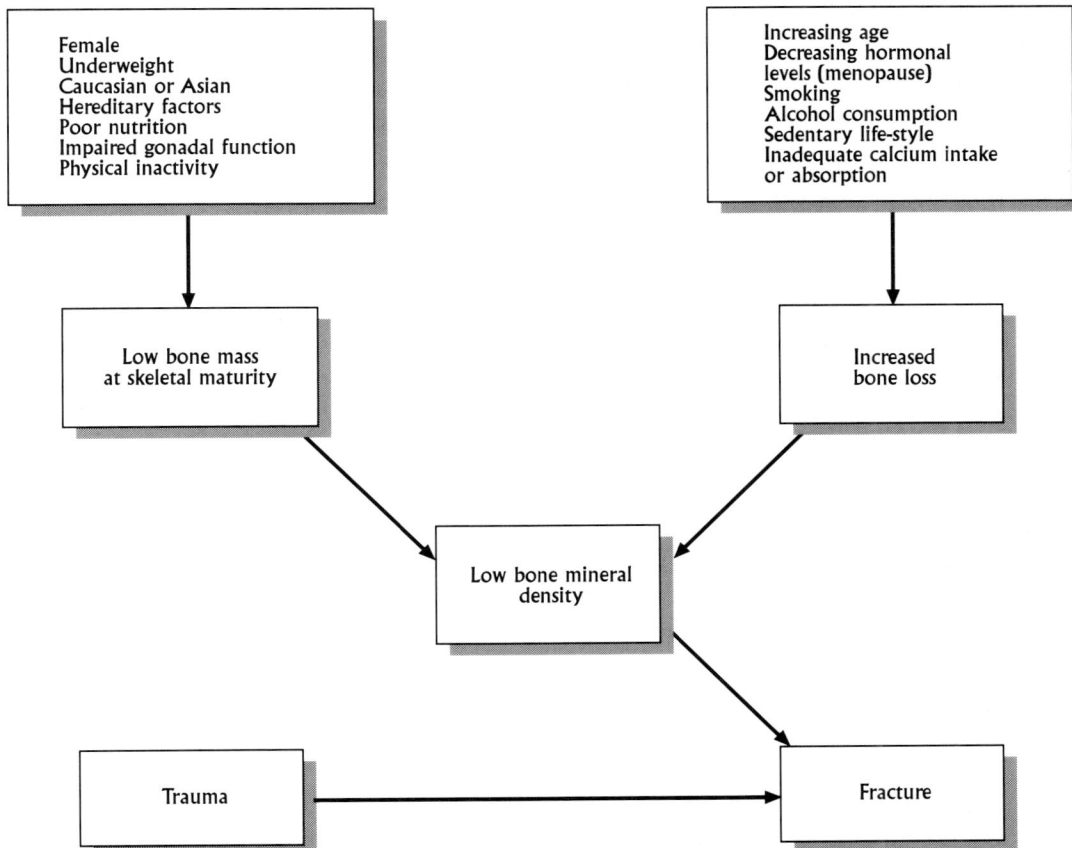

```
┌─────────────────────────────┐        ┌─────────────────────────────┐
│ Female                      │        │ Increasing age              │
│ Underweight                 │        │ Decreasing hormonal         │
│ Caucasian or Asian          │        │ levels (menopause)          │
│ Hereditary factors          │        │ Smoking                     │
│ Poor nutrition              │        │ Alcohol consumption         │
│ Impaired gonadal function   │        │ Sedentary life-style        │
│ Physical inactivity         │        │ Inadequate calcium intake   │
│                             │        │ or absorption               │
└─────────────────────────────┘        └─────────────────────────────┘
              │                                      │
              ▼                                      ▼
   ┌──────────────────────┐             ┌──────────────────────┐
   │ Low bone mass        │             │ Increased            │
   │ at skeletal maturity │             │ bone loss            │
   └──────────────────────┘             └──────────────────────┘
              │                                      │
               ╲                                    ╱
                ╲         ┌──────────────────┐    ╱
                 ╲───────▶│ Low bone mineral │◀──╱
                          │ density          │
                          └──────────────────┘
                                   │
                                    ╲
   ┌──────────────────┐              ╲      ┌──────────────────┐
   │ Trauma           │──────────────▶──────│ Fracture         │
   └──────────────────┘                     └──────────────────┘
```

Age

Age is the most important determinant of bone mass. Up to 95% of the peak bone mass is deposited during childhood and adolescence prior to closure of the epiphyses. This growth phase is followed by a 10–15 year consolidation period during which bone mass increases further, resulting in achievement of peak bone mass in the early- to mid-30s. Bone loss begins once skeletal maturity has been achieved. This is a universal phenomenon, occurring in both males and females regardless of race, geographical location, occupation, exercise and dietary habits. Generally, females lose bone more rapidly than males and onset of loss, at least of trabecular bone, occurs earlier. Over a lifetime, women lose about 35% of their peak cortical bone and 50% of trabecular bone. Men lose approximately two-thirds of these amounts (Riggs and Melton, 1986) (see also Chapter 6).

Gender and Hormonal Function

Osteoporosis primarily affects women. Bone mass is lower in women than in men at skeletal maturity and with bone loss in later life women are more likely to reach fracture threshold. Second, lowered levels of oestrogen at any time in a woman's life affects bone mass. Young women who become amenorrhoeic due to intense physical exercise have significant bone loss. Similarly, other conditions which affect menstrual function in young women (see Chapters 12, 13), such as eating disorders and late onset of menarche, have a detrimental effect on bone mass. More commonly, decreased oestrogen levels related to natural or surgically induced menopause, is often associated with a period of accelerated bone loss in women. Oestrogen deficiency affects bone mass by decreasing efficiency of intestinal calcium absorption and enhancing the ability of osteoclasts to resorb bone (Slemenda, 1994).

The role of androgens on bone loss in women has been studied less extensively. However, there is evidence that postmenopausal women with higher androgen levels lose bone at lower rates than other women. Testosterone levels are also an important determinant of bone mass in men; influencing both peak bone mass and rate of bone loss (Slemenda, 1994).

Genetic/Ethnic Determinants

Bone mass in all age groups is strongly influenced by genetic factors. Less variability in bone mineral density (BMD) is found between monozygotic compared with dizygotic twins. Similarly, BMD of adults correlates with that of their children and daughters of mothers with spinal fractures have lower BMD than control subjects. These findings may be due in large part to similarities in body composition, bone size and endocrine function. Children also are likely to adopt the life-style habits of their parents which may contribute to the similarities in bone mass found in families.

Racial or ethnic differences in bone mass have also been identified. Caucasian, Hispanic and Asian women are at greatest risk for osteoporosis due in part to lower bone and muscle mass in these individuals. In the USA, hip fracture rates are approximately twice as high in the Caucasian versus the African–American population. Differences in bone mineral density between ethnic groups may be related to genetic or dietary and other life-style factors that are similar within an ethnic group (Bachrach, 1994).

Body Mass

Low body weight is associated with low bone mass and fracture risk. Thin women of smaller stature have a greater fracture risk than obese women. Obesity may protect women from bone loss following menopause by increasing the amount of biologically available oestrogen or by providing a greater stimulus to bone formation due to weight bearing forces (Scott and Hochberg, 1993). Low body weight has also been found to be a risk factor for vertebral fracture in men.

Life-style Factors

A sedentary life-style is a risk factor for osteoporosis (see Chapter 6). It has been well established that immobilization and bed rest lead to bone loss. Significant bone loss has been reported in young people placed on bed rest following spinal fusion and Harrington rod instrumentation and in individuals placed on bed rest for low back pain. Similarly, healthy, young men placed on bed rest lose bone. Exercise while in a recumbent position did not prevent bone loss;

however, quiet standing for several hours a day was effective in preventing bone loss in these individuals (Vargo and Gerber, 1993).

High levels of physical activity in childhood are positively correlated with bone mass at skeletal maturity. Similarly, it has been demonstrated that more physically fit and active adults have significantly greater bone mass than those who are more sedentary and athletes have significantly greater bone density than subjects who do not exercise regularly (Vargo and Gerber, 1993). The positive association between bone density and physical activity in young women is found until such time as the intensity of exercise becomes sufficient to interrupt menstrual function.

Other life-style risk factors for primary osteoporosis include inadequate calcium, and cigarette and alcohol consumption. Low dietary calcium intake, particularly during the years of bone development, affects peak bone mass and appears to be a risk factor for the later development of osteoporosis. Adequate dietary calcium continues to be important for maintenance of bone density in later life, particularly in the elderly. Cigarette smoking is clearly detrimental to skeletal health in both men and women. Women who smoke experience menopause an average of 1.2 years earlier and have greater bone loss in the postmenopausal period than non-smokers; possibly due to the detrimental effects of smoking on oestrogen metabolism. However, male smokers also lose bone at a greater rate than non-smokers suggesting that smoking is a risk factor independent of its effect on oestrogen metabolism. Moderate alcohol consumption is associated with bone loss in men but not in women. Chronic alcoholism is often associated with poor nutrition and decreased calcium absorption and is a risk factor in both men and women (Slemenda, 1994).

Diagnostic Tests

Osteoporosis has been called the silent thief. Significant bone loss (osteopenia) may occur without any clinical signs or symptoms and many individuals with bone loss may never experience osteoporotic fractures. Current diagnostic tests for osteoporosis consist of radiographs and bone density measures. Bone loss must exceed 30–40% before it is detected on standard radiographs. However, vertebral fractures associated with spinal osteoporosis are usually readily distinguishable on lateral spine radiographs.

Bone mass can be measured *in vivo* using a variety of techniques. Single photon absorptiometry (SPA) is used to evaluate primarily cortical bone mass in the appendicular skeleton. Dual photon absorptiometry (DPA) and dual energy X-ray absorptiometry (DXA), are useful for evaluation of both trabecular and cortical bone in the appendicular and axial skeleton. Bone mass measures are expressed as bone mineral content (BMC), the total grams of bone mineral within a given area of bone or bone mineral density (BMD), the bone mineral content per square centimetre. Quantitative computerized tomography (QCT) provides accurate measures of trabecular bone within the vertebrae but is associated with higher radiation exposure than other techniques. The preferred technique currently in use is DXA, because of ease of measurement, precision and low radiation exposure.

Bone density measurement techniques aid in diagnosis and are useful for determining long-term efficacy of treatment. However, osteoporotic fractures are related to bone strength, the determinants of which include bone mineral density, geometry or structure and material properties (brittleness). *In vivo* measures of the latter two parameters are not currently available. Measures of BMD provide an estimate of bone strength only, and therefore, have some limitation in ability to accurately predict future fracture risk.

Prevention and Treatment

Prevention Strategies

Osteoporosis is largely preventable through a reduction in the risk factors previously outlined. Preventive strategies are aimed at attaining maximal peak bone mass at skeletal maturity, maintaining bone mass during young adulthood and middle age, and minimizing the decline in bone mass with ageing and during the postmenopausal period in women.

The greater the bone mass at skeletal maturity the less likely the individual will reach fracture threshold with loss of bone in later life. The peak bone mass that an individual will achieve is in part dependent on genetic factors. However, environmental and life-style factors, which can be modified, also play a role. Thus, life-style habits which facilitate bone mineral acquisition need to be encouraged throughout the childhood and adolescent years. Maintenance of adequate intake of daily calcium is essential for bone development and maintenance of mass in adulthood. The daily calcium requirement during childhood and adolescence is 1200 mg. Calcium supplementation has been shown to have the greatest effect on bone mass when administered to children in the prepuberty period. The daily calcium requirement in the women during the postmenopausal years increases to 1500 mg. Dietary inadequacy of calcium intake has been demonstrated in individuals over 70 years of age and supplementation is recommended if diet fails to provide the age appropriate amount.

Maintenance of adequate body weight is also important during the years of bone growth and consolidation. Thus, the promotion of extreme thinness as the ideal body type, particularly in young women, needs to be discouraged and good nutritional habits need to be encouraged throughout life. Recognition and management of eating disorders is essential to minimize the detrimental effect of these disorders on skeletal health.

Physical activity should be encouraged throughout childhood and during adulthood (see Chapter 12). Any sports and activities which promote weight bearing and enhance cardiovascular fitness would appear to provide an adequate stimulus for bone formation. Programmes designed to prevent or reduce smoking and alcohol consumption in young people would be of benefit in the prevention of osteoposoris in addition to the other potential health benefits of such programmes.

Oestrogen (estrogen) replacement therapy (ETR), also termed hormone replacement therapy (HRT) in postmenopausal women is effective in slowing or stopping bone loss. In addition, oestrogen replacement has been shown to be effective in reducing the incidence of hip and vertebral fractures in Caucasian women. It is estimated that widespread long-term oestrogen use could reduce hip fractures by approximately 50% (Scott and Hochberg, 1993). Beneficial effects of oestrogen on skeletal health have been documented even in women who first used HRT more than a decade after the onset of menopause. Muscle mass and strength are also enhanced by HRT. Since reduced muscle strength is a risk factor for falling, oestrogen may help lower the risk, particularly of hip and forearm fracture, through decreased risk of fall episodes. However, HRT is not without risk. Unopposed oestrogen use increases the risk of uterine cancer, although this risk is minimized by the simultaneous administration of progestins. Long-term use of oestrogen may also increase the risk of breast cancer and therefore may be an inappropriate choice of treatment for a women with a family history of this condition. Problems of compliance with long-term oestrogen use have also been reported.

Other anti-resorptive drugs may also be of benefit in the prevention of osteoporosis. Both calcitonin and bisphosphonates (etidronate disodium), have been found to decrease overall bone loss. Long-term studies need to be completed to determine efficacy of these agents in reducing fracture incidence.

Management of Acute Fractures

The most common osteoporotic fractures are of the vertebrae, the proximal end of the femur and the distal end of the radius. With increasing age, fractures of the ribs, pelvis, proximal end of the humerus and tibia occur more frequently.

VERTEBRAL FRACTURES

Vertebral fractures are the most common osteoporotic fractures. However, since these fractures can occur without significant symptoms, afflicted individuals may not seek medical attention; as a result many fractures go undiagnosed and the true incidence of fracture is difficult to ascertain. It is estimated that 25% of women over the age of 50 in the USA will have one or more vertebral fractures (Lukert, 1994).

Decreasing bone mass and changes in trabecular architecture lead to vertebral fractures often with little or no apparent associated trauma. Often vertebrae may fracture during normal daily activ-

ities such as rising from a chair, making a bed or opening a window. Three types of fractures have been described: 1. compression fractures when there is collapse of the entire vertebral body; 2. wedge fractures when only the anterior cortex collapses resulting in a reduction in anterior height with maintenance of the posterior height (Figure 2); and 3. biconcave fractures (concave or codfish vertebrae) in which there is collapse of the superior and/or inferior endplates resulting in a concave deformity of the upper and/or lower margin with relative maintenance of both the anterior and posterior height. The lower six thoracic vertebrae and all the lumbar vertebrae are commonly involved, whereas the upper thoracic and cervical vertebrae are almost never affected (Lukert, 1994).

Approximately 80% of vertebral fractures result in symptoms of acute pain at the fracture site associated with paravertebral muscle spasm and loss of flexion. Radicular pain may also be present due to nerve root irritation. Pain is aggravated by motion and many patients find weight bearing difficult or impossible initially. The acute pain

Figure 2   An anterior wedge fracture of the vertebral body, often associated with osteoporosis.

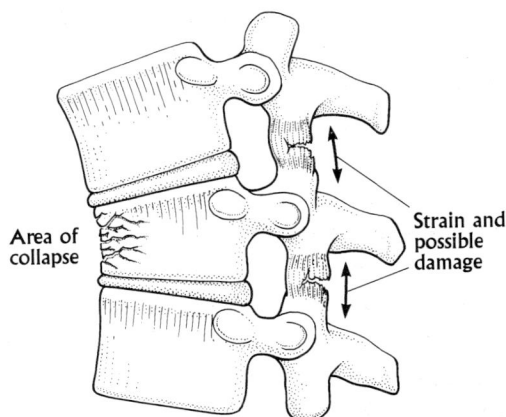

Area of collapse

Strain and possible damage

gradually subsides within a few days but discomfort often persists for several months and single or multiple fractures can lead to chronic pain and spinal deformity.

Fractures of the vertebrae frequently require bed rest and analgesic medication initially. Prolonged bed rest is discouraged because of the detrimental effects on bone health and general deconditioning. Some individuals are actually more comfortable sitting and walking which is an acceptable alternative to bed rest. Patients usually remain at home unless they have associated neurological or bowel or bladder problems. Fractures generally heal within 2–4 months and patients are able to resume normal activities.

Physiotherapy intervention during the acute phase focuses on patient education, relief of pain and increasing mobility. Patients need to be reassured that the acute pain will subside and that they will be able to gradually resume their previous activities. If the diagnosis of osteoporosis has recently been made, education about the syndrome is also appropriate. Patients should be given the opportunity to ask questions and have their concerns addressed. Advice regarding positioning to minimize pain is important during the early postfracture period. Patients are generally most comfortable lying on their side with hips and knees flexed. The mattress should be firm and a pillow placed between their knees to minimize stress on the spine due to thigh adduction. Some patients prefer supine lying with pillows under the knees. Sleeping in a recliner chair is an acceptable alternative for those who are uncomfortable lying down. Instruction in log rolling with knees flexed towards the chest in preparation for sitting up from the lying position will reduce pain associated with changing position. Safe transfers are taught from bed to chair and weight bearing and ambulation are gradually increased as toler-

ated. A walker or a cane may be required initially. Instruction in the principles of good spinal posture in all positions may help minimize the development of spinal deformity.

Local measures such as ice massage over the fracture area may provide pain relief. The area is massaged with ice for 5–10 minutes, until local numbness is produced. The effect may last up to 2 hours at which time the treatment can be repeated (Lukert, 1994). Transcutaneous electrical nerve stimulation may also be of benefit for pain relief. Moist heat, in the form of a warm bath or hot water bottle, may alleviate paravertebral muscle spasm.

Bracing may also be an effective means of reducing pain following vertebral fracture. Pain related to fractures of the lumbar spine may improve with the use of a wide lumbar corset or belt. Several types of braces and body jackets are available to support the thoracic spine. Generally they function to restrict mobility and to promote extension of the thoracic spine, therefore reducing compression forces on the anterior vertebral body. They are generally bulkier and more difficult to apply than the lumbar corsets and are less well tolerated by patients. However, if fitted properly, they can provide significant pain relief. The stabilization of the spine provided by bracing during the early postfracture period allows patients to be mobilized more quickly.

Extension exercises should be started as soon as tolerated to relieve pain, strengthen and increase endurance in the back extensors and retard the progression of kyphotic deformity. Initially, if pain is acute, exercises may simply consist of active spinal extension performed in a comfortable position such as supine or sitting. Spinal extension should be accompanied by deep breathing to elevate the ribs, maintain rib mobility and facilitate extension of the vertebral column. In many exercise programmes, recommended for persons with spinal osteoporosis, vertebral extension is often combined with bilateral scapular retraction. The important component of the exercise must be extension of the spine; the addition of scapular retraction may result in the exercise being done incorrectly and is of questionable value. Prone lying for a short period several times daily may help maintain extension and relieve pain. Once the acute pain subsides, prone lying can be progressed to prone position with forearm support, and extension exercises in prone lying can be initiated (Figure 3).

FRACTURES OF THE PROXIMAL FEMUR

Fractures of the proximal femur are common in older individuals and are associated with high mortality, morbidity and enormous economic cost. The incidence of hip fracture increases with age in individuals over the age of 50 years and is twice as high in women. Physiotherapists can expect to deal with more and more patients with hip fracture as the number of older people in the general population rises in the future.

Although less common than vertebral fractures, fractures of the proximal femur result in greater morbidity and mortality. It is estimated that 15–20% of patients with hip fracture will die within one year of hip fracture. Of those who survive, 50% will require long-term nursing care (Riggs and Melton, 1986).

Hip fractures are primarily attributable to Type II osteoporosis which affects trabecular and cortical bone. It has been established that density of the proximal femur is less in subjects with hip fractures than in individuals of the same age without hip fracture. However, whereas vertebral fractures can occur spontaneously, 80–90% of hip fractures generally occur as a result of a fall (Chapter 15), suggesting that balance impairment

is also a dominant risk factor for hip fracture. Recent data support the view that both bone density and fall characteristics are important determinants of hip fracture risk (Greenspan et al., 1994). Fractures are more likely to occur when the fall is to the side, resulting in impact on the hip or side of the leg. Muscle mass and soft tissue padding around the hip are reduced with age making the hip less able to withstand the impact of a fall. Protective reactions are also diminished with age; thus the older individual who falls may be less likely to extend their arm to break the fall. This decrease in reaction time may account for the higher incidence of hip versus forearm fractures in older individuals.

Fractures may involve either the femoral neck or trochanteric region. Femoral neck fractures may be further classified as intracapsular (subcapital or transcervical) or extracapsular (basilar). Intracapsular fractures commonly result in an interruption in the blood supply to the femoral head resulting in a high incidence of non-union and necrosis. Complications occur less frequently with extracapsular fractures as the blood supply to the femoral head is less likely to be impaired. Trochanteric fractures involve fractures through (avulsion), or between (intertrochanteric) the femoral trochanters. These fractures generally unite without difficulty because of good blood supply and the large volume of trabecular bone in the area.

Surgical intervention is the treatment of choice for all elderly subjects with hip fracture as the risks of surgery are lower than those associated with the prolonged immobility required by conservative management. Fractures of the femoral neck are managed with internal fixation with various pins, nails, plates and compression screws or by prosthetic replacement. Replacement of the femoral head with a hemiarthroplasty avoids the complications of ascetic necrosis and non-union in intracapsular fractures. A total hip replacement is indicated in patients with degenerative changes affecting the acetabulum. Trochanteric fractures are commonly managed with internal fixation. Surgical repair is generally done within 24–48 hours of the fracture. Physiotherapy seldom plays a role in the preoperative period.

The primary objectives of physiotherapy in the postoperative period are to regain range of motion, and regain pain free and independent ambulation. In the immediate postoperative period it is important that the patient be positioned in supine-lying with no pillows under the knee for a period of time each day to prevent the development of hip and knee flexion contractures. Frequent alteration of the patient's position from supine to side-lying will aid ventilation and help prevent skin breakdown. An overhead trapeze will facilitate independence in bed mobility and use of the bed pan. Active assisted hip range of motion exercises and isometric quadriceps and gluteal muscle contractions are initiated in the early postoperative period. Active ankle exercises are encouraged to minimize the risk of venous thrombosis. Patients are mobilized as soon as possible to minimize the potential complications of bed rest. Ambulation is initiated early in the postoperative period, using a walker or crutches as appropriate (see also Chapters 7, 25 and 26). Weight bearing is progressed from feather touch to partial weight to weight bearing as tolerated over the next 12–16 weeks depending on the degree of stabilization achieved at the time of surgery and radiographic evidence of healing. The patient is progressed from crutches or a walker to a straight cane as tolerated. The postoperative physiotherapy programme is similar following a femoral head or total hip replace-ment. Weight bearing may not be allowed for 6 weeks following surgery depending on the type of prosthetic replacement used.

FRACTURES OF THE DISTAL RADIUS

Fractures of the distal forearm (Colles' fractures) are common in persons over 50 years of age and occur more frequently in women. The incidence of forearm fracture exceeds that of hip fracture in the early postmenopausal years. The incidence rises until approximately age 65, after which rates tend to remain constant. There is a relationship between bone density of the distal radius and forearm fracture risk. However, fractures generally occur as a result of a fall on the outstretched arm.

Colles' fractures are rarely fatal and they result in less morbidity than hip fractures. Generally, neither hospitalization or extensive rehabilitation is required. The fracture is reduced and a plaster applied from the elbow to the metacarpal phalangeal joints for 4–6 weeks. Reflex sympathetic dystrophy and shoulder hand syndrome are both potential complications of this type of fracture. To minimize this risk, the patient is encouraged to exercise the fingers and shoulder while the cast is on. Following its removal, the objectives of physiotherapy are to regain pain free wrist and finger motion, grip strength and hand function (see Chapters 8 and 9).

Long-term Management Strategies

The long-term goals of physiotherapy, whether or not the individual has sustained a previous fracture, are to prevent fractures and the development of spinal deformity (see also Chapter 13). These goals are achieved primarily through exercise and education programmes. Physiotherapy treatment strategies in three main areas will be discussed: 1. the role of exercise in increasing or maintaining bone mass; 2. treatment specific to prevention of vertebral fractures and spinal deformity; 3. strategies to minimize injury risk among older adults.

EXERCISES AND BONE MASS DENSITY

Most fractures in elderly people are related to low bone mineral density. Data from cross-sectional studies demonstrate that activity level, aerobic fitness and muscle strength all correlate significantly with bone density. There is also scientific evidence that both aerobic and muscle strengthening programmes are effective in increasing bone density or at least in reducing the rate of bone loss in older individuals including those with osteoporosis. However, the role of exercise in maintaining or improving bone mass is controversial as not all studies have demonstrated a beneficial effect of exercise on bone. It is unclear which types of exercise best protect against bone loss and optimal intensity and duration parameters have not been clearly established. Several principles are considered important when designing an exercise programme to regain bone or prevent loss of bone and are outlined below.

Exercise intensity Exercises must be of sufficient intensity to cause a change in bone mass. It has been demonstrated in animal models that the intensity of the mechanical load applied is more important than the number of load cycles for stimulation of bone formation. Two primary factors affecting exercise intensity are weight bearing and strong muscle contraction. Compression forces through the bone provided by weight bearing appear to be necessary to stimulate bone remodelling. The fact that bone density in swimmers is not higher than that found in non-athletes supports the concept of importance of the weight bearing component of the exercise.

Theoretically, forces exerted by contracting muscles during resisted exercises should produce a similar mechanical stimulus to bone as that provided by weight bearing. The significant relationship between both muscle strength and muscle mass and bone density that has been reported in several studies lends support to this hypothesis. However, studies investigating the effect of resisted exercise programmes for the trunk, performed in a non-weightbearing position, reported no change in the BMD of the lumbar spine or hip as a result of exercise. Conversely, bicycle ergometry programmes, which are considered to be non-weight bearing, have been found to improve BMD of the lumbar spine but had no effect on the proximal femur. Similarly, a high intensity, low repetition, muscle strengthening programme on Nautilus equipment in conjunction with oestrogen replacement was found to be more effective in improving BMD of the lumbar spine and distal radius in surgically menopausal women than oestrogen therapy alone (Notelovitz *et al.*, 1991). A Nautilus strength training programme may be preferable to an aerobic programme (treadmill walking and bicycle ergometer) for protection against bone loss.

For increases in bone mass to occur the loads applied must exceed those to which the bone is normally exposed during daily activity. Thus, to some extent, programmes must be individually tailored, with age, health and ability of the person taken into consideration. A walking programme may provide sufficient stimulation for bone formation in previously sedentary individuals but is unlikely to result in change in bone mass in persons with a more active life-style. It is necessary to establish baseline levels of activity and design a programme which exceeds these levels.

Site specificity The effect of exercise on bone tends to be site specific; that is changes in BMD occur in bones subjected to load. Tennis players have greater BMD in the humerus of the playing arm compared with the non-playing arm. Similarly, an exercise programme which focused specifically on training of the forearm resulted in increased bone density of the distal radius, whereas, no change was observed at this site following a general aerobic exercise programme. In addition, most aerobic and weight training programmes that have been studied, have a greater effect on the axial than on the appendicular skeleton; a finding which may be related to the greater metabolic activity of trabecular bone. To be effective, a programme designed to improve bone density must incorporate exercises which will stress the skeletal sites most prone to fracture, i.e. spine, forearm and proximal femur.

Diversity Diversity in the direction and type of the forces applied is important to obtain maximal increases in bone mineral density. A programme designed to apply compressive, tensile and bending forces in different planes, as well as torsional force, to the forearm was effective in increasing the bone density of the distal radius in postmenopausal osteoporotic women, whereas, a unidirectional strength training of the lower limb in young women failed to alter the BMD of the exercised limb.

Programme duration Bone mass density reverts back to baseline levels once exercise is discontinued. Thus, if exercise programmes are to be of long-term benefit they must be continued indefinitely. Currently, few older adults partici-

pate regularly in physical activity programmes. Efforts need to be directed toward the education of older adults about the benefits of physical exercise. A lifelong commitment to regular exercise is more likely to occur if the individual chooses activities which they enjoy (Chapter 12).

Summary Exercise has a beneficial effect on the growing skeleton and is important in maximizing the development of peak bone mass. There is also scientific evidence that physical activity in later years is important for the prevention of bone loss with ageing and exercise may help replace bone already lost in some cases. To be effective, exercise must be of sufficient intensity, provide diversity in the forces applied to the skeleton and stress skeletal sites most prone to fracture. If the benefits of exercise on bone are to be sustained exercise must become a lifelong habit. The ultimate goal of any management strategy in osteoporosis is to reduce the incidence of fracture. The efficacy of exercise programmes in meeting this goal has yet to be determined.

PREVENTION OF VERTEBRAL FRACTURES AND SPINAL DEFORMITY

Accumulative fractures and soft tissue contracture, together with normal flexion forces on the spine due to daily activities, lead to a gradual loss of height and an increase in kyphotic curvature of the spine. The location of the apex of the curve and the resulting postural abnormality is dependent on where the fractures occur. Fractures of the mid thoracic region commonly lead to an increase in the thoracic kyphotic curvature and a compensatory increase in the lumbar lordosis. Fractures of the thoracolumbar junction or lumbar spine are more likely to lead to a thoracolumbar kyphosis or total kyphotic curvature of the spine. With this type of deformity, there is a forward lean of the trunk above the apex of the curve and hip and knee flexion angles in standing may be increased in order to compensate for the kyphotic spinal curvature. For further detail regarding these postural deformities see Chapter 7.

The alteration in the shape of the thoracic cage in either posture type may lead to restrictive lung disease. The abdomen tends to protrude and patients may complain of distension and early satiety (MacKinnon, 1988). As the spinal deformity progresses the ribs may begin to rest on or overlap the iliac crests causing further pain. Deformity of the thoracic and lumbar spine commonly lead to a forward head position which may contribute to chronic neck pain and stiffness. In addition, abnormalities in sagittal plane alignment of the spine have been shown to be associated with balance in older women. Thus, the postural deformity, resulting from vertebral fracture, may increase the risk of falls in older individuals.

The physiotherapeutic goal of reducing risk of fracture and subsequent spinal deformity is achieved through patient education, postural training and exercise. Patients need to understand the causes and consequences of fracture including the need for avoidance of single or repetitive flexion forces on the spine. A primary component of the education programme is teaching correct lifting techniques, utilizing the lower extremities and maintaining a straight spine throughout the lift. Individuals with osteoporosis should seek assistance with lifting heavy items; it has been suggested that persons with spinal osteoporosis lift no more than 10 pounds (Aisenbrey, 1987).

Patients need to be provided with information regarding correct alignment of the spine in sit- ting, standing and lying. A lumbar roll to maintain the lumbar curvature in the sitting position, is appropriate in patients with loss of lumbar lordosis. Neck retraction exercises (chin tucks) may help correct the forward head position and alleviate chronic neck pain common in patients with a more caudal spinal deformity. Avoidance of flexed postures for prolonged periods should be emphasized to minimize the development of deformity.

Extension exercises for the spine are often prescribed to minimize the development of deformity and to strengthen the back extensor musculature. The patient's level of pain and mobility must be considered when prescribing exercises. Exercises in sitting and supine lying are appropriate for subjects with pain. Positioning in prone lying and trunk extension exercises in prone lying are generally recommended for those patients who are able to assume and tolerate this position. Extension exercises in prone lying need to be modified according to the location of previous fractures and the deformity present. A pillow should be placed under the stomach for a patient with a thoracic kyphosis and compensatory increase in lumbar lordosis such that the exercise results in strengthening of the back extensors without further accentuation the lumbar curvature (Figure 3). For patients with a kyphotic curvature of the lumbar spine or thoracolumbar region a smaller pillow or no pillow under the stomach would be more appropriate to facilitate extension of the lumbar spine.

Flexion exercises are contraindicated in patients with osteoporosis as they have been shown to cause an acceleration in vertebral fracture rate in osteoporotic subjects (Sinaki and Mikkelsen, 1984) (Figure 4). Fifty-nine patients, aged 49–60 years, with spinal osteoporosis were allocated to one of four groups. Group one subjects ($n =$

Figure 3   Positioning and appropriate exercises following vertebral fracture, introduced in the early postfracture period and progressed as acute pain subsides. a) Prone lying to relieve pain and minimize development of spinal deformity; a pillow should be placed under the abdomen for patients with exaggerated lumbar lordosis. b) Prone position on elbows to facilitate passive spinal extension. c, d) Spinal extension exercises in supine and sitting accompanied by deep inspiratory effort. e) Active spinal extension in prone position.

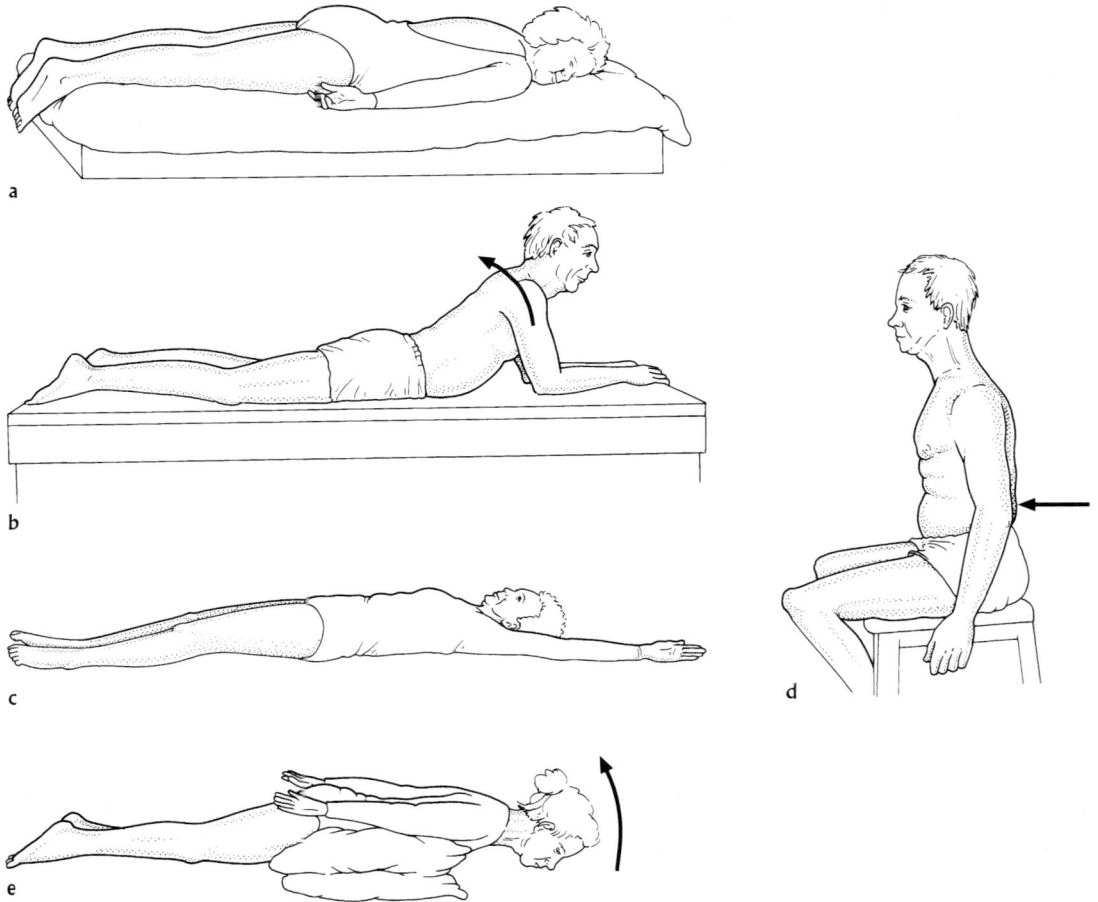

25) performed spinal extension exercises, group two subjects (n = 9) did spinal flexion exercises, group three subjects (n = 19) did a combination of flexion and extension exercises and group four subjects (n = 6) did no exercise. Incidence of spinal compression or wedge fracture on X-ray was recorded at the beginning of the study and at the end of the exercise period. In the group performing extension exercises, 16% of the subjects had further wedging or compression of vertebrae at the end of the study (mean follow-up = 1.4 years). In the flexion exercise group, 89% and in the combined flexion and extension exercise group 53% of the subjects had further vertebral wedging and compression following the exercise period. In the no exercise group, 67% of the subjects had an increase in fracture. It was concluded by the authors that exercises which

Figure 4 Contraindicated flexion exercises which may contribute to wedge and compression fractures of the vertebrae in patients with spinal osteoporosis.

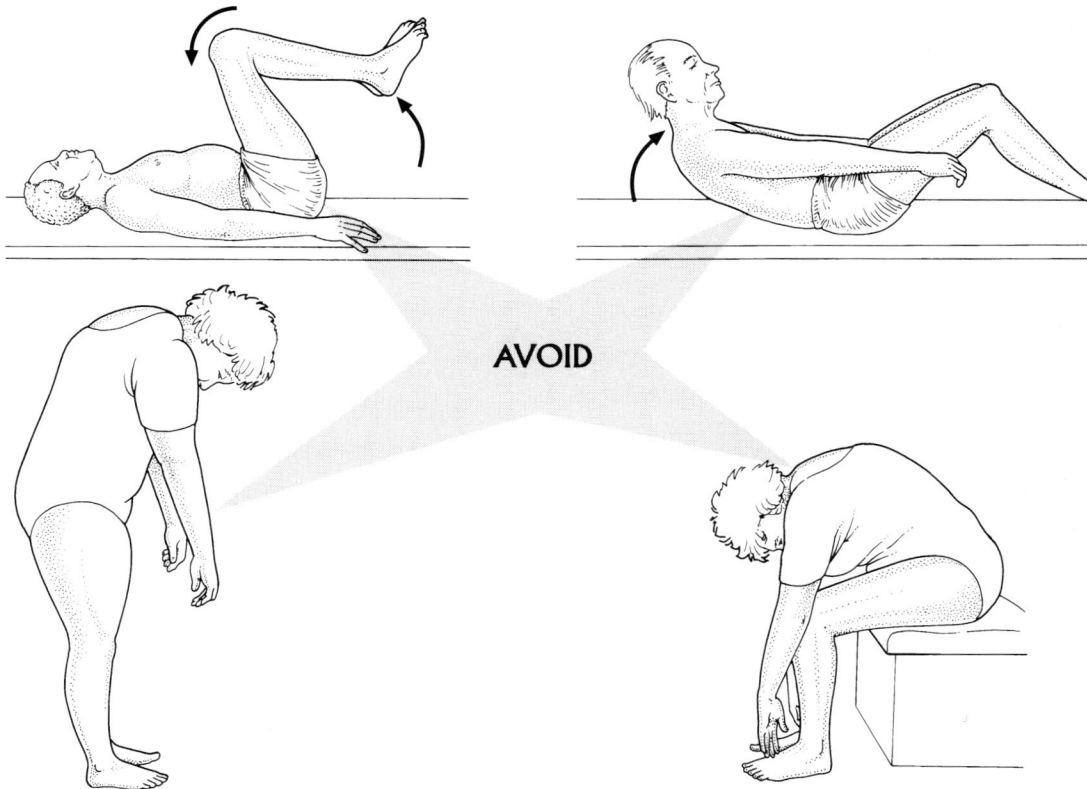

AVOID

increased flexion forces on the vertebrae were inappropriate for subjects with osteoporosis. Thus, sit ups should not be encouraged as a method of increasing abdominal muscle strength. Similarly, the posterior pelvic tilt is rarely indicated. Fractures commonly involve the lower thoracic and lumbar vertebrae resulting in a loss of lumbar lordosis. The pelvis is already tilted posteriorly. The pelvic tilt exercise would be encouraging development of the deformity and bring the anterior rib cage into closer proximity with the pelvis, a problem that needs to be prevented. Osteoporosis and possible vertebral fracture must be suspected in

postmenopausal women and older individuals presenting with back pain, in which case pelvic tilt and flexion exercises may only serve to aggravate the condition. Abdominal strengthening exercises need to be carried out isometrically, keeping the spine straight and without increasing compressive forces on the vertebrae.

Spinal orthoses may be beneficial for patients experiencing chronic pain or discomfort in the spine due to previous fracture or deformity. Use of long-term spinal bracing is controversial. Braces may be of benefit in relieving pain, reducing fatigue in the back musculature and improving function. However, spinal bracing may lead to reduced use of the back extensor muscles and contribute to increased weakness and loss of their stabilizing function. Few studies have investigated use of spinal orthoses in long-term management of osteoporosis. Kaplan and Sinaki (1993) evaluated the use of a posture training support in 30 patients with spinal osteoporosis. This simple device consisted of a pouch containing a weight of 794 g (1.75 lb). This pouch was positioned posteriorly below the scapula and was supported by shoulder straps. It was designed to promote extension of the spine and relieve pain by applying a force below the scapulae. Effects were postulated to occur through either reduction of force on the anterior vertebral bodies or proprioceptive reinforcement of good postural alignment. Of 23 patients who had significant pain prior to use of the device, 17 reported pain relief. Subjective reports of improved posture were also noted and it was suggested that patient acceptance of this device may be superior to that of more conventional spinal orthoses.

INJURY PREVENTION

Osteoporotic fractures commonly occur as a result of an injury in older adults with skeletal frailty. Vertebral fractures are more likely to occur with lifting particulary if the movement combines flexion and rotation of the spine whereas hip and forearm fractures most commonly occur as a result of a fall. Balance impairment and fall frequency increase with age. It is estimated that one in three community-dwelling older people will fall each year. Falls are more likely to result in injury among frailer older adults than healthy, more mobile individuals. Fractures resulting from falls cause physical morbidity or death in some cases. In addition, falls can also have serious psychological consequences, including fear of future falls which leads to loss of confidence, limitation of mobility and social isolation.

Impairments in the musculoskeletal system, including lower extremity muscle weakness, decreased flexibility and spinal deformity are among several intrinsic factors which increase susceptibility to falls in older people. These impairments can be improved with exercise. Individuals with osteoporosis, however, may be reluctant to participate in exercise programmes because of fear of new fracture or aggravation of pain from a previous fracture. Health care workers may reinforce a pattern of inactivity by discouraging physical activity in order to minimize the risk of falling and likelihood of fracture. Lack of activity ultimately leads to further muscle weakness, loss of mobility and general de-conditioning contributing to balance impairment and increased susceptibility to falls. This cycle must be broken through education regarding the rationale for, and importance of, physical activity and through the provision of safe and appropriate exercise programmes for persons with osteoporosis (McClung, 1994). Also, older people, particularly those with osteoporosis, may need a home environmental assessment and assistance with physical adaptation of the home including installation of hand rails on stairs and in the bathroom, improvements in lighting, and repair of worn flooring.

In addition to decreasing the incidence of falls, attention has also been directed toward reducing the consequence of falls. Loss of muscle and soft tissue padding around the hip has been implicated as a causative factor in hip fractures. The wearing of protective padding over the hips of frail elderly nursing home residents has been found to reduce the incidence of hip fractures. Although further research is required the results indicate that this may be an effective preventive strategy, at least in the frail elderly population.

Summary

Osteoporosis is a common problem in older people and it has been suggested that incidence has reached epidemic levels in North America and northern Europe. The number of people sustaining osteoporotic fractures is predicted to increase as the population ages. These fractures can lead to chronic pain and considerable impairment in mobility and function. Pain, immobility and fear of falling frequently lead to a reduction in activities outside the home which in turn contributes to social isolation, depression and an overall decrease in quality of life.

Physiotherapists have a role to play in primary prevention, in management following skeletal fracture and in prevention of subsequent fractures and associated deformity. Primary prevention begins in childhood and aims at achieving maximum peak bone. Physiotherapists need to become involved in education programmes focusing on the importance of physical activity, good nutrition and avoidance of life-style which can impair skeletal growth or contribute to bone loss. Decreasing pain, improving mobility and independent function and prevention of deformity are the goals of rehabilitation following fracture. Long-term objectives for individuals with osteoporosis include preventing fractures and the development of spinal deformities.

References

Aisenbrey, JA (1987) Exercise in the prevention and management of osteoporosis. *Physical Therapy* **67**: 1100–1104.

Bachrach, LK (1994) Bone acquisition in childhood and adolescence. In Marcus R (ed) *Osteoporosis*, pp. 69–106. Oxford: Blackwell Scientific Publications.

Greenspan, SL, Myers, ER, Maitland, LA *et al.* (1994) Fall severity and bone mineral density as risk factors for hip fracture in ambulatory elderly. *Journal of the American Medical Association* **271**: 128–133.

Josse, RG (1989) Osteoporosis, a modern plague: Widespread, expensive and too often deadly. *Canadian Pharmaceutical Journal* **122**: 460–468.

Kaplan, RS, Sinaki, M (1993) Posture training support: Preliminary report on a series of patients with diminished symptomatic complications of osteoporosis. *Mayo Clinic Proceedings* **68**: 1171–1176.

Lukert, BP (1994) Vertebral compression fractures: how to manage pain, avoid disability. *Geriatrics* **49**: 22–26.

MacKinnon, JL (1988) Osteoporosis: A review. *Physical Therapy* **10**: 1533–1540.

McClung, M (1994) Nonpharmacologic management of osteoporosis. In Marcus, R (ed) *Osteoporosis*, pp. 336–353. Oxford: Blackwell Scientific Publications.

Notelovitz, M, Martin, D, Tesar, R *et al.* (1991) Estrogen therapy and variable-resistance weight training increase bone mineral in surgically menopausal women. *Journal of Bone and Mineral Research* **6**: 583–590.

Riggs, BL, Melton, LJ (1986) Involutional osteoporosis. *New England Journal of Medicine* **314**: 1676–1686.

Scott, JC, Hochberg, MC (1993) Prevention of osteoporosis. *Bulletin on the Rheumatic Diseases* **42**: 4–6.

Simon, L (1993) Pathogenesis of osteoporosis. *Bulletin on the Rheumatic Diseases* **42**: 1–3.

Sinaki, M, Mikkelsen, BA (1984) Postmenopausal spinal osteoporosis: Flexion versus extension exercises. *Archives of Physical Medicine and Rehabilitation* **65**: 593–596.

Slemenda, CW (1994) Adult bone loss. In Marcus, R (ed) *Osteoporosis*, pp. 107–124. Oxford: Blackwell Scientific Publications.

Vargo, MM, Gerber, LH (1993) Exercise strategies for osteoporosis. *Bulletin on the Rheumatic Diseases* **42**: 6–9.

17

Incontinence

G ELIZABETH TATA

Scope of the Problem
•
Prevalence of Urinary Incontinence
•
Physical, Psychosocial and Economic Implications of Incontinence
•
Age Changes Affecting the Lower Urinary Tract and Bladder Function
•
Types of Urinary Incontinence
•
Assessment of Incontinence
•
Overall Goals of Management
•
Physiotherapy Management
•
Conclusion

Scope of the Problem

Urinary incontinence is defined by the International Continence Society as a condition in which the involuntary loss of urine is a social or hygienic problem and is objectively demonstrated (Abrams *et al.*, 1988). Rectal incontinence is the involuntary loss of rectal contents. Both conditions affect males and females for different anatomical and physiological reasons. Urinary incontinence is more common and is the focus of this chapter.

Incontinence is a major problem for older people, their families and for professional caregivers in community or institutional settings. The deci-

sion to place an elderly relative in an institution is strongly influenced by their continence status and the burden of care placed on the family (Johnson and Werner, 1982). However, in many instances, it can be managed in the same way as in the younger adult because the causes of incontinence are the same.

Physiotherapists must be prepared to address the multifactorial nature of the problem. Standard methods of treatment, including bladder training, pelvic floor exercise and control of caffeine intake, may be successful for the majority of older clients in achieving a cure or improvement, and should be offered also to those who are receiving drug or surgical management for their incontinence. When incontinence is part of a more complex picture of physical or cognitive disability, the approach must be adaptable and comprehensive and may involve working with family caregivers and other health care professionals.

Prevalence of Urinary Incontinence

The prevalence of urinary incontinence among older adults living in the community may be as high as 30%. However, reported incidence of urinary incontinence varies widely depending on the population of older people studied, from $12\frac{1}{2}$% of those living in the community, through 50% of nursing home residents to 80% of patients in psychogeriatric facilities (Tobin, 1992).

Principal risk factors for urinary incontinence are gender, age, childbirth, menopause, smoking and obesity (Walters and Karram, 1993). Urinary incontinence is more common in women than in men, due to anatomical differences and the effects of childbirth (nulliparous women have a lower incidence) and menopause. Changes in bladder function directly related to ageing increase prevalence, and the presence of acute or chronic illness, physical disabilities and cognitive impairment further exacerbate the problem. The prevalence of incontinence in older people living at home is relatively low compared with those in residential care.

Physical, Psychosocial and Economic Implications of Incontinence

Among concommittents of incontinence, are problems directly related to leakage of urine or faeces: perineal skin irritation, chapping, sores and urinary tract infections. Besides the physical impact, elderly incontinence sufferers, fearing accidental leakage and the embarrassment it might cause, lose their self-esteem and become depressed.

Wet pads and clothing are extremely uncomfortable and the odour that arises very unpleasant for both the incontinent person and others. As a result, social interaction may be curtailed, particularly intimate relationships, as well as participation in physical activities such as walking, exercise classes and dancing.

Caring for a person with incontinence requires compassion, patience and understanding, yet it may become an intolerable physical and emotional burden, causing strained family relationships. Likewise quality of care in residential facilities depends on the professional staff's knowledge and technical skill in managing incontinence as well as on them behaving in a positive and caring manner toward these clients (see also Chapter 3).

Diagnostic costs, medical and surgical treatment, rehabilitation, nursing care, institutional care, equipment and supplies such as pads and protective garments all make incontinence very expensive for patients, their families and the health care system. The indirect costs of unpaid caregivers and loss of productivity of the individual also accumulate. A 1984 survey of the economic impact of urinary incontinence estimated that direct and indirect costs totalled $8.1 billion annually in the USA (Hu, 1986).

Age Changes Affecting the Lower Urinary Tract and Bladder Function

Several age-related changes in the lower urinary tract (all organs below the ureter) affect bladder function and may contribute to voiding difficulties and incontinence among elderly people.

Most measurements of bladder function are lower in elderly people (Feneley, 1986). Normal voiding frequency and the amount voided depend on several factors including the capacity of the bladder, fluid intake, and time of day or night. The ability of the bladder to stretch and hold urine (compliance) allows for bladder filling without an appreciable rise in pressure until near capacity. Voiding normally occurs four to six times during the day (every 3–4 hours) with 240–450 ml of urine being passed each time. In old age capacity, compliance, and the ability to postpone voiding all decrease in both sexes whereas the number of uninhibited bladder contractions seems to increase. Thus voiding frequency may rise and uninhibited, accidental voiding may occur.

People are normally able to start voiding without strain and then to pass urine in a steady stream without pain until stopping completely with no post-void dribble. In old age flow rates decrease, possibly due to weaker contractions of the smooth, non-striated detrusor muscle in the bladder wall. Furthermore, men may experience increased outflow resistance due to prostate gland hypertrophy. Post-void residual urine volume in the bladder increases with age.

Although it is common for adults to get up once during the night to void, elderly people may have to do so more often.

Urethral closing is important in maintaining continence. In women, it is affected by the decreased availability of oestrogen following the menopause. Ability to maintain closure and resist the urge to void that increases as vesical pressure rises during bladder-filling depends partly on pressure generated by the muscular wall of the urethra compressing the mucosal folds which line it. Oestrogen receptors have been found in the trigone muscle at the base of the bladder, the urethra and the periurethral muscle. Oestrogen facilitates alpha-adrenergic stimulation and is important for maintaining the vascularity of the urethral mucosa, and elasticity of connective tissue in the urethral wall. Lack of oestrogen is associated with atrophy of the vaginal and urethral mucosa, reduced vascularity and elasticity, and decreased periurethral smooth muscle tone. This produces a low urethral closing pressure and a reduced functional urethral length. The urethra is already shorter in women (4 cm compared with 8–20 cm in men).

Urinary and faecal incontinence can result from an incompetent pelvic floor. In both men and women, a general decrease in connective tissue elasticity can affect support given to the pelvic contents by the three layers of the pelvic floor (Wall, 1994). This loss of elasticity especially affects women when compounded by oestrogen deprivation and the effects of earlier pregnancy and childbirth. Stretching and trauma of the pelvic floor and pudendal nerve, which innervates the levator ani muscles, can result in permanent weakness and partial denervation with loss of urethral and bladder neck support. Decrease in pelvic floor muscle strength in both sexes probably parallels the general decline of body muscle strength that occurs with advancing age.

Types of Urinary Incontinence

Urinary incontinence is a problem of the bladder filling and storage phases of micturition. The commonest dysfunctions are urge incontinence and genuine stress incontinence.

Urge Incontinence

Urgency (a strong desire to void) characterizes this type of involuntary loss of urine (Abrams et al., 1988). Older people may experience sudden overwhelming feelings of urgency at lower than normal bladder capacity and urine leaks because of their inability to inhibit detrusor contraction before reaching a toilet. The detrusor, which has become overactive and uninhibited, contracts spontaneously during filling or on sudden increases in intra-abdominal pressure. Other terms used for this condition include, unstable bladder, uninhibited bladder and detrusor instability.

Motor urgency is associated with detrusor instability. Sensory urgency is urgency at abnormally low bladder volumes, associated with bladder hypersensitivity, but without detrusor instability. In people over 75 years of age with symptoms of urinary dysfunction, the incidence of detrusor instability has been reported as high as 75–85% in women and 85–95% in men (Malone-Lee, 1994). It may be precipitated by pelvic or bladder inflammation, infection or outflow obstruction due to faecal impaction, neoplasm or prostate hypertrophy. In many cases the cause is unknown. Caffeine drinks, especially coffee and tea produce increased urgency, voiding frequency and may precipitate incontinence through a direct excitatory effect on the detrusor. Also urge incontinence may partly be a learned response as it is often brought on by behavioural situations such as hand-washing, hearing the sound of running water, or placing the key in the door on arriving home. Going suddenly from a warm to a cold environment may also produce incontinence. Voiding more frequently than every 2 hours can become a habit, resulting in low functional bladder capacity and voiding of small volumes.

Motor innervation of the bladder and urethra is by efferent parasympathetic and sympathetic nerves (Feneley, 1986). The pathophysiology of detrusor instability is unknown but the underlying cause may be a disorder of intrinsic inhibition or neuromodulation within the bladder. Enhanced sensory innervation of the detrusor and alterations in chemical neurotransmitters have been implicated (Moore et al., 1992). Detrusor instability occurring with bladder outflow obstruction, as with prostate hypertrophy, may be due to increased sensitivity to the neurotransmitter acetylcholine as a result of partial parasympathetic denervation. Incontinence following surgery for prostatic hypertrophy may also be due to detrusor instability (Tobin, 1992). Over activity due to loss of central nervous system control is known as detrusor hyperreflexia.

Genuine Stress Incontinence

Stress incontinence is the involuntary loss of urine that occurs on a sudden increase in intra-abdominal pressure (IAP). Precipitating activities include coughing, laughing, sneezing, lifting, walking, dancing, running, or getting up from sitting in a chair to standing. Genuine stress incontinence (GSI) is more explicitly defined as 'the involuntary loss of urine occurring when intravesical pressure exceeds maximal intraurethral pressure in the absence of detrusor contraction' (Abrams et al., 1988). It is important to establish during assessment whether urgency is also present, as increases in IAP may stimulate uninhibited detrusor contractions and urge incontinence. Careful questioning determines whether a feeling of urgency was felt on the precipitating activity; if so detrusor instability may be the cause.

Causes of GSI are a loss of anatomical support of the bladder and urethra, and incompetence of the urethral sphincter. Continence is normally maintained because urethral closure pressure is higher than vesical (bladder) pressure. Thickness and elasticity of the urethral mucosa and wall is important in maintaining closure but, as has been noted above, closure is less effective in older women due to postmenopausal atrophy. The endopelvic fascia and the levator ani muscles normally keep the bladder, bladder neck and proximal urethra positioned above the inferior margin of the pubis and within the abdominal cavity. Pressure in the urethra is augmented by IAP as long as the proximal urethra is located within the abdomen. In females, one-half to two-thirds of the urethra is intra-abdominal; this is very important in maintaining continence. Childbirth may damage muscle, fascia and the nerve supply of the pelvic floor muscles resulting in weakness and prolapse which is compounded in later life by a continuing decrease in muscle strength and loss of connective tissue elasticity. Incompetence of the pelvic floor results in obliteration of the posterior urethro-vesical angle which is formed between the base of the bladder and the urethra (Figure 1). This angle is normally between 90°–100° wide. The proximal urethra descends and is no longer subject to IAP

Figure 1 Pelvic anatomy in woman showing the urethro-vesical angle.

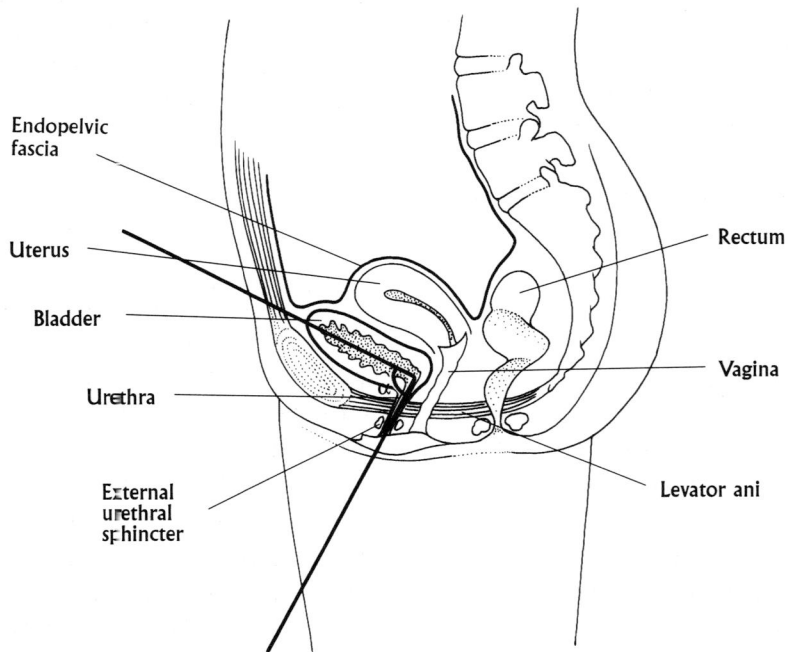

α = urethro vesical angle

increases. Intravesical pressure exceeds intraurethral pressure and leakage of urine results on sudden IAP increases. Uterovaginal prolapse, cystoceles or rectoceles may be compounding factors, as well as obesity.

Stress incontinence is less common in men but may occur with urinary tract infection, papilloma, chronic inflammation, radiation damage, urological surgery or from severe neurological disease (Williams and Panill, 1982). There is a 1–5% incidence of stress incontinence in men after transurethral or radical prostatectomy (Tobin, 1992).

Women, having just a few outer circular smooth muscle fibres around the urethral wall, lack a true internal sphincter (Gosling, 1979) whereas in men it is formed by smooth muscle fibres which encircle the preprostatic urethra distally. Stress incontinence may result from incompetence of these structures that leave the bladder neck and proximal urethra open at rest rather than maintaining a tight seal. Cauda equina lesions may lead to this incompetence, also lumobsacral spondylosis or peripheral neuropathies which damage the sympathetic supply to the urethra. Previous surgery for GSI may leave scarring which interferes with closure.

Overflow Incontinence

Overflow incontinence occurs following retention of urine when intravesical pressure exceeds maximal urethral pressure due to outlet obstruction or an under active detrusor. Common causes of outflow obstruction in men include benign prostatic hypertrophy, prostatic cancer and faecal impaction. Outflow obstruction is less common in women but may be caused by uterovaginal prolapse, cystocoele, and more rarely, fibroids or a large ovarian cyst (Williams and Pannill, 1982; Tobin, 1992).

Inadequate detrusor contraction may also lead to retention and overflow incontinence. Although this may be idiopathic, it is usually of neurological aetiology such as lower motor neuron lesions of the sacral cord or cauda equina. Other causes are diabetic autonomic neuropathy, alcoholic neuropathy or the use of muscle relaxant drugs. Diabetes or tabes dorsalis may impair bladder sensation so that there is no awareness of the need to void before overflow occurs.

Neuropathic Incontinence

There are many neuropathic causes of voiding dysfunction and incontinence (Table 1). Signs and symptoms may be complex and variable depending on the exact location and severity of the disorder. The most common lesions causing neuropathic bladder dysfunction in the elderly are cerebrovascular disease, Parkinsonism, Alzheimer's disease, diabetes mellitus and multiple sclerosis.

Functional and Transient Incontinence

Physical and cognitive impairments may lead to incontinence in elderly people who would normally be continent whereas transient incontinence may be induced by acute illness. Musculoskeletal, cardiorespiratory and neurological disease or visual loss may cause difficulties with ambulation and undressing which increase the chance of accidental urine loss before reaching the toilet. Older people are also more susceptible to urinary tract infection which can precipitate incontinence. Medications prescribed for other problems can affect bladder

Table 1
Neuropathic Bladder Disorders in Older People

Level of lesion	Symptoms	Causes
Cerebral cortex	Loss of detrusor inhibition Detrusor hyperreflexia Urge incontinence Loss of social concern re: incontinence	Cerebrovascular disease; tumours Alzheimer's disease Parkinson's disease; multiple sclerosis
Suprasacral spinal cord	Involuntary reflex voiding Loss of bladder sensation Detrusor/sphincter dyssinergia Urine retention Overflow incontinence	Traumatic spinal cord injury; tumour; cervical myelopathy; multiple sclerosis
S2–S4 spinal cord cauda equina	Loss of bladder sensation Weak detrusor contractions Urine retention Overflow incontinence Pelvic floor weakness/paralysis S2–S4 dermatome sensory loss	Diabetes; lumbar disc lesion; multiple sclerosis; tumour; spinal/pelvic trauma
Pelvic plexus (parasympathetic and sympathetic nerves)	Detrusor hypoactivity Sphincter incompetence Diminished bladder sensation Incontinence Difficulty initiating urination	Pelvic surgery (colorectal, gynaecological)

function; the combination of poor mobility and some types of diuretic is particularly hazardous.

Psychological difficulties including depression, hostility or anger, may reduce motivation to remain continent or incontinence may be used as an attention seeking device (Tobin, 1992). An elderly person with cognitive impairment and confusion may not recognize the need to void and the social requirement to maintain continence may have been forgotten. Thus incontinence in patients with senile dementia such as Alzheimer's disease may be a combination of an uninhibited neurogenic bladder, lack of awareness of bladder filling and inability to find a toilet.

An older person who is admitted to a hospital or nursing home for short-term acute care or long-term care is at risk for developing incontinence. The environment and personnel are unfamiliar and lack of privacy interferes with normal toilet behaviour. Clients can be restricted to bed-rest and left to calling a busy nurse to assist with an unfamiliar and uncomfortable bed-pan or to access the bathroom — if the wait is long involuntary voiding may occur. In these circumstances any person, of whatever age, is likely to suffer acute embarrassment and humiliation.

Assessment of Incontinence

Assessment involves taking a history of the presenting complaint, then a physical examination, including observation of related functional activity, followed by an internal, pelvic examination.

Figure 2   Scheme for recording a history.

HISTORY

Name _____ Age/Date of Birth _____   M   F

Occupation/activities _____
Social/lifestyle

Presenting symptoms & _____
Duration of incontinence

Urinary Incontinence: Voiding frequency: day____ night____Max/min vol voided___ml/___ml

Fluid intake (ml):   water_____   coffee/tea_____   other_____

Number of incontinent episodes: per day   _____   Amount of leakage: few drops _____
                                     per night _____   < tablespoon (damp)   _____
                                     per week   _____   > tablespoon (wet)   _____
                                                                        soaking   _____

Pads/protection: no pads   _____
                     pads as precaution   _____
                     small pads/liners   _____
                     large pads   _____

Activities/stress causing leak: _____   Urgency(excessive)   _____
        cough/laugh/sneeze   _____   Urge leakage:occasional _____
        bending/lifting   _____   usual   _____
        fast walk/run   _____   always   _____
        other   _____

Dysuria   _____

Faecal incontinence _____
Constipation _____

Relevant History:
Female: obstetric history/parity   _____   vaginal delivery   _____
                menstrual status   _____   prolapse   _____
                gynaecological/surgery   _____

Male: prostate hypertrophy/surgery _____

Past treatment for incontinence:conservative _____   surgery _____
other abdominal/pelvic surgery: _____

Urodynamic tests: _____

Medical History:
smoking   _____   cardiovascular _____   respiratory _____
diabetes   _____   cystitis   _____   neurological _____
musculoskeletal _____
medications

Because of the sensitive nature of the pelvic examination certain legal issues have to be addressed.

Legal Issues

Patients with incontinence are commonly referred for physiotherapy by the family physician, urologist, gynaecologist, or geriatrician. However, current legislation in Australia, Canada, the UK and USA permits direct access to physiotherapy for assessment and treatment. Physiotherapists have responsibility for undertaking a comprehensive assessment within the legal guidelines of the scope of physiotherapy practice. Scope of practice legislation may vary and physiotherapists should be aware that in some places vaginal and rectal examination may be permitted only as designated by a referring physician. Physiotherapists must ensure that informed consent is obtained from the patient (see also Chapter 27).

History

A scheme for taking a history from an incontinence sufferer is set out in Figure 2. In addition a voiding diary records pattern of voiding, number of incontinent episodes and average fluid intake. The scheme provides a systematic way of recording the severity of the problem as well as activities which may exacerbate incontinence such as smoking and certain medications.

During the interview the physiotherapist notes the client's cognitive status and ability to answer questions. It is very helpful if people with mental problems are accompanied by a relative or other advocate who can substantiate the client's responses and elaborate when these are sparse or uninformative.

Physical Examination

Certain measurements are recorded, and the client's ability to get to and use a toilet is ascertained, by observation if necessary (Figure 3).

Walking speed and use of walking aids is noted together with balance ability, safety when negotiating doors and stairs, ability to get up and down from a sitting position and to manage clothes and fastenings. A home visit may be required to assess the client's usual environment and to advise on removal of barriers to safe mobility and to recommend adaptations or alterations and appropriate assistive devices.

Pelvic Examination

The procedure determines whether pelvic floor function is satisfactory and detects problems, such as anatomical prolapse, which may require surgical intervention.

A woman may have a cystocele or rectocele which protrudes into the vagina. In order to ascertain the position of the bladder neck which normally lies above the inferior margin of the pubis, the client is helped into crook lying, then the bladder neck is palpated by placing two overlapping fingers into the vagina, palm downwards, then turning the fingers to place them each side of the urethra. Bladder neck descent may be felt as pressure on the finger tips when the patient coughs. Urine leak is noted on coughing. Sphincter tone is assessed by vaginal palpation. To assess pelvic floor muscle strength the patient is asked to tighten the muscle or 'pull up and forward as if you are trying to stop urine flow'. The contraction is graded on a scale of 0–5 (Table 2). To apply resistance and assess bilateral symmetry, the two fingers may be separated slightly and pressure applied to the lateral and posterior vaginal wall.

Figure 3   Scheme for recording the physical examination.

PHYSICAL EXAMINATION

Height_____metres   Weight_____kg   Body mass index_____(BMI=ht/wt;20-25 acceptable)

Mental orientation: _____

Physical mobility/mobility aids: _____

Dexterity/dressing/ADL: _____

Lower extremity scan(ROM,muscle strength,neurological) _____
Skin sensation S2-S4_____   Anal reflex_____

Abdominal palpation(suprapubic tenderness, bladder fullness) _____

Pelvic Examination:
Female:
Perineum/vulva/vagina _____
(trophicity, skin condition)

Prolapse(cystocele,rectocele,uterovaginal) _____

Bladder neck descent and/or leak on Valsalva:_____ on cough:_____

Pelvic floor strength grading:(Gd 0-5)_____   hold time(secs)_____

                                       number of repetitions: slow_____ fast_____

                                       perineometer reading:_____
Male:
Skin condition_____

Anal sphincter tone/contractile capacity (Gd 0-5)_____   perineometer reading:_____

DIAGNOSIS/PROBLEM LIST
Urinary Incontinence (SI, UI, mixed stress/urge)_____

Faecal Incontinence

Manual grading of pelvic floor contractions is only loosely standardized and specific definitions of grades, particularly the amount of resistance offered and duration of contraction vary between practitioners. Contraction of the pelvic floor compresses the urethra and lifts the bladder neck. The efficiency of this should be noted on assessment.

A pressure-sensitive vaginal perineometer (water or air-filled) gives an objective measure of contractile ability (Figure 4) whereas an electromyographic (EMG) perineometer provides a profile of pelvic floor muscle activity via surface perineal electrodes, vaginal or rectal electrodes.

Table 2
Manual Testing of Pelvic Floor Muscle Strength

Grade 0	No contraction
Grade 1	Flicker, unable to sustain contraction
Grade 2	Weak contraction, no resistance, held < 3 s
Grade 3	Moderate contraction, against slight resistance, held 3–6 s
Grade 4	Good contraction against moderate resistance, held 6–10 s
Grade 5	Strong contraction against resistance held > 10 s

Figure 4   A pressure perineometer.

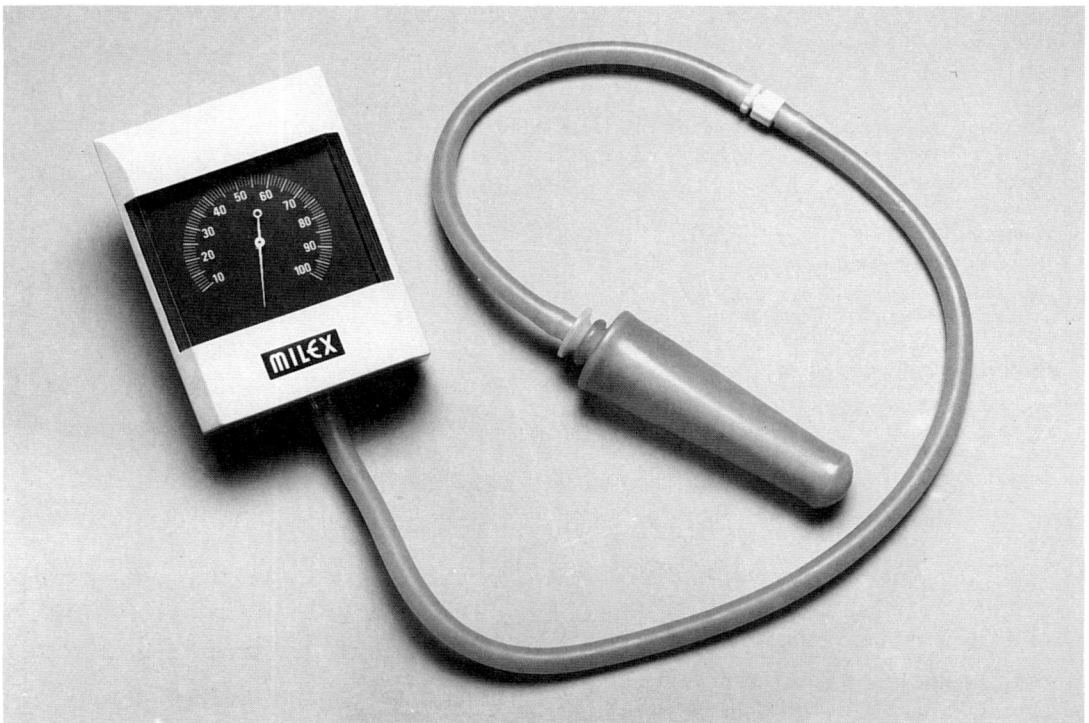

Overall Goals of Management

Ideally management should first be preventative, and then rehabilitative. Objectives are:

1. to promote continence and prevent incontinence,
2. to restore continence in an incontinent person.

The first of these goals apply to people at risk for developing incontinence. In old age, people with impaired mobility are particularly at risk, whereas younger women are especially vulnerable during pregnancy, after childbirth and at menopause. Increased public awareness about the nature of incontinence and how it can be managed together with education of community health practitioners who come into first contact with potential sufferers are key factors in continence promotion (Chapters 5 and 31). Family doctors, nurses or physiotherapists who see people at risk should, tactfully, ask questions about any continence difficulties and suggest preventive measures if appropriate.

The second goal applies to people who are incontinent. Management involves patient and caregiver education as well as treatment techniques tailored to clients' own individual problems.

Physiotherapy Management

Physiotherapy objectives for the management of urinary incontinence are:

1. to inform clients of factors which may provoke or aggravate incontinence;
2. to promote optimal bladder control, voiding frequency and volumes;
3. to improve pelvic floor function;
4. to inform clients about treatment possibilities and to refer for assessment and treatment when clients' problems are beyond the scope of physiotherapy, e.g. to a urologist or a urogynaecologist.

Individual goals should be specific and personalized – directed at the client's particular pattern of incontinence. They should be negotiated and agreed by both physiotherapist and client. Besides individually tailored education in continence promotion there are several other treatment options including: alleviation of constipation, mobility restoration, which may include appropriate adaptations to the client's environment, behavioural techniques, pelvic floor exercises including use of biofeedback, electrical stimulation; also drug regimes, surgery, and the provision of protective garments and appliances. Except for drug regimes and surgery physiotherapists use any or all of these approaches.

Client and Caregiver Education

Management of incontinence is most successful if the patient participates in the process: people need to know how the bladder works and what causes incontinence before they can fully appreciate the techniques used to promote continence. Specific problems found on assessment are discussed, including details of the voiding diary and factors that precipitate leakage. Illustrations can help to explain the factors which upset normal voiding patterns and habits, paying particular attention to the client's own situation.

Caregivers must be involved when clients, because of mental or physical disability are unable to take charge of their own treatment programme. They may be family members, friends or professionals visiting clients at home or caring for them in nursing homes. Physiotherapists discuss with them the causes of clients' problems and plan management strategies.

CHRONIC COUGHING

Chronic coughing from smoking or respiratory disease aggravates stress incontinence. Possible causes of the cough should be explored with the client and if necessary the client is referred to a physician. Stopping smoking is something the patient needs to deal with; all the physiotherapist can do in this respect is draw attention to the smoking as precipitating factor for incontinence and encourage the patient to stop.

EXCESS BODY WEIGHT

Excess body weight places extra pressure on the bladder and increases stress on the pelvic floor therefore the client is advised to lose weight (Chapter 12).

CHRONIC BACK PROBLEMS

Chronic back problems involving sacral nerve roots may be a less obvious cause of pelvic floor weakness and detrusor dysfunction. It is not known whether conservative management of lumbar spine problems can change bladder and bowel symptoms but the possibility of this should not be ruled out. When a client does have disabling chronic low back pain, physiotherapy may be suggested.

DRUGS

Drugs that may cause incontinence should be reviewed by the client and physician. It may be possible to discontinue a drug, alter the dosage, substitute another without the disagreeable side-effects, or change the time at which it is taken. Sedative-hypnotic type drugs may cause confusion and a depressed ability to inhibit bladder contractions. The client may be taking drugs with a diuretic action which increases urine output and urgency. Caffeine is present in tea, coffee and cola drinks. Intake of this drug should be reduced or eliminated; doing so can have a dramatic effect on reducing frequency and urge leakage. Clients with stress incontinence may also benefit from reducing their caffeine intake. Once the effect of caffeine has been demonstrated patients can control caffeine intake themselves but a return to drinking large amounts may exacerbate the symptoms. Habitual tea and coffee drinkers often drink several cups per day thereby increasing fluid intake above what is necessary. Similarly advice to reduce alcohol intake may be indicated.

EXCESS FLUID INTAKE

Excess fluid intake can aggravate incontinence. The body needs about 2 litres of water per day and, with a healthy diet, about half of this comes from food. Up to 2 litres in drinks is usually suggested, but thirst should be the guide, although this may be less reliable among elderly people. Fluid requirements vary depending on the temperature and humidity of the environment and the client's habitual activity level. Nevertheless, adequate fluid intake should be ensured and even supervized when a client is confused. Fluid restriction for incontinence management is not usually suggested, but some people drink excessively large amounts of water, being under the impression that six to eight glasses of water a day, in addition to other drinks, is healthy and will help with weight loss. There is no scientific basis to support this, and the excess water further compounds an incontinence problem. When nocturia is a problem, the last drink of the day should be not less than 3 hours before going to bed.

Physical Mobility and Adaptations to the Environment

Impaired mobility results in incontinence if the person is unable to get to the toilet in time and poor manual dexterity makes removing clothes difficult. Physiotherapists should ensure that all these clients attain their optimal mobility, even to the extent of providing wheelchairs. They make certain that the clients can stand up from chairs and toilet seats with minimal effort, advising on height and appropriate adaptations, possibly recommending seats that raise and lower electrically, toilet raisers and grab rails (Chapter 25). A commode may be necessary in the home or residential care facility, where the toilet is too far away or up stairs which the patient cannot negotiate. Some people who have only one toilet which is upstairs benefit from having a commode downstairs so that they only have to negotiate the stairs to retire at night. At night it may be convenient to have a commode placed next to the bed allowing the client to transfer independently or with the help of a caregiver. Whenever clients are likely to require assistance, they should be confident of getting it promptly. They should be able to summon their caregiver easily either because the caregiver is within calling distance or because a call system has been installed. If a commode transfer is out of the question urinals may be useful. Designs for men are usually satisfactory but those for women are much less successful. They are often difficult to position and there is risk of leakage.

Older people with incontinence need clothing which can be quickly and easily removed, especially if they have poor manual dexterity or lack good inhibitory control so they have to hurry to the toilet. Clothing may be made easy to manage by using elasticized waist-bands to trousers and pants, velcro fly fastenings instead of zippers (although some men find velcro too scratchy), and looser clothing in general, especially avoiding panty-hose or tights.

Behavioural Approaches

Learned responses may give rise to urge incontinence associated with loss of inhibitory control over the detrusor muscle. Going to the toilet before the bladder is full, for example before an outing or going very frequently 'just in case' to guard against the possibility of leaking are habits which may give rise to incontinence (see Chapter 9). Other causes of urgency such as cystitis or bladder infection should be ruled out or treated before starting a programme to retrain inhibitory control.

The first step is to ask clients or their caregivers to complete a voiding diary for one week. A person with urge incontinence might record hourly or even more frequent visits to the toilet and more than one at night. The goal of bladder retraining is to reduce voiding frequency to once every 3–4 hours i.e. four to six times a day (7 am–11 pm) and no more than once at night. Bladder drill and bladder training are two approaches to regaining inhibitory control that are commonly used with clients who can take charge of programmes themselves.

BLADDER DRILL

Bladder drill aims to train clients to remain dry for predetermined voiding intervals which are lengthened as success is achieved. Rate of progression varies and will depend also on factors such as caffeine intake and pelvic floor control. Clients are instructed to go to the toilet, whether they feel the need to or not, at regular intervals, usually starting with 1 hour and progressing by half hour increments toward the goal of 3–4 hour intervals, and check off their toilet visits on a chart. Episodes of leakage are also recorded on the same chart. This record is reviewed with the physiotherapist at each visit. The emphasis is on deferring voiding for the required length of time and on overcoming urgency in that period. Techniques to resist voiding include:

1. Contracting the pelvic floor muscles. Doing so should inhibit detrusor activity, but may increase urge for some people by simultaneously increasing pressure on the bladder, especially if the abdominal muscles also contract.
2. Relaxation. Urge increases general body tension thus adding to the problem. Clients are trained to reduce intra-abdominal pressure by relaxing the abdominal muscles.
3. Distraction. Clients are encouraged to think about or to do other things to take their

attention off the urge sensation. Consciously following a regular breathing pattern or walking briskly may help some people.

4. Perineal pressure. Exerting pressure on the perineum, by hand or by sitting on a firm rolled up towel inhibits detrusor contractions.

A combination of these methods may help. Physiotherapists encourage clients to find their own best way of inhibiting detrusor contractions. Once the strong urge has passed, clients may be able to resist voiding until the end of the current interval is reached. Clients who know that they are susceptible to certain environmental triggers such as running water or approaching their front door, should prepare themselves in advance and use these urge quietening techniques before detrusor contractions become uncontrollable.

Older people can follow bladder drill while at home, or away from home on outings such as visiting relatives or day centres or even shopping. Naturally, it is easier to do at home with a convenient toilet. Some people find it difficult to maintain the regime away from home if no toilet is available or because of social restrictions.

BLADDER TRAINING

Bladder training has the same goals as bladder drill but, rather than adhering to pre-set voiding intervals, clients wait for the urge sensation and then try to defer voiding for increasingly longer periods. Deferral of voiding uses the same techniques as for bladder drill; clients try to defer voiding at first for 5 minutes, progressing to 10, 15 minutes and so on until normal voiding intervals are achieved.

Both bladder drill and bladder training have been successful in managing urge and mixed incontinence. However, these regimes are unlikely to be successful with clients suffering from neurological impairment, confusion or dementia, as they require clients to have normal urge sensation, motor innervation and the motivation to achieve the set goal. Some clients do not experience urgency, cannot interpret it correctly or may be unaware of when they are wetting themselves.

HABIT TRAINING

Habit training or timed voiding is a schedule for telling clients at regular intervals when to void and then assisting them to the toilet if necessary. Timing is based on the patient's normal voiding pattern and no effort is made to retrain this by suppressing urge or delaying voiding. Habit training has led to a reduction in incontinence among nursing home residents.

PROMPTED VOIDING

Prompted voiding is similar to habit training and may be used in conjunction with it. At regular intervals clients are asked whether they need to void but they are only taken to the toilet if they feel any urgency. This method teaches awareness of the need to void and encourages clients to request assistance. The success of habit training and prompted voiding depends on the constant availability of caregivers or nursing staff. It places a heavy burden on them, both in terms of patience and time so, if they are under pressure, their adherence to the regime may be poor.

Pelvic Floor Exercises

Pelvic floor exercises can improve and often cure both genuine stress incontinence and urge incontinence. Older people have as much potential to improve voluntary control of the pelvic floor muscles (PFM) and to improve their strength as for other muscle groups, although their rate of response may be slower than in younger people.

OBJECTIVES

Objectives of pelvic floor muscle exercise training are to:

1. Improve coordination, strength and endurance of the PFM.
2. Increase PFM cross-section area.
3. Increase urethral closing pressure.
4. Improve the ability to recruit the PFM during times of sudden increased intra-abdominal pressure.
5. Facilitate detrusor inhibition through the pudendal-pelvic reflex.

TEACHING METHODS

Clients are asked whether they can stop or slow the flow of urine during voiding. If they can, this is drawn to their attention as an indication of their ability to work these muscles. If they cannot stop the flow or have never tried, it is suggested that they try this occasionally to assess the ability to perform an isolated pelvic floor contraction. They are advised however, not to repeatedly do this every time they void as it may promote an abnormal voiding pattern. With the client in a half crook lying position, the physiotherapist observes and palpates the pelvic floor contraction as previously described under Assessment. The client pays attention to the feeling of the contraction, assisting with self-palpation or by using a mirror as necessary. Some women are reluctant to try vaginal palpation, but may be assured that it is a helpful and acceptable way of feeling and giving resistance to the contraction. A woman can feel PFM contractions by inserting her first and second fingers inside the vagina as well as palpating externally over the perineum and around the anus. She is encouraged to resist the contraction by separating her fingers to exert pressure on the vaginal walls laterally and posteriorly. A man

may palpate over the perineum around the anus, externally. The buttocks, adductors and abdominal muscles should be relaxed and the physiotherapist discourages breath holding as it increases intra-abdominal pressure. The PFM contraction should be described and felt as a sensation of squeezing around the fingers (for women), pulling forwards from the tailbone and anus to the pubic bone and upwards into the pelvis.

TYPES AND PARAMETERS OF PFM EXERCISE

Pelvic floor muscles should be trained for sustained contractions and endurance as well as for the high tension, fast contractions which are required for stress activities. Parameters of PFM training which must be considered are:

1. Fast and slow contractions.
2. Number of repetitions.
3. Duration of contraction and relaxation (seconds).
4. Tension level (client awareness, proprioception or instrumentation).
5. Frequency of exercise (number of sessions per day).

A variety of PFM exercise programmes have been advocated (Laycock, 1987; Dougherty, 1994). Recommended exercise frequency varies from hourly, to three times daily, to three times per week whereas the recommended number of contractions per session varies from five to 45; number of contractions per day from 15 to 300 and the duration of contraction from 2 to 30 seconds. No comparisons of the efficacy of these different exercise regimes have been reported. Nevertheless, the following scheme is suggested.

First a baseline from which to start the exercises has to be established (Chiarelli, 1991; Laycock,

1987). The client attempts a series of contractions and relaxations (1 or 2 second contraction, 4 second relaxation). The number of contractions that can be accomplished without fatigue becomes the baseline number. It may vary from two or three to over ten. In the latter case, ten remains the starting number and the quality of contraction can be worked on. Next a baseline duration of contraction is established. The contraction is held at a steady tension ending with a clearly felt relaxation. Often the initial contraction is felt, but is gradually lost so that by the end of the hold-time there is no clear distinction between the states of tension and relaxation. The longest period for which a distinct contraction followed by a discernible relaxation can be felt is timed.

Tension level of contractions can be varied from low to high, but the aim should be to increase them. However, excessive effort introduces associated muscle activity so it may be advisable for the client to consciously relax the whole body, then start with low level PFM contractions while maintaining abdominal relaxation, gradually increasing the tension level to the maximum required to improve muscle strength.

An example of an exercise regime is given in Figure 5. It shows three types of PFM contraction:

1. Fast contractions which develop control and the ability to contract and relax quickly. They may be performed at both low and high tension levels.
2. Sustained contractions which start at the baseline number of seconds and progress to a 10 second hold.
3. Augmented contractions which encourage progressively increased tension development. A minimum of five to a maximum of 20 contractions of each type is recommended, to be repeated six times per day.

Exercises regimes may be carried out in association with regular daily activities: after voiding, during household activities, when driving the car or sitting reading. PFM exercises should also be practised in the different positions that the PFM are required to work; sitting, standing, bending, lying and on position change from sitting to standing. Practice of strong, fast contractions in conjunction with lifting and coughing is particularly encouraged to retrain reflex function of the PFM. Fatigue, muscle soreness and back pain are initial problems occasionally associated with intensive exercising and the programme is adjusted accordingly. As with any continence programme physiotherapists reassure clients and try to prevent them from being discouraged by setbacks which are not uncommon and are associated with fatigue, catching a cold and emotional stress. People who are not overweight and whose general fitness level, body awareness and motivation to exercise are good, tend to respond best to PFM training.

Once the exercise programme is established, and continence has improved, PFM exercises should be continued on a maintenance basis five to ten times per day usually when cued by various activities such as voiding, washing dishes, taking a shower.

INSTRUMENTATION

Vaginal cones can be used to apply resistance to PFM contractions (Figure 6). They are weighted and available in sets of 20–100 g. A client attempts to hold a cone in the vagina while standing and walking for 10 minutes once or twice a day. Another method of resistance is to use an inflated cuffed catheter in the vagina, with the client gently pulling on this, while contracting the PFM in order to hold it in the vagina. Feedback about the contraction is given verbally with digital

Figure 5   Example of a pelvic floor exercise regime.

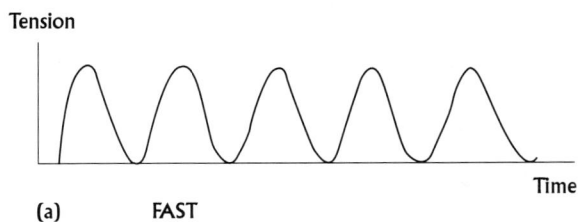

Tension

(a)   FAST

- Tighten and relax
- Repeat 5–10 times

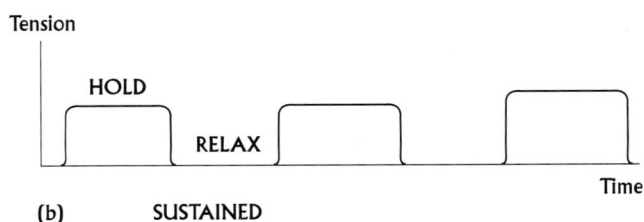

Tension

HOLD

RELAX

Time

(b)   SUSTAINED

- Tighten
- Hold 2–10 seconds
- Relax 10 seconds
- Repeat 5 times

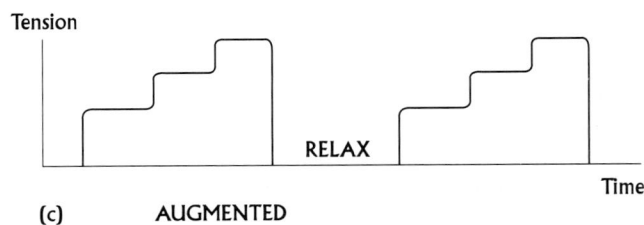

Tension

RELAX

Time

(c)   AUGMENTED

- Tighten
- Hold up to 3 seconds

↓

Tighten more and hold up to 3 seconds

↓

Tighten more and hold up to 3 seconds

- Relax 10 seconds
- Repeat up to 5 times

Figure 6   A set of weighted vaginal cones.

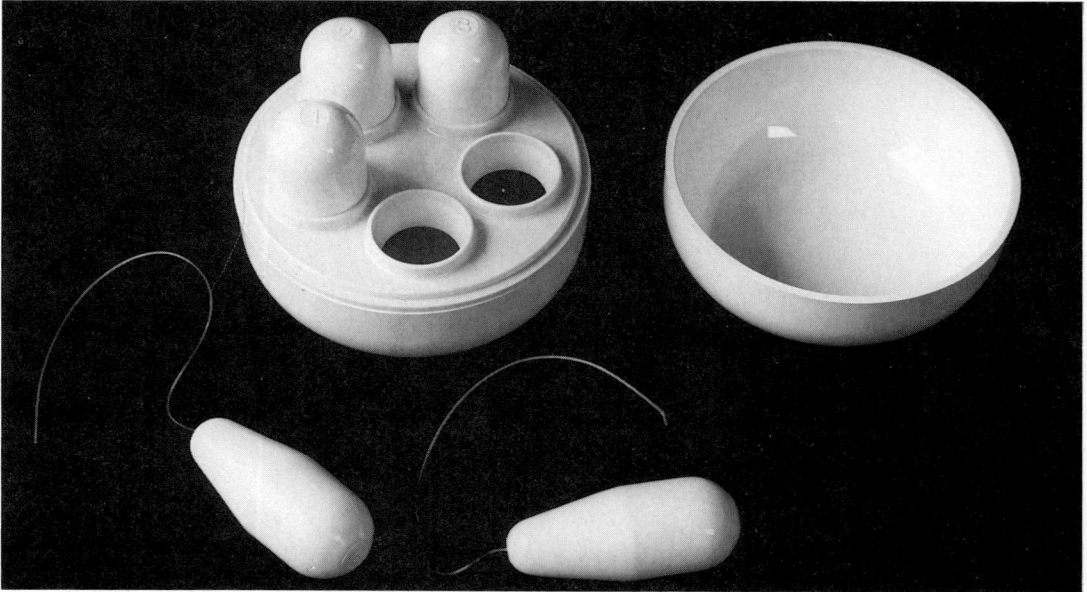

Figure 7   A portable EMG biofeedback unit.

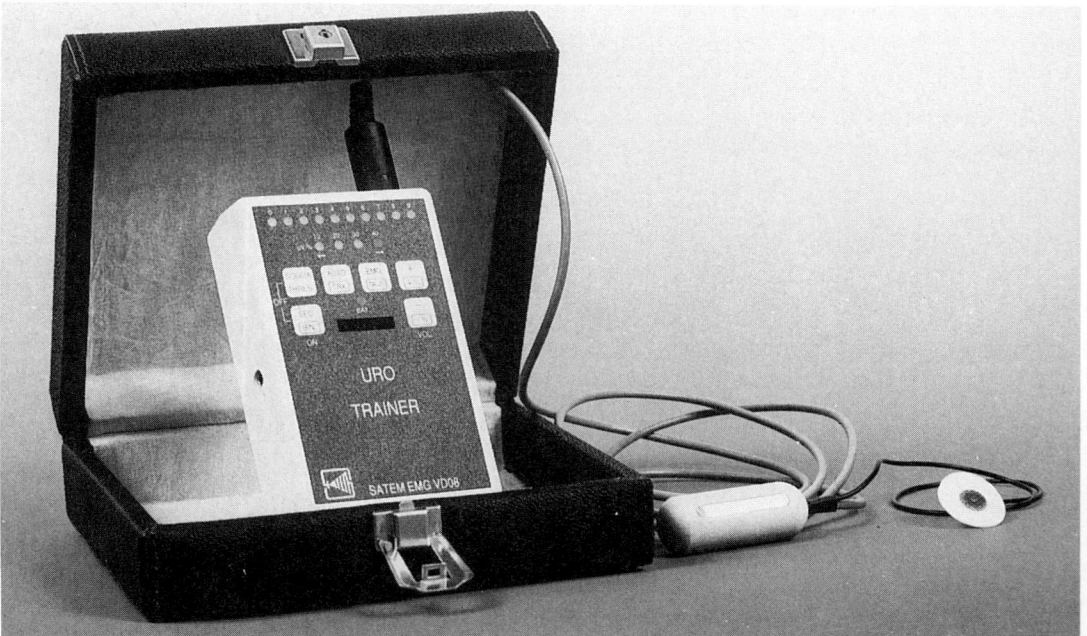

palpation, visually by a mirror, or by the ability to retain the vaginal cones.

Biofeedback is more accurate and can be given by a pressure device or by an electromyographic (EMG) recording device inserted into the vagina. Pelvic floor exercises are often called 'Kegel exercises' as the first pressure biofeedback device (perineometer) for use in pelvic floor muscle training was devised by Kegel in 1948. There are several varieties of perineometer which are helpful for training clients both in the clinic and at home.

An alternative method of providing immediate knowledge of results is by EMG biofeedback. A vaginal sensor picks up muscle activity of the PFM and shows this to the patient in the form of light array on a portable feedback unit (Figure 7) or a graphic display on a computer screen. A second set of electrodes may be used to monitor abdominal muscle activity so that excessive activity there can be reduced. Surface perianal or rectal electrodes may be used for men, and surface electrodes for women if a vaginal electrode is difficult to insert. There is evidence that instrumental feedback is superior to verbal feedback and PFM exercise alone in improving continence but further research is needed (Knight and Laycock, 1994).

The EMG biofeedback equipment is expensive, so clients may be unable to afford to rent the unit or to purchase single user electrodes for home use. Extreme caution must be taken in sterilizing multiple-user equipment; disinfection fluids such as Cidex and Milton are used and pressure probes are covered with a condom. Because the PFM are less accessible than other muscles for observation and measurement of activity, biofeedback instrumentation is particularly helpful for assessing baseline muscle function, setting goals, monitoring progress and improving patients' awareness

Figure 8   An EMG biofeedback display of (a) a series of fast contractions; (b) sustained 10-second contractions; (c) augmented contractions of the pelvic floor.

(a)

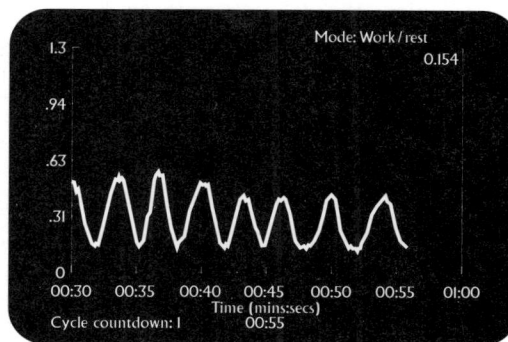

(b)

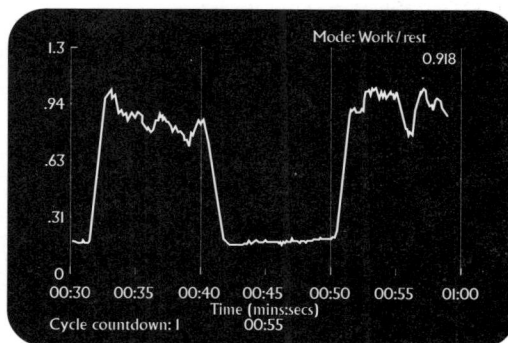

(c)

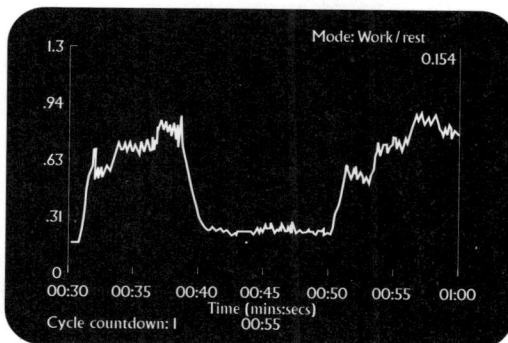

and motivation. Acceptance of instrumentation is variable. Some people like using gadgets, others dislike the idea of having them inserted into the vagina or rectum.

Electrical Stimulation

Electrical stimulation is used for stress and urge incontinence. Various approaches have been described, using different types of current (interferential or pulsed), different current parameters (intensity, frequency, phase duration) and different electrode placements (Figure 9). It is suitable for clients who have the necessary physical and cognitive abilities and who are likely to tolerate it. Urgency, frequency and retention associated with multiple sclerosis have been shown to respond well to electrical stimulation, as well as urgency and stress incontinence in men following prosta-

tectomy. One or two daily treatments for 15–30 minutes are recommended.

GENUINE STRESS INCONTINENCE

Stimulation of the pelvic floor muscles via the pudendal nerve improves urethral closure. Vaginal, rectal or surface perineal electrodes can be used. Surface electrodes give a strong sensory stimulus which may not be tolerated at intensities in the range required to produce an adequate contraction. Vaginal and rectal electrodes should be fully inserted so that the muscle contraction is felt without the sensation of the current. Laycock and Green (1988) recommend the following surface electrode placements for interferential current; these can also be used for pulsed current:

1. Bipolar, one electrode each side of the anus.
2. Bipolar, one electrode each side of the gluteal cleft just anterior to the anus.

Figure 9   A portable electrical stimulator with vaginal electrode.

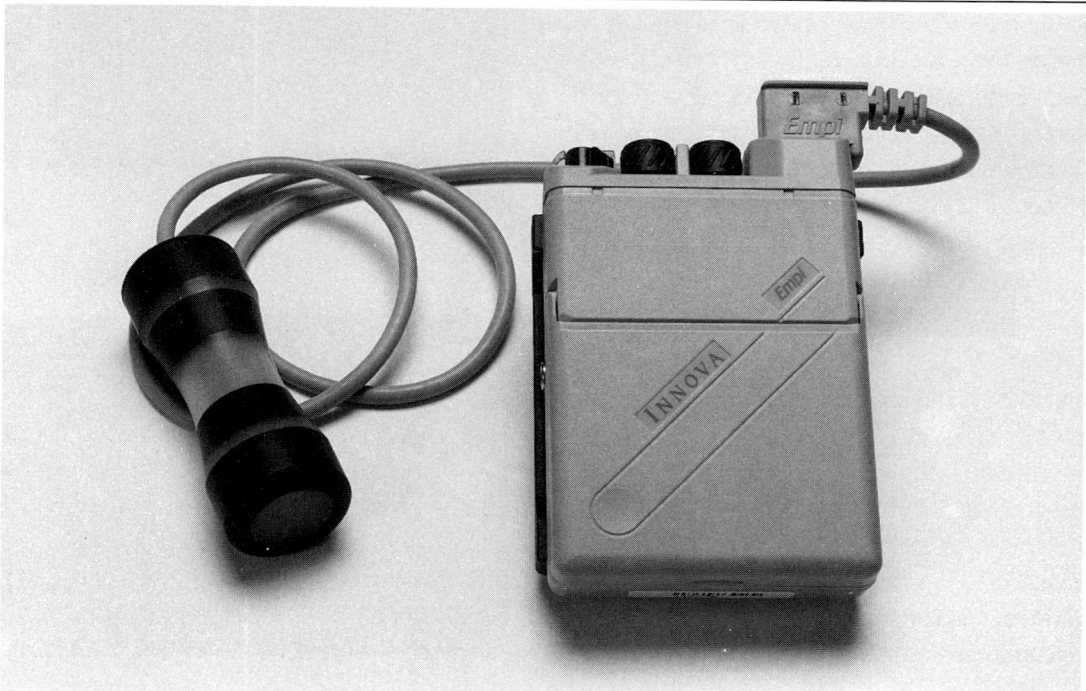

3. Bipolar, one electrode over the anus, one electrode anteriorly on the perineum.
4. Quadripolar (interferential current), two electrodes under, or medial to the ischial tuberosities, two electrodes anteriorly on the perineum or over the obturator foramina.

Depending on the location, self-adhesive electrodes may be used, or electrodes requiring conductive gel, water soaked gauze or sponge pads that can be secured with tape or body weight.

Recommended current intensities vary between 35 and 80 mA and depend on the type of current and its phase width. To produce strength gains of any skeletal muscle by electrical stimulation, current intensity must be sufficiently high to produce at least 65% of maximal voluntary contraction, therefore motor level stimulation must be used. Choice of current frequency is based on the muscle type. The levator ani and external sphincter muscles are composed of slow twitch and fast twitch motor units which respond best to 30–60 Hz and 10–20 Hz respectively. Laycock and Green (1988) suggest a range of 10–50 Hz when using interferential units which provide for an automatic sweep through a frequency range. An upper limit of 35 Hz is probably adequate and fatigue will be faster as frequencies increase. There is no evidence that interferential current is any better than pulsed currents, but it does have the advantage of the automatic frequency sweep. Phase durations of 80 µs to 1 ms are commonly used. Longer durations are more effective for stronger stimulus but must be balanced with patient comfort. Portable electrical stimulation units such as the pulsed current stimulator shown in Figure 9 are convenient for home use.

Electrical stimulation is most useful for stress incontinence when voluntary contraction is absent or extremely weak and is used as a facilitation technique to increase awareness of PFM contraction. Once good voluntary contractions are achieved, PFM exercises can be continued without the stimulation as long as the patient is well motivated and consistent with the exercise.

URGE INCONTINENCE

Afferent stimuli from the pudendal nerve have been shown to have an inhibitory effect on the detrusor via the pudendal to pelvic nerve spinal reflex pathway. This reflex is active during PFM exercises and may account for improvement in urge incontinence with such exercises. The same electrode placements may be used as listed under stress incontinence and both sensory and motor level current intensity may be successful although motor level stimulation will produce a greater afferent input. Detrusor inhibition is best achieved with lower frequencies for stimulation of the smaller diameter myelinated pudendal afferents. Laycock and Green (1988) suggest 5–10 Hz, but up to 25 Hz has been reported. Phase width also varies, durations of 250 µs–1 ms usually being recommended.

Drugs Used to Treat Incontinence and their Side-effects

Physiotherapists working with incontinence sufferers are advised to recognize and understand the side-effects of any drugs that may be prescribed for their clients.

The rationale for drug use in stress incontinence is based on the high concentration of sympathetic alpha-adrenergic receptors in the trigone muscle at the base of the bladder, in the bladder neck and the proximal urethra. Alpha-adrenergic agents increase muscle contraction of the internal sphincter and increase bladder outlet resistance.

Side-effects of alpha-adrenergic agents include hypertension, cardiac arrythmia, anxiety, tremor, headache, insomnia and sweating.

Drugs for urge incontinence act by reducing unstable bladder contractions. Anticholinergic agents inhibit transmission at the neuromuscular junction on the detrusor muscle cells. Calcium antagonists are smooth muscle relaxants which act directly on the smooth muscle cells. Clients may report side-effects such as dry mouth, blurred vision, confusion and constipation. Anticholinergic agents and muscle relaxants have side-effects of fatigue, dizziness and postural hypertension and may therefore increase the risk of falling. Physiotherapists should advise clients who report any of these symptoms to consult their physician about drug usage in order to minimize side-effects and maximize benefit.

Oestrogen may be helpful for both stress and urge incontinence by its effects on urethral mucosal proliferation and alpha-adrenergic responsiveness.

Surgical Management of Incontinence

Various procedures are used to manage genuine stress incontinence (GSI) in women and incontinence secondary to outflow obstruction in men (Tobin, 1992; Walters and Karram, 1993). Being familiar with these surgical procedures allows physiotherapists to discuss their implications with clients who are considering surgery. Surgery is not always successful and does not necessarily eliminate the need for the conservative treatment approach of physiotherapy.

The objective of surgery for female GSI is to raise the bladder neck and proximal urethra to a high retropubic position, so that increases in intra-abdominal pressure are more normally transmitted to the urethra to maintain closure. The surgical approach may be vaginal, suprapubic or a combination of these. Cystocele and rectocele may require surgical repair.

Another technique involves injection of Teflon or collagen into the periurethral tissues. It stimulates fibrosis and increases periurethral support. Injections may be used for women with GSI and for men with postprostatectomy stress incontinence due to sphincter damage, but results may not be longlasting. Postprostatectomy stress incontinence may also be helped by the insertion of an artificial sphincter (an inflatable cuff) placed around the urethra.

Protective Systems

Protective systems do not treat the problem, but reduce the social side-effects and the cleaning burden, and allow the patient to cope with it. In desperation, people resort to some sort of absorbent pad as a firstline management of their incontinence problem, if they are unaware of the professional help available or are too embarrassed to seek it. Strips of old hand towels may be stuffed inside knickers and women commonly make use of menstrual panty-liners and other sanitary pads to absorb urine. However, specialized pads worn inside retaining pads are available for clients of both sexes (Chapter 25).

A modern incontinence pad has a thin, non-absorbent surface next to the skin through which urine flows, keeping the skin dry, a highly absorbent centre and a waterproof backing. Pants may be disposable or reusable, and it is important that the correct pad and pant are used together as systems are not always interchangeable. One pad-pant system has a washable polyester pant with a permeable lining incorporating a pouch from front to back into which a pad is inserted. The pads may be changed without the need to change the pants and there are versions for men and for women. Another system consists of elasticized pants which hold absorbent pads with waterproof backing securely in place, they can also cope with faecal incontinence. Dribble pouches for men are available.

Bed pads and draw-sheets may be used to protect mattresses and furniture. The most satisfactory type of draw-sheet or pad incorporates a hydrophobic surface layer, absorbent middle layer and waterproof outer layer. Both disposable and reusable types are available.

Skin care and odour are controlled by careful attention to cleanliness, with the help of disposeable wipes, cleansing agents, barrier and healing creams, and deodorants.

Catheters and Collecting Devices (see Chapter 25)

Indwelling catheters are a final option for both men and women. Catheters are indicated for urinary retention which cannot be adequately managed by other methods (including intermittent self-catheterization) and in the cases where severe incontinence causes skin irritation and sores or makes care very complex. Indwelling catheters are retained in the bladder by a water-filled balloon and are connected to a drainage bag, forming a closed, sterile system. Straps and pockets are available for securing the collection bag to the leg or thigh or within pants. Night drainage bags are necessary for the collection of larger volumes of urine.

Complications of catheter use include leakage and bypassing of urine due to catheter blockage or involuntary detrusor contractions. Confused patients may pull the catheter out. Bacteruria develops within 2–4 weeks but treatment by antibiotics is indicated only if there is systemic infection. Changing the system too frequently and bladder irrigation tend to promote further infection. Indwelling catheters are changed about every 30 days. Crystallization of urine with encrustation around and within the catheter is managed by bladder washouts or use of Teflon catheters. Other problems of indwelling catheters are pain, urethritis, periurethral abscess, haematuria, bladder spasms, chronic renal failure and fistula (Tobin, 1992; Urinary Incontinence Guideline Panel, 1992).

Penile sheaths are used by males as external collecting devices, secured by adhesive or straps which must be correctly applied to prevent damage to the penis, but external devices for females are much less successful as design is a problem.

Conclusion

For most older people, incontinence is highly amenable to conservative treatment and hence can be very satisfying for physiotherapists to treat. Moreover, physiotherapists are not only very well qualified to provide individual client care but also to be proactive in community education about continence and incontinence.

References

Abrams, P, Blaivas, JG, Stanton, SL et al. (1988) The standardization of terminology of lower urinary tract function. *Scandinavian Journal of Urology and Nephrology* 114 (Suppl):5.

Chiarelli, PE (1991) *Women's Waterworks: Curing Incontinence*. London: Gore & Osment Publishing (distributed in the UK by the Incontinence Advisory Service at the Disabled Living Foundation, 380–384 Harrow Road, London W9 2HU, UK).

Dougherty, M (1994) Pelvic floor exercise. In Laycock, J, Wyndaele, JJ (eds) *Understanding the Pelvic Floor*, pp. 55–68. Dereham, UK: NEEN HealthBooks.

Feneley, RCL (1986) Normal micturition and its control. In Mandelstam, D (ed) *Incontinence and its Management*, pp. 17–34. London: Croom Helm.

Gosling, J (1979) The structure of the bladder and urethra in relation to function. *Urologic Clinics of North America* 6: 31–38.

Hu, TW (1986) The economic impact of urinary incontinence. *Clinical Geriatric Medicine* 2: 673.

Johnson, MJ, Werner, C (1982) We had no choice – a study of familial guilt feelings surrounding nursing home care. *Journal of Gerontological Nursing* 8: 641–645.

Knight, SJ, Laycock, J (1994) The role of biofeedback in pelvic floor reeducation. *Physiotherapy* 80: 145–148.

Laycock, J (1987) Graded exercises for the pelvic floor muscles in the treatment of urinary incontinence. *Physiotherapy* 73: 371–373.

Laycock, J, Green, RJ (1988) Interferential therapy in the treatment of incontinence. *Physiotherapy* 74: 161–168.

Malone-Lee, J (1994) Recent developments in urinary incontinence in late life. *Physiotherapy* 80: 133–134.

Moore, KH, Gilpin, SA, Dixon, JS *et al.* (1992) Increase in presumptive sensory nerves of the urinary bladder in idiopathic detrusor instability. *British Journal of Urology* 70: 370–372.

Tobin, GW (1992) *Incontinence in the Elderly.* London: Edward Arnold.

Twible, R, Beukers, M, Chiarelli, P (1992) *Continence promotion seminar: a wee look at a big problem.* Canberra, Australia: The Veteran's Quality of Life Program (VQLP), Department of Veteran's Affairs, (and Continence Foundation of Australia, PO Box 311, Kippax ACT 2615).

Urinary Incontinence Guideline Panel (1992) *Urinary Incontinence in Adults: Clinical Practice Guideline.* AHCPR Pub. No. 92–0038. Rockville, MD: Agency for Health Care Polity and Research, Public Health Service, US Department of Health and Human Services.

Walters, MD, Karram, MM (1993) *Clinical Urogynecology.* St. Louis, USA: Mosby-Year Book Inc.

Wall, LL (1994) Anatomy and physiology of the pelvic floor. In: Laycock, J, Wyndaele, JJ (eds) *Understanding the Pelvic Floor*, pp. 7–21. Dereham, UK: NEEN HealthBooks.

Williams, ME, Pannill, FC (1982) Urinary incontinence in the elderly. Physiology, pathology, diagnosis and treatment. *Annals of Internal Medicine* 97: 895–907.

18

Stroke

KAREN BRUNTON, CAROLYN McCULLOUGH

Much has been written about the management of stroke. However, despite the majority of patients with stroke being over the age of 65 and half of this group being over 75, few authors, with the exception of Bohman (1987), have addressed specifically the physiotherapy management of older people with stroke. The proportion of older people in the global population is rising (Chapter 2), so that physiotherapists will be managing an increasingly older group of stroke survivors in the future (Kelly-Hayes *et al.*, 1988). Assessing and treating this older population is extremely challenging to physiotherapists as they must inevitably deal with a multitude of psychological factors and social problems besides the physical consequences of the cerebral vascular accident (CVA); they must also take account of changes associated with normal ageing and the increased likelihood of coexisting health problems.

In this chapter we profile the needs and progress of the older person with stroke, give guidelines for physiotherapy assessment and provide management schemes and treatment suggestions appropriate for this client group.

Short-term and Long-term Outcome of Stroke Among Older People

Results of stroke rehabilitation programmes highlight prognostic indicators and likely functional outcomes for this age group. Following a

255

CVA, mortality may be as high as 38% (Stineman and Granger, 1991). Survivors may go directly home with little to no treatment or may be discharged home after a comprehensive rehabilitation programme. Other patients will require long-term institutional care (Chapter 30). Kalra et al. (1993) found a similar pattern when looking specifically at stroke patients over the age of 75.

Age alone does not determine rehabilitation outcome. However, it is one of the adverse prognostic indicators of function following stroke. Other negative indicators include prior CVA, incontinence of bowel and bladder, cognitive impairment and perceptual problems: denial, neglect, visuospatial deficits, inattention, apraxia (Jongbloed, 1986). After stroke, older people were able to return home at 3 weeks if they had no cognitive impairment, good motor recovery, no sensory or inattention deficits and no incontinence (Kalra et al., 1993).

The Framingham study (Kelly-Hayes et al., 1988) showed that stroke patients who required institutional care were older and more likely to be women. Social factors also influenced institutionalization patterns. Older women, single or married, with moderate to severe residual impairment and minimal education were at greatest risk, whereas married men of similar age and functional status were likely to live at home. Most older people with stroke who live in institutions have low functional ability and some degree of cognitive impairment (Kalra et al., 1993) (Chapter 8). Those people who need to use wheelchairs for mobility after stroke, either because they cannot walk or because walking is not functional, are usually in care (Thorngren and Westling, 1990).

Stineman and Granger (1991) extensively reviewed the stroke rehabilitation outcome literature. In general, they found that clients treated in comprehensive rehabilitation programmes were more often discharged home with better functional skills and in less time than clients treated in other settings. Nevertheless, even after comprehensive rehabilitation, 29–50% of patients with stroke have some degree of dependency in activities of daily living (ADL). As clients' age increases, a greater proportion are women and their dependency increases (see Chapter 22). Functional improvement appears to peak between 3 and 6 months after stroke. Functional ability scores on admission and on discharge are correlated but the middle ranked group in terms of function at the time of admission improve the most, while the highest and lowest functioning groups change less. Any delay between CVA and the commencement of rehabilitation has a detrimental affect on eventual functional outcome, especially for ambulation and transfer status.

Rehabilitation for elderly stroke clients can be very successful. Kalra et al. (1993) reported that 80% of stroke survivors over age 75 were discharged home: 32.7% of these by 3 weeks post-onset and 67.3% after 3 months of rehabilitation. The remaining 20% had cognitive impairment with poor functional status and were discharged to institutions. Among clients discharged home after rehabilitation, 66% walked independently with or without walking aids, 23% used wheelchairs, 11% needed assistance for mobility and transfers – and all needed additional community support services. The success of rehabilitation for stroke survivors over 75 years of age was related to cognitive status and the ability to learn new techniques.

Long-term follow-up reports provide physiotherapists with expectations about long-term functional status (Greveson et al., 1991; Reutter-

Bernays and Rentsch, 1993). Most older people with stroke who are discharged home after rehabilitation are still there at follow-up. Only when there is a major deterioration in health status or social situation is a person with stroke placed in an institution. Greveson et al. (1991) followed-up survivors at 3–5 years post CVA, and found mortality to be 27% and that 19% had suffered a second CVA. Using a follow-up time of 2–5 years, Reutter-Bernays and Rentsch (1993) reported similar figures: 38.2% mortality and a second CVA in 22% of survivors. Functional scores at long-term follow-up were close to discharge scores with small decreases being attributed to ageing and the presence of other disease processes (Reutter-Bernays and Rentsch, 1993). At just 1 year post-stroke, Thorngren and Westling (1990) found that 81% of their sample could walk independently but only 69% could use stairs by themselves. Sadly, despite survivors being capable of performing many functional activities, they rarely actually did so and socialization outside of the home was severely restricted (Greveson et al., 1991). Moreover, depression was identified in 28% of survivors and was more likely to occur in those with functional dependency.

Physiotherapists should be prepared, not only to treat the stroke survivor, but also to take account of the caregivers' concerns, as the ability of the person with a stroke to remain at home in the long-term is linked to the presence of a caregiver. A caregiver is usually a female spouse, and is commonly living at home with the client. Caregivers may carry a great deal of burden. Greveson et al. (1991) found that they had greater emotional, sleep, and social problems than age and sex matched controls and 30% of them suffered marked strain after 3 years. Surprisingly, community support services were underutilized and were poorly coordinated to meet needs.

Stroke survivors who live in institutions do not do as well as those who live at home. Not only are they likely to be older, but after the same follow-up interval, stroke survivors in institutions are found to have significantly more cognitive impairment and be more functionally dependent. Their ADL scores may show marked decline toward total dependency compared with their discharge scores. These changes may be attributed to comorbidity, low functioning before the CVA, greater likelihood of another CVA and decreased stimulation (Kalra et al., 1993; Reutter-Bernays and Rentsch, 1993). Their poor functional status means that most of these people need to be cared for in long-term or chronic hospitals which can provide for their heavy nursing care needs.

Clients whose function is fairly good may, nevertheless, have to be cared for in a residential home or a nursing home that provides light nursing care if they have significant cognitive impairment (Greveson et al., 1991). They are usually independently ambulatory but require constant supervision for their own safety. They cannot be left unattended and require direction to complete ADL and other tasks.

Some older clients with stroke need to continue physiotherapy after discharge, to continue the rehabilitative process if further benefit is anticipated, to provide preventative maintenance therapy or to upgrade functional status several years post CVA.

Table 1 summarizes older patient characteristics and ongoing treatment needs by discharge placement. Table 2 presents characteristics and treatment needs at follow-up, 2–5 years after discharge. The treatment needs identified are intended to guide physiotherapists when plan-

Table 1
Older Patients with Stroke – Characteristics at Discharge and Ongoing Treatment Needs

Placement	Characteristics at discharge	Ongoing treatment (Tx) needs
Home directly from acute care	Good early recovery, few residual motor deficits No cognitive, perceptual or sensory deficits Continent Independent, residual disability unlikely No community support services	Medical management of risk factors to prevent subsequent CVA No Tx implications for physiotherapy
Home following rehabilitation	More married males Walks independently (± aids), may not climb stairs Continent Lives with caregiver Requires community support services	Day hospital Tx to maximize functional status Community activities to maintain function and provide socialization Patient and caregiver education Caregiver support to reduce stress
Residential care/nursing home	Older, more females, males likely single Mild to moderate functional disability along with cognitive impairment Cannot be left alone, needs supervision for tasks, has the physical capacity to walk	Supervized activities to maintain function and provide socialization; groups are suitable Tx delegated to PTAs PT consultant role, PRN active intervention Recreation therapy programmes
Long-term care/chronic hospital	Older, more females, males likely single ADL dependent, possible prior impairments Cognitive, perceptual and/or sensory deficits Uses wheelchair for functional mobility Incontinent, possible prior CVA, comorbidity	Improve or maintain assisted functional status Maintenance activities delegated to PTAs Preventative intervention to offset complications from residual deficits Wheelchair seating and mobility with occupational therapy

Abbreviations: Tables 1 and 2:
PT: Physiotherapy.
PTA: Physiotherapy assistant.
Tx: Treatment.
PRN: As needed or when required.
ADL: Activities of daily living.
CVA: Cerebral vascular accident.

ning management. General areas of treatment are outlined according to the patient's care setting and length of time post CVA. Physiotherapists can expect to be involved with the treatment and management of older patients with stroke in various community and institutional settings during the acute, the rehabilitative, and the chronic post-stroke phases.

Table 2

Older Patients with Stroke – Characteristics at Follow-up and Treatment Needs at 2–5 year Follow-up

Placement	Characteristics at follow-up	Treatment (Tx) needs at follow-up
Home directly from acute care	At home unless ageing, comorbidity and/or social/economic factors cause change No functional change related to initial CVA	None related to initial CVA
Home following rehabilitation	Home with caregiver. More married males Slight ADL decline but functional, still walks Limited activities out of home, depression and social isolation may occur Caregiver stress, support services minimal	Upgrade functional skills at day hospital Link with community activities and programmes Utilize support services for caregiver relief Patient and caregiver education to prevent inactivity, functional decline and institutionalization
Residential care/nursing home	Older, more females, males likely single Significant cognitive impairment Mild to moderate functional impairment Slight ADL decline, still walks, supervision and direction for tasks	Supervized maintenance programmes (PTAs) and leisure activities (recreation) Upgrade any ADL and functional declines Address age-related changes and comorbidity affecting mobility status
Long-term care/chronic hospital	Older, more females, males likely single Cognitive, perceptual and/or sensory deficits Complications arising from residual deficits Significant ADL decline, total dependency Wheelchair user, functional mobility declining Incontinent, subsequent CVA, comorbidity	Upgrade to assisted functional status Maintenance activities delegated to PTAs Address complications due to residual deficits Revise seating and wheelchair mobility with occupational therapy Address age-related changes and comorbidity affecting mobility status

Physiotherapy for Stroke

There is an extensive body of work on stroke rehabilitation, but few studies have investigated the physiotherapy component of rehabilitation programmes. Ashburn *et al.* (1993) have reviewed the literature looking at specific physiotherapy treatment approaches and parameters. Therapeutic approaches such as neurodevelopmental treatment (NDT) developed by Bobath, proprioceptive neuromuscular facilitation (PNF) based on the work of Kabat and motor relearning developed by Carr and Shepherd all aim to improve function to as near normal quality of movement as possible. All may lead to functional improvements, but no one approach has been shown to be superior to the others; however, functional outcome measures show that some kind of physiotherapy is preferable to no physiotherapy at all. Ashburn *et al.* (1993) noted that the published comparative studies have a number of methodological difficulties: details of treatment content may be either lacking or vary considerably between study groups; delays between CVA onset and treatment initiation, which are known to have a negative impact on ambulation and transfer outcomes, often occurred; the skill level of the physiotherapists providing treatment was not taken into account and it was rarely possible to separate the physiotherapy component from the therapeutic intervention provided by other disciplines. Critically, patients' ability to perform functional activities with near normal quality movement was not used as the principal outcome measure in any study; instead an ADL index, lacking any motor performance indicator is commonly used. It is not surprising, therefore, that the relative efficacy of the various approaches has not been established.

As for treatment parameters, it seems that early intervention has a positive effect on functional independence and mobility status (especially ambulation) and that more intense therapy, i.e. more treatments per week, may be of greater benefit than less intense therapy. However, based on the current literature, only these generalizations can be given to guide therapists when planning treatment programmes.

Assessment

Assessing an elderly person with stroke takes place within a framework of normal movement but also against a knowledge of age-changes that may already have restricted functional mobility (see Chapters 6, 7, 9 and 12).

Normal Movement

All movement requires a base of support appropriate for the activity and alignment of the body's centre of mass over the base. This alignment comprises the relationship of head, trunk, pelvis and limbs to each other and to the base. During movement, the base of support and the alignment will change from the initial to the final posture, as when rising from a bed or a chair (see Chapters 7, 15). Movement also requires a sequence (order and timing of events) as the movement transpires. Inherent in the ability to perform controlled movement is stability as well as mobility within the body. In any functional activity some muscles must provide stability i.e. postural support, while others act as prime movers. In rising to standing, after the point of lifting off the surface, the head and trunk are reasonably stable while the lower extremity joints move through a considerable range from flexion to extension (Nuzik *et al.*, 1986). These four components – base of support, alignment, sequence, stability and mobility – interact to promote efficiency of movement and variety in movement patterns (Fisher and Yakura, 1993).

Premorbid Age-changes in Functional Mobility and the Impact of Stroke

Age-related changes in the musculoskeletal, neurological and cardiorespiratory systems mean that some mobility tasks have already become rather difficult for older people, causing them to reduce their functional status even before the additional impact of a stroke (Chapter 6). Considerable flexibility is required in the spine and lower extremity joints in order to roll onto their side or rise from a bed. Elderly people may require relatively more strength for tasks such as rising from sitting, walking, climbing stairs, and bending to pick up an object from the floor to overcome their increased stiffness.

Elderly people with knee flexion contracture

(KFC) approaching 20 degrees should be given high priority for intervention since they appear to be on the brink of a change in ambulation status. The point at which joint restriction begins to interfere with functional mobility interested Mollinger and Steffen (1993), who followed 112 nursing home residents, mean age of 83, over a 10-month period. Most of their sample showed KFC of 10 degrees or less, and it was observed that increases in KFC were associated with decreased walking ability. Whereas residents with less than a 20 degree KFC varied from independent to non-ambulatory, most with KFC of 20 degrees or greater were non-ambulatory and all subjects with KFC greater than 33 degrees were non-ambulatory. Thus KFC greater than 30 degrees should be classified as severe. A cerebral vascular accident has a profound additional impact on existing mobility problems. Movement becomes yet more difficult, due to altered alignment over the base of support that results from muscle imbalances secondary to the hemiparesis and to abnormal muscle tone. Problems with timing and firing of motor units and an inability of muscles to act in their normal synergistic fashion mean that sequencing of movements may change. Stability and mobility are reduced as mobility declines through inactivity, and muscles are unable to provide postural support or produce movement.

With endurance already reduced, the deconditioning effects of bed-rest following stroke and the increased energy demands associated with a hemiplegia, it is understandable that the older person becomes less tolerant of activity after a stroke (Mol and Baker, 1991). Prolonged inactivity may explain in part why delays in starting rehabilitation are related to poorer functional outcome for ambulation and transfer status, as well as increasing the potential for the development of joint contractures, pressure ulcers and other complications.

Observation and Measurement

In view of the high probability of premorbid health problems and functional difficulties, it is crucial that during the assessment of older persons following a stroke physiotherapists record enough information to be able to determine which problems are stroke-related and amenable to rehabilitation, and which are long-standing and less likely to change.

Assessing elderly people, like assessing younger people with hemiplegia, includes taking a detailed history of the client's pre-stroke status in terms of social situation, lifestyle and activity level. The nature of the home situation and any adaptations already made receives detailed attention. Current status is examined in relation to communication and mental state, sensation, tone, range of motion of the trunk and limbs, motor recovery and active movement, gross motor ability, balance and gait (see Chapters 7 and 15). However, neurologically oriented assessment skills are not enough. Physiotherapists working with elderly people often need to use their orthopaedic and cardiorespiratory assessment skills as well. All three systems must be assessed as changes in any one will impact on functional mobility.

Objective measurement of the client's baseline status are taken using standard procedures. Several of the most commonly used are described in Cole et al. (1994) and in Wade (1992). Responsive measures are selected to record progress over time and client's status and progress can be monitored against recovery milestones (Partridge et al., 1993).

Management and Treatment

Motivation is known to be an important factor in learning (Chapter 9), and older people and their caregivers are more likely to be motivated to work towards a goal in which they have a vested interest. With older people, as with all clients, physiotherapists should strive for the highest attainable level of independence. Whereas some clients can realistically aim to regain independent ambulation in the community, for others the highest level of function may be the ability to roll over in bed without help or to get around independently in a wheelchair.

Management and treatment procedures for problems of trunk mobility, trunk stability, balance, limb and gait dysfunction will be outlined. They are based on neurodevelopmental treatment concepts and many of the techniques described have been developed by Bohman and Utley (1983–1994).

Trunk Mobility

Functional movement is largely dependent on adequate trunk mobility. During relaxed sitting, the spine is normally in a slightly flexed or 'slumped' posture. To initiate any functional activity while in this position a person normally sits up straight by moving the pelvis from a posteriorly tilted to a neutral or slight anterior tilted position and aligns the shoulders over the hips. This movement lifts the body weight off the sacral area and establishes a base of support through the feet and ischial tuberosities. When the spine is flexible, this change in pelvic position is accompanied by extension throughout the spine which establishes the centre of mass over the base. By maintaining this posture and elevating

the pelvis on one side, weight is shifted to the contralateral buttock. This allows postural adjustments to be made in sitting while still keeping the centre of mass over the base and thus maintaining balance.

Postural changes associated with ageing may result in decreased trunk mobility and interfere with the ability to achieve the posture and movement described above. Older people are often somewhat kyphotic which, together with loss of mobility in the lower back, tends to make them move the upper trunk and shoulders on the pelvis instead of initiating the movement at the pelvis. These changes may interfere with balance reactions. As the shoulders move beyond the base, the centre of mass is also transposed thereby exaggerating the potential to lose balance. Premorbid loss of range of movement may be compounded by prolonged inactivity associated with hemiplegia.

People with stroke who are stiff in their low back need to increase their range of movement (Fisher, 1987). One way by which this can be attempted is with the person sitting, a position from which many functional activities can be initiated. The physiotherapist gradually applies very firm pressure in the midline of the low back, at the same time stabilizing the upper trunk to isolate movement to the lower lumbar region (Figure 1). The pelvis is rotated out of a posterior tilted position towards an anterior tilt and the lumbar spine towards extension. The thoracic spine may also need to be mobilized towards extension but the immobility of the lumbar spine is addressed first.

Because older people are prone to osteoporosis (see Chapter 16) such mobilizing techniques must be carried out with care. Pressure must be applied slowly at first, only gradually increasing. The physiotherapist observes the client's facial expression for signs of discomfort and moderates treat-

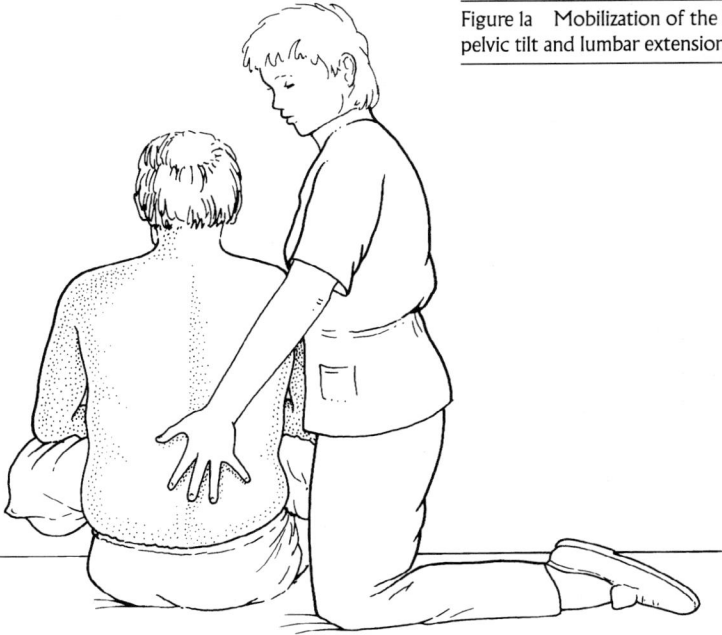

Figure 1a   Mobilization of the low back towards anterior pelvic tilt and lumbar extension.

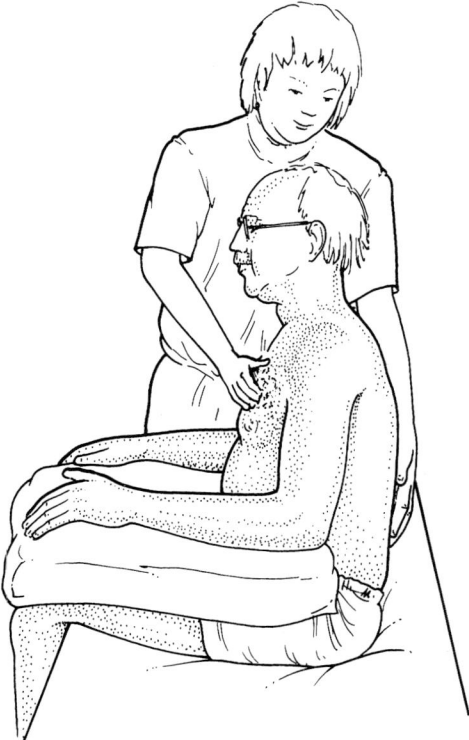

Figure 1b   If necessary, the physiotherapist places her hand on the upper chest for stabilization.

ment or stops it all together if necessary. Any small increase in spinal extension facilitates better functional alignment over the base of support. With increased range, treatment can be targeted at improving sitting balance and functional movement.

Trunk Stability

Approaches to neurological physiotherapy such as NDT, PNF, Rood usually emphasize proximal control and the need for postural set or stability as a background to limb function. Fisher (1987) reviewed several studies which confirmed this view by demonstrating electromyographic activity in the trunk prior to limb movement.

Trunk stability is frequently compromised follow-

ing CVA due to unilateral loss of muscle control. Inability to initiate and/or sustain muscle contraction on the hemiplegic side creates problems when co-contraction of muscle groups is necessary for trunk stability. Therefore physiotherapists need to facilitate active lower trunk movement (Bohman, 1987; Davies, 1990; Fisher, 1987). There are several ways that this can be done. One of them is for the physiotherapist to sit beside the patient, stabilizing the upper trunk with one hand and with the other placed in the midline of the client's low back (Figure 2). Pressure from the physiotherapist's hand is directed forwards and slightly upwards to assist the pelvis to rotate towards an anterior tilt. In applying this pressure, the physiotherapist's hand stays in contact with the client's body but the forearm moves from a neutral to a slightly supinated position in

Figure 2   Facilitation of active lower trunk movement towards anterior pelvic tilt.

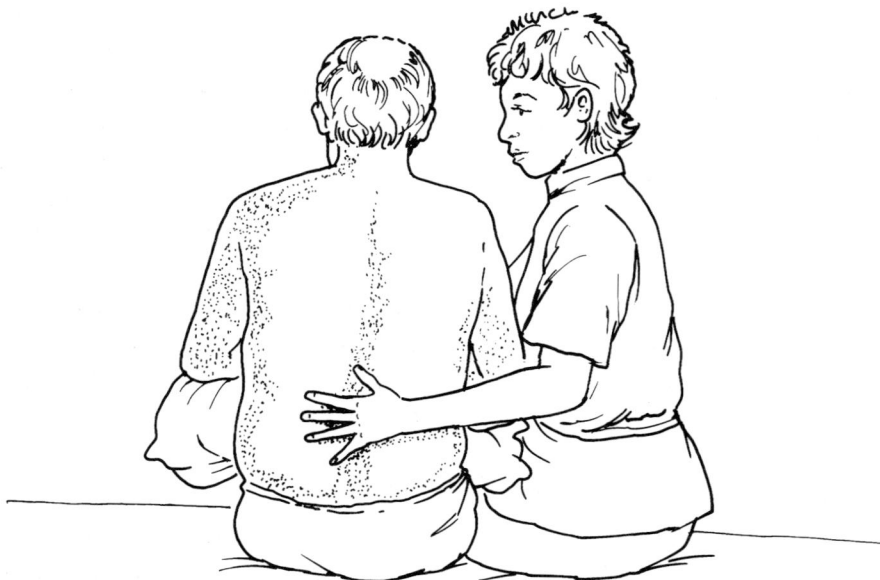

Figure 3   Facilitation of active lower trunk movement – lateral weight shift to the right hip. Arrow indicates direction of pressure.

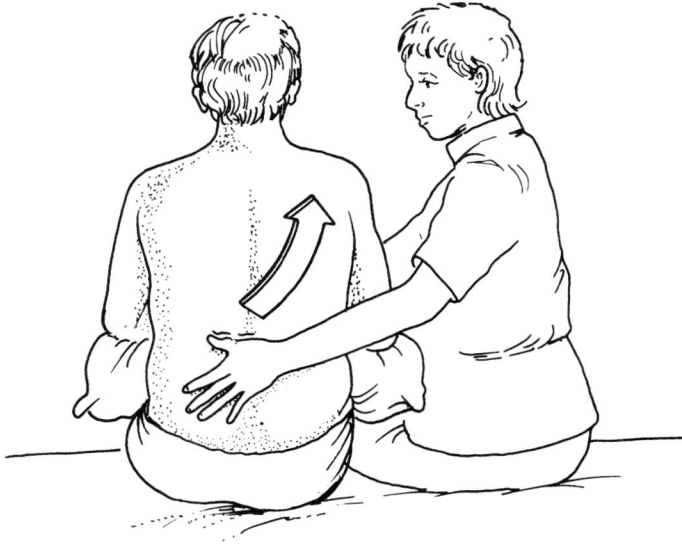

order to apply the pressure firmly in the required direction. Some clients will respond better to a pressure slightly higher in the thoracolumbar area. If the physiotherapist is sitting on the client's right, pressure is given with fingers of the other hand against the lateral edge of the left erector spinae muscle just above the pelvis. This pressure is directed toward the right to facilitate a lift of the left pelvis and a weight shift to the right hip (Figure 3). By using the ulnar border of the hand against the lateral edge of the right erector spinae muscle a similar pressure directed to the left can facilitate a weight shift to the left hip (Figure 4). By placing a hand lightly over the patient's sternum, the physiotherapist can stabilize the patient's upper trunk while facilitating these low back movements. The amount of pressure varies depending upon the assistance required to achieve movement of the lower trunk. More pressure may need to be applied on the hemiplegic side than the sound side.

As muscle control is gained, the physiotherapist gradually decreases the pressure to allow the client to assume control of the movement. These trunk movements are incorporated into a variety of functional situations, in order to improve the individual's overall functional mobility. The physiotherapist might help the patient maintain a slight anterior tilt and extended thoracic spine while facilitating lateral weight shifts to allow the person to adjust his or her position in the chair. This same anterior tilt and extended trunk must be maintained while flexing forwards at the hips to transfer weight to the feet and lift the buttocks off the seat to come to standing or to transfer.

BALANCE

While treating trunk mobility and stability, the physiotherapist also begins to address the client's balance problems (see Chapters 7 and 15). In order to balance, a symmetrical alignment over

Figure 4   Facilitation of active lower trunk movement — lateral weight shift to the left hip. Arrow indicates direction of pressure.

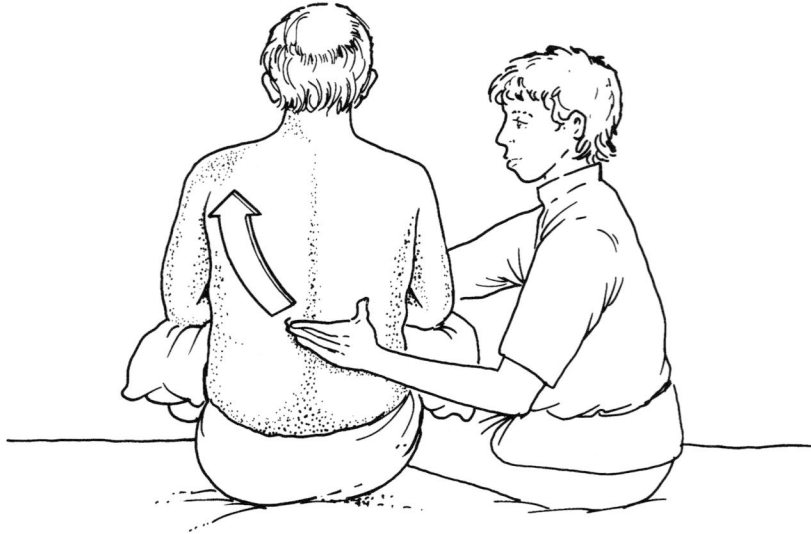

a base of support must first be achieved before working towards controlling movement over the base. As the physiotherapist works on facilitating an anterior tilt and extended upright sitting posture with clients, work is also started on controlling greater and greater ranges of movement in all directions away from and back to midline. In this manner equilibrium reactions are incorporated into the treatment programme.

Many older people have problems when standing because of decreased strength in the antigravity muscles (see Chapter 6). Often, they assume a kyphotic posture with flexed hips and knees. Standing alignment problems need to be addressed before working on the standing balance itself. Alignment is symmetrical when the centre of mass is central over the base of support so that shoulders, hips and knees are aligned over the ankles. Work on trunk mobility, so far addressed in sitting, prepares the client to

achieve better alignment in standing. Once standing, the physiotherapist, using hand pressure, gives tactile input to the hip extensors and/or knee extensors to facilitate appropriate standing alignment. Some clients may need preparatory joint mobilizations and/or soft tissue stretching to ensure sufficient range at the hip and knee. With hemiplegic patients, more input will need to be given to the hip extensors, abductors and/or quadriceps on the involved side (Figure 5). Once a more extended posture is achieved, the physiotherapist may need to add light pressure over the patient's abdominal muscles to achieve muscle co-contraction and the stability required in the trunk to maintain a symmetrical midline oriented standing posture (Figure 5). Treatment progresses to facilitate the client moving with control through greater and greater ranges of motion in all directions around the midline while facilitating the trunk

Figure 5 Physiotherapist provides input to right hip extensors, abductors and the abdominals to achieve a midline, symmetrical standing posture.

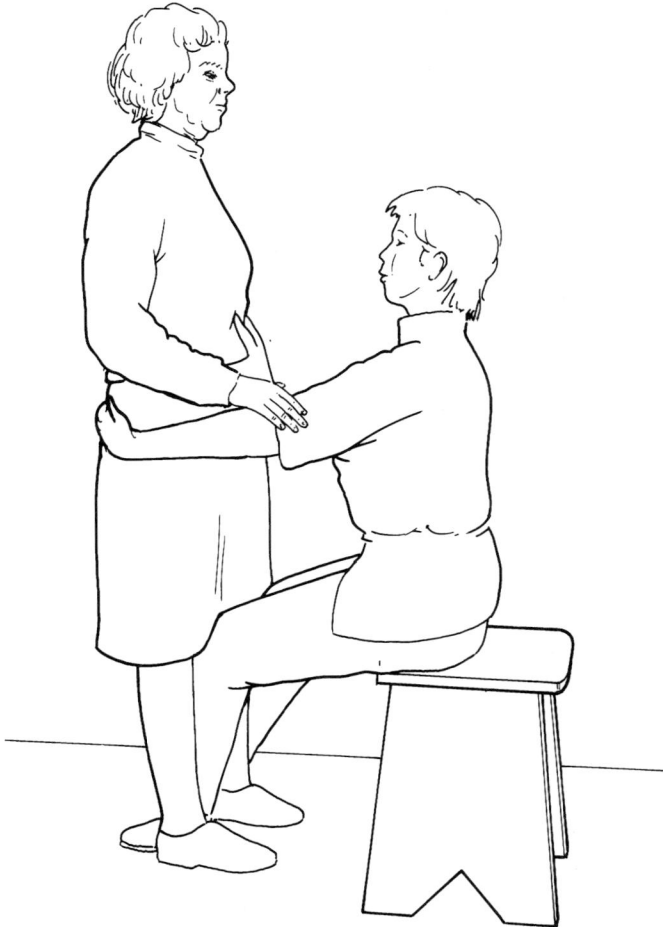

and lower extremity on the involved side to accept weight appropriately.

LIMB FUNCTION

As trunk control improves, the limbs are gradually included in the treatment session. Both upper and lower limbs have two functions: ability to weight bear and ability to move, with control, through space. A prerequisite for moving the upper limb in a skilled manner is not only the ability to stabilize the trunk but also the ability to stabilize the upper limb. Weight bearing through the arms assists trunk stability as well as improving proximal stability in the limb itself, i.e. stability of both the glenohumeral joint and the shoulder girdle on the thorax.

These concepts underpin management of upper limb problems in hemiplegia. If the person with

Figure 6   Alignment and positioning, of the involved upper extremity, in weightbearing to promote shoulder girdle stability.

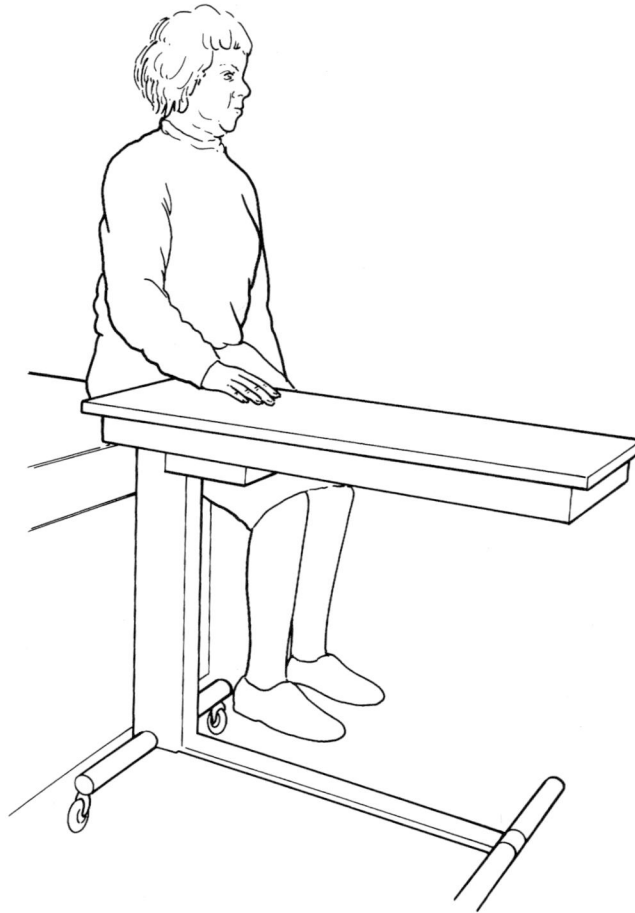

stroke has a flaccid arm, it should be supported on a firm surface with the shoulder positioned in slight lateral rotation, the elbow slightly ahead of the shoulder and the hand slightly lower than the elbow when the patient is sitting (Figure 6). Weight bearing and approximation through the appropriately aligned hemiplegic arm stimulates shoulder girdle stability. It also decreases the likelihood of shoulder subluxation, and goes a long way to preventing the excruciating shoulder pain which often arises from tissue overstretching when the heavy, unsupported, flaccid arm drags heavily on the shoulder and shoulder girdle structures.

Careful arm positioning is an integral part of every treatment session. It may be achieved in a variety of ways when the client is sitting. The arm may be placed on pillows on the lap, beside the person's hips on the edge of the sitting surface or on a table placed in front of the patient (Figure 6).

When working on postural control in sitting, having the table in front of the patient may be ideal; however, when the patient moves from sitting to standing a table in this position may be an obstruction, and placing the hands along the edge of the high mat by the patient's side may be more appropriate. In standing, a hospital overbed table, raised to an appropriate height, becomes a good weight bearing surface for the arm. The physiotherapist maintains the upper extremity in weight bearing throughout treatment and facilitates movement of the body over the limb. Movements of the body over the limb might include facilitation of an anterior pelvic tilt, lateral weight shifts, reaching activities in sitting, coming to standing and/or transfers. These movements, with weight bearing maintained, put the upper extremity joints through a functional range of motion, establish a better tone quality in the arm and develop proximal stability, all of which provides a foundation for re-education of selective arm movement. A wheelchair-bound patient can use a lapboard or arm trough to gain satisfactory positioning.

The same principles can be applied to the lower extremity. Treatment emphasizes weight bearing through the involved leg. In sitting with the feet on the floor, the feet are an integral part of the base of support, but the proportion of weight passing through them varies with body movements. It increases as the pelvis rotates forward at the hips and then is transmitted more to one foot and then to the other as bodyweight is shifted from buttock to buttock. Patients with hemiplegia are not always able to accomplish this weight transference. As they lean their bodies forward or shift their weight from side to side, the involved foot may slide or may pull up off the floor.

Throughout treatment, the entire plantar sur-faces of both feet should be kept in contact with a firm surface. During sitting activities, the feet should be positioned so that the heel is under the knee. If the patient is going to stand or transfer, the foot position must be adjusted. A position with the ball of the foot underneath the knee is more conducive to performing these transitional movements. The physiotherapist's foot (with shoe removed) is placed over the patient's foot to stabilize it during treatment. With hand pressure above the knee, and over the distal end of the patient's femur, the physiotherapist may give an approximation cue down into the foot. The approximation, appropriately timed, increases weight bearing into the foot and maintains foot placement.

Older people with severe hemiplegia frequently overuse the sound side. In extreme situations, the sound limbs are fully extended which moves the patient's centre of mass over the hemiplegic side. In sitting, these patients will fix or hold with the sound arm in attempts to balance. During transfers or in standing, they will often push themselves completely off balance to the hemiplegic side. Davies (1985) allocates an entire chapter to the problems and treatment of these 'pusher' patients. The essence of treatment is to maintain the hemiplegic limbs in weight bearing while facilitating body movements. Initially, clients with this problem are encouraged to move toward the sound side in order to re-establish a midline alignment. Doing so requires the trunk muscles on the hemiplegic side to act and also requires limbs of the sound side to move out of their fixed, extended posture. Treatment progresses by moving beyond the midline to the sound side, returning to the midline and then moving to the affected side. Moving to the affected side must be accomplished without excessive pushing of the sound limbs. The movement of the body while maintaining the involved limbs in weight bearing not only facilitates trunk muscle activity but also, because of the approximation, increases the awareness of the hemiplegic arm and leg and facilitates limb muscle activity. Successful treatment results in decreased overuse of the sound limbs, muscles on the hemiplegic side become more active and a symmetrical midline posture begins to develop.

PRE-GAIT AND GAIT ACTIVITIES

While performing sit to stand, transfers and midline oriented standing, equal weight bearing through the legs is stressed. The hemiplegic arm should be maintained in a weight bearing position, possibly using a hospital overbed table, which should enhance the client's trunk stability. An added advantage of the table is that it can move as the patient progresses into pre-gait and gait activities (see also Chapter 7).

Pre-gait activities emphasize weight shift to the involved leg. The physiotherapist chooses hand placements, often referred to as key points of control, according to the client's standing alignment problems. The trunk must be a stable unit during standing and gait. To this end tactile input over the trunk extensors and abdominals may be required. Weight shift to the hemiplegic leg may be accompanied by gradual increase in hand pressure in order to further facilitate activity in the trunk musculature and thereby enhance stability. Alignment of shoulders, hips and knees over the ankles is critical to stability in standing. The physiotherapist may apply hand pressure over the hip extensors, abductors, and/or the quadriceps to facilitate activity in these muscles and ensure loading of the leg in the correct alignment. The hand placements used and the amount of pressure from the physiotherapist will vary with the needs of the patient and the demands of the activity. Generally more facilitation is required during single limb support on the involved leg than during double limb support, with the least facilitation during single limb support on the sound leg.

Treatment logically progresses from facilitating weight shift onto the hemiplegic leg to stepping forwards and backwards with the sound leg. Frequently, clients lean forward at the trunk and hip and lock the knee of the hemiplegic leg in hyperextension. The physiotherapist must anticipate these tendencies and use hand pressures to maintain the correct alignment between the trunk and lower extremity.

Stepping is followed by forward weight shift of the body over the advanced foot. Patients with hemiplegia are often reluctant to weight shift forwards and backwards over the base of support, preferring to adopt a wide based stance and weight shift from side to side. However, the wide base means that the smooth forward progression of gait is interrupted. Following facilitation of forward weight shifting onto the sound leg, the client is encouraged to take a step with the hemiplegic leg. Frequently this will result in rotation of the trunk, hip hiking and circumduction of the leg. To avoid these abnormal patterns, the physiotherapist maintains correct trunk and hip alignment and may assist in advancing the hemiplegic foot. Treatment then progresses into reciprocal stepping. The amount of time spent on gait training per session will depend upon the patient's motor control and tolerance. With some patients, gait training may consist of taking only a few steps; in other cases, it may include the challenges of stair climbing and community ambulation.

The prescription of walking aids for people with stroke is controversial (see Chapters 25 and 26). In our opinion, it may not be realistic to expect older stroke patients to walk without walking aids. The choice of device will depend upon premorbid status, present level of motor control and balance, and expected place of residence. If the return of function in the involved arm is sufficient to grasp, then a front wheeled walker may be the aid of choice. The walker promotes a more symmetrical alignment over the base, and because it is in front of the person, forward weight shift is promoted. A wheeled walker versus a lift one is more conducive to a smooth flowing reciprocal gait pattern. However, the patient must not be allowed to push the walker so far forward that the elbows become fully extended. This would result in unwanted forward flexion of the trunk and hips with knee hyperextension. If the client requires less support, a long stick, resembling a shepherd's staff, promotes a more extended upright posture than a traditional stick or cane. The long stick also provides less stability than a quadripose cane. A disadvantage of quad or walk canes is that they extend the person's base of support laterally to the sound side. The patient, now leaning towards the cane, is likely to weight bear more on the sound leg, be less likely to use the hemiplegic leg and lapses into a lateral lurching step or gait. This is not to say that the walking aid alone makes or breaks the gait pattern, but consideration should be given to devices that will promote more normal movement patterns. Gait training with the device should incorporate appropriate alignment and weight shift. In this way the components emphasized in treatment will carry over into independent ambulation with the walking aid.

TREATMENT IN THE VERTICAL VS HORIZONTAL POSITION

We have stressed treatment in vertical postures. This is advantageous, since the focus of neuror-ehabilitation is on the retraining of functional skills; therefore relearning of these activities should be done with a functional orientation. Treatment in the vertical position becomes particularly important with older people, who may find supine and prone lying very disorienting due to information processing problems related to the CVA, and visual and somatosensory changes associated with ageing (decreased transmission of light through the eye, reduced proprioceptive input, etc.).

The horizontal position should not be ignored, but incorporated into treatment as it would be used functionally (rolling supine to side lying, adjusting one's position in bed, getting from supine to sitting). When requiring patients to practise these activities, physiotherapists should consider the age appropriate movement patterns and variations. During treatment, activities may need to be broken down into their subcomponents. For example, while working on rolling, the head and trunk component or the lower extremity component may be practised separately. However, the complete activity should always be included in the treatment session.

Therapeutic Bed Positioning

Bed positioning needs for stroke patients will vary according to the care setting and the length of time since onset of CVA. Careful positioning in the acute phase immediately post CVA protects and supports the flaccid, paralysed limbs, prevents the development of contractures and breakdown of the skin, and reduces the risk of respiratory complications.

Clients with stroke who remain immobile for a prolonged period or who are functionally dependent with residual deficits will require ongoing therapeutic positioning. Ideally positioning needs should be addressed continuously whether the patient is up in a wheelchair or resting in bed. In this way, appropriate alignment of the limbs, trunk and head will be maintained at all times and especially between treatment sessions. Consistent, good positioning provides sensory feedback, promotes body-awareness and reduces the risk of joint deformities occurring.

Therapeutic bed positioning is a process whereby external devices provide support, and skilled handling is used to align patients' limbs and trunk in bed. External devices may be prefabricated commercial products, or more likely are custom-fabricated rolls produced out of foam padded tubing of varying diameters depending on the body part to be supported and the degree of deformity present. When deformity and/or tone abnormalities are severe and longstanding, the physiotherapist may need to be very creative in the design of these rolls.

A non-ambulatory patient with bilateral hip and knee flexion contractures will need an appropriately sized roll placed under the knees, to support the deformity and prevent further hip and knee flexion from occurring by blocking movement into flexion. When positioned over the roll, the legs can be placed in a neutral rotational position wth the hips, knees and ankles aligned with the shoulders. A smaller pad or roll placed between the knees will prevent hip adduction and relieve pressure. If therapeutic positioning is not carried out then it is likely that the hip and knee flexion deformity will progress. When placed supine without positioning devices in place, a rotational movement of both lower extremities together to one side ('wind sweeping') will occur due to the effects of gravity on the unsupported deformity. This position, if allowed to become fixed, will prevent turning to the opposite side in bed,

increase the risk of pressure ulcers and prevent the patient from being seated in a wheelchair in an aligned, functional upright posture. The use of low load, long-term elongation of muscle and connective tissue to reduce contractures may be incorporated into the individualized bed positioning programme. Mogensen (1994) describes a positioning education programme for staff, providing hands-on care designed to train them in strategies and techniques to manage challenging positioning needs. Physiotherapists have the expertise and skills to provide education and consultation to caregivers (staff and/or family) on appropriate alignment and handling techniques to manage these difficult positioning problems.

Wheelchair Seating and Positioning

Wheelchairs with seating components should be viewed as treatment interventions to enhance and maximize clients' movement potential and function in sitting. They may provide non-ambulant people with the only option for functional independence whereas people who can walk short distances independently or with assistance may use wheelchairs to extend their independence over longer distances and into the community. Caregivers of fully dependent people use wheelchairs to provide transportation and passive mobility.

At least in western-style societies, the majority of people with stroke who are wheelchair users reside in institutions. This group of people tend to suffer from additional cognitive and perceptual deficits that affect their ability to learn independent and safe wheelchair propulsion about their environment. Physiotherapists and occupational therapists collaborate and reinforce safe wheelchair management.

Although occupational therapists are often primarily responsible for prescribing wheelchairs, physiotherapists ensure that clients' trunk control is satisfactory during functional activities in sitting and that transfers in and out of the wheelchair are of optimal quality. Wheelchair users must be able to accomplish a variety of functional activities while seated. Success depends on movement and control of the trunk, head and extremities interacting appropriately. Sitting is not a static activity, so provision of therapeutic seating, and ability to modify it as necessary is the background to optimal function.

The four components of movement described above under 'Assessment' also apply to functional movement in a wheelchair. First there must be a base of support with an alignment over the base, then movement occurs in an ordered sequence with different areas of the body providing stability and mobility. The wheelchair seat provides the base of support with additional components inserted to enhance stability and support the appropriate alignment about which functional movement will occur. In this way a wheelchair contributes to the rehabilitation goals between treatment sessions.

Body alignment in a wheelchair should incorporate midline orientation with the shoulders aligned over the hips, the head centered in both the frontal and sagittal planes, right/left symmetry through the trunk, pelvis and limbs and an even distribution of body weight over the base of support. Alignment correctly maintained by a tailored wheelchair provides positive reinforcement of functional sitting posture through proprioceptive and other sensory feedback.

A wheelchair can provide additional support and supplement postural control for trunk and extremities. This support offsets fatigue and allows a comfortable sitting position to be maintained, thereby increasing tolerance and lengthening the time the user is able to remain in the wheelchair. Appropriate alignment and support in the wheelchair should assist in preventing secondary complications such as contractures and skin breakdown in the most dependent clients.

THE SEAT

The seat should offer a firm base of support. The height and depth should be sufficient to provide full thigh contact especially for the hemiplegic leg. This distributes pressure over a larger surface area and controls alignment of the hip and knee. Many hemiplegic wheelchair users can transfer either independently or with assistance and can reposition themselves in the wheelchair. For these patients, the choice of cushion should not impede their movement. Maximum stability will be provided by a fixed base component attached to the wheelchair frame. An unfixed cushion is less stable and may slide during movement. Wedged or contoured cushions may make it difficult to move forward in the wheelchair for transfers or for reaching activities with the upper extremities. The physiotherapist balances clients' movement needs and abilities against their positioning, pressure relief and comfort needs. Dependent patients who are unable to reposition themselves or to transfer need cushions to meet their greater pressure relief and comfort needs. No patient should be left without an appropriate cushion and especially not in a chair with a slack canvas seat, as sitting on such a concave surface promotes internal rotation and adduction at the hips.

THE BACK

Patients who spend most of their day sitting in a wheelchair should have a supportive back component added to the chair to support spinal curves and maintain alignment. Excessive slackness in the back upholstery will align the shoulders behind the hips, promote a kyphotic trunk posture and a posterior pelvic tilt. Over time this slumped, reclined, sacral sitting posture may lead to restricted movement in the low back. The ability to move the upper body forward in the wheelchair for functional activities will be reduced. When mobilizations of the low back are being included in a treatment programme, an appropriately aligned back component will help maintain spinal range by preventing unwanted movements that lead to sacral sitting between treatment sessions. Back components may be flat or curved. A slightly contoured back may be more comfortable as it allows more extensive contact with the person's back. Increasing the curvature of the back component allows a fixed thoracic kyphosis to be supported, and may also provide additional lateral trunk support and stability. Lateral supports at the level of the thorax or pelvis may be needed with more severely impaired clients, to increase stability in the upright posture, help maintain midline orientation and enhance upper extremity function. A disadvantage of this added stability is that trunk movement may be impeded.

RELATIONSHIP OF THE SEAT AND BACK

The final position of the seat and back must be determined in relationship to each other. The fixed angle chosen is usually set between 90 to 100 degrees to obtain an aligned, upright sitting posture with the shoulders over the hips. Reclining the back so the angle between seat and back is greater than 100 degrees will result in the shoulders being positioned behind the hips. This posture impedes forward movement of the trunk for transfers, displaces weight from the thighs and ischial area to the coccyx and sacrum and promotes sliding forward in the wheelchair. If the patient then attempts to self propel the wheelchair from this slumped, reclined posture using the uninvolved leg and arm, additional sliding will occur, often accompanied by an unwanted backward thrust of the shoulders. Installing a wedge shaped seat cushion will not correct the poor body alignment or the backward thrusting during wheelchair propulsion. The back position should be adjusted out of the reclined position. A seat/back angle of greater than 100 degrees should only be used to accommodate fixed hip or pelvic deformities.

If slide-down occurs with a correctly aligned back, a positioning belt aligned across the pelvis or the upper thighs may be required to keep the patient well back in the wheelchair. The attachments of the positioning belt to the wheelchair seat frame should not be at the posterior corners of the seat but should be slightly more anterior. A belt attached at the posterior corners runs across the abdomen and tends to slide upwards toward the axilla and does not prevent sliding forward in the wheelchair. It acts only as a restraint without having any positioning benefits.

Dependent patients with severe hemiplegia may not be able to sustain an aligned, upright posture over a reasonable sitting time. In this situation, the back of the chair may be angled backwards with an accompanying upwards tilting of the front of the seat to maintain the seat/back angle between 90 to 100 degrees. The upward tilt of the seat may be accomplished by using a wedged seat cushion or by adjusting the mounting position of a base component. This fixed tilt position provides postural stability and reduces sliding while increasing sitting time and comfort. However, weight bearing transfers and foot propulsion will be compromised by this chair position.

FOOT SUPPORT

Full plantar contact on the foot plate is desirable for the involved foot and usually requires an upgrade to a larger foot plate size. Foot contact is part of the base of support and helps provide stability over which movement occurs (see also Chapter 26). Both the angle of the foot plate with the footrest and the distance of the footrest from the wheelchair need to be considered in order to achieve correct alignment of the hemiplegic lower leg. The height of the footrest should be adjusted to obtain full thigh support with weight bearing maintained through the foot. The knee should not be aligned higher than the hip.

ARM SUPPORT

Adjustable height armrests will allow the hemiplegic arm to be aligned in weight bearing. A half laptray or trough may assist in positioning the upper extremity appropriately and provide support to prevent or manage glenohumeral subluxation. Trays are preferred to slings which tend to immobilize the limb in a non-functional position. Trays should not be so close to the abdomen that an upright sitting position is restricted. Where the ability to voluntarily reposition or move the arm is impaired, padding under the elbow area may be required to prevent pressure on the ulnar nerve.

Seating needs require ongoing monitoring and reassessment. As treatment goals are achieved or if medical status changes, then alterations to seating may be necessary. Through this process, seating and positioning will complement overall patient management and assist in maximizing functional status for wheelchair users.

Patient and Caregiver Education and Support

Client and caregiver education is an essential part of all management for patients with stroke (see also Chapter 3). Early education in the physical, psychological and behavioural effects of stroke prepares the caregiver to understand the patient's problems. Education by the rehabilitation team prior to discharge will ensure that the caregiver is trained to provide assistance or supervision appropriate to the client's functional level. This is critical if the client is to maintain his or her discharge level of function. If the patient requires substantial assistance, caregiver education in proper body mechanics and lifting techniques is important to prevent injuries.

On discharge, the client and caregiver should be linked with community services providing emotional and physical support. Homemaking services, day care programmes and periodic respite care may be options for alleviating caregiver stress. Patient and caregiver education should be continued by the team providing follow-up care. This will allow the caregiver to continue to match provision of assistance to the patient's changing function. Follow-up services to maintain the patient's functional status and the caregiver's physical and emotional well-being are critical if the client is to avoid future institutional placement.

Education continues to be important for the patients and caregivers after institutionalization. Family as well as staff care for and assist the client with functional activities. The physiotherapist provides education on ambulation, transfers, seating and/or positioning as appropriate to each individual's level of function and care setting. In this way functional mobility and quality of life are enhanced through a collaborative approach.

Summary

Elderly individuals recovering from stroke should be given adequate opportunity for rehabilitation as it is clear that age alone does not determine functional outcome. Physiotherapy assessment and treatment of the older person with stroke may be more complex due to the increased likelihood of age-related changes, multisystem involvement, prior cognitive impairments and prior dependencies in functional mobility. The emphasis of physiotherapy at any time after the stroke is to enhance functional mobility. Active treatment in conjunction with other management (therapeutic seating, bed positioning, education) complement each other so each person's maximum potential is reached.

Many people are left with residual impairments and mobility deficits following a stroke. It is important that physiotherapy not be restricted to the acute or rehabilitative phase of recovery but continue following discharge from hospital. For the person discharged home, ongoing or periodic treatment may be indicated to maximize or maintain functional mobility. This should assist the individual to lead a more active lifestyle and prevent depression, social isolation and future institutionalization. For those individuals discharged to institutions, perodic physiotherapy intervention may be indicated to upgrade or maintain functional mobility status. In this way, secondary complications should be minimized and quality of life enhanced.

Numerous opportunities exist for physiotherapists to be involved with older persons recovering from stroke, and when dealing with the complex needs of this patient population will be both challenging and rewarding.

References

Ashburn, A, Partridge, C, DeSouza, L (1993) Physiotherapy in the rehabilitation of stroke: a review. *Clinical Rehabilitation* 7: 337–345.

Bohman, I (1987) The Bobath approach and the geriatric stroke patient. In: Jackson, OL (ed) *Therapeutic Considerations for the Elderly*, pp. 183–195. New York: Churchill Livingstone.

Bohman, I, Utley, J (1983–1994) NDTA Inc. (Bobath) Courses in the Management of Adult Hemiplegia, The Queen Elizabeth Hospital, Toronto, Canada.

Cole, B, Finch, E, Gowland, C, Mayo N (1994) *Physical Rehabilitation Outcome Measures.* Toronto: Canadian Physiotherapy Association.

Davies, PM (1985) *Steps to Follow*, 300 pp. Berlin: Springer-Verlag.

Davies, PM (1990) *Right in the Middle*, 277 pp. Berlin: Springer-Verlag.

Fisher, B (1987) Effect of trunk control and alignment on limb function. *Journal of Head Trauma Rehabilitation* 2: 72–79.

Fisher, B, Yakura, J (1993) Movement analysis: A different perspective. *Orthopedic Physical Therapy Clinics of North America* 2: 1–14.

Greveson, GC, Gray, CS, French, JM, James, OFW (1991) Long-term outcome for patients and carers following hospital admission for stroke. *Age and Ageing* 20: 337–344.

Jongbloed, L (1986) Prediction of function after stroke: A critical review. *Stroke* 17: 765–776.

Kalra, L, Smith, DH, Crome, P (1993) Stroke in patients aged over 75 years: Outcome and predictors. *Postgraduate Medical Journal* 69: 33–36.

Kelly-Hayes, M, Wolf, PA, Kannel, WB et al. (1988) Factors influencing survival and need for institutionalization following stroke: The Framingham study. *Archives of Physical Medicine and Rehabilitation* 69: 415–418.

Mogensen, CL (1994) PEP – Positioning education programme: A transdisciplinary programme to assist in the management of hypertonicity and immobility related problems. *Canadian Physiotherapy Association Gerontology Division Newsletter* 28: 9–10.

Mol, VJ, Baker, CA (1991) Activity intolerance in the geriatric stroke patient. *Rehabilitation Nursing* 16: 337–343.

Mollinger, LA, Steffen, TM (1993) Knee flexion contractures in institutionalized elderly: Prevalence, severity, stability and related variables. *Physical Therapy* **73**: 437–446.

Nuzik, S, Lamb, R, VanSant, A, Hirt S (1986) Sit to stand movement pattern: A kinematic study. *Physical Therapy* **66**: 1708–1713.

Partridge, CJ, Morris, LW, Edwards, SM (1993) Recovery from physical disability after stroke: profiles for different levels of starting severity. *Clinical Rehabilitation* 7: 210–217.

Reutter-Bernays, D, Rentsch, HP (1993) Rehabilitation of the elderly patient with stroke: An analysis of short-term and long-term results. *Disability and Rehabilitation* **15**: 90–95.

Stineman, MG, Granger, CV (1991) Epidemiology of stroke-related disability and rehabilitation outcome. *Physical Medicine and Rehabilitation Clinics of North America* 2: 457–471.

Thorngren, M, Westling, B (1990) Rehabilitation and achieved health quality after stroke: A population-based study of 258 hospitalized cases followed for one year. *Acta Neurologica Scandinavica* **82**: 374–380.

Wade, DT (1992) *Measurement in Neurological Rehabilitation*. Oxford: Oxford University Press.

19

Psychiatric Problems

SANDRA KUNANEC, JANET M SIMPSON

Introduction
•
Groups of Psychiatric Conditions
•
Organic Mental Disorders
•
Delirium
•
Schizophrenia
•
Mood Disorders
•
Mobility Problems Associated with Dementia
•
Interactions with Older People with Dementia
•
Physiotherapy Assessment of People with Cognitive Difficulties
•
Working with People with Cognitive Difficulties
•
Working with Depressed People
•
Summary

Introduction

Dementia is one of the most common problems of old age but is not the only psychiatric condition confronting physiotherapists who work with older people. As there is a greater likelihood of psychiatric illness among older people than among younger people it is essential that physiotherapists who work with them learn how to cope and how to achieve the rehabilitation goals despite their clients not always being able to cooperate fully with them. In this chapter the main groups of psychiatric conditions affecting older people will be outlined, then each of them will be considered in more detail. Then mobility problems associated with dementia will be discussed, before strategies for conducting an assessment and for organizing treatment are examined. The focus will then shift to suggestions for working more effectively with people who have cognitive and mood problems.

Groups of Psychiatric Conditions

Terminology in this field is confusing. 'Psychiatric disease' and 'mental illness', for example, seem to be used interchangeably and 'intellectual impairment' and 'cognitive impairment' also seem to mean the same thing. Generally throughout this chapter we shall refer to psychiatric conditions and cognitive impairments. The classification of psychiatric conditions in old age has presented many difficulties, but the current World Health Organization classification (ICD-10) seems to be useful (WHO, 1992). In old age the main problems are: organic mental disorders leading to dementia; delirium or acute confusional states; schizophrenia and related disorders; mood disorders or affective disorders; neuroses.

This chapter will only be concerned with the first three of these groups, it will not address problems of schizophrenia and neurotic problems such as obsessional disorders, phobias and hypochondriasis that feature in old age. This is not to say that physiotherapists may not face clients whose management is complicated by neuroses but in old age most difficulties are likely to arise in association with organic and mood disorders. Further details of all these conditions may be found in Wattis and Martin (1994), and an in-depth coverage is given by Copeland *et al.* (1994).

This chapter focuses on the difficulties that may be encountered during the physiotherapy assessment and treatment of older people who present with psychiatric problems in addition to mobility difficulties; most of those who are severely affected will be cared for in institutions. People with these diagnoses present with varying degrees of cognitive impairments that potentially pose obstacles to the attainment of physiotherapy management goals.

Organic Mental Disorders

Organic disorders are believed to arise from structural changes in the brain and probably affect about 10% of people over 65 years old, rising to about 20% of people over 80. They may be subdivided into two syndromes according to the likely outcome: dementia and delirium.

Dementia is defined as: 'a decline in both memory and thinking which is sufficient to impair personal activities of daily living' (WHO, 1992). It is irreversible at the present state of knowledge and has been identified as a major cause of disability in old age (Jorm, 1994). Poor memory means that sufferers become increasingly unable to make sense of what is going on in the world around them, so people with dementia may become very anxious or even aggressive. They fail to recognize where they are in time and place, getting lost easily and possibly mistaking receptacles such as waste bins for toilets. They may fail to recognize people, eventually even their close relatives. The process of transformation of a loved one into a stranger can be extremely distressing to carers.

A psychosocial model of dementia has been developed which shows how an elderly dementia patient's behaviour affects the way other people react to them. This, in turn, may lead to greater deterioration in their functional state than is warranted by the objective level of impairment (Pomeroy, 1995).

Several conditions give rise to dementia. The most common is Alzheimer's disease (AD) which also occurs, though more rarely, in middle-aged people. It has an insidious onset, at first sufferers and relatives may attribute increasing forgetfulness to old age until independent living for that person is recognized as hazardous, and supervision becomes necessary. The anatomical and biochemical pathology are only partly understood, and the cause remains elusive, although there is evidence for a genetic component, especially for early onset AD.

The next most common cause of dementia is vascular: multiple-infarct dementia (MID) associated hypertension and stroke. It has a relatively sudden onset and a step-wise progression. Physiotherapists working with stroke patients should be prepared for the difficulties to which dementia can give rise, as well as to the possibility of post-stroke depression. Some patients may have problems arising from a mixture of the vascular causes and AD. Less frequent causes of dementia include nutritional disorders such as Korsakoff's syndrome as well as Jacob-Creuzfeldt disease, Pick's disease, cerebral tumours.

Delirium

Delirium is 'a transient organic mental syndrome characterized by global disorder of cognition and attention and reduced level of consciousness' (WHO, 1992). It has a sudden onset and perceptual distortions; even hallucinations are common. It is more often encountered in acute settings, as elderly people, especially if they already have a mild dementia, can become delirious as the result of intercurrent infections, cardiac problems or when recovering from an anaesthetic. Dehydration, various drugs, and metabolic disorders such as thyroid deficiency can also give rise to delirium. For this reason and because it will dissipate once the underlying cause has been identified and treated the term 'acute confusional state' is commonly used.

Schizophrenia

This condition is thought to have a biochemical basis and affects about 1% of old people. It is characterized by formal thought disorder and auditory hallucinations (hearing voices). Formal thought disorder includes thought-blocking, when clients' thoughts end abruptly, thought withdrawal when the clients feel that thoughts are withdrawn from their head and thought insertion. Auditory hallucinations, or 'hearing voices' occur in several psychiatric illness but predominantly in schizophrenia. Clients may hear a voice repeating their own thoughts or several voices talking about them in the third person often in a derogatory way. Clients with severe depression may have similar experiences. Many people with schizophrenia which began earlier in life survive into old age. Increasingly they will be cared for in the community and need help when the problems of old age are added to their existing illness. Late-onset schizophrenia (often called paraphrenia) takes the form of a paranoid illness. It develops mostly in women who have had schizoid premorbid personality and is characterized by paranoid delusions with or without auditory hallucinations.

Mood Disorders

Mood disorders or affective disorders are characterized by disturbance of mood which can be elevated (manic) or depressed. Recent classification of the various forms of mood disorder has generated over 30 categories of depression and at least eight for elevated mood! Mania can vary from expansive or irritable syndrome to agitation and excitement. These episodes are accompanied by increased energy, decreased need for sleep, decline in normal social inhibitions and sometimes by grandiose delusions. Elderly people are more likely to suffer 'irritable' or 'angry' manic episodes.

People afflicted with extreme depressive mood may neglect their own basic needs, they become mute and unresponsive to their environment and they may suffer delusions. A delusion is a false but unshakable belief out of keeping with the person's cultural background; for example, severely afflicted people may believe that they are dead or that their bodies are rotting away. When the condition is less severe they may have delusions of guilt, unworthiness, poverty, or ill-health. Wattis and Martin (1994) warn that depression may emphasize the least attractive aspects of a person's personality. They advise helpers to beware of relatives who claim the person has 'always been like this' for what they really mean is that the person has had similar tendencies e.g. towards excessive dependency, but these have now got worse.

Reactive depression occurs in response to life circumstances and usually recovers as the person adjusts to them. In old age severe depression may be a reaction to bereavement and the person may need a great deal of help to recover. Understandably, stroke is commonly accompanied by psychological distress in part as a reaction to loss of abilities; but it may also be related to the site of the lesion (Allman, 1991). Physiotherapists working with stroke victims need to be aware of the strong possibility of psychological distress and be prepared to develop strategies to cope with it.

A depressed older person may have been so throughout life but the condition may also appear first in old age when it is termed late onset depression. The later depression appears, the less probable is any genetic influence, and more likely that the cause may be an imbalance among cerebral neurotransmitters. Older people lacking a close confiding relationship are thought to be particularly vulnerable to depression. The concept of 'learned helplessness' might provide an explanation for the remarkable association between depression and physical illness in old age (Wattis and Martin, 1994) (Chapter 8).

Most of the signs and symptoms of these conditions may be regarded as problems in cognitive functioning: reduced attention span, poor concentration, reduced ability to learn and recall new information, and increased reaction time. They demand an imaginative approach from physiotherapists who work with these clients. Although most research has been done in connection with dementia, the same principles of management apply to most elderly people with any psychiatric problem (Simpson, 1992).

Mobility Problems Associated with Dementia

Older people with dementia, like other older people, may have impairments and injuries that affect their mobility. A weak association exists between the severity of AD and various parameters of gait and balance and occurs in roughly half of those with severe AD. Pomeroy (1995) explored the extent to which pathological changes in the nervous system could reduce the capacity of persons with AD for appropriate motor behaviour, regardless of any other pathology. Any such effect might be exacerbated by the side-effects of neuroleptic drugs used in AD and in MID and the secondary effects of inactivity. She concludes that increased sensory input would lead to improved functional ability among those with dementia.

Interactions with Older People with Dementia

For the purposes of the rest of this chapter dementia, schizophrenia and delirium are covered together, as the behavioural problems associated with these conditions are similar.

Drawing on the psychosocial model of dementia, Pomeroy (1995) listed the consequences of inappropriate (but all too common) interactions between people with dementia and others: disempowerment — not being allowed to complete tasks for oneself because staff find it easier and quicker to do it instead; infantilization — being talked to like a child; intimidation — not being given the chance to understand what is being done to oneself; labelling — the self-fulfilling prophecy of being labelled as demented; outpacing — being outpaced during task performance because of not being allowed enough time; objectification — being treated not as a person but as an object or source of tasks to be completed.

This problem has been addressed in various ways. A set of principles of good practice when providing services to people with dementia has been drawn up and formalized communication approaches have been elaborated: Reality Orientation, Validation Therapy, and Reminiscence (Holden and Woods, 1995).

The service principles are based on the normalization concept, first elaborated for services to people with learning difficulties (King's Fund, 1986): that people with dementia have the same human value as other members of society irrespective of their degree of dementia; that they have the same varied human needs; and the same human rights.

Simpson (1992) described two strategies for working with older people based on psychological concepts of reduced information processing capacity and reduced resources available for mental activity. The two basic strategies are to allow the older person enough time to complete the task and not to ask older people to do more than one thing at a time. Although these two principles seem rather obvious, they need reinforcing with inexperienced staff, even more so when clients have memory problems.

Reality Orientation (RO) was the first approach reported and although originally exaggerated claims were made about its ability to improve memory, it awakened professionals out of their nihilist state, and at the very least it reintroduced norms of good manners and courtesy (Simpson, 1982). The underlying concept was that all interactions with people with memory problems should be used to help the person regain or maintain orientation. Thus 'Hello' conveys less information than 'Good morning' and 'Good morning Mrs Jones, it is time for you to practice your exercises' conveys even more. As is so often the case, aspects of RO were misinterpreted to the extent that clients were 'examined' about information that was not of any practical use to them — knowing the day of the week has little meaning to someone in an institution. A practical aspect of RO is using the environment to support failing memory. Remnants of RO may be recognized in RO boards displayed around wards and day units. All too often they disorient when not kept up to date. However, using signposts and training clients in ward-orientation can be very effective in helping people to find their way about (Lam and Woods, 1986). It can be built into physiotherapy sessions very fruitfully.

Validation is a form of counselling for elderly people with advanced dementia (Feil, 1993). Its purpose is to enhance communication with very confused people by emphasizing active listening — trying to recognize the emotions that are being expressed as well as noting the actual words. The techniques have become very popular with carers and professionals seeking to understand the world of people with dementia; especially the ideas for group work and the helpful insights into the possible meaning of confused behaviour. Although many psychologists have reservations about some of the elaborate claims made for validation therapy, physiotherapists may find the basic technique of active listening very useful.

Reminiscence work can also usefully be built into interactions with elderly people with dementia. It aims to stimulate recall of past events which may be better preserved than recent events. Just showing an interest in people's jobs and the things they did at the most active period of their lives can enhance client's self-esteem and elicit cooperation.

Physiotherapy Assessment of People with Cognitive Difficulties

During the assessment process, a conventional physiotherapy approach may lead to difficulties. Physiotherapists should be prepared to make use of alternative strategies as necessary.

The main difficulty is that people with dementia have some degree of memory problem. It is advisable to get an objective measurement of the severity of the problem as it can easily be disguised during everyday conversation. Socially skilled people are especially adept at filling gaps with polite but bland remarks so that observers may be misled to think that the problem is very minor or even non-existent. This can be very unfortunate if the observer is a powerful professional. For example a mentally alert elderly woman, living in London UK, was unable to walk more than a few yards because of severe osteoarthritis in both knees whereas her husband, who had a military background, was fully mobile. However, he suffered from AD and was incapable of doing the shopping. His wife asked her local social service department for assistance with the shopping. The professional who assessed the need was impressed by the husband's smart military appearance and apparent ability to converse sensibly. She did not objectively test his ability to learn and retain new material and was misled into thinking he was capable of doing the shopping. She refused the request for help.

Physiotherapists who lack a clear idea of an older person's learning and memory ability may not adopt the appropriate techniques when teaching the person a new skill such as how to use a walking aid or to propel a wheelchair.

Several brief tests of mental ability have been published. Many are interpreted in terms of the total score across several sub-tests. These tests usually tap a variety of abilities whereas physiotherapists wish to know how easy it is for a client to learn and retain new information. They also need a test which is quick and non-threatening to administer and very easy for them to interpret. Learning a fictitious name and address appears in several screening tests. It has face validity for clients and provides physiotherapists with a clear idea of the client's ability. Advice for conducting the test, best described as a memory exercise for client's benefit, is shown in Figure 1.

Eliciting an older person's cooperation is not so straightforward as with younger people, and even

Figure 1 A memory exercise to check an elderly person's ability to learn and retain new information. From Hodkinson (1973).

Sit down, introduce yourself, establish rapport.
Then say something along these lines:

'I am going to give you a memory exercise . . . most patients do it'

'I am going to ask you to remember something, then after 5 minutes we are going to see how much you can still remember'

'It is an imaginary address. Please repeat this after me
   MR JOHN BROWN
<patient repeats>
   42 WEST STREET
<patient repeats>
   GATESHEAD'
<repeats>

Ask the patient to repeat the whole address.
If she makes a mistake, correct it and request another repeat.
Engage the patient in conversation to prevent rehearsal.
   After 5 mins say:

'Five minutes ago I asked you to remember something, can you remember what it was?'

Record your patient's response

Score one point for every item correctly recalled
Ignore MR,
Count 42 as one item
Normal old people recall everything correctly
Accept 4, but if the score is less than 4, repeat the test in a few days with a different address but with the same number of syllables and of similar familiarity.
If the score is still less than 4 watch for further evidence of memory problems.

less so if the person has memory problems. Oddy and Taylor (1988) made the point that it is wise, as well as courteous, to use the person's surname, at least initially, as elderly people are probably unaccustomed to being addressed by their forenames – unless they have been in an institution for some time. They also suggest that this sign of respect may give a boost to the flagging self-esteem of a person with depression.

Poor memory means that history taking is often difficult and to obtain a clear idea of the presenting problem may require tenacity and patience. Often clients cannot recall how long they have had the pain or physical problem, perhaps not even when they were injured, or indeed that they were injured at all. Physiotherapists need to recognize confabulation which is when clients fill gaps in their memory with apparently fabricated information – a more severe problem than just filling the gaps with bland but apparently appropriate remarks. Sometimes this process is so severe that it sounds like nonsense. But people who confabulate are unaware of their memory gaps, and their responses may be due to misuse of environmental cues, failure to inhibit incorrect responses, or be drawn from a store of earlier, still accessible memories (Whitlock, 1981).

To overcome these difficulties, information may have to be gathered over several sessions. It is advisable to read the client's records or charts before the interview, but if the client is in a psychiatric facility background information on physical problems may be sparse.

During the interview it is best to avoid open-ended items which allow clients to become distracted. Instead, pose short, closed, directive questions and repeat them politely, in the same format, as often as necessary. If they wander off the topic encourage them to return to it: 'That is interesting but can we get back to . . .'

Repetition is also useful when assessing pain. Disturbed sensory integration can give rise to vagueness about the presence of pain. This may lead a client to report pain when being moved through a range but the pain may not reappear when the movement is repeated. Often, clients are unable to report whether their pain has been better or worse since treatment, or whether their pain is increased or decreased by stress or anxiety. The apparent vagueness or inattention of older clients should never be interpreted to mean they do not have a serious problem. Useful information about pain can be inferred from careful observation. Altered postures, decreased function and agitation may signal the presence of pain that the patient is unable to describe.

Clients may also appear non-communicative because they are unable to speak or because they are unwilling to do so, as their 'voices' warn them against it or because they lack trust. Again, careful observation of clients' postures and movements must be relied upon to supply information not otherwise available. Clients may be encouraged to perform specific functional activities so that pain-free ranges of motion and functional inabilities can be determined. Hands on palpation is a good way to assess problems but some clients do not tolerate it.

Many clients have a short attention span and become agitated or want to leave if questioning is prolonged. Therefore, physiotherapists are advised to plan each client's assessment session in advance. More than one session may be necessary. If physiotherapists spend too much of the session measuring and questioning, clients may fail to keep the next appointment. It is essential that some treatment be given at each session, either to ease pain or increase function.

Touching a person during assessment could be construed as an assault if the client does not understand what is taking place and misinterprets the physiotherapist's intentions as intimidation (Pomeroy, 1995). It is also advisable, as far as possible, to make eye contact on an equal level or even on a 'submissive' level rather than looking down on the client, although there are occasions when it may be appropriate to take a more authoritative stance.

Pomeroy (1995) stressed the value of functional assessment and the need to establish achievable, measurable goals when working with older people with dementia. She developed a functionally oriented assessment of mobility scale suitable for use with these clients (Pomeroy, 1990). Information obtained at the assessment may have to be supplemented with information supplied by carers who know the client well.

It is good practice to ask clients to state what they understand to be their problem and what activities they wish to regain. Goal identification is particularly important with this client group. It shows a genuine interest in them and can inspire their trust and reveal the extent to which they have insight into their problems. Even more than with others, it is important that physiotherapists pay full attention to what these older people are saying, and not allow themselves to be distracted or to appear insincere or insensitive.

Also, by paying attention to clients' moods and emotional reactions, physiotherapists can get a good idea of how best to approach them, and how to plan their treatment programme.

Working with People with Cognitive Difficulties

Besides restoration or maintenance of optimal function, common goals include easing the carers' physical handling problems, and providing suitable seating. The same physiotherapy techniques are used with people with dementia as are used with other older people, but special skill is required in one's approach to clients.

Initially, clients may not appear very interested in the way lack of joint flexibility, lack of endurance, weak muscles or oedema affects them, or they may be unable to understand the connection. The order of goal priority for clients is usually: resolution of pain, improvement of function, restoration of mobility. Their interest is most likely to be aroused if their own goals are shown to be clearly linked to the means needed to resolve the various impairments.

The severity or acuteness of clients' psychiatric problems, especially their ability to concentrate, affects the frequency, duration and location of treatment. Clients needing intense physiotherapy, for example, to deal with muscle weakness associated with a fracture might attend for only a few minutes each week. Physiotherapists may have to be content with this schedule when clients are anxious, are distrustful or because their 'voices' are out of control and do not allow them to concentrate for longer periods. If poor concentration is a consideration, clients are seen for shorter but more frequent sessions in order to achieve management goals. Short attention span may indicate the need for individual treatment, even when the physical problems are less severe. Simple exercise programmes cannot be left unsupervised — a physiotherapist or attendant needs to be there to ensure clients fulfil the exercise requirements. Individual sessions also suit very anxious older people. A distraction-free treatment environment is important so it is not advisable to treat these clients in the wards. A quiet physiotherapy department or treatment area well away from other clinics is most suitable.

Anxiety may mean that clients do not tolerate being touched. However, they may be amenable to using equipment such as a restorator bicycle, an arm ergometer, slings and springs, although they may require supervision. These machines allow familiar, repetitive movements and are very useful for people with dementia, high anxiety, and poor concentration.

Allowing clients choices about aspects of their treatment is good practice (King's Fund, 1986); doing so often helps to elicit their cooperation. Very anxious people should be allowed to choose the timing of their treatment sessions regardless of how inconvenient this may be in a busy situation. Once the patient is more relaxed and has acquired greater trust, a more convenient schedule may be negotiated. Aggressive patients may choose to spend a session either riding the bicycle or practising climbing stairs. If their aggressive behaviour begins to escalate they can be given the choice of either staying and exercising correctly or leaving. Challenging behaviour in all its aspects has been examined by Wilson (1995).

Preparation of treatment plans in advance of each session is not only good practice, but it avoids the physiotherapist appearing indecisive. It also enables clear, simple, instructions to be prepared which are more likely to be successful with confused elderly people. Once formulated, an instruction should be repeated in the same way because using different wording can be confusing. Similarly, it is unwise to indulge in unnecessary talk as this can muddle an already confused person. Gesture and physical cuing are used to clarify and reinforce instructions and requests.

Altered sensation is common, so treatment modalities must be chosen carefully. It is best to avoid traction, electrotherapy and equipment that requires cooperation and subjective input. Hot packs should only be used with clients who can be relied upon to recognize and say when the packs are too hot.

Poor memory means that clients often forget appointment times. Clearly written appointment cards and diaries are advisable and the ward staff need to be informed. However, it is necessary to be as flexible as possible about scheduling, to accommodate those who arrive at an unplanned time. Clients who are asked to return at the correct time are unlikely to do so, not because they are disinterested or being difficult but because they cannot remember the new instruction or because they feel too embarrassed to return. The existence of memory problems also makes it unlikely that these clients will, on their own, follow a home programme once they have been discharged. If there is no carer to ensure that the programme is followed alternative arrangements will have to be made.

Pomeroy (1995) detailed an intervention programme designed to increase functional mobility among elderly people with dementia. It comprises body awareness training, music and movement, functional mobility training, seating and positioning for activity and comfort, and advice and training for carers. Preliminary work indicates that physiotherapy for $1\frac{1}{2}$ hours per week for about 10 weeks may be required to obtain optimal functional mobility in people with severe dementia.

Behavioural techniques can be very useful to physiotherapists. Setting achievable mobility goals comes under this heading. Clients are not going to participate willingly in an activity at which they know they will fail or that will be painful or frightening. Even the smallest achievement should be rewarded with congratulations and showing an interest in the person, perhaps by some comments on a success in middle-age or youth. In contrast attention-seeking or other undesirable behaviour should not be rewarded with attention but just ignored and the withdrawal of the (hopefully normally rewarding) presence of the physiotherapist.

The role of physiotherapists caring for people with dementia is explored further in Taira (1986) and Everett et al. (1995).

Working with Depressed People

Telling people with moderate depression to 'try harder', being assertive, or trying to distract or amuse them rarely helps. However, when lack of stimulation is suspected as being at the root of the depressed mood rather than some intrinsic cause an enthusiastic, assertive approach may help to improve the situation. By offering an older person something to do that is highly likely to interest him and that he would normally want to do, a positive response is usually obtained.

Genuinely depressed people may feel very vulnerable so that physiotherapists need to be sensitive to their needs and wants, telling them not to be 'blue' is unhelpful. Depression can be successfully treated but medication usually takes about 2 weeks to begin to work.

Summary

Older people with psychiatric problems may have additional physical problems meriting the same high quality physiotherapy available to people of any age who are fortunate enough not to have psychiatric problems. The physiotherapy skills used to solve their physical problems are no different to those used with client groups elsewhere; the challenge to physiotherapists is to learn specialized communication techniques in order to engage these elderly people in their rehabilitation programmes. Recent research shows that the physiotherapist's role can extend in a theory-based manner into the prevention of inactivity-related impairments among people with dementia who might otherwise suffer further decline in functional disabilities.

References

Allman, P (1991) Depressive disorders and emotionalism following stroke. *International Journal of Geriatric Psychiatry* 6: 377–383.

Copeland, JRM, Abou-Saleh, MT, Blazer, DG (eds) (1994) *Principles and Practice of Geriatric Psychiatry*. Chichester: Wiley.

Everett, T, Dennis, M, Ricketts, I (eds) (1995) *Physiotherapy in Mental Health: a Practical Approach*. Oxford: Butterworth–Heineman.

Feil, N (1993) *The Validation Breakthrough*. London: Health Professions Press.

Hodkinson, (1973) Mental impairment in the elderly. *Journal of the Royal College of Physicians of London* 7: 305.

Holden, U, Woods, RT (1995) *Positive Approaches to Dementia Care*. Edinburgh: Churchill Livingstone.

Jorm, AF (1994) Disability in dementia: assessment, prevention and rehabilitation. *Disability and Rehabilitation* 16: 98–109.

King's Fund (1986) *Living Well into Old Age*. London: King's Fund.

Lam, DH, Woods, RT (1986) Ward orientation training in dementia: a single-case study. *International Journal of Geriatric Psychiatry* 1: 145–147.

Oddy, R, Taylor, M (1988) Mental state and physical performance. In Squires, AJ (ed) *Rehabilitation of the Older Patient*. London: Croom Helm.

Pomeroy, VM (1990) Development of an ADL-oriented assessment of mobility scale suitable for use with elderly people with dementia. *Physiotherapy* 76: 446–448.

Pomeroy, VM (1995) Dementia. In Everett, T, Dennis, M, Ricketts, I (eds) *Physiotherapy in Mental Health: a Practical Approach*. Oxford: Butterworth–Heinemann.

Simpson, JM (1982) Reality orientation in Tuscaloosa. *Nursing Times*, May 26: 876–877.

Simpson, JM (1992) Growing older: changes in mental performance. In French, S (ed) *Physiotherapy: a Psychosocial Approach*. London: Butterworth–Heineman.

Taira, ED (1986) (ed) *Therapeutic Interventions for the Person with Dementia*. New York: Haworth Press.

Wattis, J, Martin, C (1994) *Practical Psychiatry of Old Age* 2nd edn. London: Chapman & Hall.

Whitlock, FA (1981) Some observations on the meaning of confabulation. *British Journal of Medical Psychology* 54: 213–218.

Wilson, J (1995) Challenging behaviour. In Everett, T, Dennis, M, Ricketts, I (eds) *Physiotherapy in Mental Health: a Practical Approach*. Oxford: Butterworth–Heinemann.

World Health Organization (1992) The ICD-10 Classification of Mental and Behavioural Disorders and Diagnostic Guidelines. Geneva: WHO.

20

Pain

EDITH HERMAN, ROGER SCUDDS

The Prevalence of Pain in Older People

Defined as 'an unpleasant sensory and emotional experience associated with actual or potential tissue damage, or described in terms of such damage' (Merskey, 1986), pain is the most commonly encountered symptom of disease. In older people, because of their increased vulnerability, persistent pain takes a particularly heavy toll in terms of human suffering. Frequently afflicted with numerous coexisting pain-producing ailments, physical function and quality of life may be seriously affected during the later years of life.

The prevalence of specific diagnoses and asso-ciated patterns of pain seems to change with age. Most common are disorders of the musculoskeletal system; more than 50% of people over 65 experience pain from arthritis. Other frequently encountered conditions include rheumatoid disorders, fibromyalgia and myofascial pain syndromes, as well as neck and back pain as a result of degenerative disorders or osteoporosis-induced fractures. Lack of adequate rehabilitation or malnutrition can lead to more pain and physical problems from disuse. Disorders of the peripheral or central nervous system (CNS) may produce neurogenic pain, deafferentation pain, or thalamic pain.

Among pain problems of vascular origin, the incidence of migraine headaches decreases sharply with age but is countered by increased incidence of temporal arteritis, anginal discomfort and intermittent claudication. As might be expected from the more frequent occurrence of neoplastic diseases in older age groups, the prevalence of cancer-related pain also increases. The majority of cancer patients suffer pain before death.

Considering the wide spectrum of age-related painful disorders, it is not surprising that older people experience a great deal of pain. Unfortunately, it is often inadequately controlled. An accurate estimate of the prevalence of persistent pain problems among older people is difficult to determine from the scant epidemiological data available at present. In community-based populations prevalence rates of chronic pain sufferers have been estimated at between 30 and 40%; however, the rates in nursing home residents have been reported as between 45 and 83% (Crook *et al.* 1984). While reports of temporary pain episodes do not seem to differ significantly between younger and older individuals, reports of persistent pain increase in proportion to advancing age. Older people may underreport pain, or are led to believe that pain is an inevitable part of ageing. As a result, older people's pain may be under-treated – with detrimental effects on their quality of life.

Is pain perceived differently or communicated differently by older people? What age-related changes occur in the pain-signalling systems? How do these changes affect the perception of pain? Do older people require different methods of assessment and treatment of pain? Unfortunately, the answers to these perplexing questions are still elusive.

The Nature of Pain

General Concepts

Pain is a complex perceptual experience based on the interaction of signals from various systems. Sensory, emotional, cognitive–behavioural, and social–cultural factors are inextricably interwoven in pain states. Nociception (the perception of noxious stimuli) produces an affective reaction (an emotional experience). The resulting perception of pain may be embellished by the meaning ascribed to it, and be accompanied by behavioural changes. Pain, therefore, is not a mere consequence of somatic input but is determined by the modifiable interaction of multiple systems in a complex neural circuitry of ascending and descending pathways. We are never treating the 'pain' that happens somewhere in neural structures; we are always dealing with an individual who consciously experiences and suffers the pain in a highly personal way.

Pain can be an aid or a barrier to rehabilitation. Acute ('nociceptive') pain has adaptive value as a biological warning signal of tissue damage. since it is typically well localized, pain is also a useful guide for monitoring a client's progress; diminutution of pain suggests that the treatment strategy selected was effective. The longer the pain persists, the more likely it may become dissociated from its original cause. Chronic pain tends to radiate and spread, so that it is a less reliable guide to diagnosis. Treatments usually effective for acute pain may be ineffective in dealing with chronic pain states. The expression of pain is – at least in part – a conditioned i.e. learned, behaviour which may become a barrier to rehabilitation. To be effective, treatment of chronic pain may need to be set within a behavioural model.

Characteristics of Pain

Pain occurs when something impinges upon a pain-sensitive structure. For example, malignancies do not cause pain until they invade pain-sensitive tissues. However, perception of pain is subjective and can only be inferred from a client's self-report. In order to interpret and understand each client's pain, physiotherapists learn to help clients describe their pain and the effect it has on their functional activity. Specific patterns of location and distribution characterize different types of pain (Bonica and Loeser, 1990).

Localized pain is restricted to its site of origin, as is arthritis, bursitis or tendinitis. Tissue damage may produce a state of sensitization, called hyperalgesia. Hyperaesthesia refers to cutaneous pain in response to non-noxious stimulation, such as touch and heat stimuli. Allodynia is pain which occurs in response to non-noxious stimuli which do not normally produce pain. Any cutaneous hyperalgesia and hyperaesthesia are confined to the affected area.

Radicular pain is projected along the course of a nerve in the corresponding dermatome. Post-herpetic intercostal neuralgia, sciatic pain, trigeminal neuralgia and meralgia paresthetica are examples of radicular pain.

Referred pain is deep pain originating from a somatic or visceral structure and referred to another region within the same segment. Referred pain is usually accompanied by hyperalgesia, reflex muscle spasm, deep tenderness, and autonomic hyperactivity. Examples are pain referred to the right shoulder area from cholecystitis, or to the left shoulder area from myocardial infarction. Referred pain may also be related to the presence of myofascial 'trigger points' that produce pain in a non-dermatomal pattern at areas away from the source.

Reflex sympathetic pain does not follow dermatomal pattens and typically presents as hyperalgesia and/or hyperaesthesia, associated with vasomotor and trophic changes. Examples are causalgia and reflex sympathetic dystrophy.

Psychogenic pain is pain for which somatic or visceral causes have been ruled out, and which does not fit any recognizable neuroanatomical pattern. However, purely psychogenic pain is far less common among older people than among younger chronic pain sufferers.

Sensitization is a state of enhanced sensitivity due to continuous activation of the small, unmyelinated C fibres which become hypersensitive. When pain seems to be getting worse without any discernable reason, central sensitization in the dorsal horn neurons should be considered.

Psychophysiological Basis of Pain

An understanding of the pathophysiological basis of pain underpins appropriate pain management. Many in-depth reviews of the neurophysiology of pain are available, such as those in Bonica (1990). Current conceptualization of pain is based on the gate control theory (Wall and Melzack, 1984). The pivotal concept of this theory is that noxious impulses are not simply transmitted but interact with the input from other afferents, with input from spinal interneurons and with input from descending control systems; thus the nociceptive message is modified. 'Closing the gate' refers to the operation of a negative feedback loop in the dorsal horn where the nociceptive transmission by small fibres is modfied by large fibre activity at the segmental level. Heuristically rich, the 'gate control theory' inspired a flood of research which revealed many more complexities, and led to discovery of the endogenous opioids and the formulation of specific pain modulation systems (Fields, 1987).

Pain typically generates emotional arousal in the form of fear, anxiety, and motivation to escape the source of pain. These symptoms are the psychological correlates of the sympathetically mediated 'fight and flight' response. Release of norepinephrine at the sympathetic nerve endings can sensitize nociceptors and enhance pain transmission and perception of pain. The anxiety experienced in acute pain states usually abates with explanation, reassurance and treatment of the underlying cause. When pain persists, however, the negative affect may produce a mood of depression, as a result of changes in the monoamine metabolism in the brain. Catecholamine systems (nor-epinephrine and dopamine) and serotonin metabolism are also vulnerable to ageing. The functional consequences of reduced serotonin levels may include disturbed sleep patterns and depression, both of which are prevalent in older people, as well as having an influence on pain (Georgotas, 1983).

Age-related Changes in Sensory and Pain-control Systems

Details of the characteristic patterns, mechanisms, management and prognosis of various pain syndromes are to be found in Wall and Melzack (1984), Bonica (1990), and a summary of musculoskeletal pain syndromes frequently found in older patients in Payne and Pasternak (1990, p. 590).

The gradual decline of sensory function has been accepted as inevitable part of ageing. Alteration in receptor function and a general slowing of transduction processes seem to underlie the functional

deterioration of the sense organs (Harkins et al., 1990).

Theoretically, decrements in pain sensibility should result in a gradual decrease in the perception of pain with concomitant rise of pain thresholds in old age. There is some indication that this may, in fact, be the case. For example, the occurrence of painless myocardial infarctions (MI) seems to increase with advancing age (Bayer et al., 1986). It is unclear to what extent such observations reflect age-related physiological changes, psychological factors, or biased study samples. Many studies on older people are carried out in nursing homes, so the findings may be derived from groups of people with a greater incidence of mental impairment. A clear pathophysiological explanation of the phenomenon has yet to be offered.

High cutaneous thermal pain thresholds found in patients with silent MIs suggest changes in the sensory dimension of pain. Other explanations attribute the phenomenon to older clients' personality characteristics, their interpretation of pain, or problems they may have with communication (Harkins et al., 1990).

Structural changes in the peripheral nervous system have also been demonstrated in the skin. Marked degenerative transformations occur in touch receptors; Meissner's corpuscles undergo progressive atrophy (including the neural element within the receptor organ), until their density in the skin is markedly reduced. Up to 90% of these corpuscles may be lost in old age, and those which do survive change their form and take on an irregular shape. However, since similar patterns of degeneration have been observed following prolonged periods of inactivity at any age, these changes may also be due to reduced levels of stimulation of these receptors. Other manifestations of ageing in the skin result in reduced thermal pain sensitivity, reduced vibrotactile sensitivity and reduced two-point discrimination ability. In contrast, the less differentiated 'free' nerve endings remain relatively unchanged. Stimulation of skin receptors and nerve fibres may delay their atrophy.

In terms of the gate control theory, pain is not merely a function of increased input from nociceptive fibres but also the result of lack of input from large diameter fibres. The relative imbalance of sensory input from small and large diameter fibres not only results in less efficient modulation of nociceptive signals but may also account for some protracted pain problems characteristic in elderly people, such as post-herpetic neuralgia. A clinical example may illustrate the importance of sensory input for pain relief.

Case Study

A 76-year-old man was referred to the pain clinic because of excruciating pain from intercostal post-herpetic neuralgia which crippled his entire life. Since he could not tolerate the slightest touch to the right side of his chest, he would not even wear a shirt, hence was home-bound. Drugs did not control the pain. Sensory input in the form of TENS [transcutaneous electrical nerve stimulation] warm showers [via a hand-held shower attachment with adjustable pressure], firm brushing and rubbing with different types of cloth [thereby recruiting different types of fibre populations] ameliorated his pain within a couple of weeks. Achieving pain relief by his own efforts improved his outlook significantly.

Changed activity and metabolism of neurotransmitters may also affect pain modulation in old age. Central changes include changes in the balance between the biological amine neurotransmitters involved in the modulation of pain, e.g. serotonin and intrinsic opioids (endorphins, enkephalins). These biological amines normally undergo metabolic deactivation by the enzyme monoamine oxidase (MAO), which increases with age, especially in women. The resulting depletion of brain serotonin levels may account not only for persistence of pain but also for depression.

At present, no conceptual model exists which can completely account for the interrelationships between ageing and the perception of pain. Our knowledge is restricted to empirical findings which are not always congruent. The evidence needed to link pain complaints in elderly people to structural and physiological changes in the nervous system is sketchy and controversial. Among some individuals, sensitivity to pain may remain unchanged over their lifetime, among some it may increase, and among others decrease. Reports of acute pain problems do not seem to differ significantly between young and the old people (Crook *et al.*, 1984). The increased prevalence of pain among older people is possibly related to the multiplicity and chronicity of their physical problems, as well as to psychological factors.

Psychological Issues

Pain is a perceptual event. What an individual in pain feels and thinks and does profoundly affects the experience and magnitude of pain. Older people are a very heterogeneous group, and their individual responses to pain vary considerably. They may also differ greatly from younger people in their emotional, cognitive, and behavioural responses to pain and pain treatments.

Affective Factors

One of the most frequent emotional disturbances among older people is depression. Symptoms of chronic pain frequently mimic depression to such a degree that depression rating scales cannot distinguish between depressed individuals and patients with chronic pain. Whether depression is primary or secondary to pain is unresolved. Depression can interfere with rehabilitation outcome, therefore its treatment is a necessary component of pain management.

Even among individuals free of illness, at least 10% of people over 65 suffer from depression, an estimate that increases to 30–50% among elderly people with some concomitant illness (Wasylenki, 1987). Among populations with chronic pain, estimates of depression range from 10 to 83%, depending on the stringency of the criteria used to assess both depression and pain. Older patients are often reluctant to describe their emotional distress, and for many a 'physical' cause for the pain is more understandable, more acceptable and 'treatable'.

Cognitive–Behavioural Aspects

How people construe their pain profoundly affects not only the magnitude of perceived pain but also the likely outcome of interventions. The meaning ascribed to the pain and expectations about the ability to control it can amplify or diminish the associated distress. Cognition and behaviour are opposite sides of the same coin. Just as thoughts influence feelings and behaviour, behaviour can influence feelings and thoughts. Increasingly, pain is conceptualized in a learning model. What is learned over extended periods of unremitting pain are pain behaviours, that is the way people communicate their pain (verbally or non-verbally) to the world around them.

Personality Factors

Personality traits are relatively enduring mannerisms or habitual behaviours that are characteristic for a particular individual. Clinical observations suggest that differences in personality traits between individuals contribute to differences in their responses to pain. Emotional disturbances and personality changes occur in all individuals if pain persists over prolonged periods of time.

We can understand human reactions to the dual threats of pain and helplessness in terms of the individual's pre-existing (premorbid) personality traits. Personality not only colours the presentation of a clinical problem, it also determines the way a person copes with it. While some people will become hypervigilant to the presence of pain stimuli, others will repress attention to painful events and will not attempt to cope with them in any direct way. Such premorbid traits may be exaggerated in advanced age. A client's usual habits of perceiving and reacting to environmental cues have to be considered in the management of their pain. The success of individual coping strategies may very well depend on the success with which these can be adapted to the person's mode of functioning.

For example, a person with pre-existing histrionic tendencies may greatly exaggerate symptoms in a hypochondriacal way, whereas those with a narcissistic personality may become highly manipulative. A dependent person who has always lacked self-confidence, is likely to be a very passive patient; conversely, a compulsive type of person may become very demanding. It may be difficult to establish a trusting therapeutic relationship with a client who has already shown premorbid paranoid tendencies and who is likely to become even more suspicious and reclusive with advancing age. Physiotherapists who exercise interpersonal skills and pay attention to their clients' idiosyncracies can enhance compliance and collaboration with the treatment programme.

Psychosocial Influences

The most significant influence on the prognosis of physical and emotional illness is the social support system available to the patient. People with strong social ties to family and friends usually find it easier to reinterpret the pain experiences, and to adapt cognitively to altered circumstances in a more positive way. Absence of social supports often means isolation and loneliness, which may engender feelings of uselessness, worthlessness and helplessness. Seen from a behavioural perspective, in an environment in which pain behaviour was originally learned, the individual is surrounded by cues which elicit, maintain and strengthen pain behaviour and do not reinforce the display of 'well behaviours'. Psychosocial factors have been related to the client's pain reactions through uncertainty, perceived loss of control, social isolation, and social modelling (Chapman and Turner, 1990).

UNCERTAINTY

We fear most what we do not know. Lack of relevant information generates misconceptions and erroneous beliefs, and reinforces the myth that pain is the inevitable companion of old age. Unless corrected, these maladaptive thoughts constitute a continual source of stress which can undermine coping and sabotage treatments targeting a physical cause. Explanations and reassurances can dispel some myths and reduce fears. Moreover, verbal interchange in itself has therapeutic value as it competes with negative thoughts, encourages problem-solving and often increases self-confidence.

PERCEIVED LOSS OF CONTROL

Treatment sessions should provide opportunities for the client to experience mastery. Giving the client an active role in his rehabilitation programme and making the outcome contingent on his own efforts will restore some sense of personal control. Conversely, being the recipient of passive treatment perpetuates the perception of dependency and 'uselessness'.

SOCIAL ISOLATION

Loneliness leads to ruminations, depression, and 'giving up'. Pain behaviours are often the way a patient attempts to draw attention to his predicament. Gathering older clients together in groups for physiotherapy is not only a good way to make optimal use of staff resources, but also provides human contact and mutual support and frequently gives these clients a positive emotional experience.

SOCIAL MODELLING

Continually observing pain behaviours in other people not only engenders anxiety, it also has detrimental effects on a client's own pain behaviour. The impact of modelling on pain tolerance may be even stronger than that of personality factors. Conversely, extremely positive effects on pain sufferers may be achieved when optimistic attitudes are 'modelled' by physiotherapists and others.

An astute physiotherapist will integrate these principles into the rehabilitation programme by (a) imparting information about the treatment programme; (b) providing opportunities for the client to experience control and mastery; (c) encouraging social contact; (d) being a good and optimistic model. All these strategies are likely to reduce the perception of pain.

Assessment of Pain

Preliminary Considerations

The overall goal of rehabilitation for older people is to assess, maintain, and to improve function within appropriate levels of expectation. Once pain has been identified as a factor limiting function and a barrier to rehabilitation, it warrants assessment and treatment in its own right as well as interpretation in the context of the total clinical picture.

Since pain is not a function of age the principles of pain assessment are the same for young and old people (Helme and Katz, 1993). However, the format of the assessment process might differ substantially depending on individual problems which are frequently more complex and varied in advanced age. Older people commonly present with multiple problems of a biomedical, psychosocial and behavioural nature. Differential diagnosis, traditionally considered the *sine qua non* for planning appropriate treatments, is difficult because any one of the coexisting pathologies might account for, or contribute to, the presenting pain syndrome. To ascribe symptoms of an underlying disorder to 'normal' ageing processes may lead to undertreatment whereas treatments based on erroneous diagnoses may not only be ineffective but also discouraging for patient and physiotherapist.

Assessing a frail elderly person may be more multi-facetted and time-consuming than assessing a younger person. Although physiothera-pists are crucial to successful management of the problems of frail elderly people, they may find that complete assessment requires interprofessional team work to avoid duplication of effort and to develop a coordinated treatment plan tailored to a particular client. There should be a specialist in pain management in the team. Clients, and possibly their carers, should be full members of the team, not merely passive recipients of care.

Assessment Objectives

As with people of all ages, conducting an assessment yields the opportunity to establish rapport with clients and build their confidence. Creating favourable expectancies builds the basis for a placebo effect, an essential ingredient of any successful therapy, but perhaps even more important when dealing with pain. Physiotherapists have the same objectives when assessing the pain problems presented by older people as they do when assessing younger people:

1. To identify causative factors as far as possible, i.e. biological sources of pain and impairment.
2. To identify any contributory factors, such as the effects of pain on clients' mood and personality which perpetuate the pain, or psychosocial problems that may exacerbate the problem.
3. To judge the impact of pain on clients' physical function by observation and quantification of pain behaviours, e.g. medication intake, number of rests taken, degree of restriction of activities etc.
4. To understand clients' perception of their problems as well as strengths and resources.
5. To facilitate treatment planning in a problem-oriented approach.
6. To provide a basis for measuring treatment outcomes.

Problem Identification

During a pain assessment the physiotherapist should elicit information about the qualitative and temporal properties of the pain by allowing clients to describe their complaints in their own words. These properties include:

- duration, i.e. acute or chronic
- location and distribution
- any precipitating event
- quality (burning, stabbing etc)
- intensity / severity
- pattern (fluctuations)
- course (getting worse or better?)
- effect on functional activities
- impact on personality
- exacerbating and relieving factors
- temporal relationships (worse at night etc)
- effect on sleep
- contributory factors (stress etc)
- use of medication

Physiotherapists should be alert to intellectually impaired older people confabulating in order to camouflage their cognitive loss. Confabulation is verbose and circuitous speech with a semblance of fluency but lacking coherence and intelligibility. In these cases the questions should be particularly clear and to the point. If the answers are ambiguous, they should be repeated in a rephrased form, possibly during a subsequent session. Frequent 'don't know' answers, however, may be indicative of depressive pseudodementia which may improve with treatment of the underlying depression.

Physical Examination

It is wise to assess clients who have multiple problems over more than one session. The relevant examination procedure needs to be adapted to the condition of the older patient: appearance, posture, mobility, motor strength, neurological signs, dermatomal pain referral, sensory disturbances, reflexes, appropriate tests, balance, gait, and the role of pain in functional activities. As early as possible in the process it should be established whether the client's pain is associated with cancer.

The type and direction of movements which cause pain is very useful in identifying lesioned structures in musculoskeletal pain which is typically brought on by weight-bearing and relieved by rest. Pain that occurs only with activity suggests mechanical or vascular causes whereas pain on activity and rest may indicate inflammation. Nocturnal pain is characteristic of tumours, infections, neoplasms and neuritis.

Palpation may reveal areas of hyperalgesia or hyperaesthesia. If mental impairment has been identified, gentle squeezing of tissues, or other tactual stimuli, while observing the person's facial expression may be used to determine if and where pain is felt. Skin sensation should be tested for touch, prick and heat perception.

Measurement of Pain

A range of simple instruments should be used to measure pain distribution and intensity in older people especially if there are signs of mental impairment. This range may include: pain drawings, visual analogue scales, numerical scales and Faces scales. The first three of these procedures are described in Cole et al. (1994).

PAIN DRAWINGS

Pain drawings are useful to document the spatial properties of pain. The client indicates the location and distribution of his pain by shading the corresponding areas on the chart whereas the severity can be indicated by darker or lighter shading. This task involves clients actively in their rehabilitation and lets them talk about their pain. The chart provides useful information, can validate verbal description, and draw attention to inconsistencies. It is well to remember that the longer pain persists, the farther away it may be referred from the original site because of sensitization of nociceptors and other pain-sensitive structures.

VISUAL ANALOGUE SCALES

Visual Analogue Scales (VAS) are used to determine the intensity of pain. If the scale is a vertical, as opposed to horizontal, line (the anchors of which are defined as 'no pain' or 'worst pain imaginable', respectively) it can be compared to a thermometer which can aid administration and comprehensibility. At the initial assessment, the client marks two VAS lines corresponding to his pain level at 'best' and 'worst' times. For very sick people, the physiotherapist may run a pencil along the line and place the mark indicated by the person's nod. Pain fluctuations ('best' and 'worst' times) may indicate the extent of normal pain modulation, as well as the effect of medication and treatment strategies. Antecedent circumstances of 'best' and 'worst' pain can provide clues as to whether the pain is 'respondent' or 'operant' (see p. 302), or due to depression. Furthermore the effect of a single treatment can be assessed on two scales — before and after the intervention.

NUMERICAL SCALES

Numerical scales are useful when an older person has difficulty with the abstract concept of space and hence with understanding visual analogue scales despite likening it to a thermometer. A numerical scale (from 1–5 or 1–10) may be used.

Matching responses on this type of scale with those made on a visual analogue scale can be a useful check on the reliability of clients responses.

THE FACES SCALE

The Faces scale may be the solution when elderly clients continue to have difficulty in responding. The Faces scale consists of a series of schematic faces showing a range of moods from smiling (happy) to crying (sad) (Ferrel, 1991).

The multidimensional experience of pain, however, cannot be measured with a single instrument. Other dimensions such as sadness, inner tension, bodily discomfort, concentration difficulties, memory disturbances, unpleasantness of pain, fear, and worry may also be assessed by a VAS or a variety of specialized instruments. However, collecting large amounts of data burdens clients and should be avoided. For example, daily monitoring of pain may reinforce preoccupation with pain in some people. For the same reason, completing daily pain diaries are contraindicated in people with obsessive-compulsive or hypochondriacal tendencies.

Indices of pain can be objectively quantified once pain is operationally defined as behaviour. Three categories of pain behaviour can be scored in terms of frequency of the verbal and non-verbal expressions of pain; medication use; and activity level.

Principles of Pain Management Among Older People

Treatment goals may change with the patient's condition. Towards the end of life, when pain at times sems to erode the will to live, relieving the suffering is the overriding, and perhaps only goal of treatment. Unfortunately, no data exist at present about the best approach to ease suffering in confused and demented patients. Older people with chronic pain should be discouraged from expecting a complete cure. Instead, physiotherapists help them to understand that physiotherapy is to help them to become, or to remain, as active and independent as possible by optimizing their capacity to cope with the pain problem.

As with assessment, the basic principles of pain management are similar in young and old patients (Helme and Katz, 1993) and the challenge of managing pain problems in elderly clients similarly lies in multidisciplinary teamwork and integrated care.

Therapeutic methods may have to be adapted to accommodate any general age-related physiological and emotional changes or any additional specific problems revealed during the assessment. The physiotherapist must take into account the client's total bio-psycho-social and cognitive-behavioural profile, as well as any concurrent treatments, especially medications, that are being used.

Immediate short-term pain relief is typically achieved by analgesic drugs. However, despite the convenience and relative reliability of analgesics, drugs have an increased potential for toxicity in old age (Ciccone and Wolf, 1990). Various age-related changes mean that many drugs reach higher blood concentrations in older people. Also, this effect coupled with polypharmacy because of multiple pathology greatly increases the risk of drug interactions. Therefore non-pharmacological treatment may offer an equally effective and much safer method of pain control.

Physiotherapy

When selecting a pain control strategy, physiotherapists consider six questions:

1. What is the goal to be achieved?
   - amelioration of pain to enable the client to engage in functional activities?
   - symptomatic relief as an end in itself?
   - other?
2. In what way will the strategy contribute to the goal?
   - neuromodulation?
   - enhancement of self-esteem?
   - other?
3. Will any special precautions have to be taken?
   - are there any contraindications?
   - are there likely to be any interactions with other treatments, e.g. drugs?
   - how likely is the client to comply with the physiotherapy intervention?
4. What indices will show whether the client benefits from the physiotherapy intervention?
   - subjective? objective? observable evidence?
5. What other factors might be contributing to the pain and hence might influence the client's response to physiotherapy?
   - anxiety, lack of sleep, malnutrition, depression, pain behaviours, personality, psychosocial issues?
   - how can these concerns be integrated in the treatment plan?
6. How is pain controlled at present?

Physiotherapy can be used either as an alternative or as complement to drugs, thus permitting a reduction in the drug dosage. The aim of non-drug methods of pain control is to maintain or restore normative function in peripheral nerves and pain-modulatory systems. Apart from using injections, nerve blocks and medication, balance in pain transmission pathways can be restored either by decreasing or abolishing nociceptive input, or alternatively by increasing or changing sensory input to stimulate pain-modulatory systems. Many manual, mechanical, electrical, thermal and cryotherapies are available to physiotherapists, all of which can provide pain relief. The physiological effects of these modalities and techniques seem to be much clearer than the mechanism of their action on pain. Their common feature is that they produce different types of sensory input, generating nerve impulse patterns which enter the spinal cord, reach the brain in form of epicritic information, and influence the complex pain modulation processes. Electroanalgesia, heat and massage are the foremost examples of providing altered neural input that results in pain relief. These treatment options together with exercise and cognitive behavioural techniques will be discussed.

Electroanalgesia by Transcutaneous Electrical Nerve Stimulation (TENS)

Direct electrical stimulation of sensory nerves can be an extremely valuable addition to the therapeutic regimen of selected older patients, especially when used in conjunction with an active exercise programme. TENS is the application of low-voltage electrical pulses through the skin to nerves or spinal roots supplying the painful area. Based on the gate control theory of pain (Wall and Melzack, 1984), the underlying rationale is that selective fibre activation results in modulation of the transmission and perception of pain signals.

Although TENS has been reported as being less effective with elderly people, it still has considerable value. However, just as age-related changes may require much *smaller* doses of pharmacological agents in older than younger people to achieve comparable pain relief, TENS may require much *longer* periods of sensory stimulation. Hours rather minutes may be required to correct for imbalanced neural input due to loss of touch receptors, slower conduction, diminished large fibre input, increased firing of nociceptive afferent and sympathetic efferent fibres in the affected nerve. By the same token, TENS may have reduced ability to provide stimulation aimed at the release of endogenous opioids as decline of endorphinergic systems has been demonstrated in old age. Opiate medication may also affect TENS efficacy.

Sharing common neurophysiological underpinnings, such as the route of transmission, both TENS and physical exercise are capable of correcting neural regulatory defects in the modulation of pain. In acute pain states, TENS has been found as effective as oral analgesics (such as acetaminophen with codeine), but without any side-effects; in chronic pain states, the response rate is lower. Acupuncture-like (low-frequency) TENS is a method of 'counter-irritation' and may activate endorphinergic pathways unless the patient is on opiate medication.

TENS should not be used: over the carotid sinuses where a hypotensive response may lead to cardiac arrest; when a cardiac pacemaker has been fitted; or when the client suffers from dementia or is otherwise confused. If the client has a history of cerebral vascular accidents, transient ischaemic attacks, or epileptic seizures, TENS should only be used with very careful monitoring (Mannheimer and Lampe, 1984).

TENS is a passive modality which may increase the patient's dependency, unless integrated in an active treatment package. By involving patients actively in their treatments and teaching them how to apply TENS to themselves may give a sense of increased control and responsibility.

Case Study

A 70-year-old woman was referred to the Pain Clinic because of severe osteoarthritic pain in both knees. She was intelligent, bitter, angry, controlling and manipulative. Asked what she missed most in her present life style, she replied 'my daily walks'. After breaking down this client's problems into all its components, each became the target of focussed but integrated intervention. Her response to TENS was excellent; she learned how to pace her weight-bearing activities and intersperse them with periods of relaxation; faithfully adhering to a regular exercise programme increased her muscle strength considerably; she always met her exercise quotas and exerted considerable effort to change maladaptive habits. Her medication [NSAID] was changed. Gradually, she became less hostile, and soon took daily walks using one or occasionally two canes and with four TENS electrodes firmly attached over the joint spaces of her knees, the unit being attached to her belt. She enjoyed life again and seemed a much happier person.

Heat

The analgesic, antispasmodic, and sedative effects of any form of heat make it a particularly useful method of treatment for older people. When judiciously combined with other treatments such as massage or pool therapy, it can often considerably enhance treatment effects. As with TENS, there are few differences in the contra-indications between young and old people although for older clients certain age-related factors and disease carry increased risk such as reduced thermal sensation hence increased risk

of burns; changes in vascular perfusion where heat may exacerbate oedemas or areas of ischaemia; higher risk of malignancy; a history of cardiac disease may be a contraindication to pool therapy because of the large area of the body that is warmed and subject to peripheral vasodilatation; being on a vasodilator drug regime may similarly be a contraindication to pool therapy.

Exercise

Exercise is the single most important remedial strategy in the rehabilitation of any person with pain, and especially so with older people, to prevent or counter the deteriorative effects of disuse. Older clients may have reduced their physical activities not only because of progressive disability, but also because they have experienced or anticipate pain on exercise. Avoidance of activity may be more related to anxiety and fear than to actual impairment. Physical exercise can reduce pain and anxiety, as well as change the client's belief of self-worth and ability to cope.

Exercise gives the patient an active role in his rehabilitation and some responsibility for the outcome, which may have beneficial psychological effects (one of which is a better body image). As in younger persons, the actual exercise regimen is determined by the specific pathology, and progresses gradually from the most basic and specific exercises to more vigorous regimes. The older the client, the more important it becomes to adapt the exercise regimen to avoid excessive fatigue and the risks of injury. Exercise programmes also need to be tailored to the person's idiosyncratic characteristics and always be given within a behavioural framework (Chapter 12).

In order to reinforce 'well behaviour', the task demand should always be within a person's capability to avoid experience of failure. Experimental evidence suggests that perceived failure can lead to an increase in perceived pain (Chapter 13).

Before beginning a behaviourally oriented regimen, its purpose is explained to the client who might want to decide on a desirable long-range goal ('what would you like to do most?'). The goal has to be specific, realistic, objectifiable and measurable. After the long-term goal has been broken down into small achievable intermediate stages, a contract confirms the patient's agreement. A baseline of what the patient is capable of doing at present is established, and small incremental quotas set for each week. Non-achievement of the set quota is ignored, while the therapist's attention and praise are contingent on the client's performance. Performance of the agreed activities can often provide a distraction from the pain.

Cognitive–Behavioural Strategies

During the past few decades, chronic pain has been treated very successfully within a framework of operant conditioning developed from learning theory (Fordyce, 1976). Within this behavioural framework, the aetiology of pain is relatively unimportant. The objective is to modify the learned pain behaviour, such as complaining, moaning, groaning, guarding, grimacing, limping, and avoidance of activities. These illness behaviours are assumed to reflect not solely underlying pathology but rather – at least partially – conditioned responses, habitually emitted because they had been strengthened by either positive reinforcement (attention, sympathy, praise etc), or negative reinforcement (encouragement of avoidance behaviours).

Behavioural approaches are being used with increasing success in the management of pain in older people, as well as to increase their activity level and prevent immobility. Behaviour modification is indicated in cases of excessive use of medication, expression of excessive illness behaviour, reduced activity levels (deconditioning), or excessive concern with pain and illness. Treatment goals should not be limited to the symptom of pain but rather focus on the person resuming as active a lifestyle as possible.

Most clients with persistent pain will present with a mixed picture of responses to tissue damage (respondent pain) and illness pain-behaviour that has been conditioned by subtle reinforcement (operant pain). While respondent pain is managed within the medical model by identifying the cause and treating it, the way in which clients express their pain is dealt with in an operant framework. Clients who complain excessively, demand more medication, spend most of the time resting, avoid exercise, limp more than considered justified, and want to talk only about their illnesses might be expressing conditioned pain behaviour. If a client is given attention and sympathy only when pain behaviour is expressed, this will strengthen the illness behaviour, and will eventually result in more pain, increased dependency and loss of self-esteem. Rewards should be made contingent on the display of 'well behaviour' such as improved self care, or an increase of exercise quotas, smiling, or social interaction. Pain medication should be given on a fixed schedule (not on demand) to avoid drugs becoming reinforcers for pain.

Pain behaviours can be unobtrusively 'shaped' and diminished by appropriate reinforcement contingencies. An overly dependent patient, for example, might need a great deal of reinforcement for performing independent actions such as applying TENS electrodes to himself, while excessive demands of another patient can be gently discouraged by withholding reinforcement, or perhaps by cooly ignoring them.

Regardless of the underlying pathophysiology, psychological strategies such as teaching relaxation, using behavioural methods to discourage inappropriate behaviours, and teaching clients appropriate coping strategies should be part of the management of chronic pain in elderly people (Helme and Katz, 1993). Dispelling negative thought patterns by encouraging their replacement with more realistic and optimistic ones is an effective way to restore self-esteem and to maintain motivation.

Relaxation therapy has beneficial physical and psychological effects. Increased sympathetic activity in pain states resulting in sensitization and spontaneous activity of nociceptors, interference with blood supply, production of muscle spasms, and magnification of pain may be reduced by relaxation therapy. This has proven to be one of the most effective and inexpensive treatments to restore homeostasis in the autonomic nervous system, and to reduce the subjective experiences of pain and emotional distress (Tunks, 1988). Relaxation procedures can lead to learned control of autonomic responses, to self-regulation of neurophysiological processes and to a change in patterns of brain processes. Physiological and psychological processes (placebo effects) can be maximized with autogenic suggestions to expect pain relief.

Cognitive coping strategies are techniques that, once acquired, can be successfully integrated into physiotherapy. They include: thought monitoring and changing one's 'internal dialogues'; reconceptualizing one's problem by dispelling certain 'myths' about pain through information and education; discussions; engaging in problem-solving; and stress management.

Older people respond as well as younger chronic pain patients to these strategies. Middaugh et al. (1988) compared outcomes of older people (55–78 years) and younger people to a multi-disciplinary chronic pain rehabilitation programme, and found no significant differences in benefit between the age groups. Older patients benefitted at least as much, if not more, from a behavioural approach consisting of physiotherapy, occupational therapy, biofeedback, relaxation, psychology (cognitive strategies) and medical management.

Summary

Successful management of older clients with pain depends on the optimal combination, appropriate timing, skilful application and careful evaluation of convergent therapies. The concurrent use of several procedures: exercise, TENS or massage, and relaxation all embedded in a behavioural framework is likely to produce better results than those produced by the serial application of each procedure in isolation. It is also important for physiotherapists to have an optimistic outlook and encourage positive feelings of control and of being valued in their older clients.

References

Bayer, AJ, Chadja, JS, Farag, RR, Pathy, MSJ (1986) Changing presentation of myocardial infarction with increasing old age. *Journal of the American Geriatric Society* 34: 263–266.

Bonica, JJ (1990) Anatomic and physiologic basis of nociception and pain. In Bonica JJ (ed) *The Management of Pain* 2nd edn, pp. 28–94. Philadelphia: Lea & Febiger.

Bonica, JJ, Loeser, JD (1990) Medical evaluation of the patient with pain. In Bonica JJ (ed) *The Management of Pain* 2nd edn, pp. 563–579. Philadelphia: Lea & Febiger.

Chapman, CR, Turner, JA (1990) Psychologic and psychosocial aspects of acute pain. In Bonica JJ (ed) *The Management of Pain* 2nd edn, pp. 122–132. Philadelphia: Lea & Febiger.

Ciccone, CD, Wolf, SL (1990) *Pharmacology in Rehabilitation*, 524 pp. Philadelphia: FA Davis.

Cole, B, Finch, E, Gowland, C, Mayo, N (1994). *Physical Rehabilitation Outcome Measures*. Toronto: Canadian Physiotherapy Association.

Crook, J, Rideout, E, Browne, G (1984) The prevalence of pain complaints in a general population. *Pain* 18: 299–314.

Ferrel, BA (1991) Pain management in elderly people. *Journal of the American Geriatric Society* 39: 64–73.

Fields, HL (1987) *Pain*, 354 pp. New York: McGraw Hill.

Fordyce, WE (1976) Behavioral concepts in chronic pain and illness. In Davidson, PO (ed) *The Behavioral Management of Anxiety, Depression and Pain*, pp. 147–188. New York: Brunner/Mazel.

Georgotas, A (1983) Affective disorders in the elderly: diagnostic and research considerations. *Age and Ageing* 12: 1–10.

Harkins, SW, Kwentus, J, Price, DD (1990) Pain and suffering in the elderly. In: Bonica, JJ (ed) *The Management of Pain* 2nd edn, pp. 552–559. Philadelphia: Lea & Febiger.

Helme, RD, Katz, B (1993) Management of chronic pain. *The Medical Journal of Australia* 158: 478–481.

Mannheimer, JS, Lampe, GN (1984) *Clinical Transcutaneous Electrical Nerve Stimulation*, 636 pp. Philadelphia: FA Davis.

Merskey, H (1986) Classification of chronic pain. *Pain* (Suppl.) 3: S217.

Middaugh, SJ, Levin, RB, Kee, WG *et al.* (1988) Chronic pain: its treatment in geriatric and younger patients. *Archives of Physical Medicine and Rehabilitation* 69: 1021–1026.

Payne, R, Pasternak, GW (1990) Pain and pain management. In Cassel, CK, Riesenberg, DE, Sorensen, LB, Walsh, JR (eds) *Geriatric Medicine* 2nd edn, pp. 585–606. New York: Springer.

Tunks, E (1988) Behavioral interactions and their efficacy. In Dubner, R, Gebhart, GF, Bond, MR (eds) *Pain Research and Clincial Management* Vol 3, pp. 298–309. (Proceedings of the Vth World Congress on Pain) Amsterdam: Elsevier.

Wall, PD, Melzack, R (eds) (1984) *Textbook of Pain*, pp. 717–750. Edinburgh: Churchill Livingstone.

Wasylenki, DA (1987) Depression. In Wasylenki, DA, Martin, BA, Clark, DM *et al.* (eds) *Psychogeriatrics: A Practical Handbook*, pp. 41–58. London: Jessica Kingsley.

21

Palliative Care

LYDIA GILLHAM

What is Palliative Care?

Medical Measures and How they Can Affect Physiotherapy Management

Making Decisions about Physiotherapy – Some of the Difficulties

Thinking Through The Situation – Rehabilitation or Active Re-adaptation

Common Problems which will Affect Physiotherapy Treatment

Practical Clinical Examples of Disabilities Encountered in Palliative Care

Conclusions

To many people the words 'palliative care' convey the impression of a speciality which is all about dying and death. In practice, professionals working in this area find their attention is focused mainly on the living and the ways in which, with professional help, patients can achieve the best possible quality of life. The majority of patients encountered in palliative care are older (Greer, 1983), often with advanced cancer. This means that physiotherapists in these units encounter death and bereaved friends and relatives much more than in other specialities.

When working in palliative care physiotherapists work alongside professionals whose efforts are directed particularly to helping patients and their relatives, cope with the process of dying and afterwards with bereavement. Not suprisingly, some physiotherapists choose to extend their training and move into this phase of care but when operating in their own professional capacity as physiotherapists their contribution to the final stage of dying is small. It is likely to involve procedures which contribute to the comfort of the patients such as positioning, turning, gentle relaxing massage and passive movements.

The majority of physiotherapists' time in palliative care is given over to very active and practical work. Frequently it can be very similar to working in neurology, orthopaedics and surgery. Indeed many of the patients eventually referred to palliative care units have been in such units previously. Physiotherapy is most likely to help when an improvement in function can be anticipated following recent medical or surgical treatment.

This chapter concentrates on palliative care provided for patients who require from physiotherapists a different approach to treatment. It is concerned with patients who have advanced malignant disease and whose abilities are likely to deteriorate regardless of treatment. Those people constitute the majority of patients needing palliative care – although a small proportion of patients with other conditions such as motor neurone disease and AIDS may also be helped by a palliative approach to their management. Whilst older patients are likely to be in the majority, a palliative care unit will also cater for younger people.

What is Palliative Care?

The word 'palliative' is not new to physiotherapists. It has always been used to describe treatments which will relieve and alleviate symptoms but will not lead to cure. Some people involved in health care believe that curing patients is their prime concern, but even with conditons where patients are not deteriorating there are often symptoms which require palliation.

The term 'palliative care' is now conventionally used to describe the management of patients with advanced incurable and deteriorating disease, especially cancer. The efforts of all health professionals involved are dedicated to relieving of symptoms, and improving the quality of life, of dying people and supporting those they leave behind. Palliative care of this kind requires a team of different professionals to cater for the patients' varied needs. A physiotherapist is only one member of this team. The team is likely to include professionals less frequently represented in other areas of health care – bereavement counsellors, chaplains and complementary therapists. These specialists are needed because the psychological, emotional, social and spiritual needs of patients are felt to be as important as their physical needs. Older patients cared for in palliative care will benefit from this interdisciplinary holistic approach (Greer, 1983). In most countries hospices have been the organizational units primarily involved in the development of palliative care. However in the UK an increasing number of hospital and community units are beginning to establish palliative care teams and units applying the hospice philosophy, ethics and expertise in these settings also. In North America the emphasis is more on palliative care in the community setting.

A useful definition of palliative care is:

> The active total care of patients whose disease is not responsive to curative treatment. Control of pain, of other symptoms, and of psychological, social and spiritual problems is paramount. The goal of palliative care is achievement of the best quality of life for patients and their families. Many aspects of palliative care are also applicable earlier in the course of the illness in conjunction with anti-cancer treatment.
> (Doyle *et al.* 1993)

There is a need to distinguish between palliative care and palliative medicine. Palliative care is a broad field involving many specialists which nevertheless involves all the necessary components of any medical speciality including matters such as education, research and clinical audit. Palliative medicine on the other hand is a narrower term which is used to describe the speciality as practised by physicians.

Terminal or Dying?

Patients being treated in palliative care units are frequently near the end of their lives and are often described as being terminal (see also Chapters 3

Figure 1 Putting palliative care in context.

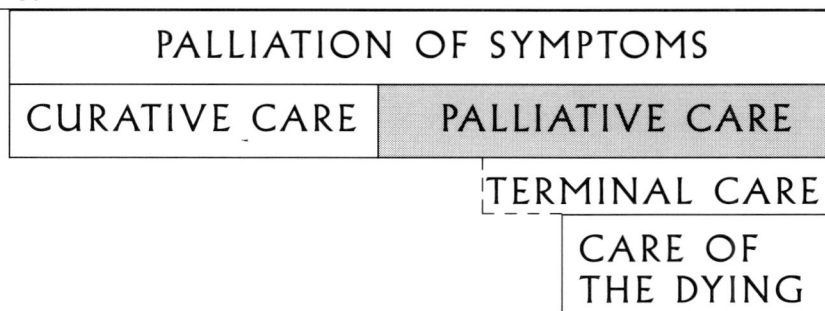

PALLIATION OF SYMPTOMS	
CURATIVE CARE	PALLIATIVE CARE

TERMINAL CARE

CARE OF
THE DYING

and 5). In his research study on the rehabilitation of 301 patients with advanced cancer Yoshioka (1994) defined terminal as having a remaining life span of 6 months. 'Terminal' is a word which professionals in palliative care are very reluctant to use for several reasons. It certainly has negative connotations which risks attaching a label to patients. It might well induce a less active and, less positive attitude on the part of all concerned. The words we use are important because they provide information about how we think and feel, they communicate our attitudes and encourage consensual approaches in those offering treatment. In dealing with advanced incurable disease a positive yet realistic approach is required (Gray, 1993). Physicians are fequently asked 'how long' a patient has to live, but this is a quesiton which is almost impossible to answer. When, against their better judgement, they are persuaded to do so, they are frequently proved to be wrong. The phrase terminal care certainly conveys the impression that the patient is dying. However once symptom control is established such prognostications can frequently be proved wrong. These perceptions can have implications for the physiotherapy which is provided. Sometimes in so called 'terminal' cases physiotherapy may be considered inappropriate, and patients are then denied skills and knowledge which could make them more comfortable. The word 'dying' is usefully confined to describing the stage when physiological changes such as peripheral shut down of circulation, and Cheyne Stokes respiration herald the final event.

Philosophical and Ethical Issues

(see Chapter 27)

It is a basic human right that when cure is not possible patients should be assisted in achieving the best possible quality of life, free of pain and distressing symptoms. It is important for the professional involved in helping to achieve this, not to feel that this outcome is 'second rate' compared with procedures which lead to cure. Therapy which contributes to comforting the patient and relieving symptoms in a caring way is intrinsically valuable in its own right. A thought widely quoted in the literature, sometimes attributed to Hippocrates, provides a powerful motto for those working in palliative care: 'To cure sometimes, to relieve often, to comfort always'.

Physiotherapists working in palliative care spend a considerable time in working closely with individual patients. Consequently they are often drawn into conversations which involve answering very difficult questions:

Have I got cancer?

Will I ever walk again?
Am I dying?

Early professional training in physiotherapy rarely provides an adequate preparation for responding to such questions. Professionals may be beset by feelings of inadequacy as they struggle for an appropriate response and inevitably this adds to the stress of working with people who are very ill. Many physiotherapists respond by extending their skills, for example by training in counselling. However, it is important to appreciate the diversity of training courses available, both in terms of duration and content.

Training in counselling is likely to benefit a physiotherapist in many ways, for example by improving the skills of listening and attending, and in enhancing the ability to reflect. Reflection involves reflecting back to the patient what they have been saying. It doesn't involve simply repeating the patient's words but also involves signalling what is being conveyed by the emotions they display and the language they use. This process reminds the physiotherapist that a counsellor is not engaged in solving the patient's problems. Rather, the physiotherapist is using skills which clarify situations so that patients can help themselves.

Acquiring counselling skills also raises the physiotherapist's awareness that the mode and style of communication which they adopt with the patient needs to be adjusted to suit the situation. For example there are many times when it is counter-productive to be directive and be telling the patient what to do. On other occasions it is perfectly appropriate to simply tell the patient what the best line of action will be. In practice success depends on using the right approach, at the right time, with the right person.

There is a considerable body of literature dealing with the counselling of patients with cancer (Maguire and Faulkner, 1988). However, physiotherapists need to bear in mind that they are much more likely to be using a counselling approach with a small 'c' during their day-to-day management of patients reather than being a 'Counsellor' with a capital 'C'.

Maguire and Faulkner's work (1988a,b) on counselling cancer patients contains much very practical advice useful to a palliative care physiotherapist. For example they point out that in breaking bad news to a patient that there are 'first liners' and 'second liners' involved. The 'first liner' in this example will probably be the doctor whose job it is to inform the patient of their diagnosis. The physiotherapist is a 'second liner' because they have to deal with the patient after the initial bad news has been delivered. In this situation the patient may well ask the physiotherapist questions like – 'Have I got cancer?' or 'Will I walk again?'. Physiotherapists might respond by reflecting the questions back to patients, asking them what they have already been told or why they are asking the question. It will then become apparent that the patient has already been told the bad news. As second liners physiotherapists will simply be providing confirmation of what the patient has already heard and already knows.

Medical Measures and How they Can Affect Physiotherapy Management

Whilst physiotherapists are never involved in prescribing or giving medicines a clear understanding of their contribution to the care of the patient is essential. Medical intervention can affect physiotherapy management in both positive and negative ways and therefore the physiotherapy given must match other treatment appropriately in order to get the best result.

Admission to palliative care units such as hospices is not arranged solely because the patient is dying. Indeed the majority of patients with advanced cancer will not die in a hospice but in a hospital or at their own home. In fact a common reason for involving a specialist palliative care team is to bring about relief from pain and unpleasant symptoms and improve the patient's quality of life. Consequently patients may be encountered a long time before their death. Palliative care units are also used to provide respite for carers and psychological, social, spiritual and rehabilitation care for the patient.

Often it is the very symptoms which have precipitated the involvement of the specialist unit which pose the main problems for the physiotherapist. For example, pain can be so dominating that it makes physiotherapy assessment and treatment difficult or even impossible. Extreme dyspnoea can make active therapy inavisable as it would increase demands on an already overtaxed respiratory system.

Sensitivity and timing of the initial physiotherapy assessment can be crucial. A patient who is wracked with pain may, if assessed too soon, can give a false impression of immobility. Conversely such pain may mask important problems like muscle weakness and joint stiffness. Therefore because of this it is often better to delay active physiotherapy until a pain relief regime has been established and the patient's condition is more stable. At this point patients can often demonstrate dramatic improvements in function.

Controlling the Pain

USING DRUGS

Most cancer patients have a variety of pains, some of which are not attributable to the cancer. They may experience pain from problems which are regularly encountered during normal physiotherapy practice. For example pain resulting from arthritic conditions, recent injuries, skin disorders, infection, pressure sores co-existing can often be overridden by cancer pain. These 'lesser' pains become more troublesome once a patient's cancer pain has been relieved. Unbearable pain is one of the symptoms patients expect and fear most in cancer. If it isn't controlled it can be 'all consuming'. However, around one-third of all patients with cancer are pain free, and of the remainder 90% have their pain successfully relieved.

When assessing the impact of pain another important factor needs to be considered. Fear, anger, feelings of isolation and other psychological and social factors all build up the 'pattern' of pain presented by the patient. Pain is a 'whole person' experience and it needs to be considered in this context.

Operation of an established sequence is one of the key features in administering drugs for pain relief. The Cancer Pain Relief Programme of the World Health Organization recommends the use of a three-step analgesic ladder. Unless the pain is extremely severe it is suggested that one of the drugs from the bottom step, the non-opiates is tried first. If unsuccessful then a drug from the second step — the weak opiates — is selected. If necessary this is followed by a move to the third step — the strong opiates.

Another key feature is the maintanence of pain control throughout 24 hours. This is achieved by finding the lowest effective dose to prevent breakthrough pain for each individual patient. It also needs to be administered regularly enough to avoid leaving the patient unprotected. The time interval between doses depends on the length of action of the nature of the drug. A physiotherapy programme should not be allowed to interfere with this regular medication.

Weak opiates and strong opiates are drugs made from morphine which has very potent effects — both positive and negative — which must be taken into account by physiotherapists (Thompson, 1994).

On the positive side the powerful analgesic effects of morphine often make it possible for the physiotherapist to consider active physiotherapy. However, it is important to remember that the cause of the pain is still there and that caution must be exercised by avoiding excessive or inappropriate exercises or activities. For example it is possible for the pain from a cancer in the bone to be masked enough to allow the patient to bear their full weight on the bone even though it may not be strong enough to do so.

On the negative side nausea, vomiting, constipation, sedation and dizziness are all likely to affect physiotherapy. These side-effects can often be relieved by other drugs. In addition many patients are afraid that they will become addicted to morphine, but experts in palliative medicine believe that dependance on this drug for pain relief is not the same as addiction. In the case of addiction, patients crave drugs for psychological reasons in a way unrelated to their use for pain relief.

When patients are taking their drugs orally, rectally or by injection it does not complicate physiotherapy. But other modes of administration may do so. For example poor handling of the patient or inappropriate activity can be responsible for dislodging a needle or a catheter. Pain relief drugs are commonly introduced in to the subcutaneous tissues via a butterfly needle which is left in place indefinitely. Doses of medicine are then given continuously by using a battery operated 'syringe driver', often with a 'boost' facility. The physiotherapist must have a clear idea of the context within which they are working in order to avoid problems.

Spinal Analgesia

Another route increasingly used for the introduction of opioids is the spinal route. It is chosen when simpler approaches have not provided pain relief or they have been associated with unacceptable side-effects. A catheter is introduced into either the epidural space or, more commonly, into the subarachnoid (intrathecal) space in the lumbar region of the spine. If it is brought directly to the surface in the lower back it can only be left in place for 3–4 days, otherwise the body would start to react to the 'foreign body' implanted in it and begin to reject it. Importantly, the catheter can provide direct access to the spinal canal for infection. Therefore, the catheter is tunnelled into the subcutaneous tissues, away from the site of entry, before exiting from the skin usually over the anterior chest wall. In this position the patient is able to lie comfortably without pressure on the exit site.

One or two bacterial filters are frequently introduced into the system with regular changes at set intervals. Sometimes these are external filters, sometimes they are implanted. In order to deliver the pain relief drug regularly into the spinal line some palliative care centres prefer continuous infusion using a reservoir system. The reservoir system and continuous infusion means the patient is less restricted in their movements and rehabilitation becomes easier.

Disease Modifying Measures in Palliative Care

PALLITATIVE CHEMOTHERAPY

Powerful drugs are used widely in cancer treatment but their contribution to palliative care is less well accepted. Unpleasant side-effects such as nausea and vomiting are feared by most patients. These negative effects together with problems like bone marrow depression and secondary infection, must be balanced against the positive effect which chemotherapy can have on reducing tumours. Indeed many of the unpleasant symptoms of the disease, such as pain and dyspnoea, can be relieved or palliated for a while thereby improving the patient's quality of life.

Physiotherapy for patients receiving chemotherapy is likely to be most useful when the worst side affects have begun to wear off and some of the benefits have become apparent.

CORTICOSTEROIDS

Malignant tumours comprise a central mass of cancer cells surrounded by a zone of chronically inflamed oedematous tissue. This non-cancerous outer zone contributes significantly to the overall size of the tumour and therefore increases the pressure on other tissues such as nerves and organs. High-dose steroids are used to shrink this area. The two principal steriods used are dexamethasone and prednisolone. The useful effects of these drugs depend on which tissues have been under pressure and the response is usually appreciable within 24–48 hours. Unfortunately the tumour shrinkage achieved in this way is temporary although the effect can last for weeks or even months.

This is often a good time for physiotherapists to take action which will improve the patient's func-tion. Unfortunately, some of the side-effects make the management of physiotherapeutic measures more difficult. Patients easily put on weight around the face the so called 'moon face' effect and on the abdomen. In addition mobility may be affected by osteoporosis and proximal myopathy involving the muscles of the limbs. The legs are usually most affected and consequently activities such as rising from a chair or going upstairs can be difficult.

PALLIATIVE RADIOTHERAPY

When radiotherapy is used locally to achieve a 'cure' it is called radical radiotherapy. Palliative radiotherapy is used to reduce the size of localized tumours and to alleviate the accompanying symptoms. However once the cancer has metastasized and spread to many sites in the body it is less useful. In these circumstances a larger field is irradiated, for example in hemibody irradiation half the body is irradiated. Radiotherapy is very effective with bone mestastasis where the success rates in reducing pain is around 80%. This treatment is often given when bones are in danger of a pathological fracture. When the vertebrae are affected by cancer the spinal cord can be compressed either by tumour or by collapse of the affected vertebrae. The physiotherapist is in a good position to identify early signs of cord compression – such as muscle weakness and back pain. Emergency treatment can be provided in the form of radiotherapy alone or accompanied by surgical decompression.

Another area where radiotherapy is often used is in treating brain tumours. In this case physiotherapy becomes most effective approximately 6 weeks after treatment when the effect is likely to be at its maximum.

SURGICAL PALLIATION

Physiotherapists may be involved in the palliation of symptoms in the surgical wards of general hospitals after patients have undergone surgery. Later these patients may be transferred to palliative care units. General surgical procedures used involve excisions, reconstructions, colostomies, draining of abscesses and the insertion of cannulae of shunts. Orthopaedic surgery is required to fix pathological fractures and stabilize bones with a high risk of fracture. Neurosurgical techniques applied to these patients include surgical cordotomy and decompressions. Post-operative physiotherapy is provided in the way most appropriate to each speciality.

Making Decisions about Physiotherapy – Some of the Difficulties

Predictability and Unpredictability

One of the distressing features of cancer is that it may not remain confined to the site of the primary lesion and may spread to the rest of the body. The fact that the malignant cells will be carried to other parts of the body in the blood and lymph provides an explanation for the variety of tissues and areas involved and for the extent of the body which can be affected. The scope for spread is potentially enormous and unpredictable. Nevertheless patterns can be identified in clinical practice. Malignant tissues with a similar histology and a similar site of origin are likely to spread in a similar way. Predictability therefore co-exists within apparent unpredictability. This situation can make long-term goal setting particularly difficult.

Complex Realities and the Therapeutic Limitations of Simple Treatment Models

In palliative care the physiotherapist is usually dealing with malignant disease at such an advanced stage that the patient is rarely afflicted with one single disability or one single clinical problem. The example which follows is not untypical of the level of complexity presented to the physiotherapist:

Marion a 76-year-old woman is admitted to the hospice 5 years after having a mastectomy for breast cancer. The cancer has metastasized to present the following problems:

- *Thoracic and lumbar spine metastases resulting in paraparesis and back pain.*
- *Metastases of the femur in both legs and humerus in both arms.*
  In the past year all but the right humerus have been fractured. She has now arrived at the hospice following a further recent fracture of the left femur which could not be fixed internally, this involved traction only to provide pain relief. This fracture is not expected to heal.
- *Mild lymphoedema in the right arm.*
- *Skin on the thorax has multiple skin metastasis*
- *Secondary tumour behind the right eye – leading to loss of vision.*
- *Dizziness*

Thinking Through the Situation – What Kind of Assessment?

In many areas of physiotherapy a problem-oriented approach is advocated. The problems presented by the patient and the situation are carefully identified and the physiotherapy goals and programme are developed from that point. In a complex case like Marion's the list of problems may seem too long to manage effectively. However a lot of these problems will never be relieved or improved. It may therefore be more realistic to start with the patient's goals and what they want to be able to do at the time. Goals which are realistic and identified by the patient themselves, coupled with a calculated professional input from the physiotherapist are more likely to improve quality of life (Yoshioka 1994). When the situation is dominated by the physiotherapist there is a danger of imposing what is seen as 'suitable' for their patient.

So, one approach for the physiotherapist could be to start with the patient's needs and goals. The assessment then takes place with these in mind and the programme can be worked out in detail. For example in the above example of Marion.

Suppose that her main personal goal is to attend her granddaughter's wedding in 1 month's time. This will lead the physiotherapist into assessing all the factors which will make this possible.

- *How will she transfer?*
- *How long will she be able to sit?*
- *What kind of wheelchair and cushions will she require?*
- *Which carers will need to be available and how will they be prepared for helping her?*

- *Is the church and the reception area accessible?*
- *How can the wheelchair and any treatment devices be camouflaged?*

This careful assessment of the context will lead to the physiotherapy programme necessary to achieve the goal.

This example illustrates the three stage nature of the process:

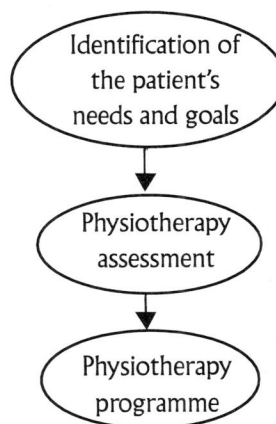

The Pain and Pleasure of Professional Duty

In practice in any area of work the physiotherapist experiences a range of emotions from pain to pleasure, comfort to discomfort, hope to despair, usefulness to a feeling of helplessness. In palliative care these emotions may be experienced by the physiotherapist in an extreme form. This is a natural consequence of working with such a concentrated group of patients and their relatives who are aware all that the patients are living out the last 'chapter' of their lives. The physiotherapist has to learn to work reasonably comfortably with the certain knowledge that patients are likely to decline during the period

Figure 2   Making decisions about physiotherapy in advanced malignant disease.

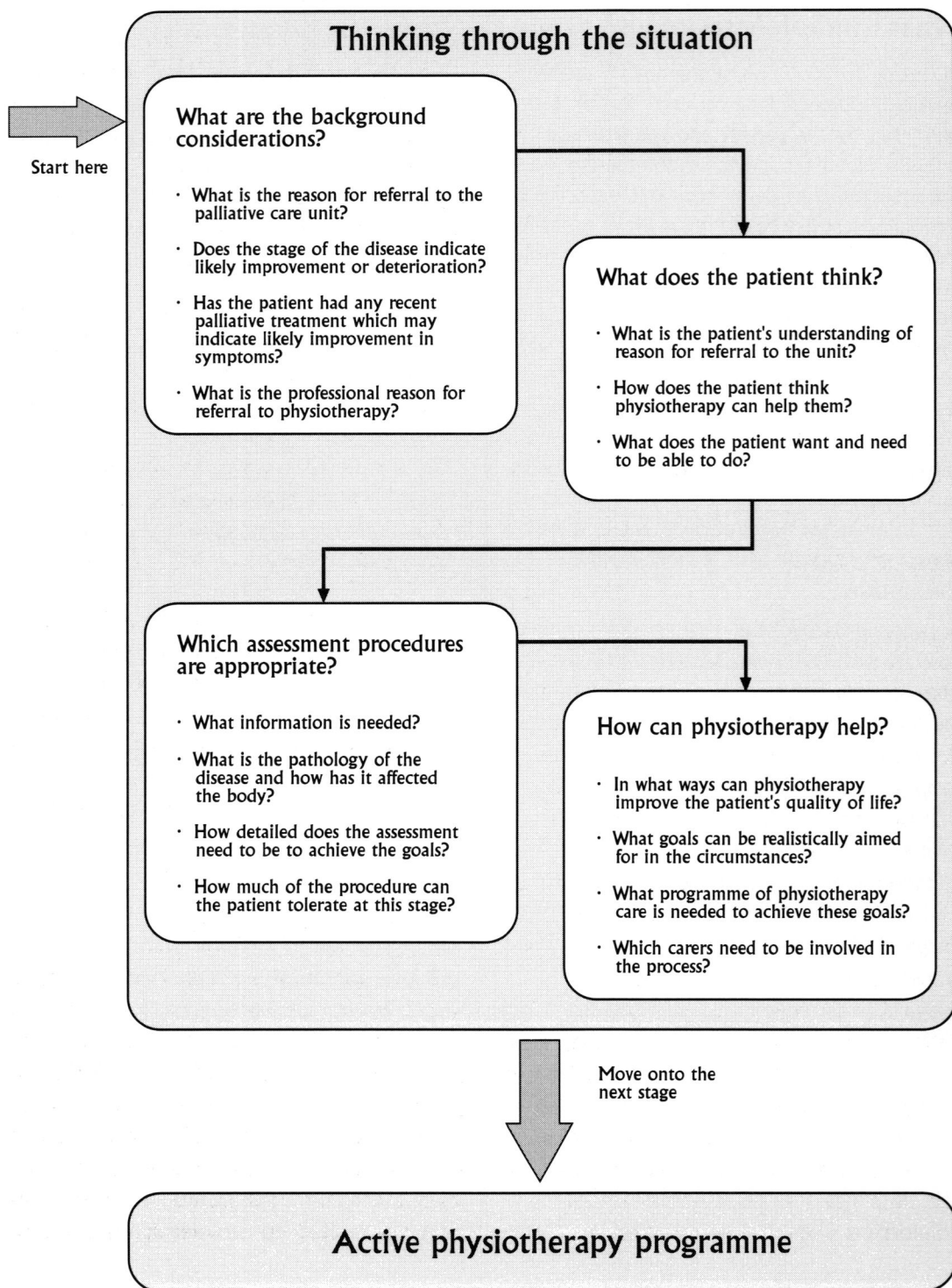

of care. Whilst this deterioration in patient health exists in many areas of physiotherapy work, in palliative care it works at a more accelerated rate. To survive this experience without emotional 'burnout' and to achieve job satisfaction physiotherapists must be aware of the very natural human reactions and be honest about them. Acting otherwise is likely to create additional stress. It is however important that a mental frame is developed in which physiotherapists can employ an approach which is constructive, professional, positive and flexible and yet retains the 'human touch'.

Thinking Through the Situation – Rehabilitation or Active Re-adaptation?

Rehabilitation

The use of the word rehabilitation in patients who are not only elderly but also obviously so ill and deteriorating may at times seem strangely inappropriate. The difficulty lies in the connotation that this term has for patients, their carers and professionals. In the minds of many people rehabilitation means restoring and regaining abilities previously lost whilst for others it conjures up an image of very active hard and tiring work which would clearly be too much for such people who are so ill. In the wake of this linguistic confusion patients may therefore be denied physiotherapy because they are 'too ill for rehabilitation'. In addition when the length of survival time is thought to be short it may be felt that a word which implies restoration and a return to a former self does not fit the real circumstances very comfortably. The words people use can radically

affect practice, and also the way people think, communicate and act.

Dietz (1981) strongly recommended the use of this dynamic word in the treatment of cancer patients because he considered it powerful in fostering a positive and hopeful approach to the planning of an active programme. Dietz proposes that in order to accommodate the wide spectrum of disabilities the goals set for patients with cancer should fall into the four different categories:

1. Preventative goals where disability is likely to occur and the treatment provided is designed to keep disability to a minimum.
2. Restorative goals when patients can be expected to return to normal.
3. Supportive goals where the disease is controlled, but continued support is needed.
4. Palliative goals when the patient has advanced progressive disease.

Rehabilitation is a dynamic concept and therefore goals have to be continually set and re-set, sometimes on a daily basis. These four sets of goals will help many professionals in their work in palliative care, however others will find that in some circumstances the word rehabilitation does not fit comfortably with reality, even when their goals are palliative ones.

Active Readaptation

The use of the phrase 'active readaptation' may be more meaningful for some physiotherapists faced by the problems posed by certain palliative care patients. Active readaptation would imply that the patient is encouraged to readapt to a new set of circumstances as they gradually lose abilities and function. The word 'active' emphasises that activity is needed for reassessing, readjusting, introducing new techniques and equipment. Active readaptation does not involve passive acceptance of the situation. Attention needs to be diverted away from what the patients cannot do towards what they can realistically be expected to do.

Common Problems which will Affect Physiotherapy Treatment

There are several symptoms of particular interest to physiotherapists because they affect most patients with advanced malignant disease at one time or another. These problems need to be taken into account when assessing and planning the programme of physiotherapy for individual patients.

Lethargy, Fatigue and Tiredness

I can't be bothered to do anything

These overarching symptoms may reduce the patient's ability to comply with physiotherapy and any programme of exercise will need to take account of this and be tailored accordingly. Many factors contribute to this general debility. In some cases intervention can bring relief in others not.

Blood tests frequently indicate that these symptoms are related to anaemia, increased blood calcium or electrolytic disturbances. These can often be helped by appropriate drugs or blood transfusion. Disturbances in sleep patterns caused by pain, other symptoms or psychological reasons also contribute to general tiredness. In some cases the patient may be weak as a result of poor nutrition which has been affected by nausea and vomiting or the involvement of the gastrointestinal tract in their disease (Lichter, 1990). In these circumstances the contribution of the physiotherapist is likely to involve establishing ways in which the patient can conserve energy and avoid unnecessary activity whilst avoiding the damaging affects of complete inactivity.

Muscle Weakness

Haven't got the strength to do exercise

Patients may have developed muscle weakness for all the usual reasons encountered in general physiotherapy practice – for example through muscle atrophy resulting from a lack of exercise (see Chapter 6). But a number of other explanations are possible in advanced cancer; some drugs may cause proximal muscle weakness; nerves may be compressed by a tumour resulting in weakness associated with pain. When distal muscle groups are involved there is also the possibility of a spinal cord compression (a matter we will return to later in this paper); muscle weakness may also result from the failure or reduced efficiency of organs such as the heart, kidneys and liver and there may be other systemic causes such as urinary and chest infections; many muscles may become weak or paralysed as a result of paraneoplastic syndrome when the tumour produces toxins which put neurones out of action leading to paralysis.

The important point about this list is that the physiotherapist must be fully alert to the range of possibilities and act cautiously and appropriately.

Increased Risk of Pressure Sores

I can't move and I might get a sore

Many patients with advanced malignant disease experience a period of rapid weight loss. Weight loss reduces the amount of protective fat in the subcutaneous tissue and muscles become atrophied leading to the emergence of bony points which are not only physically more obvious but increase the risk of damaging the overlying skin. The situation is further compounded because the skin is likely to be fragile, overstretched and easily damaged in any case. These factors are of particular relevance to the physiotherapist when assessing and advising on the lifting, handling and moving of such patients. Movement must avoid direct friction on the skin, which can easily occur during sliding transfers, for example. In this case a sliding mat, or piece of sheepskin, should be held directly in contact with the skin so that the friction generated during the movement occurs between the mat and the sliding board. The provision of pressure-relieving cushions can also help. This attention to pressure-relief must also extend into all of the patient's daily activities. For example toilet seats and commode seats will need to be covered in pressure relieving washable 'gel' cushions. This is particularly significant because many patients have problems with constipation – as a result of their disease or as a side-effect of drugs – and may spend much time sitting on the toilet or commode. The prevention and treatment of pressure areas is also accepted as an important part of the nurse's role, for example by the use of pressure-relieving mattresses. However, all the good work done by the health professionals can be quickly undone if the prevention 'regime' is not extended into every area of the patient's life. Relatives, carers and volunteers need to be advised to make sure that they also help the patient by using the cushions, wheelchairs and techniques of moving prescribed for the patient.

Practical Clinical Examples of Disabilities Encountered in Palliative Care

Examples are worth a thousand words in clearing the fog in complex situations. So what follows are typical examples of the sort of patients encountered by the physiotherapist in palliative care. They represent some of the common clinical patterns and disabilities where physiotherapy can make a positive contribution. As you read through what follows you must remember that many patients may because of the complexity of their condition figure in more than one of the categories below. Separating them in this way certainly helps to achieve some initial clarity and understanding. In practice higher levels of combinative complexity will have to be faced.

Paraplegia and Paraparesis Resulting from Malignant Cord Compression

Compression of the spinal cord is a rare but serious complication of cancer. It is a medical emergency. Neurological symptoms can develop rapidly over a period of hours and delay can lead to irreversible permanent paralysis (Kramer, 1992). The physiotherapist is in a good position to observe and recognize the early signs and needs to be vigilant particularly when dealing with patients with particular primary cancers.

Spinal cord compression is associated most commonly, in descending order of frequency, with cancers of the lung, breast, unknown primary, lymphoma, myeloma, sarcoma, prostate and kidney. The cord is compressed by metastasis in the vertebrae enlarging to press extradurally in approximately 85% of cases, the remaining 15% resulting from tumours pressing intradurally inside the spinal cord and its covering. The most common clinical indicators of cord compression are motor loss, urinary difficulties, sensory loss, extensor planters and significant back pain. Patients are commonly described by carers as having 'gone off their legs'.

Plain X-rays of the spine will correctly predict the presence or absence of an extradural tumour in at least 80% of cases (Kramer, 1992). This is a sobering confirmation of how important it is for physiotherapists dealing with back pain to insist on an X-ray prior to manipulation. Intractable pain particularly in the thoracic region should always be viewed with suspicion. Prompt palliative treatment such as radiotherapy or surgery may reverse the condition and patients who are ambulatory before treatment are most likely to remain so.

If paraparesis has developed, then approximately 50% of patients will regain the ability to walk and survival may be lengthy. Physiotherapy management is usually carried out in radiotherapy or neurosurgical units and involves all the usual assessment and treatment components used in these situations. Exercises to improve function and muscle power are often successful in making the patient more mobile for a period of time.

If paraplegia has developed, then only 5% will regain ambulation after surgery or radiotherapy and survival will be short (Ingham *et al.*, 1993). This group of patients poses a particular challenge for the palliative care physiotherapist. There may be a temptation to view them simply as 'paraplegics' or 'tetraplegics', thinking of them in the same way as those with traumatic spinal cord injury. There is a danger that this approach may lead to unrealistic expectations of the degree of independence which can be achieved. In reality the only factor these two groups of patients have in common is their paralysis. The 'palliative care paraplegic' will have many additional problems which make rehabilitation problematic. For example, they have a short prognosis of between 2 and 6 months, and the quality of their remaining life may be diminished by recurrent respiratory and urinary tract infections, bowel disturbances and musculoskeletal pain (Kramer, 1993). The overall aim of the

physiotherapist will be to help the patient to achieve mobility in a wheelchair whilst taking account of all the complicating factors. Patients may still have fatigue, weakness and persistent back pain. Forward flexion of the spine with the legs out straight – a position achievable and necessary for the spinal injury patient – may be not be possible for these patients. In addition, because of the progressive nature of the disease and prognosis it is unrealistic to expect these patients to increase the strength in the upper arms significantly. Consequently independent pain-free transfers may only be achievable in a small number of patients. The physiotherapist may therefore need to accept that the patient will remain wheelchair mobile for a longer period if it is electrically powered and the transfer onto it can be made comfortably using a hoist. The physiotherapy goals need to emphasise all the time what these patients can do rather than struggling in a demoralising way to achieve what they can't.

Hemiplegia and Hemiparesis as a result of a Brain Metastasis

It has been estimated that above a quarter of patients who die of cancer will have brain metastasis (Obbens, 1993) (see also Chapter 18). The primary sites which most commonly metastasize to the brain are cancer of the lung, breast and melanoma. It is usually a sign of advanced disease and because of this patients are likely to have widespread tumour deposits elsewhere.

If brain metastasis remains untreated, survival is only about 1 month. Steroids are used frequently before other treatment and when used by themselves can extend survival to 2 months. Whole brain radiotherapy is the commonest additional treatment and this can extend life for 3–6 months. Surgery is reserved for those patients — around one third — who have one deposit only. The neurological deficit which results depends on the location of the deposits. For example parietal lobe involvement will give rise to hemiparesis and hemiplegia. However, even in the most optimistic cases survival is likely to be short and the physiotherapist is once again left with decisions about how physiotherapy can best improve the patient's quality of life, for the time which is left.

It is important to recognize that some physiotherapy treatment techniques commonly used in patients recovering from strokes may not always be appropriate to these cases. For example techniques which hold back weight-bearing in order to minimize spasticity, may need to be rejected here in favour of early ambulation using walking aids and splints.

Bone Metastases and Pathological Fractures

Skeletal metastases can potentially occur with any malignant tumour but is most common in breast cancer or myeloma. These secondary tumours may be osteolytic causing destruction of the bone. In those cases treatment is aimed at pain relief and the stabilization of bones to prevent pathological fractures (see also Chapter 14). Long weight-bearing bones are at a particularly high risk of fracture. Radiotherapy is the first choice treatment and will often give pain relief within 1–4 weeks.

In patients with metastases of the spine, the collapse of individual vertebrae may occur. Patients will experience excruciating pain associated with movement and are in some cases only comfortable when lying still. Orthopaedic stabilization may be carried out using decompression if the cord is compressed as well. Once again

this will be followed by radiotherapy. The physiotherapist may become involved in supplying walking aids or wheelchairs to relieve the pain during weight-bearing. When the spine is involved reclining wheelchairs are often more comfortable because less weight is directed through the vertebral bodies.

Pathological fractures may occur spontaneously when the patient is involved in normal everyday activity. Where this is the case orthopaedic operations such as internal fixation and replacement arthroplasty may be carried out in order to ensure early mobilization. Once the wound has settled down postoperative radiotherapy is essential.

A particularly difficult challenge for physiotherapists is the group of patients with cancer which is so advanced that no stablization of the pathological fractures is possible. Such patients still have to be toileted and carers will certainly require lifting and handling advice. The amount of lifting may be reduced by using urinary catheters. However, bowel movements still cause difficulties. Using a hoist may cause stress on the fracture site, making lifting the patient on and off a bed pan a problem. Pain relief in the form of a spinal line may be necessary to improve the situation.

Swollen Arm or Leg as a Complication of Cancer

A physiotherapist will encounter swollen limbs in a variety of clinical situations. In patients with cancer this swelling may well be due to lymphoedema. In this condition, swelling occurs in a limb as a result of damage to the lymphatic drainage caused either by the tumour, the surgery or follow-up radiotherapy. In patients who have had a mastectomy following breast cancer approximately 30% will develop lymphoedema. During treatment the axilliary glands are often removed and the area treated by radiotherapy. Postradiation fibrosis can cause damage to the lymphatic system at a later stage, in some cases this can be even after several years. Swelling of the legs may occur following operations for tumours which are low down in the pelvis which have been treated by radiotherapy.

The physiotherapist must recognize that there is no cure for lymphoedema. The swelling can only be controlled. Experience and research shows that treatment using compression for short periods of time — for example using a compression pump — only has limited value. The fluid will simply be pushed to the root of the limb where the drainage is already compromised. A combination of treatments is likely to be necessary including the wearing of compression sleeves and stockings particularly during exercise and daily truncal message to move the fluid into unobstructed drainage territory (Casely-Smith, 1994). Skin care in the form of skin hygiene, moisturising and prompt remedial treatment of infections has to become a way of life. If cellulitis is allowed to develop it can progressively damage the lymphatic system and exacerbate the condition.

Swollen Abdomen as a Result of Malignancy

The presence of intra-abdominal tumours will undoubtedly increase the size of the abdomen but the commonest cause of this distension is ascites. Ascites is the accumulation of fluid within the peritoneal cavity, usually caused by pressure on the venous or lymphatic system either in the region of the liver, or in the peritoneum, or more rarely, behind it.

The fluid is high in protein and readily re-establishes itself after it is 'tapped'. This procedure is called paracentesis and involves withdrawing the fluid through a cannula introduced through the abdominal wall. Removing too much fluid can result in protein depletion and a rapid deterioration in the patient's general condition. An alternate treatment involves the introduction of a shunt to carry the fluid from the peritoneal space to the internal jugular vein.

Patients with ascites feel heavy, uncomfortable, and bloated. Cosmetically the altered body images is also difficult to accept. The fluid causes mechanical problems with movements requiring the patient to bend in the middle. In addition rising from a lying to a sitting position is difficult not only because of the mechanical obstruction of the distended abdomen itself but also because the abdominal muscles are overstretched and unable to contract efficiently. Any daily activity involving reaching the feet may be a problem and also patients may complain of being short of breath. The latter is due to the heightened level of the diaphragm resulting from that condition which means that it will be unable to descend properly. The patient may also need to be taught a variety of techniques for getting out of bed such as rolling onto their side first. In dealing with this problem mechanical aids like inflatable backrests may assist. Gentle abdominal exercises following paracentesis may help in the short-term and breathing exercises may help to reinflate the lower parts of the lungs.

Inability to Sit Because of the Presence of Tumours

Tumours can occur almost anywhere in the body, but those affecting the 'sitting areas' of the patient — as in rectal or vulval cancer — pose a particular problem. Local recurrence often means that patients are unable to sit comfortably even when using the most efficient pressure relieving cushions. They therefore alternate between walking around and lying in bed, avoiding sitting activity. If the pelvis or sacrum becomes invaded by tumours even lying on their backs can become uncomfortable. If sitting at a table to eat becomes impossible patients cannot participate socially in meals or other such activities in the same way. The physiotherapist may become involved in assessing for adaptations which will make improved functional activity possible.

Breathlessness as a Result of Advanced Disease

Although physiotherapists treat cancer patients with chest infections and chronic respiratory diseases using traditional methods, it is important to bear in mind that many causes of breathlessness originate outside the respiratory system, for example as a result of cardiac disease or metabolic acidosis. The breathing pattern may also be disturbed as a result of psychologically induced factors as in the case of hyperventilation.

Diagnosing the cause of dyspnoea is clearly the responsibility of the doctor, but, decisions about the effectiveness of chest physiotherapy is often left to the physiotherapist. In patients with very advanced cancer of the lung with associated retention of secretions the dilemma faced is whether chest physiotherapy can be given in such a way that the 'treatment is not worse than the disease'. There is no place for heavy handed methods and patients will need to be assisted in gentle ways to cough, or huff more effectively. Instruction in diaphragmatic breathing and relaxation techniques also may help. Exercise tolerance is also low in these patients, and improving the quality of their lives will involve the careful conservation of limited energy — for example by providing wheelchairs for covering any distances.

Paralysis as a Result of Motor Neurone Disease

Palliative care units often provide services for advanced deteriorating and incurable diseases, such as motor neurone disease. The disease tends to be relentlessly progressive causing paralysis in recognizable patterns. It may start with wasting in the upper limbs and spasticity in the legs. Less commonly in the bulbar palsy type swallowing and speaking is affected or rarely paralysis starts in the legs and ascends. Articles written by patients who have this disease invariably emphasize the comfort derived from daily passive movements, a skill which the physiotherapist can usefully teach to carers.

The inevitable downhill course of the disease makes an 'active readaptation' approach to care necessary. Aids and adaptations such as electric wheelchairs, page turners, communicators and remote control equipment must be very carefully and selectively prescribed. Each new aid will confront the patient with the inescapable fact that they have deteriorated further. This can be such a disturbing and distressing condition that professionals are often in danger of providing too many pieces of equipment. There is a need to supply only the equipment which is necessary at that time, ensuring it is removed immediately it becomes inappropriate or unacceptable to the patient. The professionals supplying equipment to such patients may have to cope with the rejection of some of their ideas (Chapter 25).

The Patient who is Dying

As stated earlier in this chapter the physiotherapist is likely to be less involved in this stage, while other professionals may become more involved. The Hospice movement has its roots in Christian foundations but the chaplain may not necessarily be the person most appropriate to help an individual patient. Spiritual needs will differ according to cultural background, life experiences and individual belief systems and should not be confused with religious needs. Death and bereavement is an essentially individual and unique experience for each individual.

The skills of the physiotherapist may be useful in making the dying patient comfortable with the use of strategically placed cushions. The importance of touch as a comfort and means of communication is of paramount importance here. Carers can often be taught gentle soothing massage and thereby given a more structured way of being actively involved. At this stage passive movements can ease discomfort in the joints and carers are often pleased to be given this job to do.

Lifting, handling and turning the patient has to be done safely and without discomfort. It is often difficult to do because of the presence of skin lesions, fractures, oedema and fragile skin making manual holds a problem. The use of a strong drawsheet, used like a hammock is particularly useful for moving the patient up the bed or to the side prior to turning. The lifters then hold the sheet not the patient. A polythene sheet under the drawsheet will facilitate the movement and the drawsheet can then be tucked into prevent unwanted sliding.

Conclusions

The words terminal, dying and palliative care are frequently used as though they are synonymous and yet at other times they are used to describe quite different states. This points to a confusion built into the role. These differences must be resolved if the contribution of physiotherapy in palliative care is to be effective.

The physiotherapist working in palliative care must be team-centred and is likely to find the insight, knowledge, practical assessment and treatment skills used in other specialist areas of use in their work. The necessary shift in perception is more in the way of thinking, the attitudes held, the choices made and the ability to recognize the positive contribution made by physiotherapy. For those moving from mainstream physiotherapy the situation sometimes may appear otherwise.

References

Casley-Smith, JR (1994) *Modern Treatment for Lymphodema*, The Lymphoedema Association of Australia. Adelaide: The Henry Moss Laboratory, University of Adelaide.

Dietz, JH (ed) (1981) *Rehabilitation Oncology* New York: John Wiley.

Doyle, D, Hanks, GWC, Macdonald, N (1993) Introduction. In *Oxford Textbook of Palliative Medicine*, 1st edn, pp. 3–8. Oxford: Oxford University Press.

Gray, RC (1993) Physiotherapy. In *Oxford Textbook of Palliative Medicine*, pp. 530–535. Oxford: Oxford University Press.

Greer, DS (1983) Hospice: Lessons for geriatricians. *Journal of the American Geriatric Society* 31: 67–70.

Ingham, J, Beveridge, A, Cooney, NJ (1993) The management of spinal cord compression in patients with advanced malignancy. *Journal of Pain and Symptom Control* 8: 1–6.

Kramer, AJ (1992) Spinal cord compression in malignancy. *Palliative Medicine* 6: 202–211.

Lichter, I (1990) Weakness in terminal illness. *Palliative Medicine* 4. 73–80.

Maguire P, Faulkner, A (1988a) Communicating with cancer patients 1: Handling bad news and difficult questions. *British Medical Journal* 297: 907–909.

Maguire P, Faulkner, A (1988b) Communicating with cancer patients 2: Handling uncertainty, collusions and denial. *British Medical Journal* 297: 972–974.

Obbens, EAMT (1993) Neurological problems in palliative medicine. In *Oxford Textbook of Palliative Medicine*, 1st edn, pp. 460–472. Oxford: Oxford University Press.

Thompson, JW (1994) Neuropharmacology of the pain pathway. In *Pain: Management by Physiotherapy*, 2nd edn, pp. 59–67. Oxford: Butterworth-Heinemann.

Yoshioka H (1994) Rehabilitation for the terminal cancer patient. *American Journal of Physical Medicine and Rehabilitation* 73: 199–203.

E

Handicaps of Ageing

SECTION EDITOR: BARRIE PICKLES

22

Ageing with a Disability

MARYANN McCOLL, CAROLYN ROSENTHAL, W KIRBY ROWE

Introduction
•
Method
•
Elements of Handicap
•
Discussion

Introduction

There is often an assumption that as people grow older, they experience poorer health, greater disability and more handicap (see Chapters 2, 3 and 6). While research shows that, in fact, older people are healthier than stereotypes suggest (Chappell *et al.*, 1986), it is nonetheless also a fact that an overall decline in health and a rise in rates of disability and handicap do accompany ageing. If this is true for the general population, then surely it must be doubly true for those with a pre-existing disability.

Trieschmann (1987), in a comprehensive volume addressing ageing with a lifelong disability, suggested that disability exacts a 'penalty' on individuals, in terms of the psychological, physical and economic costs of living. She illustrated with case studies how individuals with lifelong disabilities have been obliged to undertake greater efforts, costs and concessions just to get through each day, compared with able-bodied individuals. Trieschmann suggested that the combination of a lifelong disability with normal ageing caused the penalty or costs of living to increase exponentially, and finally became 'the straw that breaks the camel's back'. This idea is based on an assumption that the disabled individual's resources for coping are stretched to their limit with the demands of everyday life, and any further demands may exceed the ability of the person to cope.

On the other hand, it is possible to speculate that disabled people might possess special coping resources, developed to cope with the disability itself, that would stand them in good stead to face the changes that accompany ageing. Someone with a disability might actually be better prepared to adjust to ageing as a result of having been required to make major adjustments earlier in their lives. These two opposing views are similar to two competing hypotheses found in the literature on ageing among minority populations: the 'multiple jeopardy' hypothesis and the 'age as leveller' hypothesis (Bengtson, 1979; Dowd and Bengtson, 1978; Dreidger and Chappell, 1987; Zarb and Oliver, 1993).

Both these hypotheses have found some empirical support in research (Dowd and Bengtson, 1978). There is some indication that the 'multiple jeopardy' perspective is supported by objective indicators, such as income and health, but not by subjective indicators, such as perceived health or life satisfaction (Chappell and Havens, 1980). Thus, persons ageing with a lifelong disability are likely to experience 'multiple jeopardy' with respect to income and health, but may be either similar or even advantaged relative to non-disabled older people on other subjective indicators.

According to the World Health Organization's (WHO) definition of handicap (1980), an individual experiences a handicap when he or she is prevented, as a result of an impairment or disability, from fulfilling the roles that would be considered normal for someone of comparable age and gender in that society. Handicap is classified according to six dimensions: economic self-sufficiency, mobility, occupation, orientation, physical independence and social integration.

This chapter will examine each of these dimensions of handicap as they relate to the ageing experience of disabled people. In so doing, it may be possible to assess the potential for handicap as disabled people grow older. We will attempt to give evidence particularly of the impact of what has been referred to as the 'empirical convergence of age and disability' (Zola, 1990, p. 93).

Method

To help us explore the experience of handicap among ageing disabled adults, the results of a qualitative study with spinal cord injured men wil be used.* The study involved 70 men, all of whom were 45 years of age or older. The age range was from 45 to 73 years, with an average of 56 years. Half the sample had paraplegia and half had quadriplegia; and injury durations varied from 15 to 48 years. Approximately 50% of the sample was married, about 25% never married, and 25% was separated, widowed or divorced. Almost 40% of the sample was employed, another 40% was retired, and the remaining approximately 20% was unemployed. About 25% of the sample had incomes less than $20 000 per year, while about 33% had incomes over $55 000.

These men were interviewed once in their homes, and the conversation was recorded. The interview was guided by four questions, specified in Table 1. The transcripts of these 70 interviews provide the qualitative data that supports our discussion of handicap. In addition, the Functional Independence Measure (FIM; Keith *et al.*, 1984) was used as an objective assessment of the daily living skills of our sample. The FIM is a brief, standardized

---

* For further details and more discussion of the methods and results of this study, see McColl and Rosenthal (1993, 1994).

Table 1
Questions Used in the Interview

1. What physical, mental or emotional, and social changes have you experienced as you've grown older?
2. What are your concerns, worries, issues associated with ageing?
3. What resources do you need to have the kind of life you would like to have as you grow older?
4. How has your disability affected the process of ageing for you?

measure of activities of daily living, used widely in rehabilitation. It results in a percentage score, and normative data are available from a number of populations.

Elements of Handicap

Economic Self-sufficiency Handicap

An economic self-sufficiency handicap occurs when an individual is unable to maintain him or herself in a financial or economic sense, because of the presence of an impairment or a disability. No handicap means that the person has sufficient resources so that any impairment or disability he or she may have creates no economic disadvantage relative to others in the population. In other words, any obstacle to full participation in social roles can be overcome through the use of financial resources. Increasing levels of handicap are associated with decreasing abilities to meet subsistence needs because of the impairment or disability.

Just under 50% of the men interviewed believed that they were economically disadvantaged because of their disability:

> Of course, I'm always concerned about money. A disabled person doesn't have a lot of money, and I have financial concerns for the future. Right now I have just about enough money just to get by. I don't live fancy. You can see from my apartment. I don't have a lot of money

and how I am going to continue to look after myself in the future is a concern for me. For example, if inflation was to go up or if things started to cost more, I wouldn't have enough money to be able to deal with that.

Some referred to their relative poverty exacerbating whatever other concerns they may have had about ageing.

> Because I am disabled, I will undoubtedly experience physical deterioration and with that will be increased dependency which I will need to pay for. So I am going to put a lot of financial stress on myself in the future so I need to be prepared for that and I need to plan for that because I do not want financial stress to cause a lot of problem in my family. I do not want to be a financial burden so it is important that I plan for the future.

The need to plan for the future was mentioned by numerous respondents. This need is experienced by many people as they age and anticipate entering a phase of life with potentially greater expenses, and yet with a fixed, and usually reduced income. Concerns about future financial security among the general population are often non-specific, but are related to the potential increase in disability and increased need for formal supports and services. These concerns are often expressed in vague terms, since individuals have little experience with disability. Thus, for most people, there is still room for some optimism about a generally healthy ageing process and a relatively long disability-free period in older age. However, for the 14% of Canadians who are disabled (Statistics Canada, 1986), the realities of disability, additional expenses, needs for service and the expectation of further deterioration are real and known.

Responses to the need to plan for one's economic future in old age varied within this sample. Some subjects coped with financial difficulties by dealing only with the present:

> I just deal with today and tomorrow, and I don't worry about what's going to happen next year. You know, I'm just concerned with getting my rent paid at the end of the month and getting enough food in the fridge and those things.

Others felt the need for careful planning to ensure the availability of needed resources:

> As I grow older, I find that I prepare for my action in the future more so than I did before. Before I'd live one day, then I'd do the next day. But now I'm planning much more in advance than I ever did. Before I didn't really care what happened to me, to tell you the truth. But as you get a little bit older, you care about the rest of the picture.

Because of mistaken projections about premature mortality made at the time of injury, many participants were initially unable to see the necessity for planning and preparing for old age:

> You have to make changes for your retirement; you have to plan ahead. I never thought I'd live more than 15 years. But when I knew I was going to live more than 15 years, I had to plan. That is what ageing has done.

One man expressed his concerns for the financial security of his dependents after his death, in much the same way that an ageing non-disabled husband or father might.

> I'm concerned for the future of my family. I want them to be financially secure and of course I want their lives to be as problem-free as possible – the natural things for a father and husband to be concerned about.

Government was mentioned by several participants, in terms of its failure to provide adequate financial support to disabled people, particularly as they enter old age (for further reading see Chapter 5):

> I think the government should be doing more to assist people with disabilities – special tax breaks. Everything is so much more expensive if you're disabled. So there's got to be something, you know, costs have to come down.

> Because of my injury, I'm almost completely dependent on the state for my financial security. Because I'm always at a susbsistence level I've never been able to prepare financially for the future. Consequently, I have significant concerns about my financial security in the future.

> If my health deteriorates, I will need more money to be able to pay my bills. Right now, I don't get that kind of money from the government. I don't know where I would turn for money in these circumstances. So if things don't work out for my health, I'm going to need financial help.

Financial resources were needed to purchase other needed resources, thus underlining the handicapping effect of inadequate financial resources:

> You know, most things hinge almost directly on finances. If you've got money, you can make your life as comfortable as you want.

> I want to have enough money so that no matter what happens, I can stay home.

> If there is technology or devices or whatever to assist me, I want to be able to afford those, instead of having to ask people. Being able to afford a new chair, being able to afford a van to get around in, those kind of things – that's a big burden financially. That's the problem.

Thus, to the extent that disabled people are already economically disadvantaged relative to the Canadian population as a whole (Statistics Canada, 1986), the ageing disabled may be assumed to be in a position of multiple jeopardy (disabled, older and poor).

Mobility Handicap

A mobility handicap arises when an individual is unable to effectively move around in his or her surroundings to the extent needed to fulfil normal roles. Mobility handicaps vary from a minor, intermittent restriction of mobility at one extreme, to a total bed restriction at the other (see also Chapter 7).

All subjects in the study had a locomotor disability, and used a wheelchair to get around. However, it is entirely possible that members of our sample experience no handicap as a result of wheelchair use. They may have been capable of fulfilling all important social roles in spite of their locomotor disability. However, if age and disability converge to diminish participation in social roles, then handicap exists.

Loss of mobility was mentioned by over half the men we interviewed. Many attributed changes in mobility to loss of strength and stamina with age.

> Let's say before I would push my chair for two miles. Now I know I'm not able to , just simply because I'm older and my body strength is gone.

> I've lost the ability to transfer as easily and readily. At one time, I could have one hand on the wheelchair and I could reach a bed or a chair, but now I have to be more careful.

> I feel that I'm getting weaker in strength and getting tired. My hands don't move as easy as they did before. I can't bend down like I used to and I'm losing my flexibility. It takes longer to do things than it did four or five years ago. Even to dress myself, it takes longer, and it's because of a lack of strength.

About 25% of the respondents expressed a feeling that their bodies were 'wearing out', and 60% mentioned specific complaints, most commonly shoulder or back problems. All of these complaints were seen as being directly related to living for many years with a wheelchair, and all had a direct impact on mobility. These men referred to the unnatural strain that is placed on certain parts of the body as a result of using a wheelchair for mobility, and that the disability has disadvan-taged them in terms of mobility as they have grown older.

> You know, my shoulders have gradually worn out. I find it's getting less easy to handle day to day things.

> The general wear and tear seems to be increased - the arms and the shoulders. A part of it is ageing, and part of it is accelerated. Like I am having trouble with my hands, which is directly related to pushing my chair.

> If something was to happen to my shoulders, I mean, how will I wheel myself around? How would I go around? How would I do my transfers?

> I'm concerned that if I lose the ability to use my arms I will lose my independence.

Pain was also mentioned by close to 80% of the men in the study. Other studies too have found pain to be a complaint of persons who have lived for many years with a spinal cord injury (Pentland and Twomey, 1992). Because of the presence of pain, or the fear of anticipated pain, or of causing irreparable damage by 'overdoing it', activity levels were restricted. This restriction has its own negative effects, such as reducing fitness or flexibility.

> It's painful to do that. Flexibility is diminished quite a bit too, you know. I think it's because of the pain, because, you know, you try not to do too much, because it's painful. The more you move, the more you get pain.

> You think twice about going to some places. You have to say to yourself, 'How is the transportation? How long will we have to be in the car?' Those kinds of things. Because then I have to prepare myself, like, I have to take more pain pills.

Several participants made the relationship of mobility to handicap very clear in their comments, by linking mobility with lifestyle and independence:

> I think the loss of the mobility is related to the risk of becoming isolated. I don't think this will happen for a long time, but I associate the loss

of mobility with loss of independence and then possibly isolation.

> The implications for me are much more severe than they would be for a person who doesn't have a disability. If I continue to lose my strength and if I continue to lose my flexibility, I would lose my ability to be independent and mobile. That would have severe complications in my lifestyle, and these are not developments that I would like to think about.

This is an example of the multiple jeopardy perspective discussed earlier, whereby ageing and disability compound, either additively or multiplicatively, to disadvantage the individual in many areas of life.

Occupation Handicap

An occupation handicap occurs when an individual is unable to occupy his or her time in a manner deemed customary, given factors like age, gender, education and culture. Occupation may include play or school for children, and employment, volunteerism or domestic roles for adults. For older adults, retirement usually results in a change in occupation, usually to a greater concentration on domestic and recreational roles.

In our sample, 38% of individuals were still employed, either full-time or part-time; 40% were retired, and 22% reported that they were unemployed. Unemployment figures for this sample are in excess of the Canadian rates for men in the age bracket from 45–65 (Statistics Canada, 1991).

The relationship between employment, ageing, disability and handicap is not clear. We did not ask participants directly about whether or not they thought their disability had affected their careers or their retirement. However, the only comment that links these four ideas is the following. One participant mentioned that he had observed changes in his attitude toward his

career as time went on. While this is probably fairly common among individuals in mid-life and later life, these sentiments are expressed as resulting in some way from the experience of living with a disability:

> I was disabled, so I had to prove to everybody that I could get back and do things, that I wasn't the poor disabled person. So I had to prove that I was equal or better than everybody else. Once I felt that I had proved that, I didn't have to prove it any more. So now I'm not willing to work eighty hours a week like I did at one time. Now I want to work forty or fifty hours a week and then have some social activities, have a real life. I just want to do more for my own satisfaction.

For those who are retired, people with a disability would be able to engage in the typical occupations of able-bodied retired people. While disabled older people might be less inclined to pursue active pastimes, the variety of recreational opportunities open to them are great, since most activities aimed at seniors usually take account of the potential for some measure of disability. Thus leisure is likely to be one area of functioning where the 'age as leveller' perspective applies, in that disability acts as a levelling factor, bringing the activities of the general population and the disabled population into line with each other.

Orientation Handicap

Orientation handicap refers to a disadvantage in fulfilling normal roles because of the inability to orient oneself in the environment. This handicap usually arises when an individual has a sensory or communication disability, and so is not particularly pertinent to those with mobility limitations, like our sample. There was no evidence in our data to suggest that our group of ageing disabled men experienced any orientation handicap because of their disability. The only exception might be the small proportion of respondents (15%) who referred to cognitive changes with age, particularly worsening memory. These changes may result from the ageing process, however, and be unrelated to the spinal cord injury.

Physical Independence Handicap

Physical independence handicap refers to role limitations imposed as a result of one's inability to perform self-care and other activities of daily living. It can vary from aided independence, where a person can be fully independent in daily activities if provided with aids or assistive devices, to intensive-care dependence, where a person requires 24-hour attention. Members of the study sample inevitably experienced some level of personal care disability, as they performed their activities of daily living in a different fashion from able-bodied others. However, with the assistance of an adapted environment and subsidized attendant care, they might experience little or no handicap.

In our study, the Functional Independence Measure (FIM; Keith *et al.*, 1984) showed that 24 (34.8%) of our participants were considered dependent, in that they reported FIM scores lower than the usual cut-off score of 80% for functional independence. About 10% of the sample appear to be extremely disabled, meaning they have FIM scores less than 30%. The mean FIM score for the sample is below 80% (75.7 ± 25.7), but as the standard deviation suggests, there was considerable variation among the scores.

The loss of independence appears from the quotes to be a major source of concern among the group of ageing disabled adults:

> My greatest concern for growing older is losing self-sufficiency, not being able to dress myself, to do all the things that I do now, like going in and out of the car, the bath, this sort of thing.

> Looking after myself, my personal needs, that's my greatest concern. I hate to see somebody have to come and dress me and take me in and out of my bed, you know. My fear is that due to the disability it will come earlier than later.

Numerous respondents referred to changes of lifestyle and life roles that would accompany a further loss of physical independence.

> Well, with a spinal cord injury, any degree of the reduction of the ability to transfer or provide self care would rapidly make you depend entirely on some physical orderly care or assistance. It would be a rather traumatic change in your life.

> In many ways, you have very little control over your life when you're disabled. The slightest change in health can have significant implications for lifestyle. Consequently, there is always a degree of uncertainty in terms of what the future holds.

The idea of independence might be seen as taking on disproportionate importance for members of the sample. Comments refer to the idea of depending on someone else as being unthinkable:

> If anything was to happen to me physically, it would have a direct impact on my independence, my mobility, and my lifestyle. I do *not* look forward to the fact of depending on anyone.

> You worry that you can't look after yourself too well, you have to ride on somebody else more and more. That's kind of scary. That's my concern.

In many instances, participants already depend on someone for some aspects of their daily lives, and are concerned that with the passage of time, this arrangement will no longer be viable. Often, a spouse is the primary source of support, and concern arises that a handicapping situation may occur when the spouse is no longer able to provide the necessary supports:

> If my wife can't look after me, then we would have to hire somebody to help out, and I don't think we have enough money for that. Or if my

wife was to die and I would be by myself, I would have to get someone to help me.

I don't know what I'm going to do if I get worse. Then my wife will have to look after me all the time. She will have to quit work and that will cause us money problems. This is a concern to me. Perhaps it would be better if I was not around to cause these problems.

An individual's self-image is at risk due to the threatened loss of independence (see also Chapter 1):

If I were to become a burden on my wife or on my family, that bothers me more than anything else – more than pain, just that I would be a burden to them.

When I hurt my shoulder, I was in the hospital and I saw a lot of people in there that had lost their independence and they were just vegetables and I'm not about to become one of those.

An alternate source of support is a paid attendant, but this seems to be viewed with some scepticism and reservation, perhaps because of the extent to which it further imposes lifestyle limitations that may be considered handicapping.

If I can't wheel myself around in my chair, or I can't do my transfers or I can't take care of my bowel and bladder management, I will completely lose my independence. I am not looking forward to that. Even if I had an attendant, I am not looking forward to that either. An attendant is an intrusion on your lifestyle and that is not something that I would look forward to. Naturally it is the best alternative if my health does deteriorate, a live-in attendant is preferable over being institutionalized, but these are all things that one does not look forward to.

I will need more and more support and more and more help. If my sister and her husband are not around, then I would have to be institutionalized and depend on someone I don't know to look after me. I am very concerned about that. I have never had good experiences in hospitals or with attendants. I am used to the way my sister and her husband look after me, and I would be very concerned if that care giving circumstance was to change.

If my health ever deteriorates to the point where I am unable to look after myself, for example, if I couldn't do my transfers or my bladder and bowel treatments, I would have to depend on an attendant. At that point, I would lose much of my independence. That is a development I would not like to think about.

Several participants described a kind of snowball effect of health on other factors, specifically independence, future care and money. Concerns surrounding health usually related to issues of increased dependence, doubts about ability to work and future finances, and fears about increased need for care and the potential risk of institutionalization.

When you live with a disability, even the slightest decline in health can have a significant impact on your ability to maintain an independent lifestyle.

It will be a string of problems before it's a serious restriction. I judge that now from what I see. It will be a matter of a little bit of pain, uncertainty and awkwardness for now. My uncertainty will gradually increase and at that point I'll have to stop doing things.

To the extent that finite resources, such as time, energy and money, must be used to maintain physical independence, then functional limitations of disabled older people may be considered a source of handicap, placing these individuals in a situation of multiple jeopardy.

Because I am a paraplegic, the possibility of me experiencing physical complications in the future is fairly high, so it is important that I plan for those physical complications. I need to be prepared to deal with them as they come. So as I look ahead, I want to ensure that I have enough money put away that I can maintain my independence. I want to keep my health as stable as possible so that I can maintain my independence. And I also have to work out a 'worst case scenario': who is going to look after me, where will I live, those types of things. So I am beginning to plan for that.

Social Integration Handicap

Social integration handicap occurs when an individual is unable, because of his or her disability, to participate in and maintain customary social relationships. This may vary from a minor inhibition of somewhat indeterminate origin, to social isolation and institutionalization (Chapter 5).

In our study, a slight majority (57%) of respondents reported negative changes in their social activities with ageing. They stayed home more than they had in the past, they had fewer friends and fewer social activities. This decrease in social activity was often related to the disability.

> After my accident, once I got used to being in a chair, my wife and I were very active. But now it's very difficult to get out, especially in the winter. By the time I get dressed and get prepared to go out, and then get myself down and into the car, it takes up most of my energy and most of the morning. Because it's so much trouble, we seldom do the types of things we used to do.

Some participants pointed to concerns about continence as a socially limiting factor.

> I think that I have less friends than I did before. I lost interest in going out and I like to stay home. I don't visit as much. I don't like to go places because I'm afraid that I'll have to go to the bathroom.

> My social situation has changed greatly. Many of my old friends are no longer alive and the new friends we have don't understand my injury. So I don't feel comfortable going out with anyone in case I have an accident with my bowel.

Others referred to the increased importance of accessibility as one grows older.

> I think that they could make it a lot easier for people who are getting older, not only people in wheelchairs, but older people in general. They're slowly changing, access to some of these stores, subway stations and streetcars. I think that would be a very big improvement.

> I am very isolated because of where I live downtown, because I can't easily get around. I would like to see an improvement in my community in terms of elimination of physical barriers for the disabled.

Several individuals noted that the accessibility of their own homes was highly valued, even to the extent that they found they were spending increasing amounts of time there for sheer ease of accessibility.

> I planned a long time ago for this — I built this house to be accessible, and it has been a great factor in my life. I have everything here that I need.

> If I didn't have this apartment, I'd be in really bad shape. All my wife has to do is open the apartment door, and all the other doors have buttons. I've moved from a house to an apartment where everything is more easily accessible. Things are much better in the apartment than in the house, although it's not as friendly, you know.

Others referred to transportation as a major factor in accessibility.

> My car is my legs. Without it I would be lost. I always said to myself, if I didn't have a car, I think I would do something foolish. I don't think I would have survived as long as I have if I didn't have a car. My car is my mobility, my independence. Without it I would have been sitting at home deteriorating, and I probably would be dead.

> I think the main thing for a paraplegic is his car so that he has his freedom, to get in and go when he feels like it, and he's not going to be stuck waiting for someone else to take him. This business of depending on somebody else is the worst thing in the world.

Finally, respondents referred to financial insecurity as a barrier to social integration.

> It's very difficult to get involved in a relationship with someone if you don't have any money. What are you going to do? How are you going to take them out? It's really difficult to have a relationship with a woman when you don't have any money and basically it's also very difficult to have a relationship with friends if you don't have any money, you know, because your friends are going out to places or doing things and you're

always the one who doesn't have any money. So, you can't afford to go along with them. So, you know, part of the reason that you're isolated as a quadriplegic is not because of your physical limitations, it's because of the financial limitations and basically, because of money I'm forced to spend most of my time, to interact with other disabled people who don't have any money, so we all sit around to watch the moths grow on the trees cause we don't have money to do anything else.

For some, the ultimate loss of social integration would be the transition to institutional living. Sentiments towards institutionalization vary from resignation to fear, for a variety of good reasons.

> There are all kinds of horror stories about hospitals and the spinal cord injured. I think it's commonly acknowledged among spinal cord injured that most professionals in institutions have no clear idea of the needs of a spinal cord injured person.

> I have managed to stay out of institutions for most of my life, and I want to continue to stay out of them.

Thus it seems clear that participants identified a number of factors, some related to their disability and some related to their age, that decreased their ability to participate fully in their social and community environments. These factors are illustrative of the convergence of multiple factors to produce a handicapping or multiple jeopardy effect on older disabled individuals.

Discussion

In summary, the findings suggest that some level of handicap is experienced by ageing spinal cord injured men in five of the six areas discussed. Handicap is experienced when environmental conditions combine with disability to create a situation of disadvantage (Badley, 1993). Neither ageing alone nor disability alone would be expected to result in significant disadvantage. But, when ageing is layered over the effects of a life-long disability, handicap appears to be present, particularly in the following areas: economic self-sufficiency; mobility; physical independence; and, social integration. In addition, for those who are not retired, an occupation handicap may be experienced, according to national workforce participation rates. However, our sample did not raise employment issues in response to open-ended questions about changes, concerns or effects of the prior disability on ageing. Therefore, although it would be mistaken to suggest that no handicap exists, it is worthwhile noting that when given the opportunity, participants did not spontaneously raise employment as an issue. Thus one might conclude that it was not as important to them as other areas that were stressed, such as changes in independence and lifestyle.

For those who are retired, the ability to occupy one's time in meaningful ways is the one area of handicap that may not be affected by the presence of a pre-existing disability. Recreational activities aimed at older people often take accessibility issues into account, because of the need to accommodate disabilities of various types in the older population. However, in order to be able to participate in leisure activities, disabled older people may have to overcome handicaps in other areas, such as mobility and transportation, self-care and economics.

The present study has focused on ageing spinal cord injured men, however, the experience of handicap or disadvantage may be common to other disabled people as they age as well. For example, disabled women are at least as likely as disabled men to experience handicap, based on what we know about gender, ageing and disability

(Arber and Ginn, 1993; Fine and Asch, 1981). The literature shows that disabled women are disadvantaged relative both to disabled men and to able-bodied women (Fine and Asch, 1981), especially in the areas of employment, income, presence of a spouse and other social supports. Older women, too, have been shown to be disadvantaged economically, socially and in terms of their health (Gee and Kimball, 1987; Verbrugge, 1976). Indeed being female has been explicitly identified as a factor contributing to multiple jeopardy (Chappell and Havens, 1980). Thus older disabled women could be expected to experience handicap to at least the same extent as men, and perhaps more. Studies are currently underway to examine the parameters of disadvantage among ageing disabled women (Pentland *et al.*, 1994–6).

Those with other types of disability, besides spinal cord injury, might also be expected to experience handicap as they age, although perhaps not to the same extent as those in our sample. Spinal cord injury has been classified by Schulz and Rau (1985) as a statistically non-normative event, meaning one that occurs at a time in life when it would not statistically be expected. The statistically non-normative event requires greater adjustment than the statistically normative event (such as the onset of a degenerative disability in old age), and therefore has a more significant impact on the remaining years of life. Thus, someone with a disability that was acquired at an older age, or in a more gradual fashion, might experience less disruption to the usual process of ageing. However, for someone with a progressive disability, such as multiple sclerosis, the issues related to ageing would be magnified by fear and uncertainty about the future, and the threat of premature mortality.

With regard to the two theoretical positions proposed earlier, the 'multiple jeopardy' and the 'age-as-leveller' approaches, our results provide evidence that the convergence of ageing and disability can be viewed from either perspective. Some individuals express this notion that with age, the effects of disability are obscured. These individuals would probably subscribe to the 'age-as-leveller' hypothesis, and they would not be expected to experience handicap as ageing combines with their disability. They express comments like,

> I don't think of myself as getting older with a disability; just getting older.

> I'm immune to my disability, so I can't see it having any effect at all.

Alternatively, there were a number of possible interactions of ageing and disability suggested by the data. With each of these positions, the probability of experiencing handicap increases. Some of the comments suggest that participants believe there is a negative interaction effect between ageing and disability. In other words, when ageing and disability occur together, their joint effects are less than the sum of their independent effects. Thus there must be a cancelling out or a 'levelling' of some effects because of the presence of others. This may be another view of the 'age-as-leveller' hypothesis: not that disability totally obscures the effects of ageing, but that it hides or camouflages some of the effects. For example, several of our participants clearly indicated that they felt they had a head start on the adjustments required for ageing, because of the degree of adjustment they had accomplished so far.

> I went through the same life experiences, from marriage, to career changes, to different health problems, that I see my other friends going through. I, as a quadriplegic, was going through the same career path, the same social interactions, only at a slower rate, and of course, with a lot of support to get me there, but nevertheless,

paralleling their lives. Now, with the exception of a few who have also had very distinct health problems, I have come back. In fact, overall, physically, emotionally, psychologically, my condition resembles that of friends who have had medical problems develop in the last couple of years.

A second possible way of seeing the joint effects of ageing and disability is to see them as simply additive. The effects of ageing are simply layered over the effects of a life-long disability. This is one way 'multiple jeopardy' can occur, and represents a situation where the effects of ageing produce the context that changes disability to handicap. Particularly, it seems that handicap is experienced in the areas of economic self-sufficiency, mobility, physical independence and social integration.

Finally, some of our participants supported Trieschmann's (1987) contention that this layering does not result in a simply additive effect of ageing and disability, but rather a multiplicative or exponential effect, another type of multiple jeopardy. The effects of ageing are not only added to the effects of the disability, but somehow the two seem to aggravate each other to produce a further degree of change. As participants stated,

> There's a multiplying factor, because of having to use what's left.

> I don't think what is happening to me is unusual for a sixty year old man, but because it affects the limited areas that I can feel in, it has a much greater impact on my overall well-being.

These and many other comments cited in the chapter reveal that many of the concerns of ageing disabled people are the same in content as those of ageing able-bodied people. Worries about future dependency, being a burden on one's family, the possibility of institutionalization, and financial insecurity are all common among ageing individuals. However, when combined with a life-long disability, these concerns have the potential to create a situation of 'multiple jeopardy', or in terms of the WHO framework, handicap. Our data suggest that these concerns are more acute among disabled persons, no doubt because the odds are higher that these feared possibilities will become realities.

While the evidence suggests the 'multiple jeopardy' perspective is considerably more prevalent among our sample, the 'age-as-leveller' view may be more adaptive. As we come to better understand this latter view, it may be increasingly possible to convey it to other survivors searching for meaning in the changes that they are experiencing.

Acknowledgements

The authors acknowledge the support of the Ontario Ministry of Community and Social Services, Ontario Mental Health Foundation, Canadian Paraplegic Association and Lyndhurst Hospital. We also thank Mr R. McElroy and the seventy study participants for their reflections on ageing and disability.

References

Arber, S, Ginn, J (1993) Gender and inequalities in health in later life. *Social Science and Medicine* 36: 33–46.

Badley, EM (1993) An introduction to the concepts and classification of the international classification of impairments, disabilities and handicaps. *Disability and Rehabilitation* 15: 161–178.

Bengston, V (1979) Ethnicity and ageing: Problems and issues in current social science inquiry. In Gelfand, D, Kutzkik, A (eds) *Ethnicity and Ageing* 1st edn, pp. 4–31. New York: Springer.

Bengston, V, Rosenthal, C, Burton, L (1990) Families and ageing: Diversity and heterogeneity. In Binstock, R, George, L (eds) *Handbook of Ageing and Social Sciences* 3rd edn, pp. 263–287. San Diego: Academic Press.

Chappell, N, Havens, B (1980) Old and female: Testing the double jeopardy hypothesis. *The Sociological Quarterly* 21: 157–171

Chappell, N, Strain, L, Blandford, A (1986) *Ageing and Health Care: A Social Perspective*. Toronto: Holt, Rinehart & Winston.

Dowd, J, Bengston, V (1978) Ageing in minority populations: An examination of the double jeopardy hypothesis. *Journal of Gerontology* 33: 427–436.

Dreidger, L, Chappell, L (1987) *Ageing and Ethnicity: Toward an Interface*. Toronto: Butterworths.

Fine, M, Asch, A (1981) Disabled women: Sexism without the pedestal. *Journal of Sociology and Social Welfare* 8: 233–248.

Gee, E, Kimball, M (1987) *Women and Ageing*. Toronto: Butterworths.

Keith, RA, Granger, CV, Hamilton, BB, Sherwin, FS (1984). The Functional Independence Measure: A new tool for rehabilitation. In

Eisenberg, MG, Grzesiak, RC (eds) *Advances in Clinical Rehabilitation*, pp. 6–18. New York: Springer.

McColl, MA, Rosenthal, C (1993) *Final report: Ageing and spinal cord injury.* Ministry of Community and Social Services Ontario / Ontario Mental Health Foundation.

McColl, MA, Rosenthal, C (1994) A model of resource needs of ageing spinal cord injured men. *Paraplegia* 32: 261–70.

Penning, MJ (1983) Multiple jeopardy: Age, sex and ethnic variations. *Canadian Ethnic Studies* 15: 81–105.

Pentland, W, Twomey, L (1992). Upper limb function in persons ageing with longterm paraplegia and implications for independence. *Journal of the American Paraplegia Society* 15: 126.

Pentland, W, McColl, MA, Spring, K, Tremblay, M, Rosenthal, C (1994–6) Women with pre-existing physical disabilities: The impact of ageing (unpublished raw data).

Schultz, R, Rau, MT (1985) Social support through the life course. In

Cohen, S, Syme, SL (eds) *Social Support and Health* pp. 129–149. New York: Academic Press.

Statistics Canada (1986) *Health and activity limitations survey.* Ottawa: Minister of Supply and Services.

Statistics Canada (1991) *1991 Census.* Ottawa: Minister of Supply and Services.

Trieschmann, RB (1987) *Ageing with a Disability.* New York: Demos Publications.

Verbrugge, L (1976) Sex differences in mortality and morbidity in the United States. *Social Biology* 23: 276–296.

World Health Organization (1980) *International classification of impairments, disabilities and handicaps.* Geneva: WHO.

Zarb, G, Oliver, M (1993) *Ageing with a Disability: What do they expect after all these years?* London: University of Greenwich.

Zola, IK (1980) Ageing, disability and the home-care revolution. *Archives of Physical Medicine and Rehabilitation* 71: 93–96.

23

The Disability Rights Movement and Older People

APRIL D'AUBIN

Self-Representational Advocacy
•
The Social Situation of Seniors with Disabilities
•
The Independent Living Concept
•
Accessible Transportation
•
Conclusion

Tired of being assigned the roles of clients and patients, people with disabilities in Canada redefined themselves as consumers and advocates in the early 1970s. Patients and clients are passive and take direction whereas consumers and advocates are active initiators of change.

Consumerism, based upon the world view that a service or product user is equal to the service provider or goods producer in the economic processes of our world, provided the first theory of equality which rallied people with disabilities in the 1970s (Derksen, 1985).

To realize their aspirations for equality, people with disabilities formed the disability rights movement (see also Chapter 5). Two distinct types of organizations were established: self-

representational advocacy groups and mutual aid service organizations. Self-representational activities include: consumerism, political advocacy and public education to alter attitudes and discriminatory behaviours (see Chapter 3). Mutual aid activities involve the provision of Independent Living services (i.e. peer counselling, information and referral, individual advocacy) by people with disabilities to people with disabilities.

Some authors suggest that community based rehabilitation is a strand of Independent Living.

> Community based rehabilitation (CBR) is also a strand of Independent Living. That is, the CBR which is not just a re-forming of the old hierarchial systems — the top down approach which aims to normalize people — but the local, bottom

up approach which enables and liberates the individual . . . But the key to these CBR programmes is the self-determination of the disabled people — self determination in what rehabilitation they want and its appropriateness for them as individuals. These projects are fully sustainable, low-cost initiatives which integrate the disabled individuals and change the awareness and attitude of the community quite dramatically.

(Hurst, 1994)

The multiplicity of strands which comprise the disability rights movement indicates the growing complexity of this social movement. This chapter will describe two components of the disability rights movement: self-representational advocacy and Independent Living, and will explain the relevance of both of these to seniors with disabilities.

Self-Representational Advocacy

The Rise of the Council of Canadians with Disabilities (CCD)

Since the early 1970s, persons with disabilities in many countries at the grass roots level have organized self-help, cross-disability organizations, at the local and national levels to advocate social, economic and political change that would improve the status of people living with disabilities. This resulted in people with disabilities making their own representations to government and other decision makers. These were organizations OF, not FOR, persons with disabilities.

Typical objectives of these organizations are:

- To improve the status of persons with disabilities;
- to promote self-help for persons with disabilities;

- to provide a national democratic structure for disabled citizens to voice their concerns;
- to monitor federal legislation;
- to promote policies determined by citizens with disabilities;
- to establish a positive image of disabled Canadians in the public mind;
- to share information and cooperate with disabled persons' organizations in Canada and in other countries.

Objectives of these organizations focus primarily on self-representation advocacy activities. With the exception of information sharing, mutual aid services are not within their mandate. This is not accidental. The founders strongly held the conviction that a monitoring organization could not provide services, because this would eventually put it in a conflict of interest position as it would be unable to evaluate critically its own performance in the area of service provision.

These national bodies are cross-disability organizations. This means that they are willing to work with all people who self-define themselves as having a disability. As cross-disability organizations, they address issues which pertain to any type of disability. This is in contrast to uni-disability organizations which seek members with only specific disabilities and work solely on the issues which pertain to people with those disabilities.

Because of their cross-disability orientation, they have a very broad and varied agenda. For example, they advocate on such public policy concerns as alternate media for persons who are handicapped by print, barrier-free architectural design to eliminate barriers for people with mobility problems, plain language for persons who have been labelled mentally handicapped, integrated living arrangements rather than institutionalized care options and access to generic drugs.

People with disabilities have advanced a disability rights agenda. In Canada, for example, those with disabilities have witnessed the Canadian Human Rights Act amended to include protection for people with disabilities and the inclusion of disability in the Charter of Rights and Freedoms, Canada's constitution. These advances were achieved through the intensive interventions of people with disabilities, via CCD and other disability organizations. These protections which have been won by the disability rights movement have had long-ranging effects. The disability rights coverage in the Canadian Human Rights Act affords protection to people with AIDS, which was not recognized as a disability when the Act was amended to include disability.

Indeed, people with disabilities are beginning to transform thinking about what equality really means. In the not so distant past, equality was framed according to a same-treatment model. Through court cases and other means, disabled people have demonstrated that treating people in dissimilar circumstances the same will not result in equality. Other equality seeking groups, such as women, have also been arguing the same position. Thinking about equality has shifted and the focus is now on substantive equality in which an equality of results is the objective.

The substantive theory of equality will have a profound impact on many groups in society. A societal acceptance of this model motivates the creation of priority seating for disabled and elderly passengers in local public transit and pushes forward the redesign of jobs so they can be performed by people with varying physical limitations.

Multiple Jeopardy

The concept of multiple jeopardy was first identified in the disability rights movement by women with disabilities (see Chapter 22). Disabled feminists discovered that women with disabilities tended to occupy a lower socioeconomic position than either men with disabilities or women without disabilities (Fine and Asch, 1981). Aboriginal people with disabilities also pointed out that they experienced additional disadvantage not experienced by non-Aboriginal persons with disabilities (Demas, 1990). The personal testimonials that the disability rights movement is hearing from seniors with disabilities point to the fact that this group also experiences multiple jeopardy, because the preponderance of seniors are women (see Chapter 2). Subgroups within the population of persons with disabilities who are experiencing multiple jeopardy may require a 'special measures' approach from the disability rights movement to ensure that their issues are adequately addressed.

The Philosophy of the Disability Rights Movement

Part of the uniqueness of the philosophy of the disability rights movement is that it speaks equally to all people with disabilities — youth, working age adults, seniors and to people from different ethnic backgrounds and cultures (see Chapter 4). In that everyone has the potential to become a person with a disability, the disability rights movement also has a relevancy to all people.

The movement's philosophy reminds everyone that citizens with disabilities have the right to participate fully and equally in their society, despite the fact that discriminatory ablest attitudes and systemic barriers have served to marginalize people with disabilities limiting their access to the mainstream of society. The disability rights movement calls to action both disabled and non-disabled persons and governments for the purpose of removing barriers which prevent equitable participation in the day-to-day activities of their communities.

The Core Principles of the Disability Rights Movement

The disability rights philosophy emphasizes a number of core principles: self-identification, the dignity of risk, self-determination/consumer control, independent living, equalization of opportunities, accommodation, integration.

SELF-IDENTIFICATION

The person with the disability discloses whether or not they consider themselves to be a person with a disability. For example, the Canadian Employment Equity Act requires that individuals with disabilities, themselves, self-declare disability; the Act does not sanction this designation being made by second parties, such as employers or doctors.

SELF-DETERMINATION/CONSUMER CONTROL

1. Persons with disabilities retain majority political control in their self-representational advocacy organizations and their service delivery organizations.

2. Disabled persons, themselves, determine their own needs and identify the types of supports which are necessary to assist them and make the fundamental decisions about all aspects of their day-to-day lives.

INDEPENDENT LIVING

In Canada, this is the progressive process by which people with disabilities take responsibility for managing and developing the resources which they require to live in the community, and determine what risks are appropriate for them in any given situation.

EQUALIZATION OF OPPORTUNITIES

The process whereby the generic systems of society are made accessible to persons with disabilities.

ACCOMMODATION

The removal of barriers in systems and institutions to enable people with disabilities to participate in an equitable manner.

INTEGRATION

People with disabilities participate fully and equally with non-disabled citizens in society and receive services from the same generic service delivery systems as persons without disabilities.

Disability and Handicap

In common every day discussions, disability is viewed as an individual problem. The disability rights movement has rejected this definition of disability and in its place has developed a continuum of definitions which focuses on the individual's functioning within his/her environment and the social construction of disability. The United Nations' World Programme of Action Concerning Disabled Persons, which was heavily influenced by the international disability rights movement, provides definitions for these terms.

Impairment Any loss or abnormality of psychological, physiological, or anatomical structure or function.

Disability Any restriction or lack resulting from an impairment of ability to perform an activity in the manner or within the range considered normal for a human being.

Handicap A disadvantage for a given individual, resulting from an impairment or disability that limits or prevents the fulfillment of a role that is normal, depending on age, sex, social and cultural factors for that individual.

(UN, 1983)

Handicap is therefore a function of the relationship between disabled persons and the environment. It occurs when they encounter cultural, physical or social barriers which prevent their access to the various systems of society that are available to other citizens. Thus handicap is the loss or limitation of opportunities to take part in the life of the community on an equal level with others.

(UN, 1983, p. 3).

The disability rights movement views the disabled individual as the appropriate gatekeeper with respect to determination of disability status. Unlike other interest groups in society, the disability rights movement rejects efforts to establish doctors, or other professionals, as the determiners of disability status. In instances where disability status conveys social or economic benefits, the disability rights movement advocates that peer panels composed of persons with disabilities adjudicate disability claims, as peers will have the most accurate appreciation of the claims being brought forth (CCD, 1994).

The Social Situation of Seniors with Disabilities

Institutionalization sometimes occurs because community resources have not been deployed in a manner which enables people with disabilities, both working-age adults and seniors, to self-manage the disability resources and services which they require to live in an integrated manner in their communities. Often persons with high level needs for personal services (i.e. homemaker services, attendant services) find that such services are unavailable in the community and institutionalization is the only option which is available to them.

In Canada, the disabilty rights movement has advocated for many years self-managed personal services for persons with disabilities. (In Europe, personal services are referred to as personal assistance.) Two examples of personal services where self-management would be an appropriate option are attendant care services and homemaker services. With self-managed systems, disabled service users hire/fire, train, schedule, and pay their own service providers with funds provided to them by the government for that specific purpose. Consumers develop an employer-employee relationship with their service providers and are accountable for the funds which are entrusted to them. Many service users find this preferable to government operated service systems.

Self-managed services are an alternative to what has been termed institutional-type services. The following negative characteristics of institutional-type services have been identified:

- there is no alternative,
- the disabled person cannot choose who will assist them,
- the user has to adapt their needs to the needs of the whole scheme,
- there are written and unwritten rules regulating the assistance, rules over which the user has no control,
- the assistance is limited to certain hours, activities, locations, (for example, the consumer has to live in certain houses as opposed to living anywhere),

- the staff providing assistance is shared by several persons,
- there is a hierarchy with the user at the bottom of the pyramid (Ratzka, 1990).

Institutional-type services can be delivered in either institutions or community settings. The key characteristics of institutional-type services are that: they disempower consumers, they afford little or no opportunity for consumer control and self-determination.

Self-management is a concept which is particularly germane to seniors:

> Social policy at present is often solving [the problems of an aging population] by building more residential accommodation or providing more and more separate or special community services, over which the individual has no control. The provision of personal assistance [self-managed services] gives the individual autonomy and allows them to stay in their own homes, to use mainstream facilities and to integrate in their community. Some programmes based on self-determination are demonstrating that the progress of dementia can be slowed and contained, if the individual retains control and choice over their own lives.
>
> (Hurst, 1994)

In some parts of North America and Europe self-management demonstration projects have been established and seniors with disabilities have successfully participated in these programmes. Seniors, like their younger counterparts, appreciated the opportunity to control and develop their own service system which meet their unique needs.

Despite years of intensive advocacy on the self-management issues, personal services are still delivered primarily according to the institution-type model.

People with disabilities and seniors share similar experiences with institution-type services. Unfortunately one of these shared experiences is abuse. Acts of violence and abuse take many forms. While society has gained some familiarity with the characteristics of domestic violence, there is less acknowledgement of the violence which people with disabilities face within the social service system.

> People in positions of power (usually white, affluent men) dismiss violence done to [non-white middle class women] as insignificant . . . other forms of discrimination create special vulnerabilities. People rarely take acts of violence as seriously if the woman is poor, old, a prostitute, a lesbian, a woman with physical or intellectual limitations or institutionalized . . . Older women and disabled women are frequently raped.
>
> (The Boston Women's Health Collective, 1984, p. 101)

Institutionalization may increase the likelihood of abuse, because perpetrators, often employed in positions of trust, have ready access to a group of people who are dependent upon them.

> Among women generally, there are women even more vulnerable to violations on their person, or premises, and these are: the psychiatrically disabled, the developmentally disabled, elderly women, and the physically disabled. They are not only more vulnerable, but, in addition, very dependent on care givers in hospitals, personal care home, doctors' offices, and their own homes. These vulnerable dependency situations carry a very high potential for assault of any kind and degree. Too often, if some incident is reported, the woman is further victimized by the systems which are responsible for the situations in that either the woman accepts the care given with abuse and/or its potential of abuse, or she may have to go without the care given. As the woman cannot live independently of such care, she is then forced into situations which violate her person actually or potentially.
>
> (COPOH, 1985b)

The disability rights movement, particularly local and national organizations of women with disabilities, is working to focus attention on the situation of women who are vulnerable to violent and abusive situations. To ameliorate this situation it is necessary to increase awareness of the problem (i.e. police, service provider, community, family), improve access provisions to shelters for the abused, and sensitize the women's movement to the issues of young and older women with disabilities.

Elderly women with disabilities often find themselves incarcerated in psychiatric facilities, where their rights are frequently violated. As women tend to outlive men, the residents on psychogeriatric wards tend to be elderly women with disabilities. Those who are widows, without children or estranged from their families are particularly vulnerable to abuse.

> Patients are handled, fed and moved about roughly . . . My personal clothing was forcibly taken from me when I was admitted. I have worn pajamas, housecoat and slippers for 18 days now. This is considered a form of punishment. I saw my psychiatrist to try to find out my legal status in the hospital. When I asked him, he told me he did not know. I learned that while 'informal', and 'voluntary' I should not be on a locked ward and should have out privileges at all reasonable times.
>
> (Sawyer, 1981)

The Independent Living Concept

In addition to advocacy organizations, people with disabilities have also formed Independent Living (IL) Centres (see Chapter 24).

> Independent Living is a concept devised by disabled people for disabled people. Although the term is sometimes seen as synonymous with the disability movement, it can just as easily be applied to other excluded people who want to have a job, a home and a chance to make something of their lives. For disabled people 'Independent Living' is the practical application of our empowerment, the ability, as individuals, to get out of bed when we want, choose what

clothes to wear, to eat when we want to, have relationships, get an education, get a job, enjoy ourselves.

> (Hurst, 1994)

By focusing on some of the basic day-to-day choices which people with disabilities must struggle to maintain within their personal control (i.e. when to rise in the morning, what to eat), Hurst's description emphasizes powerfully the centrality in IL of the crucial core principles of the disability rights philosophy: consumer control and self-determination (see Chapter 11).

Independent Living reorganizes the way disabled and non disabled people think about disability. It provides new answers to old questions about disability: what is the problem, where is the problem located, what is the solution to the problem, who controls the solution to the problem, what is the desired outcome. The beginning of a paradigm shift from the traditional rehabilitation approach to the IL framework has been identified (DeJong, 1979).

The first important question that IL addresses is — What is the problem? When using non-IL thinking, some characteristic of the person with the disability is usually identified as the problem. The problem, when viewed from the IL perspective, is seen as those features of the disability service system that maintain dependency relationships in an environment which does not accommodate to the needs of the person with a disability. IL provides a method for addressing many of the problems experienced by persons with disabilities: peer counselling, individual advocacy, self-help, consumer control and barrier removal rather than by professional intervention. With IL, the desired solution is that people with disabilities achieve choice and control over their own lives.

Disabled people have used the concepts of IL to

develop a service delivery component of the disability rights movement. This component of the movement, unlike self-representational advocacy organizations, is mandated to provide direct services to persons with disabilities.

> The self-help process takes two basic forms: the most fundamental one being self-representation or expression and the other being self-help services or mutual aid . . . The Independent Living movement . . . decided that their objective was not limited to the provision of any specific service or need, but rather their objective was the provision of all resources required to achieve an equitably independent and participatory lifestyle for each disabled person desiring this and coming to them for service.
>
> [Derksen, 1985]

In this passage, Derksen identified the most fundamental aspect of an IL Centre — flexibility. Flexibility remains a primary strategy of centres, because it enables them to work with individuals toward their desired goals. Without flexibility, centres would soon lose their ability to facilitate consumer control and empowerment.

> An Independent Living Centre promotes and enables the progressive process of disabled citizens taking responsibility for the development and management of personal and community resources. A centre, while reflecting each community's unique character will be: consumer controlled, community based (local ownership), cross disability, non-profit, advocates of Independent Living, promoters of integration and full participation (via use of existing services). Essential programme components are information and referral, advocacy, peer counselling, service development capacity (via research and planning, demonstration programmes, service delivery and coordination, service networking, consumer monitoring), and including such direct services as housing assistance, attendant care, transportation, vacation relief and technical aid loans.
>
> [COPOH, 1985]

A Centre's mission is to assist people with dis-abilities transfer the right to take risks from the state to the consumer who wants to assume the risk. People with disabilities have been housed in hospitals, not community settings, to protect them from medical crises. Consequently, today many individuals with disabilities are struggling to regain the right to make the risky choices which non-disabled citizens make on a daily basis and in the process are having to learn the skills necessary to take risks in an informed manner. Independent Living Centres may assist them to acquire these skills. The methodologies used by centres include information and referral, advocacy, peer counselling, service development capacity (via research and planning, demonstration programmes, service delivery and coordination, service networking, consumer monitoring).

There is a need for people of all ages with all types of disabilities and disability experiences to participate in IL centres and the disability rights movement, in general. Older people with disabilities have unique information resources and counselling capacities which can be invaluable to others facing similar circumstances.

Accessible Transportation

Accessible transportation remains a fundamental component of independent living. As early as 1979, Frank Bowe pointed out:

> Accessible transportation serves both as a practical necessity and a philosophical basis for independent living. Without means of transportation to educational, vocational, cultural, recreational, and commercial facilities in the community it is virtually impossible for . . . disabled people to live outside an institutional environment. In this sense, transportation is the hub of independent living. Its availability expands the alternatives from which a disabled person can design his or her life . . . yet trans-

portation is a spoke in the independent living wheel, too, because it both reflects and sustains the very philosophy of living 'in' the community, providing [persons with disabilities] with the same services accessible to others ... and requiring neither obeisance to others nor dependence upon them.

(Bowe, 1979)

The fact that transportation was the issue which sparked the formation of many disability organizations, both at the national and local levels, attests to the importance of this issue (Driedger, 1984).

The need for accessible transportation spans all age groups. Youth, adults and seniors with disabilities all experience a need for accessible transportation to enable them to participate in activities relevant to their needs and interests. For seniors, accessible transportation takes on increased significance due to problems associated with mobility and agility.

People with disabilities have used a variety of stratagies to eliminate transportation barriers. The USA witnessed years of civil disobedience by wheelchair warriors, organized by the ADAPT group out of Atlanta, who disrupted the national meetings of the American intercity bus industry with sit-ins, demonstrations and other actions geared to attract media attention to the issue. ADAPT exported their brand of advocacy to Canada, when they organized a demonstration in Montreal on 1 October 1988. These transportation protests only ceased when President George Bush signed the Americans with Disabilities Act in 1990, which promised greater access to transportation for people with disabilities.

In other jurisdictions, people with disabilities and seniors interested in transportation access have focused attention upon regulatory bodies and transportation law. The transportation handi-capped have found it necessary to establish acceptance of a number of critical principles by transportation authorities: self-determination, one person-one fare, equality of access, dignity of risk, no unreasonable terms and conditions of travel.

In the area of transportation, self-determination means that carriers accept the disabled person's assessment of whether or not they need to travel with an attendant who will assist them while they are travelling, rather than this decision being made by a carrier. Prior to the 1980s, carriers frequently refused to carry wheelchair users who were not travelling with an attendant.

When an attendant is required, an extra fare should not be charged for the attendant, because this is an extra cost of disability which the individual with a disability should not be expected to bear; rather, the cost should be shared by all travellers through a percentage increase to all tickets. Greyhound Bus Company has a one person-one fare policy which enables an attendant to travel on the disabled person's ticket.

Equality of access refers to the duty which carriers bear to accommodate the needs of people with disabilities who wish to travel. Thus, carriers should design their facilities and services according to the principles of barrier-free design. While there have been some improvements for people who have mobility impairments, carriers still have a long way to go to improve access for visually impaired, deaf and hard of hearing travellers. There is little available in alternate media to assist travellers with print handicaps.

The dignity of risk principle upholds a disabled person's right to engage voluntarily in activities which others may perceive as dangerous for them. One person who used a respirator to assist him with breathing, was told by his municipal bus operator that he could not travel on the bus because city officials were concerned that his respirator would fail and his life would be in jeopardy. This was a risk which the disabled person determined to be remote, but one which he was willing to accept. He contended that it was his right, and not the right of the transit authority, to make this decision. Eventually, human rights law upheld this person's right to risk his personal safety.

On 24 April 1980, the Canadian Transport commission found in favour of a disabled person who had been denied transport by VIA Rail because she was not travelling with an attendant; this decision established disabled people's right to self-determination in the field of transportation. This decision has been referred to as the Magna Carta of disabled persons' rights in Canada (Kanary, 1985). It also served to reinforce the concepts of one person-one fare, equality of access and dignity of risk.

Through policy statements and the regulatory process, disabled people have won acceptance of the principle that carriers cannot impose unreasonable terms and conditions of travel on persons with disabilities. Thus, disabled travellers can expect such services as assistance with boarding and deboarding from carrier personnel, competent handling of mobility equipment by ground crews, and reimbursement for personal equipment damaged by carriers. Consequently travellers with disabilities can demand that dignified practices and procedures be established by carriers. In the early 1970s, disabled people were being forced to travel in the baggage cars of trains, 'manhandled' onto airplanes, forced to use escalators because some terminals were without elevators. These dangerous and undignified practices are now being replaced with equipment and procedures which respect the dignity of disabled travellers and meet safety requirements.

The gains that have been made in accessible transportations are largely due to the participation of people with disabilities in the processes affecting the administration and regulation of transportation. Since the early 1980s people with disabilities have been serving on committees and panels which establish standards and policies governing the transportation industry. In Canada, people with disabilities have been sitting on technical committees of the Transportation Development Centre, which guides research and development in the area of transportation; consumers serve on the Minister of Transport's Advisory Committee on Accessible Transportation and on committees of the National Transportation Agency. Most Canadian cities also have consumers serving on committees which oversee accessible community bus service.

Seniors with disabilities have been at the forefront of the initiatives which have led to the establishment of some important transportation milestones. A retired business woman, a wheelchair user, played a key role in Newfoundland's Roadcruiser Demonstration Project, which put the first accessible motor coach on the road in Canada. Her participation ensured that the perspective of travellers with mobility and agility problems was heard by key decision makers — industry officials, government policy makers, designers and engineers. The Roadcruiser Project proved that it was possible to operate an accessible bus as part of a generic transportation service. The Roadcruiser went into service on 1 February 1985.

Transportation continues to be an area where there is collaboration between disabled seniors and other people with disabilities. In the Province of Ontario, people with disabilities, seniors and other people interested in advancing barrier free transportation organized the Transaction Coalition to advocate for improved services on subways, rail, air and motor coaches. The coalition was governed by two co-chairs, one from a seniors coalition and the other from provincial organization of disabled persons (Arsenault, 1990).

The need for accessible transportation continues to grow and will continue to do so into the next century. Many factors contribute to the increasing demand for access: an ageing population, the expectation of seniors and people with disabilities to live in the community and participate in the activities of daily living, changes in the delivery of health care services which see more and more people receiving services on an outpatient basis. These societal factors will increase the demand for generic transportation services to be delivered according to barrier-free design principles.

Conclusion

While the issues and problems that people with disabilities face may differ from sector to sector (i.e. women, Aboriginal people, older people, visible minorities), the philosophy of the consumer movement remains relevant to people with disabilities wherever they find themselves, whatever their age, whatever their social circumstance. The theme of self-determination is one of the most consistent themes in today's political climate. Like oppressed people everywhere, disabled people are saying — 'we have a voice of our own and we will set up our own course of action'. (see also Chapters 3 and 5).

References

Adams, O et al. (1991) Profile of Persons with Disabilities Residing in Health Care Institutions in Canada. Canada: Industry, Science and Technology, Government of Canada.

The Boston Women's Health Collective (1994) The New Our Bodies Ourselves. New York: Simon and Shuster.

Bowe, FG (1979) Transportation: A key to independent living. Archives of Physical Medicine and Rehabilitation 60: 484.

Brown, SE, Conors, D, Stein, N (1985) With the Power of Each Breath. Pittsburgh: Cleis Press.

CCD (1994) Employment Committee Minutes, 31 May 1994. Winnipeg: Council of Canadians with Disabilities.

CCD (1994) Holes in the Quilt. Winnipeg: Council of Canadians with Disabilities.

COPOH (1985) Defining the Parameters of Independent Living. Winnipeg: Coalition of Provincial Organizations and the Handicapped.

COPOH (1985b) Discussion Paper on the Issues of Disabled Women. Winnipeg: Coalition of Provincial Organizations and the Handicapped.

DeJong G (1979) Independent Living: From social movement to analytic paradigm. Archives of Physical Medicine and Rehabilitation 60.

Demas, S (1990) Triple jeopardy: Native women with disabilities. Compass: Special Edition, Disabled Women and Poverty.

Derksen, J (1985) The independent living movement and the self-help process. In: Defining the Parameters of Independent Living. Winnipeg: Coalition of Provincial Organizations and the Handicapped.

Driedger, D (1984) The struggle for legitimacy: A history of the coalition of provincial organizations of the handicapped (COPOH) (unpublished).

Driedger, D (1989) The Last Civil Rights Movement: Disabled Peoples' International. London: Hurst and Company.

Dunn, A (1990) Barriers Confronting Seniors with Disabilities in Canada. Ottawa: Statistics Canada.

Enns, H (1981) Canadian Society and Disabled People: Issues for Discussion. Canada's Mental Health December.

Fine, M, Asch, A (1981) Sexism without the pedestal. Journal of Sociology and Social Welfare 8: 233–248.

Hurst, B (1994) Social Integraton of Disabled People. DPI Elaborate Paper for the World Summit on Social Development (unpublished).

Kanary R (1985) Transportation Plenary Presentation COPOH Conference Report. Winnipeg: Coalition of Provincial Organizations and the Handicapped.

Ratzka, A (1990) Tools for Power: Resource Kit for Independent Living. Winnipeg: DPI.

Sawyer, A (1981) Women's Bodies Men's Decisions. Phoenix Rising 1 (Winter): 15–18.

UN (1993) The UN World Programme of Action 1983–1992. Geneva: United Nations Organization.

24

Housing Alternatives

HOK-LIN LEUNG

Introduction
•
Planning and Design Considerations
•
General Considerations Governing Housing Choice
•
Housing Options
•
Summary

Introduction

In a typical North American urban situation, about 70% of the elderly population live in houses, 25% in apartments (including those specifically designed for older people) and the rest in boarding accommodation or rented rooms. Those most likely to live in houses tend to be homeowners, younger (under 75), mostly married, and with higher incomes (see Chapter 2).

A majority of older people live with others: spouse, children, siblings, other relatives, friends or boarders, but a significant number (from 25–33%) live alone, often in apartments. Those who live alone tend to be older and have lower incomes. Older people who live in urban areas are more likely to live alone than their rural counterparts.

Those who live in cities have lower incomes than their suburban counterparts; they are less likely to be homeowners. Their homes are more likely to be older and in greater need of repair. Their reasons for staying may have as much to do with the neighbourhood environment as with their individual dwelling. The lives of poorer inner-city older people become increasingly neighbourhood-based and they are often neighbourhood-bound. Many are more concerned about their immediate social environment than about the physical condition of the dwelling in which they live.

Of course, some older people do move – about 5% each year compared with 20% of the general population – primarily for health and financial reasons and the difficulties encountered in maintaining their home. Most of those who move are renters and most do not move very far.

The greatest number of older people want to remain at home with the assistance of some community services. The next two most popular options are moving into a housing project where home services are available and moving into a home for older persons (i.e. the 'supportive' housing arrangement option). Only a few are interested in moving in with friends or with family members, with a supportive housing arrangement being a more preferred option for apartment dwellers, those under 75 and those who are single (Minister for Senior Citizens Affairs, 1985).

The general physical quality of all forms of housing in North America has improved dramatically in the last 50 years. Today, indoor plumbing, hot and cold running water and complete kitchens are standard provisions in all housing, except in some rural areas, inner-city slums, and remote communities. Considerations have now expanded to emphasize not only dwelling quality but also affordability (how much of a person's income is spent on housing), suitability (how well the housing and its neighbourhood meet physical and service needs) and availability (whether enough units are available that are affordable and fit the needs of potential occupants).

Planning and Design Considerations

For older people, shelter quality must satisfy their special needs – physiological constraints, sensory deterioration, support services and neighbourhood services.

Physiological Constraints

Windows that are impossible for the arthritic hand to open and close, kitchen storage that takes backbreaking bending or a reaching device to access, doorknobs that are difficult to turn, bathtubs that have no grab bars, controls that are impossible to read and furniture that is difficult to enter or exit are common problems. Many of these are simply the result of a lack of attention on the part of designers and developers to heed well established research findings and good design practice.

Some of the most successful solutions are nothing more than an improvement to the appearance of standardized items, such as making the standard handrail a larger element to resemble a chair rail or a wainscot trim, or to include lighting fixtures mounted under the rail that direct light to the floor surface, where it is needed. Often, inexpensive adjustments can enhance safety for the older people. Retrofitting existing housing, especially the single-family home, in ways that support the older person's independence can have great influence on their ageing in place.

Sensory Deterioration

Ageing affects the acuity, accuracy and general functioning of sensory organs. Taste, touch, sight and hearing can all experience normal decremental losses as people age (see Chapter 6 and 8).

Sight loss is the most architecturally demanding. Low light levels and poor figure-to-background contrast in signs, labels and graphics can make it difficult and sometimes painful to read important messages. A high level of diffused light on critical surfaces is desirable, but more light can cause glare. Therefore, single light sources and major contrasts in light levels should be avoided. Instead, indirect light sources should be used to minimize glare. Food preparation counters in the kitchen, areas around the toilet and bathtub and corridor spaces where an older person can easily trip and fall are critical settings.

Hearing loss can also be a problem. Increasing the absorption of unwanted sound in spaces where conversation takes place and minimizing reverberation and background noise are common strategies. 'Redundant cuing' uses a combination of light, sound and surface texture to alert older people of an upcoming event or problem, such as the simultaneous use of a lighted button and a synchronized tone in an elevator to alert the rider when the appropriate floor has been reached. This multiple cue approach is particularly helpful to those suffering severe loss of more than one sense.

Support Services

As people 'age in place' their support service needs often increase significantly:

1. Local agencies may provide homemaking services, such as house-cleaning, meal preparation, shopping and laundry. 'Meals on Wheels' deliver a hot meal once a day, as many times during the week as needed. These visits can also encourage social interaction. User fees may be charged. Governments may provide subsidies.
2. Older people who are coping with loneliness or death of a spouse, depression, anxiety and other psychosocial problems can arrange for visits from a social worker who may provide help or a referral to an appropriate agency.
3. Personal care (non-medical) may include assis-

tance with bathing, dressing, eating and some homemaking activities, services usually provided by an agency or by direct hiring of the helper.
4. Home care (medical) may consist of visits by a nurse or other licensed caregivers who can administer medication, change dressings, assess or monitor conditions and perform other treatments. Services are usually covered by a government sponsored health plan.

Neighbourhood Services

An older person's housing needs extend beyond the physical dwelling unit. They include such diverse elements as health, security, privacy, neighbourhood and social relations, community facilities, service and transportation. Being ill-housed can mean deprivation of any or all of these dimensions and may lead to discontent. Neighbourhood safety is a paramount issue, for older people as well as for other vulnerable groups, such as women and children. The lack of services or transportation become especially salient when older persons become more frail and their home range diminishes.

There is sufficient evidence to show that a location close to shopping, recreation, services and other people will encourage older residents to participate actively in community life. This means that while land may be plentiful and inexpensive in outlying areas, these may not be suitable as housing locations for older people. Planners should ensure that each community will have adequate facilities and services to support its older population to avoid them being forced to move away from familiar surroundings in order to find suitable accommodation. On the other hand, these facilities and services should not be overly concentrated in any one area to create a 'ghetto' of older people.

General Considerations Governing Housing Choice

The significance of the housing environment for older people has been the subject of much gerontological research. The underlying assumption is that as people get older their ability to live independently becomes more reliant on environmental supports and access to services.

Attempts to evaluate the appropriate environment for individuals as they age (Kahana, 1975; Ehrlick et al., 1982; Leung, 1992) have concluded that it is necessary to examine a host of interrelated factors, from an individual's perception and attitudes, through his/her functional capacities, to the social support network and the quality of the physical environment, as well as other demographic and contexual factors. This variety of abilities, interests and concerns underlines the necessity for alternative housing environments from which an older person can choose what is most suitable for them (Table 1).

Gutman et al. (1987) have shown that while selling and renting is seen by most older people as a solution to the problem of home maintenance, they would not consider doing it themselves. Buying a smaller single-family detached dwelling was considered a viable option mostly by those under 75, who presently own large homes. There was little enthusiasm for purchase of a mobile home; many considered the generally poor location of moble home parks as the major drawback. Although a unit in an apartment or townhouse development would carry less responsibility than a single-family home, many did not like living under community regulations and giving up control over operating and maintenance costs. A unit in special retirement housing appealed to the older group who valued benefits such as companionship, social activities, possible meal availability, security and special design features, but

Table 1

Advantages and Disadvantages of Different Housing Options

Housing Options	Advantages	Disadvantages
Single-unit housing (includes single-family and semi-detached houses, accessory apartments, granny flats, and group homes)	Autonomy and privacy Ageing in place facilitated	Inappropriate designs Inadequate services Possible socialization problems Accessory apartments, granny flats and group homes need community acceptance (zoning changes, etc.)
Multi-unit housing (includes apartments, townhouses and reused buildings)	Cost-effective Opportunity for socialization	Danger of segregation and ghettoization Inappropriate designs, especially in adaptive re-use
Supportive housing (includes the full range of retirement homes and communities, and multi-level care facilities)	Specially designed Social, health, and supportive services provided on site	Expensive Heavy administration Overly supportive housing can have adverse effect on autonomy Segregation and ghettoization

many disliked the idea of a concentration of old, sick and frail people.

The remain-at-home (ageing in place) option has the strongest pull — retaining privacy, a yard or garden — and independence. However, the physical effort and financial cost of maintaining a home and garden, and the expense of property taxes are major disadvantages. Homesharing, taking in boarders or putting in a self-contained suite can provide companionship and reduce costs, but incompatibility and loss of privacy would be considered too high a price to pay by most older homeowners.

The cost of housing services constitutes a large fraction of the total expenses of living either in the community or in an institution. The quality of the home and neighbourhood environment affects whether an older person can remain in the community. For example, having or installing a bathroom on the first floor of a two-storey home may determine whether a person with severe mobility problems can remain in their home. The safety of the neighbourhood may influence a family's willingness to care for an elderly relative. The existence of complete kitchen and bathroom facilities may be essential if care providers from outside are required to come in to render services. Moreover, it is essential to recognize that the housing situation will have to be adjusted periodically over time as household composition and housing needs change.

The present state of knowledge about in-place adjustments is extremely limited. Struyk and Katsura (1987) suggest the following types of housing adjustments: changes in the use of rooms, modifications to the dwelling to facilitate its use by persons with physical impairments, taking in roomers or boarders and adjusting the amount of repairs and improvements. Both changes in the use of rooms and modifications to a dwelling are driven by the activity limitations brought about by physical impairment, especially when an older person has to rely on outside meals and transportation services. The likelihood of having boarders in the home is sharply higher when an older person has severe mobility limitations and has been receiving some help from outside the home for an extended period. Multi-person households and men living alone appear to be more willing to take a boarder than elderly women living alone. Falling income may also be a factor pushing households to accept boarders. Adjustments to the amount of repairs and improvements are not readily identifiable one-time events. The effects of such shifts only gradually become evident. The economic position of the household seems to be the chief determinant.

Much research on housing for older people has been based on what is called the 'congruence theory' — the match (fit) between needs and environment. This should not be a static concept; people may either change their environment or alter their needs in order to maximize the fit (Kahana, 1975). Changes in subjective perceptions, attitudes and motivations are as important as objective housing characteristics in maintaining this fit (Leung, 1987).

O'Bryant (1983) observed that 'a great amount of the housing satisfaction expressed by the elderly is independent from what has been defined as physical quality' and claimed that objective housing quality indicators have limited explanatory power on variance in housing satisfaction (less than 25% in most cases).

Indeed, Lawton (1980) believed that housing satisfaction seemed to be independent of physical quality, and that research must look more carefully for factors in the person or in the environment. He has also conceded that 'the most appropriate personal characteristics for which environmental congruence should be sought are essentially unknown as yet'.

Going beyond 'the conventional wisdom of the housing professional [who] tends to see physical housing for the elderly as an end in itself, rather than a means to a different end — psychological well being . . .', O'Bryant and Wolf (1983) investigated the effect of four subjective factors: status value of home ownership, traditional family orientation, cost versus comfort trade-off and competence in a familiar environment. They found that of the three types of variables — personal-demographic, housing characteristic, and subjective — the subjective variable had as much explanatory power of housing satisfaction as the other two variables combined.

In a further study of older homeowners, using a combination of a non-standardized, non-obtrusive interview method and a thematic content analysis, an added dimension was identified — ambiguity of perceptions, attitudes and behaviour (Leung, 1987). Such ambiguities may, no doubt, simply reflect inconsistencies in human behaviour in general, but they also raise important questions about the fundamental assumption in the congruence theory: that the match between the individual and the environment is definable, identifiable and achievable. Three such ambiguities are especially interesting — independence vs dependence, privacy vs social interaction, and familiarity vs change.

Independence vs Dependence

Older people seem to want to be independent as much as possible, for as long as possible. But their commitment to independence may be less than total. Often, they are ambiguous about their independence. They enjoy the self-esteem and benefits of their independence, such as 'come and go as I please', 'doing things my way', yet at the same time they realize they could not do so without being dependent on some people for assistance. While they would like to remain independent, it becomes a progressively more difficult task. For many, the attitude is one of 'I am grateful for help, but let me try it first'.

Often, independence is gained through reciprocity. Many older people are an intergral part of their community. Many of them live near their extended families. They are not just older people who need a lot of help and take up other people's time. They are grandparents, parents, brothers, sisters, friends and neighbours. In most cases it is a give-and-take situation. They would find ways to help others and show their gratitude: baking for one's children and grandchildren, helping to care for grandchildren, or being good neighbours. Sometimes, they only insist on 'buying' the services of other people, so as to make themselves feel less dependent.

> They will do it if I ask them. I pay them. I don't pay them directly, but if there is any change, I'll leave it there.

Privacy vs Social Interaction

Privacy is generally valued by older people: 'There is a difference between being lonely and being alone.' Most prefer to live by themselves (after they have lost their spouse). Even those who have misgivings about being alone do not necessarily want to live with others.

> It's funny, you know, I don't like living alone, yet I don't believe I would want to live with anyone.

Most would like to have social interaction, but they want to have it on their terms. Being a good neighbour requires also a respect of privacy.

We are very close neighbours; mind our own business, but we are there to help each other. That's why I like it here. I don't run from one house to the other. We get along well. I think that's why we get along so well, because we are not bothering anyone too much.

Familiarity vs Change

The feeling of ambiguity can be very strong when it comes to the perception of conditions in their neighbourhood. many elderly see their neighbourhood changing for the worse, yet they feel a loyalty toward it.

> I knew all the neighbours once. It's changed now. The neighbours across the street, I don't even know what their names are. But it's hard to get away from what you have been doing all your life.

A sense of place is a basic need of many older people. More than other groups, they have the need for the sense of spatial identity. In spite of great inconveniences, such as unrepaired streets, poorly lit walkways, trash and so forth – older people stay on. Many retain memories of a better past; they do not move simply because the neighbourhood has deteriorated. In the final analysis, as someone puts it, 'I know things are wearing out, but it's home'.

Housing Options

Housing is more than just shelter. Social interaction with other people, psychological effects of the physical environment on safety and comfort and financial consideration all contribute to housing satisfaction. In general, older people want to maintain a degree of independence, and to have adequate social support, health care and a sense of security. Older people live in a variety of settings, such as single-family homes, apartments, and retirement communities.

Housing choices for older people are made on the basis of dwelling types, living arrangements, and support services (Minister for Senior Citizen Affairs, 1985; National Advisory Council on Ageing, 1992; Myers, 1982).

For years, the public sector (governments as well as non-profit organizations) response has been the building of new units for the well, active, older person. Although there were initial concerns that such settings might result in older people becoming physically and socially isolated from the rest of society, research findings have now pointed to positive effects, such as improved morale and life satisfaction, greater activity, increased social interaction, better perceptions of health status and even increased longevity (Reigner and Pynoos, 1987). The private sector is beginning to provide a range of housing options, too. But still, only a small number of older people can benefit from these efforts.

Single-Unit Housing

The most common dwelling type is still the single-family home. Since older persons prefer to stay in their own homes for as long as possible, homes and neighbourhoods may have to adapt to their changing needs as they become more frail. The challenges are to promote alternative living arrangements that support older persons in their own homes and to redesign and modify existing dwellings to maintain good housing standards and improve their suitability for older people.

'Ageing in place' implies a responsibility on the part of the older people as well as communities and local governments to support such autonomy. This sometimes requires innovative approaches to zoning regulations and neighbourhood planning and development, and availability of support services, financing and design to improve the quality of life for residents. In this respect, locally administered home repair and energy assistance programmes are important to allow ageing in place.

An accessory apartment is an extra self-contained unit in a single-family home created by converting part of the dwelling or adding one or more rooms to the structure. The advantage is that an older person may be able to generate income by adding an accessory apartment and renting it to a tenant or live in the unit and rent out the house, perhaps to family or friends. Some zoning regulations make this illegal, but it is often accepted tacitly by the community as long as those living in the extra unit are related to the owner.

The 'granny flat' is an idea originated in Australia which refers to a self-contained, portable unit installed temporarily on the property of a single-unit home and sharing its electricity, water and other services. This arrangement enables older people to live in close proximity to their families and increases their mobility, independence and security of tenure, but zoning regulations may have to be revised to permit the extra unit; and neighbours may have to be convinced to accept the concept.

Accessory apartments and granny flats are more cost-effective than heavily subsidized institutional housing and meet the desire of families to assume greater obligations to their older members. The need for support services may increase as the occupant ages and becomes less independent.

As independent living becomes more difficult, the single-unit house becomes less suitable. However, instead of moving people to new settings, services can be brought to them. Homes may have to be modified to make them more supportive and appropriate and adequate services such as homemaking, home health aid and meals on wheels must be provided.

Altering the living arrangements can also prolong the stay. House/home sharing is an arrangement in which the owner and one or several tenants share the living space, but not in the same way as a rooming house arrangement. A social agency would match owners or renters who have extra space to potential tenants. For the elderly owner, or landlord, the advantages are that cost is shared and that someone else is around. Personal care or housekeeping and maintenance services may be accepted in lieu of rent.

Another living arrangement alternative is the group home where several unrelated people live together co-operatively and share the expenses and management of a house, often with the help of a salaried resident professional who provides some services. Each person's private space is usually only a bedroom; bathroom facilities may be private or shared. Kitchen and dining facilities are shared and there is usually a common living room. A non-profit organization may act as a back-up and resource group. Staff may be hired, particularly if the group determines to 'age in place'.

Group homes, however, have a perception problem. The trend to deinstitutionalization — for the mentally handicapped, juvenile offenders, or parolees — has made the location of group homes, in general, a controversial community issue in many urban neighbourhoods. Group homes for older people usually attract the least controversy, but, local zoning regulation can sometimes stand in the way and may have to be appealed.

In both home sharing and group arrangements the basic notion is to recreate, in modern communities, the type of living experienced in societies with extended families, where the aged and the young help each other. Practical benefits include shared housing costs, lessened fear of crime, companionship and assistance with household chores. With these arrangements older people can retain their own level of independence and yet remain in their own community.

Multiple-Unit Housing

These are buildings with three or more self-contained dwellings units, in the form of apartments or townhouses each made up of a private kitchen, a private bathroom and sleeping facilities. For independent-living older people, the important attributes of resident satisfaction are maintenance, management, safety and aesthetics. Design elements in these buildings should supplement losses in health status, provide support and mitigate problem circumstances in order to maximize independence (Reigner and Pynoos, 1987).

A recent development in multi-unit housing is a growing interest in renovating existing older buildings for housing for older people. The re-use of buildings no longer needed for their original purpose, such as vacant schools and industrial buildings, can have many benefits. This may be a less costly and intrusive alternative to a community than new construction. The buildings may be of significant historic or cultural local interest. Older persons often find the familiar building in the community – the school they attended or the factory where they worked – a satisfying residential environment. This option is constrained by the increasingly high cost of buying older buildings, the special physical design and other standards required to support elderly living, and the lack of experience on the part of developers (often non-profit organizations) in renovating and retrofitting old buildings.

'Supportive' Housing

There are a number of housing options for older people who need on-site services and facilities for their well-being. Retirement homes are purpose-designed apartments or townhouse-style units, private or shared, with private sleeping quarters, bathroom and kitchenette and communal dining and other facilities. Medical and non-medical care are optional. A hired administrator manages the daily operation. In some retirement communities, housing is just one part of a whole network of facilities for the older people. Units are self-contained, and designed to permit independent living, sometimes with land for private use. The community can be organized in the form of a small village, with a full range of care and support services (including shopping) under a centralized administration. In Britain, a typical set-up has 20–40 residents living in small facilities assisted by neighbourhood wardens who visit, help organize activities, and coordinate services.

Support services housing (sheltered housing in Britain and congregate housing in the USA) is another option. This can be part of an existing neighbourhood, a section of an apartment building, or a specially designed multiple-unit building. Such housing does not generally provide nursing facilities on the premises. Residents have their own self-contained unit with a call system connecting them to an administration centre. A range of non-medical support services is available and residents generally come together once a day for a meal and social activities. Fees for service are incorporated into the rental or through a monthly charge.

Multi-level care facilities are multiple-unit complexes that offer accommodation and services ranging from independent living to chronic care. Dining facilities and activity areas are shared. Different buildings or parts of buildings are devoted to particular levels of care, often permitting a couple with differing care needs to remain together. These continuum-of-care retirement communities seek to incorporate independent housing, housing with services (for example, home health, personal care units), and nursing home facilities. They aim at keeping older people in the least restrictive environment, but they can be expensive. So far, this option has been provided mainly through the private sector (with some non-profit participation) and limited to more affluent older people.

A distinguishing feature of supportive housing is that social, health and support services are provided on site. Therefore, management style and management policies become important. In some cases, these are government sponsored (funded and/or operated) projects, where the biggest problem appears to be administrative. Government departments of housing, health, and welfare have to work together to make it succeed. There is great bureaucratic and political reluctance to mix shelter with health and social services.

An increase in the over-75 segment of the older population demands a new look at supportive housing arrangements. So far, the emphasis is on housing with support services that enhance residents' feelings of security and enable them to function at their optimal level. It is important to avoid overly supportive settings, as in the UK, where the concept of supplemental care (i.e. where services are custom-fitted to individual needs) has been designed to allow older people to live as independently as their functional abilities allow, with support provided only at their margin of need.

Management policies (or regimes) can encourage or discourage activities and the use of space. Restrictive management policies contribute to depression, a sense of helplessness and accelerated physical decline. Participation in setting rules and personalizing the environment, on the other hand, seems to encourage a sense of ownership among older residents. There is need to create a balance between individual freedom and institutional order.

We know very little about how our environment can influence an older person's social activity level, which may help combat depression and lead to a higher level of life satisfaction. It appears that linking social areas with circulation routes that carry heavy traffic improves the potential for use. Similarly, making a space visible before entering (previewing) has been shown to affect the motivation for use. Socialization, however, is to be understood in relation to privacy and the need to control, manage and sometimes avoid social interaction. We have only limited knowledge on how furniture, partial partitions and screens, various amenities and activities and the ecological composition of the resident population interact and mediate the social success of purpose-built projects.

For older people, self-confidence and the level of anxiety, especially in relation to a new environment, are affected by the degree to which they can orient themselves and move from one location to another without getting lost. Disorientation is both disturbing and frustrating. The ability to find one's way in the environment is so fundamental a concept that it may even account for misdiagnosed confusion in some older people.

Good management knows how to interpret spaces as opportunities for facilitating resident activities and interaction, as well as to establish rules and policies to discourage or forbid undesirable behaviour, activities or uses. However, managers and administrators are often unaware of design intentions: how activities can be accommodated on the grounds or within rooms that have been set aside for social purposes. Better definition of how spaces are intended to function from a management viewpoint should lead to more thoughtful and careful design attention.

Summary

Most older people want to stay in their own homes, but as they grow frail many will need support to stay on and some will move to specially designed and specially serviced accommodation.

There are four general types of planning and design considerations: physiological constraints, sensory deterioration, support services and neighbourhood services. The congruence theory is most often used to explain housing choice and satisfaction. It emphasizes the importance of 'match' between individual needs and environmental attributes. The consensus is that objective measures and subjective perceptions are equally important. Many older people are ambiguous about their needs and have ambiguous perceptions of the housing environment.

Housing options cannot be considered in isolation but must combine elements of dwelling types, living arrangements and support services. Our greatest challenge is to enhance choice and autonomy.

References

Ehrlick, P, Ehrlick, I, Woehlke, P (1982) Congregate housing for the elderly. *The Gerontologist* 22: 399–403.

Gutman, GM, Milstein, SL, Doyle, V (1987) *Attitudes of Seniors to Special Retirement Housing, Life Tenancy Arrangements and Other Housing Options*. Vancouver: Gerontology Research Centre, Simon Fraser University.

Howell, S (1980) *Designing for Ageing: Patterns of Use*. Cambridge, MA: MIT Press.

Kahana, E (1975) A congruence model of person-environment interaction. In: Wendley, P, Ernest, G (eds) *Theory Development in Environment and Ageing*. Washington, DC: Gerontological Society.

Lawton, P (1980) *Social Policies and Programmes on Ageing*. Lexington, MA: DC Heath.

Leung, H-L (1987) Housing concerns of elderly homeowners. *Journal of Ageing Studies* 1: 379–391.

Leung, H-L (1992) *Elderly Homeowners Turned Renters: Reasons for the Move*. Report 22. Winnipeg: University of Winnipeg, Institute of Urban Studies.

Minister for Senior Citizen Affairs (1985) *Elderly Residents In Ontario: Their Current Housing Situation and Their Interest in Various Housing Options*. Ontario: Minister for Senior Citizen Affairs.

Myers, P (1982) *Ageing in Place: Strategies to Help the Elderly Stay in Revitalized Neighbourhoods*. Washington DC: The Conservation Foundation.

National Advisory Council on Ageing (1992) *Housing An Ageing Population: Guidelines for Development and Design* 2nd ed. Ottawa: National Advisory Council on Ageing.

Norman, A (1984) *Bricks and Mortals: Design and Lifestyle in Old People's Homes*. London: Centre for Policy on Ageing.

O'Bryant, SL (1983) Subjective value of the home to older persons. *Journal of Housing for the Elderly* 1: 29–44.

O'Bryant, SL, Wolfe, SM (1983) Explanations of housing satisfaction of older homeowners and renters. *Research on Ageing* 5: 217–233.

Reigner, V, Pynoos, J (1987) *Housing the Aged: Design Directives and Policy Considerations*. New York: Elsevier Science Publishing Co.

Struyk, RJ, Katsura, HM (1987) Ageing at home: how the elderly adjust their housing without moving. *Journal of Housing for the Elderly* 4: 1–192.

25

Assistive Devices: Aids to Independence

PAMELA J HOLLIDAY, GEOFFREY R FERNIE

Introduction

Assistive technology devices are defined as 'any item, piece of equipment, or product system, whether acquired commercially off the shelf, modified or customized, that is used to increase, maintain, or improve functional capabilities of individuals with disabilities' (Hammel and Smith, 1993). Assistive devices may be divided into several categories, although there is no universally accepted classification scheme (Hammel and Smith, 1993). Such categories may include: accessible architectural design, augmentative and alternate communication, environmental control, job accommodation, daily living technologies, neuro-muscular electrical stimulation, orthotics and prosthetics, personal care aids, seating and positioning, sensory aids, wheeled mobility.

By now the reader may already be intimidated, imagining that it may be necessary to become familiar with hundreds of devices; one database that lists commercially available assistive devices lists some 20 000 entries (ABLEDATA, 1994). Fortunately, the needs of most older clients can be met by the judicious use of very few devices. It is important to remember that the goal of assistive device use is to impact on the function (and therefore the quality of life) of an individual, and that the assistive device is merely a 'tool' to achieve this objective. Since the most common disabilities are mobility-related, the physiotherapist's focus tends to be on devices that aid safe mobility (see Chapters 6, 7 and 22). Familiarity with aids to daily living and communication, hearing and vision aids is probably less important to the physiotherapist since these are more the focus of other disciplines such as occupational therapy, speech therapy and audiology. Physiotherapists are regarded as experts in matters relating to balance, gait and mobility. The assistive devices used for the related disabilities include: grab bars, walking devices, wheelchairs (powered and manual) and transfer and lifting aids.

Grab Bars

The physiotherapist should select a range of grab bars that are suited to different purposes and locations. Rails should be circular, or near-circular, and about 38 mm (1.5 in) in diameter to allow a good grasp. If the grab bars or rails are being used to pull up on, especially in a bathroom where hands may be wet or soapy, a textured or sculptured surface is important to prevent sliding. Such a surface may not be appropriate on a stairway where the user is encouraged to walk up and down with the hands sliding on the rail in position to prevent a fall. A grab bar or rail should be securely attached to the wall. Clients should not use a towel rail, soap dish or other device that may not be strong enough to arrest a fall.

Grab bars may not provide enough assistance to enable the client to stand from a low position. Consequently the physiotherapist should become familiar with raised toilet seats, bath

seats, chair/seat lifts, and with the design features of chairs that facilitate easier egress.

Seating

Chair design features that allow for easy egress and ingress of older people include a firm, elevated seat (seat height of 470 mm [18.5 in]) with a shallow seat rake to prevent sliding forward out of the seat, yet allow movement forward in the seat for egress. Armrests are very important. They should be broad and lightly padded, straight and parallel to the seat surface, and should extend forward at least to the front border of the seat to assist in movement forward on the chair, as well as rising and sitting (Fernie and Letts, 1991). Space should be available under the front of the chair to allow the feet to be positioned appropriately during rising. Lateral 'wing' supports on chairs are often non-functional; a back support which provides lateral support in the thoracic region is preferred. Lounge chairs should have adjustable head cushions.

Walking Aids

When assistance is required for ambulation, canes or walkers may be recommended. Most commonly, walking aids are recommended for clients with joint problems (e.g. arthritis of the hip or knee), balance problems, or a combination of both. A walking aid may be required for long-term use, or temporary (short-term) use, during recovery from lower extremity surgery or fracture.

With few exceptions, the physiotherapist should be prepared to recommend a four-wheeled walker

Figure 1   Design features of a four-wheeled walker which should be evaluated prior to prescription: handgrip shape; brake function; wheel size and function; options such as seat, tray and foldability; adjustability; overall appearance.

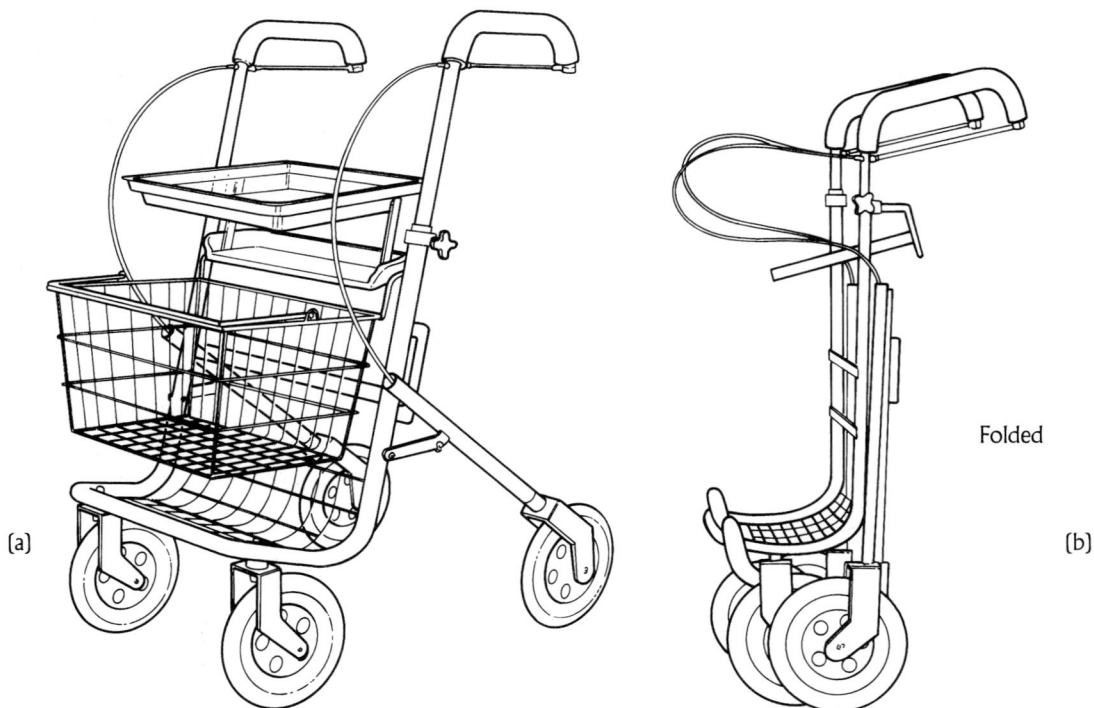

(a)

Folded

(b)

(a 'rollator'). A four-wheeled walker permits a natural uninterrupted gait and enables the older user to achieve the highest levels of independent mobility. Four-wheeled walkers often have accessories such as seats, trays and baskets and maybe used in- or outdoors. Growing numbers of older people find that these walkers increase their quality of life by enabling them to walk longer distances and to carry things (Figure 1). Walkers vary considerably in quality and price.

Training older clients for safe use of a four-wheeled walker should include use of the brakes,

stationary positioning of the walker for use as a seat and prevention of the rollator 'running away' during use on downward slopes. Four-wheeled walkers have a variety of brake actuator designs including cables, levers (bicycle), and pull-up or push-down mechanisms. Choose walkers with brakes that the client has sufficient hand function to operate. Physiotherapists should only recommend products to others that have been personally tested.

Large wheels (preferably of diameter 20 mm or 8 in) roll much more easily over obstacles. Check for annoying fluttering of the castor wheels (castor shimmy) that occurs even at low walking speeds on some models. Other questions that need to be answered include: is the seat at the right height for your client; does the walker fold sufficiently for transportation or storage; and, is there a good tray and carrying basket available? Finally, judge whether the product is attractive or whether it might have a stigmatizing 'medical' appearance that labels the user as 'disabled'.

Four-wheeled walkers may not be the best choice where: use indoors is in a very confined space; the client requires a non-moving support during gait; reduction of load on the hip is desired; or an interim device is required during (re)training. Three-wheeled walkers are more manoeuvrable but tend to be less stable. Walkers without wheels or with only front wheels (usually two wheels) may be more supportive than four-wheeled models for people who have poor balance. However, walkers without wheels must be picked up in advance of each step, breaking any natural rhythm and providing a period of instablility during which there is no support from the assistive device (Figure 2).

Crutches transfer some of the weight normally borne through the legs to the hands or forearms (axillary or forearm). Padded support for the hands or weight-bearing surface reduces user discomfort. Crutches may be prescribed for temporary use, but are rarely prescribed for long-term use for the older client. In contrast to walkers, crutches do allow use on steps and stairs.

The physiotherapist may recommend a cane or quad cane (a device held in one hand which has a base with four feet) with an ergonomically designed handle. Canes are useful for clients who require minimal support, who may only walk short distances, or where indoor space prohibits the use of a larger device. Canes usually provide support by reducing the load at the hip, contralateral to the hand in which it is held. Good hand and wrist strength are required for cane use.

Walking devices, like all assistive devices, should be regularly inspected for damage, and be repaired or replaced immediately if safety or function is impaired. All assistive devices should be free of loose and rattling parts and all points of adjustment should fit smugly. Rubber tips should be checked regularly and should be replaced if they are dry or cracked, well before the pattern on the tip bottom disappears, or before the concave surface flattens (ECRI, 1991). In cold climates special tips for gripping on ice should be recommended to users of walking aids with rubber tips (e.g. canes, crutches, walkers), because this type of walking aid is inadequate on wet and icy surfaces.

Wheelchairs

Some older clients will require a wheelchair. Although manufacturers regularly advertise the benefits of ultra-lightweight chairs for young wheelchair athletes, their benefits may be even more appreciated by older users and, especially, by their caregivers when the time comes to lift the chair into a car! Similarly, postural seating has a remarkable effect on the psychological state as well as on physical function of older persons, and yet attention to correct seating and positioning has been a focus primarily for young wheelchair users.

People tend to slide forward in chairs. This effect is particularly pronounced if the back rest is

Figure 2   Stable-base walking aids: (a) a walker showing method of advancement and its effect on the base of support (b). A quad cane also has four points of support (c).

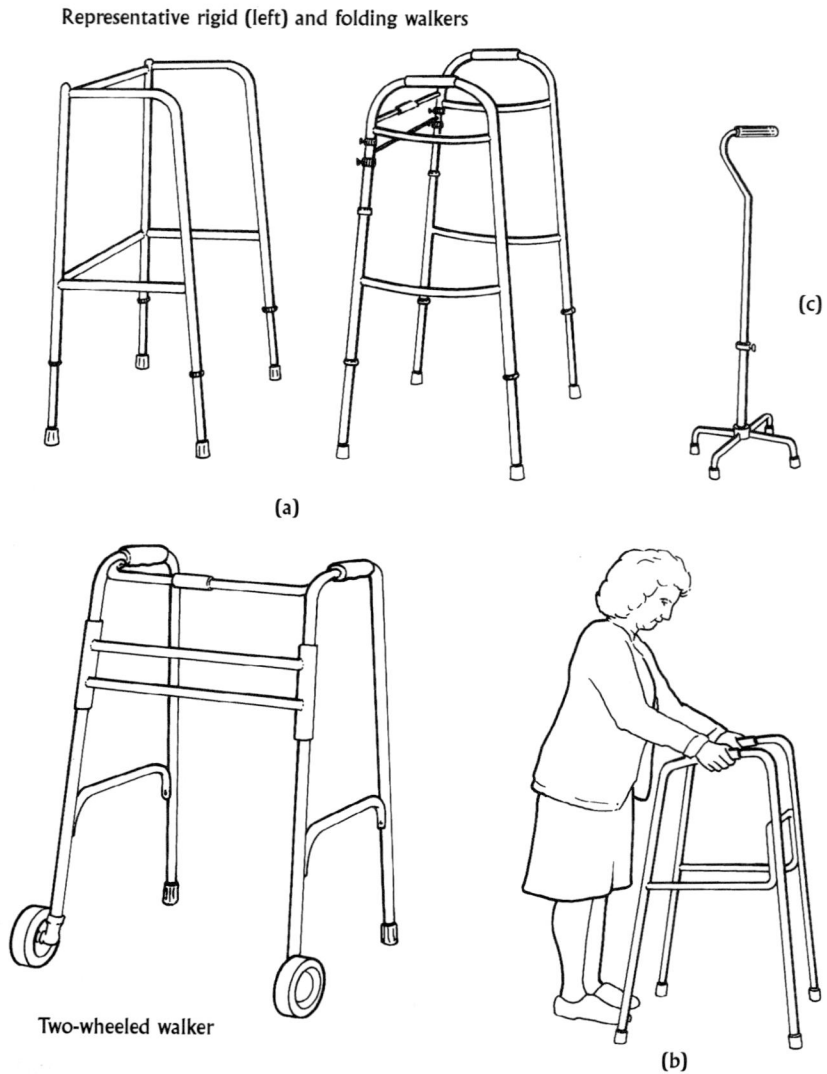

Representative rigid (left) and folding walkers

(c)

(a)

Two-wheeled walker

(b)

reclined without a coincident tilting of the seat to resist the sliding motion. Over a period of time a pattern of sliding down in the chair, with occasional active movement to restore posture, is noticeable. Caregivers spend a significant amount of time pulling (and lifting) patients from a slumped or slouched posture into the correct position. Of course, caregivers are at risk of back injuries from the heavy lifting and pulling repositioning tasks.

Figure 3   Reclining the back of the seat causes the user to tend to slide forwards, whereas tilting-in-space avoids this problem and minimizes shear forces.

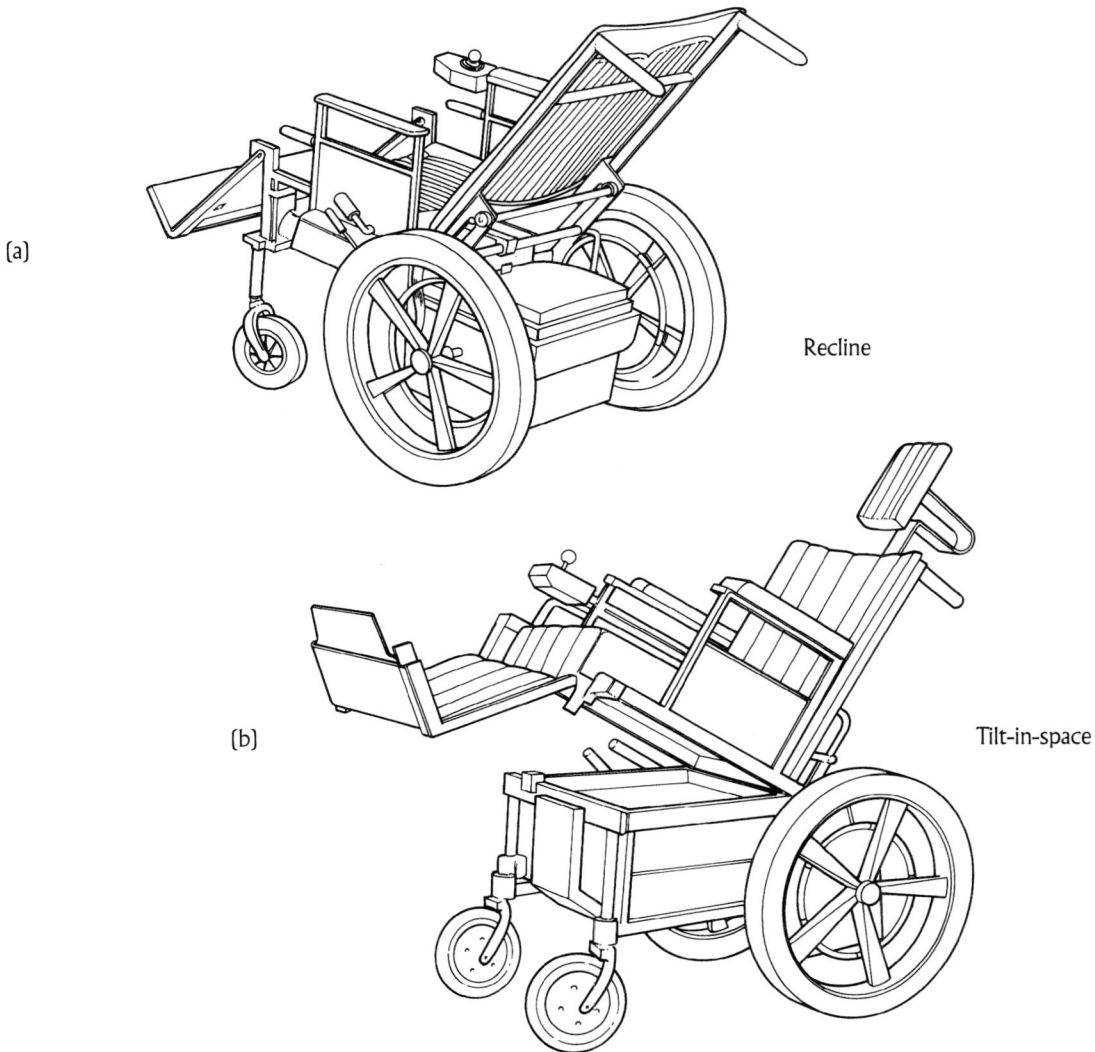

(a)

Recline

(b)

Tilt-in-space

Reclining chairs should only be recommended with caution since shear forces generated by the greater tendency to slide forward may increase the risk of decubitus ulcer formation. If a reclining option is needed, then consideration should be given to the selection of a mechanism to reduce the relative movement of the patient's back over the backrest caused by the difference in the centres of rotation of the backrest hinge and the anatomical equivalent hinge. If hip extension is not necessary then 'tilt-in-space' mechanisms are a better choice. These mechanisms allow users to change into a more restful posture without the negative effects of reclining since the seat also tips and the seat to back angle remains constant (Figure 3).

Figure 4   Scooter

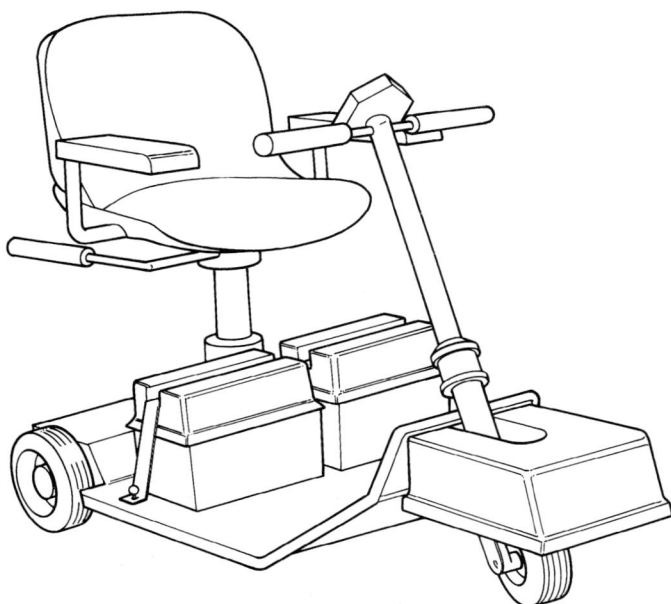

Figure 5   A power base chair

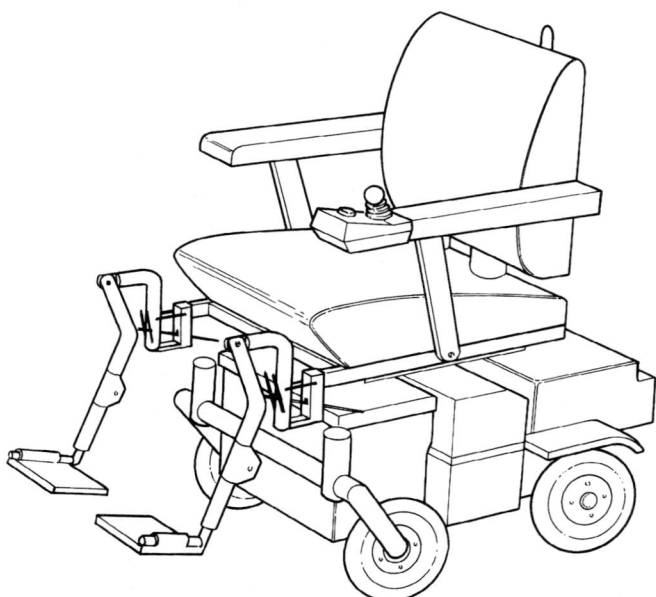

A powered mobility device might be needed either if the client does not have sufficient upper body function to use a manual chair, or if the ability to travel greater distances is desired. Most powered chairs fit into one of two general categories: scooters or power bases (Figures 4 and 5). Scooters tend to be about half the cost of powered bases but are equipped with less sophisticated seating and require sufficient upper limb function to steer using the tricycle-style handlebars. The lowest cost scooters have a motor attached to the steerable front wheel and are only suitable for fairly smooth and level surfaces. Rear wheel drive scooters are generally more powerful and can cope with rougher ground but are larger and less manoeuvrable indoors. Power base chairs are more sophisticated vehicles and generalizations about design features are less reliable. High manoeuvrability is needed for indoor function of wheelchairs, whereas stability is more important in the outdoor environment. Thus, smaller chairs may be more suitable for indoor use but a larger, less manoeuvrable chair may be needed where outdoor performance is desired. International testing standards now exist (e.g. American National Standards Institute [ANSI] in North America and the International Standards Organization [ISO] elsewhere) that specify how the performance of manual and powered chairs is to be measured. Modern powered chairs allow driving characteristics, such as maximum speed and acceleration, to be preset to match the needs and capabilities of the user. In addition, a wide range of interfaces is available including joysticks, head position sensors, puff and voice systems. Modern wheelchair controllers also have built-in capabilities for environmental control.

Transfer and Lifting Aids

It is particularly important that the physiotherapist is knowledgeable about lifting devices. Lifts may be needed to transfer patients between bed and a chair, onto a toilet, or into a bath. Some lifts are wheeled around on the floor and others are suspended from overhead tracks. Wheeled lifts avoid the expense of installing tracks (ceiling or external overhead frame) but can be very awkward to manoeuvre especially in confined spaces when carrying a person's weight. Frequently two people are needed to operate these devices to ensure safety of both the clients and the operator. Some lifts have even been perceived by users to actually increase the effort required to transfer a patient. Overhead powered lifts are less stressful and may reduce the likelihood of injury to the caregiver. They also remove the possibility of tipping accidents that sometimes occur with floor lifts. The expense of continuous tracking throughout a building or multiple overhead lift units can be reduced by the use of portable, battery-powered units that can be moved from one overhead track to another by hooking onto a strap hanging from a wheeled carriage on each track (Figure 6).

Movement between floors or over entrance steps may only require the installation of sturdy handrails for ambulatory clients but will require a ramp, elevator or stair climbing device for less agile walkers and for users of wheeled mobility aids. Optimum handrail height for stairs has been determined to be 91.4 cm (36 in) but local building codes should be followed. The Americans with Disabilities Act (ADA) (1990) and building codes elsewhere provide guidance on many aspects of environmental accessibility including acceptable ramp gradients and lengths. It is important to realize that many older clients may have difficulty managing the maximum ramp gradient of 1:12 that is specified in these standards; 1:20 may be more realistic.

Assessment

The assessment of an older person is multidimensional, and includes consideration of the individual, the environment, and the society as a whole (Holliday et al., 1992). The individual's physiologic, emotional, cultural, perceptual, cognitive and spiritual domains are all interrelated and interdependent, and are influenced by their immediate physical and social (family, friends, colleagues and caregivers) surroundings, as well as the political, cultural and economic environment within which they live. Age, social contact, and educational level have all been shown to be predictive of functional limitation (Boult et al., 1994).

The management of the older individuals who have assistive device requirements operates within the three levels of a health promotion model. Primary prevention refers to promotion of successful ageing among still healthy older persons, for example, the installation of bathroom safety equipment such as grab bars provides a 'safe' environment for all users, regardless of age and ability. Secondary prevention refers to identification of risk factors and screening of older persons, for example assessment and modification of the home, workplace and recreational sites for maximum safety and independence. A number of checklists have been devised to assess environmental risk factors; some of the available information is in the self-help format (Holliday et al., 1992). Tertiary prevention attempts to prevent further decline of existing disability and handicaps, for example

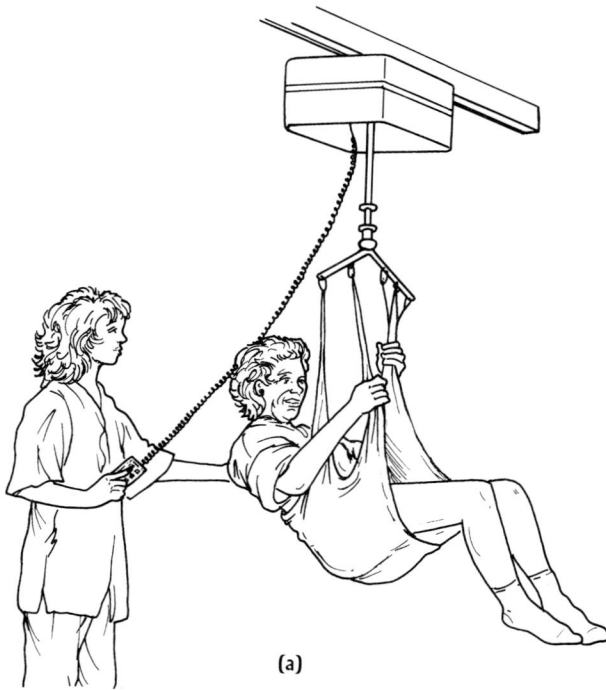

Figure 6   A typical example of a fixed (non-portable) overhead lift (a) compared with a portable overhead lift system (b) showing: 1) a caregiver retrieving a power unit from a wall storage bracket; 2) carrying it to the bedside where the strap from the unit is hooked onto a strap hanging from the overhead track; 3) a patient being lifted.

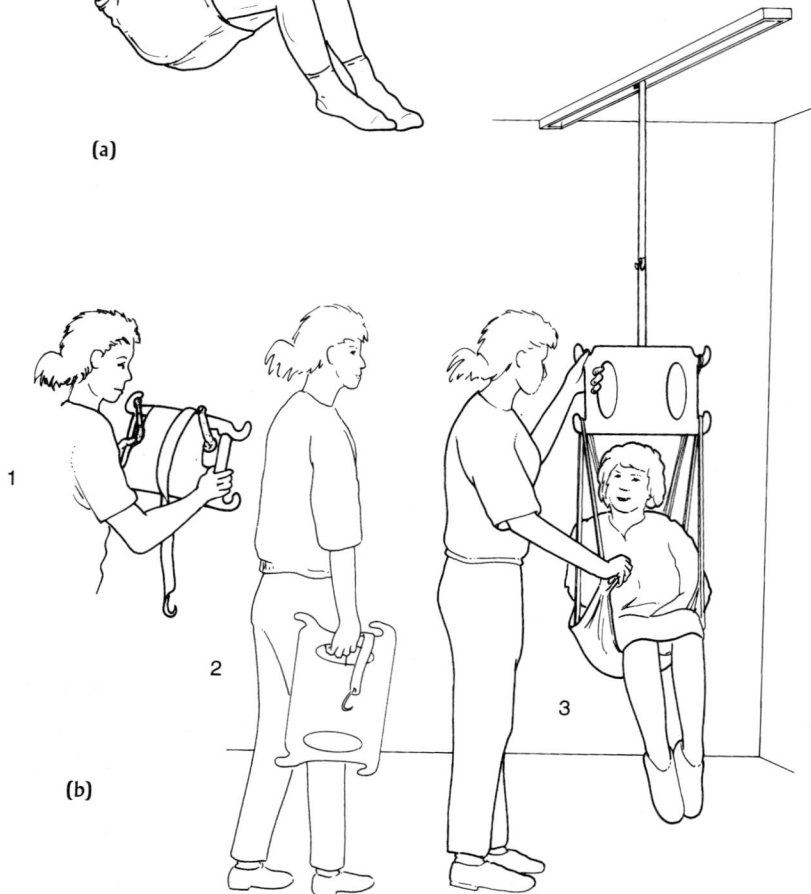

(a)

(b)

1

2

3

by using a walking aid to maintain exercise levels. Assistive devices may prevent 'impairments' from becoming disabilities or handicaps, i.e. prevent an abnormality due to physiological, psychological or anatomical loss from restricting the ability to perform everyday activities, or fulfil the individual's normal societal role (Wood, 1980).

It is most important when assessing, evaluating or monitoring function to work with the older person to understand the problem(s) in the context of the environment in which function is required or anticipated. The suitability of an assistive device is often more a function of the environment than of the characteristics of the user. While specific assessment of basic motor and sensory skills such as range of motion, muscle strength, coordination, movement dysfunction, vision, hearing, sensation, proprioception/kinaesthesis, and transfer ability may guide in the selection of the most appropriate assistive device, the extent of the social network and the availability of resources, including financial resources may be stronger influences.

Three evaluations are required: an individual assessment (e.g. 'ability' or personal characteristics of the client), an environmental assessment (e.g. bathroom and doorway size, floor coverings), and an assessment of the social network and financial resources (Figure 7). 'Environmental negotiability' describes a method of quantifying the level of function of an individual in his/her environment (Letts et al. 1994). The social/financial assessment may be completed in part, or entirely, by other team members.

The most efficient approach to the evaluation of the need for an assistive device is to identify areas of functional performance that an older person, caregiver or other person reports as: unsafe, difficult to perform, time-consuming, unable to

Figure 7 Interacting factors must be considered in the assessment of the older person for assistive devices use. The social network and financial resources provide the framework within which the overlapping functional ability of the person and the environmental milieu must be assessed.

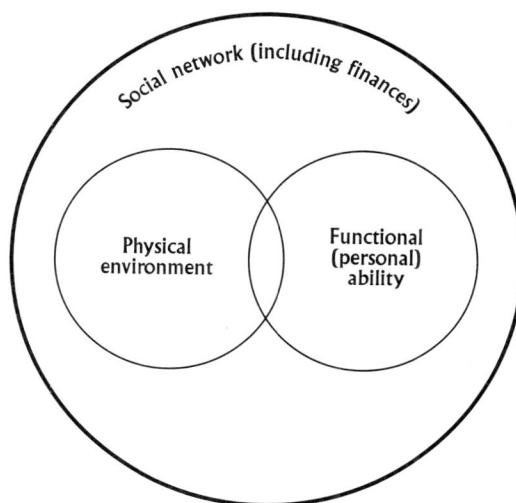

perform, avoids doing (e.g. avoid sitting in the bottom of the tub because of fear of not being able to rise), or has never done before (gender or cultural division of tasks). The distinction between capability (is the person able to do the activity?), necessity (does the person need to do the activity?), and motivation (does the person want to do the activity?) must be addressed. Identification of problematic activities may be by observation, self-report or report by caregivers or others. Functional needs are then matched against the resources (including assistive devices, help from other caregivers, and community services) to determine where assistive technology may be beneficial. Use of a checklist ensures that all domains of activity are addressed, reasons for limitation of function are evaluated, and current resources are recorded in order to assist in the selection of appropriate devices. Prioritization of need for assistive technologies (or modification of existing resources) is made by the client, in consultation with the health care professional. Computerized checklists on lap-top computers are now available.

Results from objective functional performance measures (i.e. observing someone perform an activity) and questionnaires (i.e. ask someone about performing an activity) do not always concur. Observers have been shown to underestimate the difficulty reported by seniors performing instrumental activities of daily living (IADL) tasks (Myers et al., 1993). Many instruments do not distinguish between difficulty, inability to do tasks, and capability ('can do' but may 'not do' because of division of labour between men and women, for example). Motivation and capability are not always distinguished.

In the following case, the 'Possible Solutions' sections address many generic assistive device options, while the 'Rationale for Suitability / Lack of Suitability' sections discuss a reasonable approach for the selected solutions given for the specific case.

Case Study
Mr and Mrs J

Mr J was 77 years old and had Parkinson's disease for 9 years. He had unilateral knee pain with walking and back pain especially after lying in bed. He found it difficult to rise from chairs, the bed and the toilet, and he complained about the tendency to fall backward. Bradykinesia and rigidity were managed by medication. He lived with his wife in a detached bungalow, accessible by six outdoor stairs at the front entrance and two outdoor stairs, with no handrail, at the

back door. Mr J was able to access the basement where he slept, did laundry and painted in his leisure time. A raised toilet seat (12.5 cm or 5 in) without armrests was installed on the toilet in the two-piece bathroom in the basement. He complained that the raised toilet seat was 'wobbly'. For bathing, Mr J used the bathtub on the main floor.

Mrs J who was 75 years old, had suffered from rheumatoid arthritis for 9 years. Previous fractures of both ankles and a total hip replacement made walking difficult. Active movement of her fingers, wrists, shoulders, hips, knees, ankles and feet was painful, functional range was limited and muscle strength was reduced. Although walking indoors was possible with a cane, difficulty negotiating the stairs to the outside and poor endurance limited outdoor travel. There was not enough room indoors to use a wheelchair for mobility. She had a manual wheelchair for outdoor use; it was stored on the landing at the back door, where the five indoor stairs had handrails on both sides, although the railings were not well-secured. She could not propel the wheelchair independently due to her poor upper extremity strength and pain on movement. Any outings were accompanied by Mr J, who pushed his wife in her manual wheelchair. However, he fatigued quickly.

Mrs J had access to the bathroom on the main floor of the house. It had been modified by Mr J to accommodate some of his wife's needs. A pocket sliding door replaced the hinged door. A diagonal grab bar was installed on the wall adjacent to the toilet. The toilet was above average height (45 cm or 18 in, excluding the toilet seat) to facilitate egress and ingress. A heated toilet seat that also provided wash and dry functions had been installed. Wall-mounted grab bars were installed at the entrance and interior walls of the standard bathtub and a hand-held shower was in place. Mrs J required considerable assistance from her husband to get into and out of the tub. She sat on a backless shower stool while bathing. She felt unsafe getting in and out of the tub and would have preferred installation of a walk-in shower, but financial constraints prohibited this more extensive modification.

Mr J helped Mrs J with meal preparation; he did the shopping, laundry, cleaning, and financial management for the household. Mrs J assisted with any of the IADL activities that she could manage. They did not qualify for government-supported assistance from community or social services in the home. One daughter lived close by, but her career kept her too busy to offer regular assistance. Both members of this couple were cognitively intact, although Mrs J was starting to question her husband's judgement and memory.

Prioritized Problems

PROBLEM I: INGRESS/EGRESS/TRANSFERS: CHAIRS

The most common complaint of ambulatory elderly chair users is that 'the chair is difficult to get out of'. Both the husband and wife expressed this complaint. Mrs J tried to solve the problem by purchasing office-type chairs, with a four-wheel base, armrests and height adjustment, for use in the kitchen and in the living room. These chairs were chosen because they did not require too much space (an important consideration particularly in the small kitchen), and they were higher making rising easier. The family room had a recliner lounge chair, with powered seat lift, that was used by both.

Possible Solutions for Difficulty with Chair Ingress/Egress: blocks/risers to increase the height of sofas, chairs; seat lifts and lift cushions (powered and non-powered); transfer pole/grab bar; mechanical lifting devices.

Rationale for Suitabilty/Lack of Suitability: The reclining lounge chair, that had a power-assisted seat which could be raised to assist transfers into standing, met the couple's seating needs in the family room. Although this type of chair represents a major furniture investment, the couple had already made this purchase decision. One difficulty with a reclining chair is that the solid front prevents a user from positioning his/her feet under the front of the chair to reduce the effort required when rising.

The office chair in the living room was replaced by purchase of an upholstered chair with armrests. This chair was fitted with a spring-loaded seat lift device, which is available as an add-on portable accessory (Figure 8). This device, once adjusted for the weight of the user, assists in the transfer from sitting to standing and vice versa, by lifting about 80% of the body weight. The lifting force of the seat lift device was adjusted to raise Mrs J because she was deemed to be the primary user. Only a few minutes and two trials were required

Figure 8   a) A person rising with the assistance of a spring-loaded seat lift device; b) the dominant forces during rising (reproduced with permission from Wretenberg *et al.*, 1993).

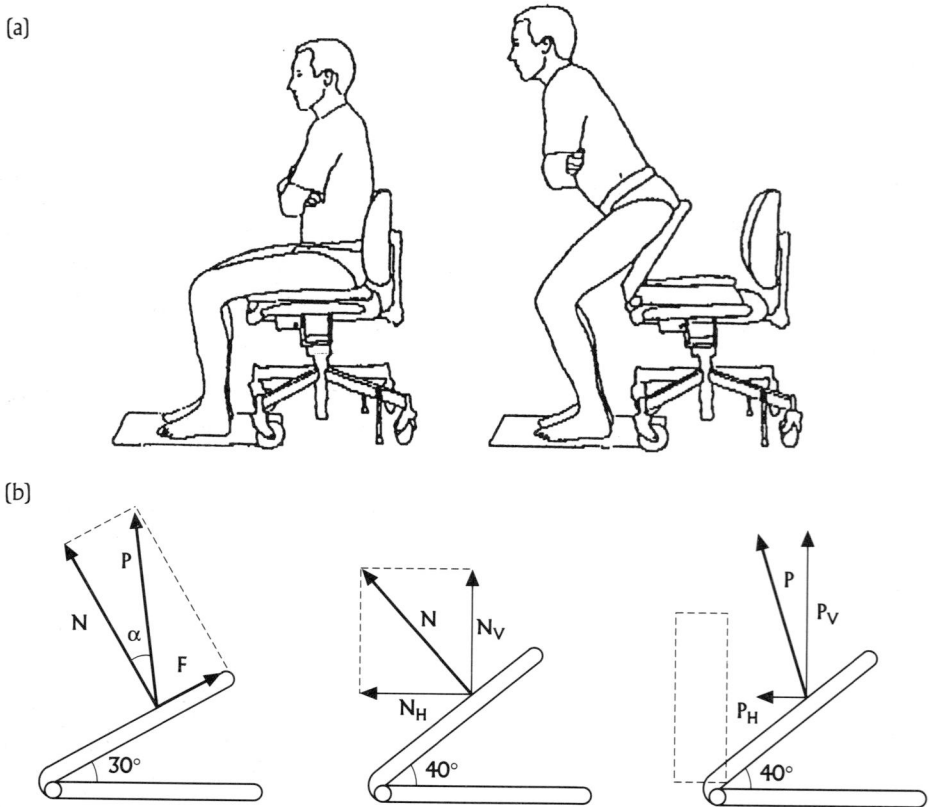

(a)

(b)

for Mrs J to become competent in its use. Seat lift devices tend to be destabilizing once the user is raised beyond 45° because the dominant force changes from vertical to horizontal; training is important. Mrs J received training to ensure that she was comfortable with the seat lift and had her walking device available for support when she got up from the seated position. Prolonged sitting on seat lift devices may be uncomfortable and as they tend to increase the seat height, the relative effectiveness of the chair armrests is reduced. They do, however, preserve the aesthetic appear-

ance of the furniture, and this was an important factor in the selection of an assistive device for this couple's home.

An alternative home-made solution to adding the seat lift would have been construction of an add-on seat. This can be made by cutting plywood to fit the seat shape, adding foam and upholstering the seat to match the chair.

Another solution to the J's problem of chair access could have been installation of a transfer pole near the 'usual' chair and

Figure 9   The main features of a transfer pole held in place by compression between the floor and the ceiling. (a) 1. Ceiling plate; 2. Spring housing and adjustor mechanism; 3. Textured (ribbed) grip surface; 4. Foot plate. The pole provides assistance for rising/sitting in locations that are not adjacent to walls (b).

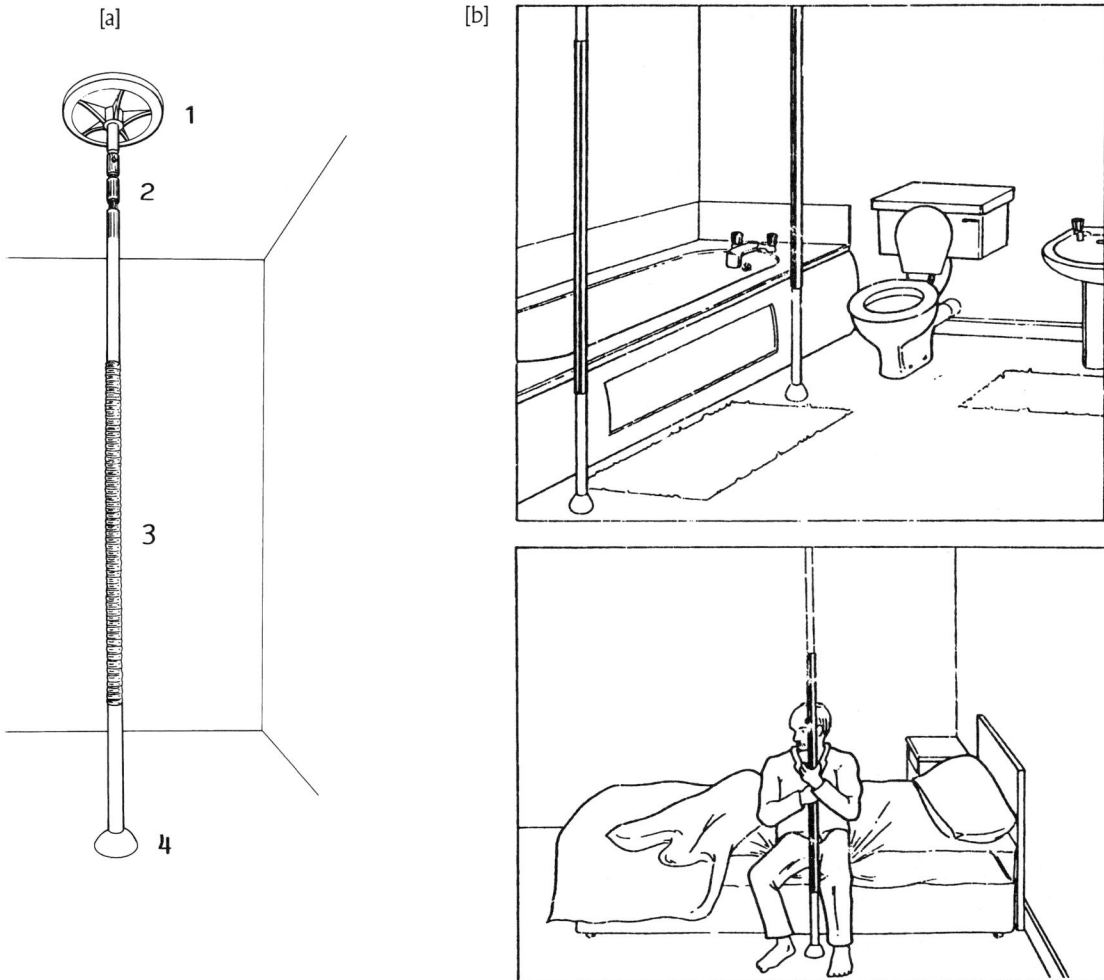

[a]

1

2

3

4

[b]

raising of the chair on blocks. A transfer pole that did not require permanent fixation would have been selected so that future changes in its location could easily be made to allow for changes in the functional status of the couple (Figure 9). These transfer poles are held in place by compression between the floor and the ceiling.

Care is needed when using blocks to raise furniture. The chair or bed may become unstable when raised, and fall off of the blocks. Floor coverings such as carpets, increase the instability. The guidelines available for the construction of blocks to raise furniture are not at all clear and have not been based on mechanical studies. Individual blocks are dangerous unless they are

Figure 10 An adjustable frame which provides stability for blocks is the safest way to raise chairs, sofas or beds (a) Note the obstruction to placing the heels under the front of the seat for easier egress.. Individual blocks may be used if they are stable and have deep holes or other means to firmly grasp the chair legs. (b) Note the less-than-ideal appearance of the device.

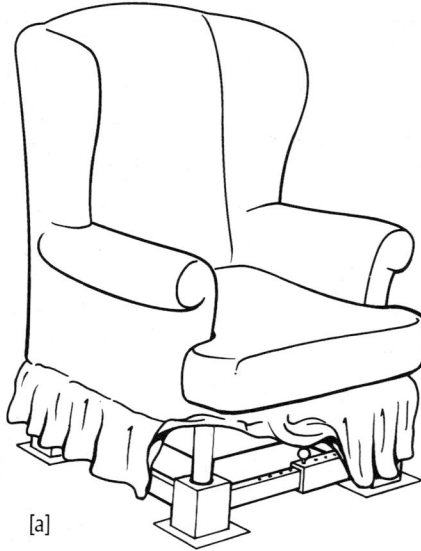

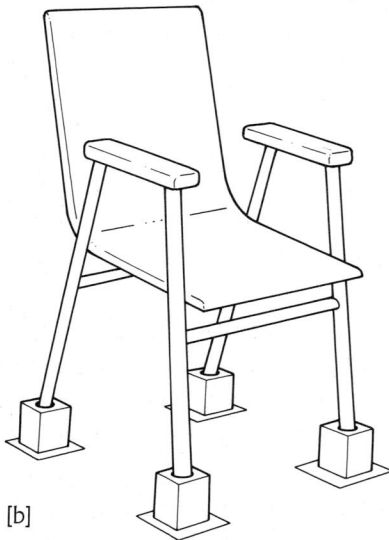

[a]

[b]

Figure 11 A portable water-powered bath seat which allows immersion in the tub. Note that the client is not lifted much above height of the side of the tub, and therefore grab bars may need to be installed for assistance to rise from the seat.

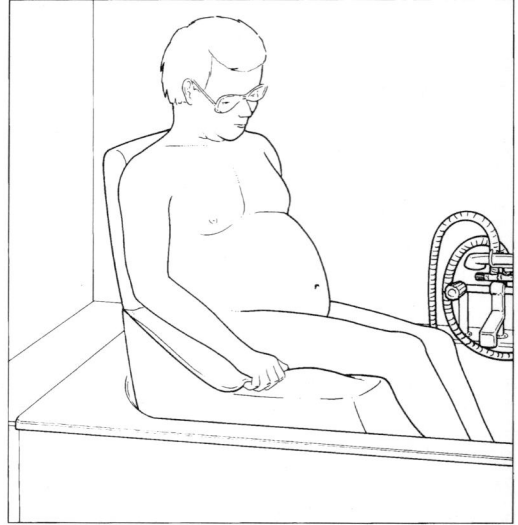

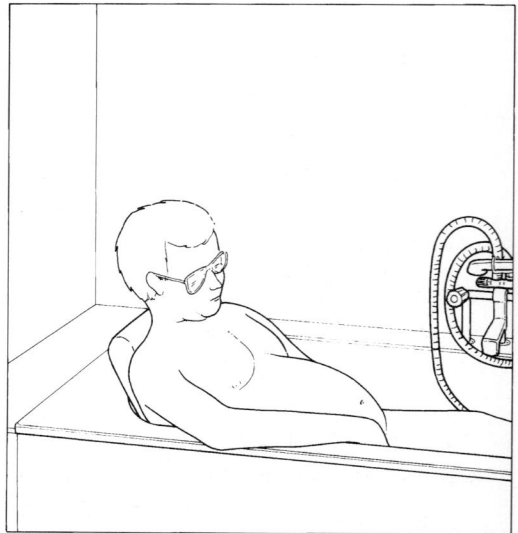

very large and have deep locations to grasp the chair legs or castors. It is preferable to construct a frame as in Figure 10. This frame joining the leg risers provides much greater stability. Mr J, although capable of constructing blocks to raise any of the chairs or sofas, did not raise any furnishings because the resulting appearance was unacceptable to him.

The castors were removed from the office chair in the kitchen to make it safer for ingress and egress.

PROBLEM 2: BATHING

Bathrooms are associated with frequent falls. Older people have particular difficulty getting into and out of the tub, and rising from the bottom of the tub once seated. In a follow-up of assistive device use by patients discharged from hospital, Finlayson and Havixbeck (1992) reported that tub transfers caused patients the greatest anxiety, regardless of the amount of training that is provided prior to hospital discharge. Mrs J required assistance to get into the bathtub and to be bathed. Mr J was able to enter the tub but felt unsteady.

Possible solutions: walk/roll-in shower (shower stall, 'barrier-free' shower); bathtub designed for ease of access (e.g. with side-opening door, integrated grab bars and seating); bath lift chair or seat (may be water-powered; some are portable); tub/shower seat or tub stool; tub/shower grab bars; tub transfer bench (board or seat); hand-held shower; rubber mat.

Rationale for Suitability/Lack of Suitability: Most residential solutions to bathing are limited by financial concerns. Major renovation is required for installation of spe-

cially-designed bathtubs or barrier-free (walk-in) shower units; for residents of rental housing units, the latter solution is not an option. A trial using a portable water-powered bath seat (Figure 11) and hand-held shower was successful for Mrs J, although Mr J needed to supervise and assist with the operation of the switch to raise and lower the seat because of Mrs J's weak finger strength and poor manual function. Mrs J enjoyed immersing in the water. One training session and one on-call follow-up was necessary for this couple to feel competent to operate the bath unit. There was sufficient space for Mr J to stand to shower with the seat in place in the tub.

PROBLEM 3: INGRESS/EGRESS/TRANSFERS: THE BED

Both Mr and Mrs J had difficulty getting in and out of bed. On both beds, the edge of the mattress, although still fairly new, was soft and did not provide support for rising. Although Mrs J had a grab bar attached to the nearby wall for assistance in getting out of bed, its location was less than ideal.

Possible Solutions for Assistance in Getting into/out of Bed: grab bars adjacent to the bed; siderails attached to the bed; free-standing transfer pole placed at any distance from the wall; transfer rail attached to the bed frame (which resembles a cane with a large loop handle); handle attached to a walking frame (the lower handle assists with the initial transfer from sitting); hospital-style bed with siderails and raise/lower functions; mechanical lifting devices.

Rationale for Suitability/Lack of Suitability: The problem of rising from a bed is made worse by soft mattresses. A good quality *spring mattress provides better support at the edge of the bed. Bedside installation of a transfer pole which was secured (non-permanently) by compression between the floor and the ceiling had the advantage that its location could be altered until optimal function was achieved (Figure 9). The vertical orientation allowed the clients to grasp the pole at their own preferred height. The ridged surface of the pole was easy to grasp and prevented slippage. The transfer pole also provided assistance for dressing, while the client was able to lean against it or circle one arm around it for support. The stigmatization associated with the use of a hospital-type bed was avoided, and the appearance of the pole was relatively aesthetic. Aesthetics were important to this couple; Mr J was a keen artist and any previous alterations in the house had been made by himself.*

Figure 12 A flat handrail is shown with the hand in 'pinch' grip (a). A round handrail allows for a 'power' grip which generates more force. Dimensions of a handrail for stairs and features for optimal function (b).

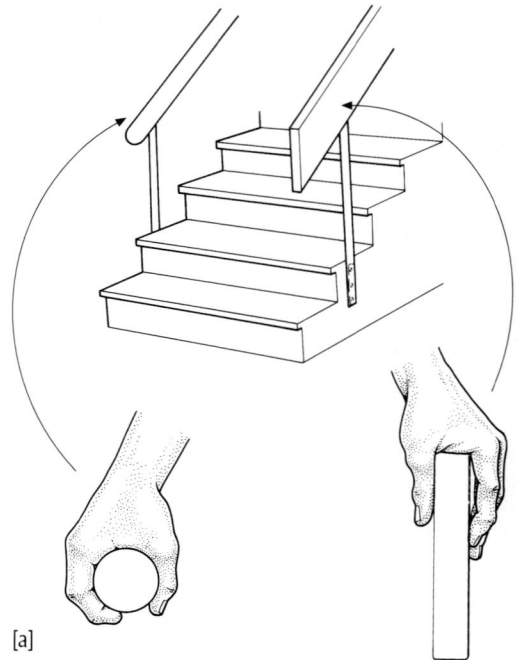

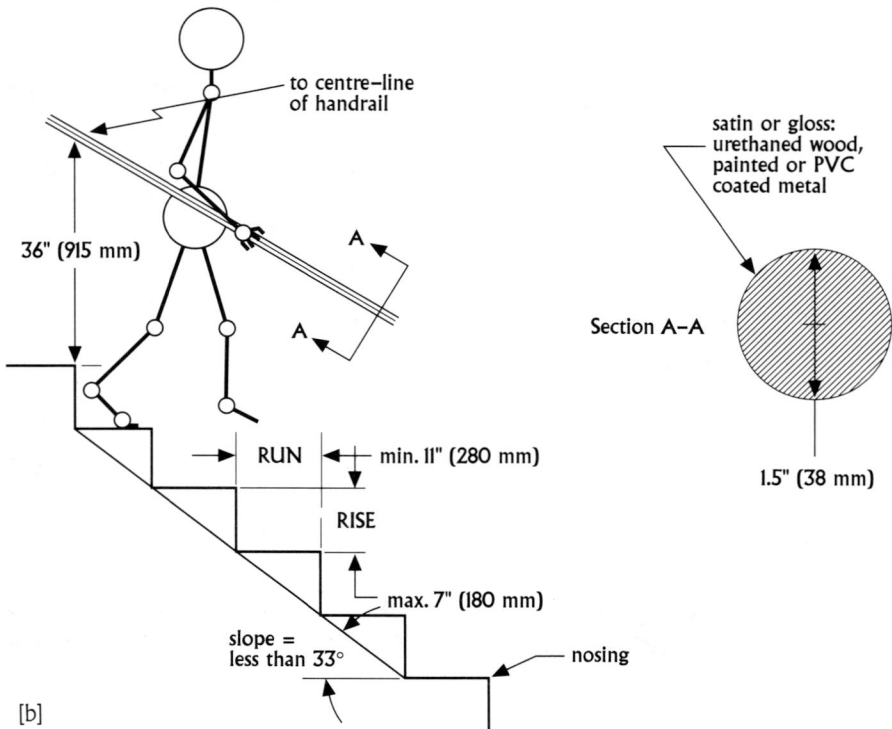

[a]

[b]

PROBLEM 4: CHANGING LEVELS INDOORS, e.g. STAIRS

The first line in defence for falls on stairs, especially during descent, is the installation of handrails on both sides. In this home, the handrails were not properly secured to the wall, and they were not of an optimum size and shape (diameter 38 mm or 1.5 in, round in shape, see Figure 12). It was difficult and unsafe for Mrs J to negotiate stairs. She could not go down the steep stairs into the basement of the house, where the laundry and storage facilities were located.

Possible solutions: *stair handrails; stair lift; stair climbing accessories for wheelchairs; residential elevator; interior ramps.*

Rationale for Suitability / Lack of Suitability: *The couple did not wish to consider moving to a home or apartment that had level access and no interior stairs. Although a stair lift was an option for the interior, the outdoor steps would still have been a problem. A ramp at the front entrance of the house was aesthetically unacceptable; labelling of the home as housing a 'disabled' person was one concern. In addition, there was insufficient room to install a ramp with even a 1:12 gradient without several switchbacks (Chapters 3, 11 and 23). The long ramp would be difficult to clear of snow. The best solution was to install a 3-stop elevator in an interior storage space and in the existing stairwell to the basement, allowing access to the main floor, outdoors onto the side walkway, and the basement. Both Mr and Mrs J were able to use the elevator without assistance. The stairs were re-configured so that they entered the basement at 90 degrees to the original location. Purchase and installation of the elevator was Can. $25,000. Stair handrails were revised to meet recommended standards of shape, size, height and secure installation (Figure 12).*

PROBLEM 5: ENTERING AND EXITING THE HOME

Getting out of the house was unsafe and difficult for Mrs J.

Possible Solutions: *keyless locks; easy-grip/turn hardware; electric door opener; stair glide, incline lift; elevator; porch lift; stair climbing accessories for wheelchairs; ramp (interior/exterior); stair handrails.*

Rationale for Suitability / Lack of Suitability: *Getting out of the home was facilitated by the installation of the elevator. Therefore, porch lifts, incline lifts, stair glides, automatic opening doors, modified door handles, etc. were not necessary. An electric door opener, altered door hardware, keyless lock, and modified keys were not required as part of this couple's solution although these devises are often helpful in other cases.*

PROBLEM 6: TRANSPORTATION

Once out of the home, Mr J had difficulty loading his wife's wheelchair into the car.

Possible Solutions: *car wheelchair carrier; adapted vehicles for drivers with disabilities; special transportation for the disabled.*

Rationale for Suitability / Lack of Suitability: *The couple agreed to book special transport for outings. A local community service was enlisted to keep the walkways clear of snow and ice in the winter. The couple kept the manual wheelchair so that independent transport was possible, if desired.*

It was not necessary to fit the car with a wheelchair transport device since only infrequent use was anticipated. A list of local grocery stores and drug stores that provided door to door delivery and shopping for customers was provided in case the couple should need them.

PROBLEM 7: MOBILITY OUTDOORS

Mobility and endurance were problems for both people. Mrs J was unable independently to propel her wheelchair and it was tiring for Mr J to push her in the chair for extended periods of time. Mr J found shopping trips had to be cut short because he felt that his left knee would give way and he suddenly needed to sit down.

Possible Solutions: powered mobility devices for Mrs J; four-wheeled walker for Mr J.

Rationale for Suitability / Lack of Suitability: Independent mobility outdoors could have been enhanced for Mrs J by using a wheelchair with a power base. However, the couple did not wish to have a powered chair (either power base or scooter) at the present time because Mrs J's outings were infrequent and use indoors was not necessary, although they held this consideration open for the future. Since Mr J was ambulatory and had good balance, a four-wheeled walker was sufficient for his needs out of doors. This walking device gave him the opportunity to sit and rest as often as required, to carry items in the attached basket, and it was collapsible for transport in the car. He received careful instruction on the need to secure the brakes on the walker prior to using the seat.

PROBLEM 8: TOILETING

The ability to get on and off the toilet is the cornerstone of independence and dignity for each individual. Mr J had difficulty getting on and off of the toilet that he used in the basement; the existing raised toilet seat was not secure. Under normal prioritization of problems, toileting would be considered as one of the highest priorities. However, in Mr J's case, the toileting priority was less important because there was a tall toilet with a grab bar on the main floor of the house, and the toilet used by Mr J in the basement merely required an upgrade of his existing assistive device.

Possible Solutions: better raised toilet seat; toilet safety frame (handrails secured to/around the toilet); wash and dry (personal hygiene) toilet seat; 'tall' toilet; toilet seat lift (mechanical lifting device incorporated into the commode seat of any toilet); reinstallation of the toilet on a raised step; commode; bedpan; urinal; adult incontinence briefs; external urinary collection device (e.g. for men, condom drainage); indwelling catheter.

Rationale for Suitability / Lack of Suitability: Commercially available raised toilet seats, with or without armrests, are the most common solution for this problem. There are, however, frequent complaints about these products. The seats tend to be unstable and users express fear of falling. Raised toilet seats 'label' the user as being disabled and do not easily encourage others to use the same toilet — frequent removal and replacement of the raised toilet seat for non-disabled users can be a nuisance. Hygiene is the major complaint of users;

Figure 13 Note the non-stigmatizing appearance of a toilet raised on a plinth (a) compared with a raised toilet seat (b).

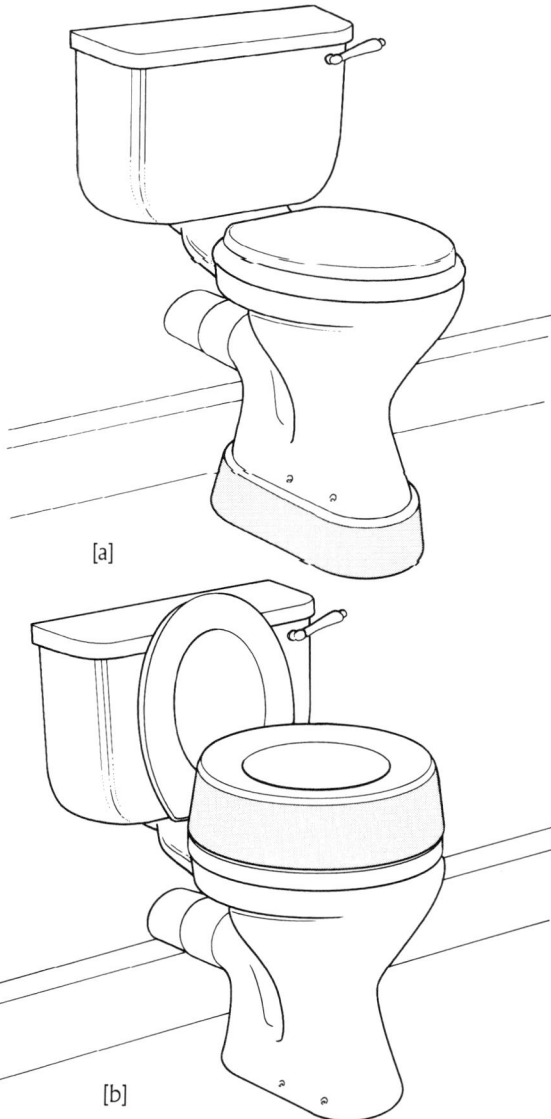

[a]

[b]

the seats soil rapidly and are hard to clean. Because Mr J used the basement bathroom for his toileting needs, his raised toilet seat was replaced by a safer model with armrests (Figure 13, raised on a plinth, armrests not shown). There still remained the main floor bathroom for use by Mrs J and guests.

The physiotherapist should not ignore other therapeutic means to manage incontinence, where appropriate. Impaired mobility is one of the biggest reasons older people do not reach the toilet in time; special attention should be given to night-time voiding since rising at this time places the older person in a particularly vulnerable state for falling.

PROBLEM 9: EMERGENCY CONTACT / BACK-UP SUPPORT

Mobility restrictions have limited the ability of Mr and Mrs J to assist each other. There was an increased risk that either person might have difficulty calling for help if an emergency occurred.

Possible Solutions: personal emergency response system (portable, wireless radio frequency transmitter and a receiver hooked up to the telephone; activated by a variety of signalling devices, e.g. a push button on the telephone, a pendant or a wrist watch call switch); environmental control unit; 'intelligent' house (centralized electronic control); security system (including keyless door lockset, light/alarm/siren activation); signal system (e.g. call bell system); auto memory dialler telephone; mobile cellular phone; tracking devices (radio transmitter and receiver).

Rationale for Suitability/Lack of Suitability: Having emergency assistance on call on a 24-hour-a-day basis was necessary for both Mr and Mrs J. An emergency call system was installed and the couple chose to wear pendant activators. The couple also located two close neighbours to be on-call should either of them need physical (non-emergency) support. At the time of the visit,

> *neither Mr or Mrs J were willing to accept any social support services or community assistance programmes.*

Concluding Comments

There has been much discussion on the issue of device abandonment (Phillips and Zhao, 1993; Gitlin *et al.*, 1993). The most frequently cited reason for failure to use assistive devices is a change of need (Phillips and Zhao, 1993). Professionals and others should realize that the level of assistance device abandonment is probably appropriate, and comparable with that of other appliances in the home, and that patients and consumers alike should be free to discard assistive devices as and when their needs change.

The use of follow-up questionnaires to clients will lead to more effective use of devices (Finlayson and Havixbeck, 1992). Client satisfaction and client perception of performance are components that need to be assessed in order to improve the performance of professionals as well as their clients. Compliance may also be improved by educating the users and allowing them more choice in the selection of assistive devices. In an uncontrolled survey of assistive device use in elderly people discharged from hospital, Finlayson and Havixbeck (1992) found that subjects who had a home visit prior to discharge were twice as likely to use all of their prescribed equipment than those who did not.

In keeping with the reduction of use of medical and professional services, more assistive devices will be purchased without professional prescription. Retail sales staff will play an increasingly important role assisting in the selection and use of technologies. An increased use of resold pro-

ducts can also be anticipated. Product rental options will be aranged through local agencies and businesses. One of the challenges to the profession is how to assist in a shift away from the medical model of service and provision of assistive devices. Consumers must be given more responsibility in the selection of assistive devices, as well as in the choice of using a device or personal assistance to optimize function. There will continue to be a need for professional/technical backup when more complex devices are required.

At the present time, there are few ways that a consumer can compare the effectiveness of assistive devices and products in a manner similar to the usual consumer practice, e.g. 'comparison shopping' for product features and price, and consumer report ratings (Post, 1993). Although sparsely distributed, several countries have 'resource' centres for the public and professionals; many of the resource centres focus on providing information on assistive technology as well as trial access to its use (Hampton, 1993).

An important factor in selecting the appropriate solution for an older persons' problem is the risk involved in the use of a particular assistive device. It must be accepted that when increasing the mobility of a person, the greater likelihood of falling accidents must be weighed against the benefits of increased mobility and improved self-confidence. Fear of falling limits the activity level of many elderly people. Interestingly, this fear itself is known to affect negatively laboratory measures of postural control in the elderly (Maki *et al.*, 1994). It has been postulated that self-confidence, or one's perception of capability, rather than actual ability is predictive of behaviour, that is, engaging in specific activities.

Finally, it is important to evaluate the effectiveness of assistive devices from a functional perspective.

Some outcome instruments penalize the use of assistive technologies by ranking function lower when such devices are used, e.g. in the functional independence measure (FIM), a lower score is given for independence where an assistive device is required to complete the activity (Hamilton *et al.*, 1987). Likewise, Boult and associates (1994) classified an individual's functional capacity as limited if they were unable to perform an activity without the help of a person or a special device. Collen and Wade (1991) used three criteria to classify mobility versus immobility in patients who survived a stroke. The use of a walking aid, other than a stick (i.e. a cane), resulted in the survivor being classified 'immobile'. The attitude that views the use of an assistive device as a disadvantage generates serious implications for the acceptance and use of assistive technologies in the health promotion model. This negative attitude allows the pepetuation of a medical model, where use of technologies labels a person as disabled and restricts the availability of assistive devices to specialty marketing and distribution. Furthermore, a negative attitude towards disability is not helped by large-scale surveys such as the United States National Long Term Care Surveys (NLTCS), which define disability as 'an inability to perform an activity without help or use of equipment, due to health or age' (Manton *et al.*, 1993). Alexandra Enders (personal communication, Milwaukee, WI, USA, July, 1994) has warned of the negative effects these scales may have on the availability of funding assistance for the purchase of assistive devices. The use of technology should not be regarded as a failure, or a second-rate solution.

References

ABLEDATA (1994) ABLEDATA Asistive Technology Information Service. Owned by: National Institute on Disability and Rehabilitation Research, Washington DC. Maintenance and information available from Silver Spring, Maryland, USA: Macro International.

Americans with Disabilities Act of 1990 (Public Law 101–336), 42 USC 12101.

Boult, C, Kane, RL, Louis, TA et al. (1994) Chronic conditions that lead to functional limitation in the elderly. *Journal of Gerontology: Medical Sciences* 49: M28–M36.

Collen, FM, Wade, DT (1991) Residual mobility problems after stroke. *International Disability Studies* 13: 12–15.

ECRI (1991) Ambulation aids: evaluation. *Health Devices* 20: 5–21.

Fernie, GR, Letts, RM (1991) Seating the elderly. In Letts RM (ed) *Principles of Seating the Disabled*, pp. 97–110. Boca Raton, USA: CRC Press.

Finlayson, M, Havixbeck, K (1992) A post-discharge study on the use of assistive devices. *Canadian Journal of Occupational Therapy* 59: 201–207.

Gitlin, LN, Levine, R, Geiger, C (1993) Adaptive use by older adults with mixed disabilities. *Archives of Physical Medicine and Rehabilitation* 74: 149–152.

Hammel, JM, Smith, RO (1993) The development of technology competencies and training guidelines for occupational therapists. *The American Journal of Occupational Therapy* 47: 970–979.

Hampton MMK (1993) An international overview of resource centers on disability. *The American Journal of Occupational Therapy* 47: 725–730.

Holliday, PJ, Cott, CA, Torresin, WD (1992) Preventing accidental falls by the elderly. In Rothman, J, Levine, R (eds) *Prevention Practice. Strategies for Physical Therapy and Occupational Therapy*, pp. 234–257. Philadelphia: WB Saunders.

Letts L, Law M, Rigby, P et al. (1994) Person-environment assessments in occupational therapy. *The American Journal of Occupational Therapy* 48: 608–618.

Maki, BE, Holliday, PJ, Topper, AK (1994) A prospective study of postural balance and risk of falling in an ambulatory and independent elderly population. *Journal of Gerontology: Medical Sciences* 49: M72–M84.

Manton, KG, Corder, L, Stallard, E (1993) Changes in the use of personal assistance and special equipment from 1982 to 1989: results from the 1982 and 1989 NLTCS. *The Gerontologist* 33: 168–176.

Myers AM, Holliday, PJ, Harvey, KA, Hutchinson, KS (1993) Functional performance measures: are they superior to self-assessments? *Journal of Gerontology: Medical Sciences* 48: M196–M206.

Philips, B, Zhao, H (1993) Predictors of assistive technology abandonment. *Assistive Technology* 5: 36–45.

Post, KM (1993) Educating consumers about assistive technology. *The American Journal of Occupational Therapy* 47: 1046–1047.

Wood, PH (1980) The language of disablement: A glossary relating to disease, and its consequences. *International Rehabilitation Medicine* 2: 86–92.

Wretenberg, P, Arborelius UP, Weidenhielm, LF (1993) Rising from a chair by a spring-loaded flap seat: a biomechanical analysis. *Scandinavian Journal of Rehabilitation Medicine* 25: 153–159.

26

Foot Problems and Footwear Prescription

OLWEN E FINLAY

Introduction

Older people, like most younger people, are unwilling to walk if their feet hurt. There is a complex interplay between footwear, walking and balance (Chapter 7); and among older people in particular, unsatisfactory footwear may hinder mobility and hence undermine health, independence and quality of life. In extreme cases, unsatisfactory footwear can so adversely affect walking that it may cause an older person to become housebound. Thus, correct fitting shoes that meet the needs of the elderly wearer are essential.

Most textbooks relating to care and rehabilitation in old age mention problems associated with inadequate footwear, but few provide advice regarding cost-effective solutions or practical tips on how to organize an efficient service.

Many variables have to be taken into account when recommending shoes for a particular person. No one shoe will suit all needs. However, in this chapter, the components of the ideal shoe will be described together with hints on modifications to suit individual requirements. Common foot problems will be described. The physiotherapist's role in the management of foot problems by provision of suitable footwear will be emphasized, although other aspects of physiotherapeutic management will be touched upon. A cost-effective footwear provision scheme will be described.

The Foot in Old Age

By old age, after many years of use and abuse, a person's foot may become unique, with deformed joints and toe nails, untended pressure points, infection beneath ingrowing toe nails, infections and poor arterial supply (Figure 1).

A clinically significant age-change is the atrophy of the pedal fat pad and plantar skin. Loss of subcutaneous tissue leads to increased local plantar pressure and increased incidence of plantar callosities. Loss of the fat pad under the heel predisposes to painful heel syndrome (Evanski, 1982).

The bony structure alone is not sufficient to ensure the ankle joint will behave as a hinge joint so additional support is provided by a strong system of ligamentous structures which pass between the tibia and fibula to the foot. Quite apart from definite disease symptoms there is often atrophy of the small muscles of the foot. As a result, the pull of the larger muscles of the foot and calf are unbalanced, leading to clawing of the toes. The reduction in support offered by the weakened intrinsic muscles permit abnormal stresses to be placed on the arches which gradually flatten longitunally and in width.

Feet are equipped to cope with enormous pressures which may be exerted in two directions, one force is at right angles to the foot and the other force parallel. It is fortunate that living tissue has a high tolerance to the force exerted, but among older people who often suffer reduced circulation, thinning of the skin, neuropathic insensitivities, and the diverse manifestations of ageing in almost all the structures, the tolerance diminishes substantially and the need to reduce abnormal stresses grows in importance (Rose, 1981).

More than 700 tons of weight is placed on each foot in the course of a day, so it is important that not only the feet, but also the footwear, can cope with these stresses. Normal pressure on the plantar surface varies between 1–7 kg/cm2 (Roggero et al., 1993), depending on an individual's bodyweight and gait pattern. A normal foot should bear 25% of the body weight on each heel during standing, the rest being equally divided and transferred from the metatarsals to the phalanges with the first toe taking double the weight of any other toe. The integrity of the medial longitudinal arch ensures that most of the body weight is transferred along the lateral borders of the foot from the heel to the toe. The arch mechanism is like a bridge and relies on inward forces generated by the plantar fascia. In severe hallux valgus however, (Figure 1) when there is angulation deformity of the great toe, weight transference is affected. Balance during walking may be threatened because the area of the sole of the foot that makes contact with the ground is decreased. In this situation the centre of load may be sited in the mid-tarsal area rather than at the heel, and such abnormal stresses may be placed on the medial longitudinal arch that heel strike and toe off are completely eliminated.

Stress on the forefoot increases with heel height

Figure 1 a) Gross onychogryphosis preventing footwear being worn. When this patient was admitted she was suffering from malnutrition as she had been unable to go out for the previous 3 weeks because she was unable to put on footwear. b) Bilateral hallux valgus. The laterally inclined great toe overrides and pushes the second, third and fourth toes towards the lateral border of the foot. c) Ulceration on the plantar surface of the foot which affected normal weight bearing.

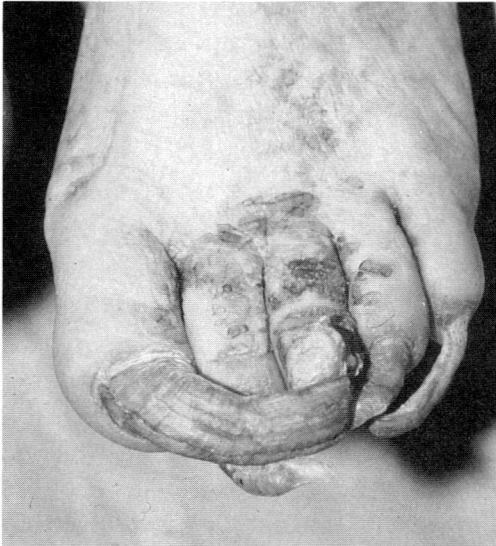

[a]

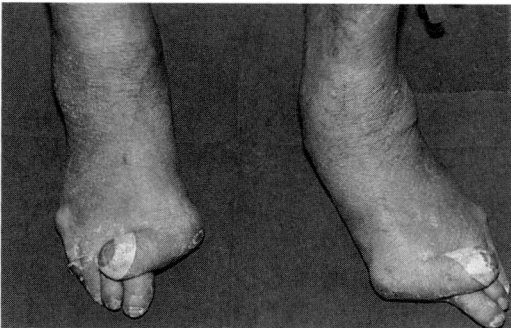

[b]

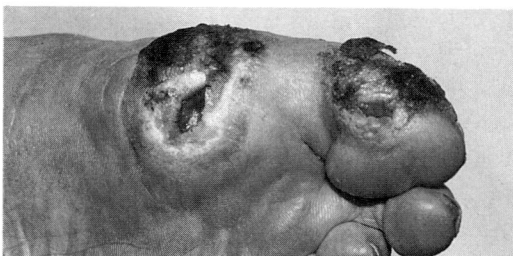

[c]

and length of stride. In older people the transverse arch may flatten out and the pads of fibro-fatty subcutaneous tissue under the metatarsal phalangeals may atrophy. The consequent loss of protection may precipitate ulceration there, one of the main weight-bearing surfaces of the foot severely affecting weight transference.

'Much foot pain is due to arthritis or rheumatism – usually mechanical in origin, the consequence of trauma or wearing inappropriate footwear earlier in life' (Dieppe, 1990). The typical deformities of rheumatoid arthritis include, pronation of the hind foot, flattening of the longitudinal arch, hallux valgus, splayed forefoot, corns, hammer and claw toes. A foot affected by rheumatoid arthritis – where the muscles are weakened, ligaments lax and cartilages and bones eroded may become deformed in a very short period of time, i.e. weeks or months, if it is crammed into badly-fitting shoes (Hart, 1983). Dieppe (1990) observed that pain and deformity are more important causes of functional impairment than loss of movement.

In older people even minor foot disorders can cause major disturbance in function whereas obesity and swollen lower limbs can also exacerbate the problem of finding suitable footwear.

People who need foot care often do not realize it, and there may be a good reason behind this behaviour. The common structural and functional disorders of the adult foot stem mainly from developmental anomalies of childhood and adolescence. If these problems are not corrected and some residual deformity results, increasing malfunction may occur. The shape of the foot may have become deformed so gradually that the client was not aware of the change. Occupational factors also contribute to the incidence of adult foot complaints (Neale et al., 1989). The majority of the elderly people present clinically with established deformities, often multifactorial in origin (for general information see Chapters 6 and 7).

Some older people neglect their feet through ignorance whereas others falsely attribute problems to the ageing process. In addition, frail old people may be incapable of carrying out the necessary self-care procedures — it can be extremely awkward to cut toe nails and wash and dry feet if the necessary trunk, hip and knee flexibility has been lost.

Nature and Size of the Problem

As people age, they become more likely to have foot problems and experience greater difficulty in finding shoes that can alleviate their suffering and promote safe mobility. A survey of men and women over 65 years of age in the USA found that almost three-quarters of the fully active older adults complained of painful feet (Evanski, 1982). Corns and calluses caused over half of these problems, painful toe nails a third, tender bunions and cold feet were present in a quarter of this group. Many presented with multiple problems and Evanski (1982) claimed that over 80% of adults in the USA will suffer at some time from at least one significant foot condition and that the majority of people attending a foot-clinic will be 65 years or older.

Old age is also likely to be accompanied by reduced financial resources as well as increasing difficulty in coping with the complex shoe market. Kwok (1994) found that older people admitted to an English hospital rarely had suitable footwear. An earlier study reported that 46% of all older people admitted to an Irish hospital were at risk due to non-existent or potentially dangerous footwear (Finlay, 1986). This figure has since risen to almost 60%.

Furthermore there are rarely any other suitable shoes at home. Clients seem to have little knowledge as to what constitutes a safe shoe and therefore they often require help in obtaining a suitable product. The shoe trade, with its strong concentration on fashion, markets little of use to older people, and as a result many are reduced to wearing shoes or slippers that fail to provide the optimum conditions for safe mobility. When moving about effectively in one's own surroundings is already difficult, unhelpful footwear can be the final straw which tips an older person into dependence.

Footwear

Although the aim of rehabilitation among older people is to maximize functional mobility, the evaluation of footwear, which is crucial for comfortable feet and willingness to weightbear, is often overlooked. In any setting, regardless of the cause of gait impairment, appropriate footwear can improve foot comfort and gait stability, whereas inappropriate slippers or shoes are a potential hazard.

Footwear may be classified as commercial, orthopaedic, or temporary. *Commercial footwear* can usually be purchased in any shoe shop.

Extra wide or extra deep styles while not defined as orthopaedic footwear, are difficult to obtain in shops, but often available from specialist mail order companies. The uppers are usually made of leather with light-weight soles, weighing approximately 300–400 g/pair and they are slightly more expensive than a similar product in the stores.

Semi-orthopaedic footwear is supplied from specialist suppliers, usually 'off-the-shelf' or in a few days. They are moulded shoes, normally made of leather but with light-weight synthetic soles and are similar in weight to the extra wide styles. Usually the cost is at least double that of the commercial extra wide or deep styles.

Orthopaedic or bespoke footwear is hand-made to suit the individual need. Delivery time is considerably longer than off-the-shelf designs, depending upon refit requirements and modifications. The uppers are usually leather or suede, and the soles either leather or synthetic. Their weight depends upon the style but are commonly two to four times heavier than moulded designs. The cost can be at least twice that of semi-orthopaedic styles.

Temporary plastazote, vinyl and tweed footwear can be made by specially trained staff. First a negative cast in plaster of Paris is made directly from the client's foot, then the shoe is made on the cast using one sheet of plastazote, $\frac{1}{2}$ metre of tweed and resin for sole. The total cost of the shoe is that of these materials plus approximately one hour of staff time. Their weight depends upon the type of sole chosen.

Regulations about the Provision of Footwear

In the UK, regulations relating to prescribed footwear indicate that where the clinical needs of the client can be met by a standard article, or such an article adapted, specially made appliances should not be supplied under the National Health Service.

In the USA health care for those people over 65 years of age falls under the Medicare Federal Health Care Plan, mandated by the Federal Government. Many of the so called 'appliances' are not covered under Medicare unless there is an absolutely clear indication for one specific appliance.

In Canada, the cost of specialist footwear, if prescribed by a physician, is borne through the Provincial Health Plan, but maybe only in part. Each province has an assistive devices programme which covers the cost of specialist footwear, as well as other devices, for those who do not have the means to pay for them. There are also many private insurance plans, mostly employer sponsored, which may pay the cost of assistive devices. If podiatrists provide a service, the client then bears the whole cost. However, the majority of older people in these countries, can be provided with effective footwear from the commercial market even when may require slightly wider and deeper styles than fashion shoes.

Acceptability and Cost

Footwear is of real psychological importance to the wearer. Shoes, which are always visible, can reflect self-image and identity. Adults who have to wear special footwear often resent these visible symbols of their disability. Whatever their age, wearers can experience real social stigma because of their 'funny shoes' with feelings of peer pressure to wear shoes that look normal. Not surprisingly, therefore, the desire to do so can be intense (Disabled Living Foundation, 1990). A survey in Northern Ireland contrasts the factors about footwear considered to be most important by the clients with those identified by therapy staff (Finlay, 1986). Ranked in order of importance to the clients were: comfort, appearance, colour, cost, and those listed by the staff were: depth, width, life-style, short-term management, deformities.

In the UK, when people have had difficulty in acquiring suitable commercial footwear and bespoke shoes appeared to be the only alternative, some apparently unnecessary and unacceptable products have been supplied leading to a high level of rejection (Herold and Palmar, 1992). The result has been a waste of £2 million per annum at national level.

The Ideal Shoe

The essential components of good shoes are that they fit well, assist the wearer to stand and to move in comfort and safety, maximize stability, protect the feet and keep them warm but not overheated, are easy to put on and off and to fasten and unfasten, and suit the individual's lifestyle (Disabled Living Foundation, 1990). In general, a balance is required between the need for fit, support, independence, ability and lifestyle, while at the same time assisting the wearer to stand, balance and move in as much comfort and safety as possible (Figure 2).

The Physiotherapist and Footwear Management

Any one of the following professionals can take responsibility for establishing a footwear provision scheme: the admission nurse, the occupational therapist, the physiotherapist or the chiropodist (see also Chapter 25). There is no real equivalent of the British chiropodist in Canada, although a training programme has been set up in Ontario; but even in the UK chiropodists do not necessarily see many of these clients.

Physiotherapists are already responsible for ensuring that a client's environment is safe, and footwear, like clothing in general, is part of that environment. Physiotherapists are in the ideal situation to evaluate the footwear, consider the fit and safety and assess clients' needs. They understand the structures of the foot and the biomechanics of gait and weight transference, as well as the movements required in the joints of the foot and ankle to achieve normal movement during locomotion. They are well-placed to identify risk factors and/or abnormalities in the feet

Figure 2   A low cost style that fulfils the criteria for safe footwear (laced, wide flat heels, firm heel counters, light-weight non-slip soles and soft supportive uppers).

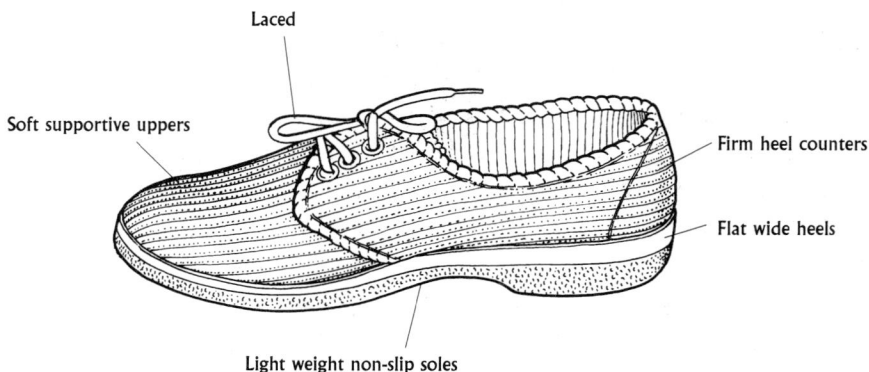

Laced

Soft supportive uppers

Firm heel counters

Flat wide heels

Light weight non-slip soles

and footwear, and to recommend any shoe modifications that may be required to re-align body weight, prevent deformity, increase the potential for mobility or improve safety.

A footwear scheme within a physiotherapy department in Northern Ireland has been described (Finlay, 1986). The experience gained has demonstrated that it is possible to have acceptable alternative cost-effective solutions to provide safe footwear.

Manufacturers were encouraged to consider the needs of older people and provide safe products on wider and deeper lasts at a reasonable cost. New, more appropriate styles were developed that have since proved satisfactory and are currently manufactured in bulk for the hospital. A wide selection of suitable products from the commercial market have been brought together in the physiotherapy department to satisfy a variety of needs and to provide clients with the opportunity of doing so effectively before the health care system sends them down the more expensive alternative route to custom-made footwear.

This scheme has provided value for money for the tax-payer as well as the client. In one year the average unit cost for custom-made footwear in the UK is about 20–25 times greater than the average cost in the physiotherapy department-based scheme. In contrast, in the same year, the rate of complaints about the local scheme were 0.3% compared with the UK average dissatisfaction rate of 17% (Herold and Palmar, 1992).

When bespoke footwear is required, joint clinics with State Registered Chiropodists or Orthotists may be advisable.

Planning and Developing a Footwear Service

Managers wishing to set up a service are advised to first define and quantify the need. Ideally, they should carry out a survey amongst the anticipated client group and identify their needs if any.

They are also advised to prepare a business plan and consider resource implications. The latter should include a location which offers privacy, staff with the necessary skills, equipment to be bought, handouts to be prepared, suitable stock to purchase, storage, stock levels, cash flow. They may also wish to seek further expert help from other professionals who may make referrals especially with respect to estimating demand, also business managers, social service workers, ward and community nursing staff, chiropodists, purchasing and finance department staff as well as local footwear suppliers and manufacturers. When plans are well advanced all relevant departments should be informed, and a date for implementation arranged.

Stock

It is important to identify suitable normal fitting, and extra-deep commercial products to provide an off-the-shelf service. A realistic target is to be able to supply off-the-shelf products within 3 working days of referral.

A variety of colours allows clients to indulge their preferences and with respect to people in hospital or resident in care-homes, it avoids increasing any appearance of institutionalization. Confused or poorly sighted clients should be supplied with a colour contrasting to the flooring, to facilitate foot-placement.

All products should be tested on various floor

surfaces (wet and dry). To facilitate stock control, stock can be coded and controlled with the aid of a computer program. Products made to the department's specifications usually require 3–4 months before delivery so accurate prediction of future need is advisable. On the other hand surplus or over stocking affects cash flow and reduces the cost effectiveness of the service. Nevertheless the service should be in a position to provide odd-sized or single shoes if required, while charging for only one pair or a single shoe.

Equipment

The following items are recommended: a standard foot measure, a small size goniometer, a fitting stool, a set of thermo-plastic bridges to measure forefoot depth, long and short handled shoe horns, scissors, a tape-measure, a set of blocks of different heights to assess discrepancies in leg length and a set of wedges ranging from 3–5 degrees, which are useful when re-aligning weight. The examiner will also find a hand-held mirror a useful adjunct for inspecting the plantar surface of the foot.

Assessment

Observation

In order to detect static malalignment and bio-mechanical abnormalities of gait, feet should also be examined during standing and walking, both with and without shoes (Chapter 7) (Thomas, 1989). Assess the alignment of hindfoot as well as that of the forefoot, as the stance of the hind-foot, especially the heel, determines the position of the forefoot (Kelihian, 1982). Hindfoot alignment is best observed from behind the client.

It may be beneficial to videotape the gait rather than ask the client to walk up and down several times. Besides avoiding overtiring a frail old person, it allows the gait to be analysed repetitively, if necessary.

Any of the following conditions should be noted and recorded: dry, flaking skin or open lesions which could lead to bacterial invasion, nail disorders, signs of circulatory disorders, deformities such as hallux valgus, bunions, claw or hammer toes, or overlapping toes, dropped or pronated feet. Actual or impending ulceration should be charted to ensure that pressure can be reduced over these points. Any swelling of the lower limbs may need further attention such as intermittent pressure therapy, with or without support stockings being recommended. Tendon sheaths, bursae and joints should be checked for localized swelling and the extent of preservation of the longitudinal arch should be observed.

Older people should be encouraged to discard tight constrictive garters or tight-banded below or above knee socks and to explain why they feel the need for any homemade 'remedies', such as newspaper insoles.

Palpation

Each foot should be carefully palpated to identify any areas of localized tenderness and swelling.

Measurements

Length and width are measured using SI units. Both these dimensions are measured while the client is weight-bearing as well as non-weight bearing as they usually increase by 1 cm when standing (Finlay, 1986). Width is taken as the circumference of the forefoot at the metatarso-phalangeal joints.

If measurements cannot be taken in standing,

then the foot should be placed on a stool with the knee flexed to 45 degrees and the foot at right angles to the lower limb. Measurements must be taken at each fitting as few adults remain the same shoe size throughout maturity, and variations can even be found at different times of the day. On rare occasions, both morning and evening footwear have to be supplied to accommodate the swelling that develops by evening e.g. with heart failure.

Thermo-plastic bridges over the foot are used at the level of the metarsophalangeal joints to establish whether the depth of the feet can be accommodated easily in commercial styles (Figure 3). If the first metatarsophalangeal joint is deviated, the angle of deviation is measured with a small goniometer (Figure 4).

When swelling is present the circumference of the ankle is measured at the level of the malleoli (or at a fixed distance from the floor if they are masked

Figure 3   Thermo-plastic bridge measures forefoot swelling. Using the bridge system one can establish in general terms what depth of feet can be accommodated easily in styles from the commercial market.

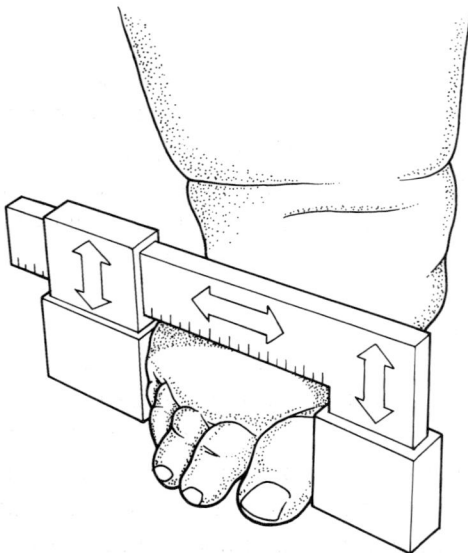

by severe swelling), the circumference of the forefoot at the metatarsophalangeal joints, and the distance from the tip of the heel passing at 45 degrees up to the front of the ankle joint. Careful records should be kept of the exact protocol followed.

Examination of current footwear

Observed wear of the sole and heel of the shoe can often verify a history of gait problems, or alert the therapist to the likely presence of one. It may indicate where excessive pressure has been exerted. Wear and tear at the tip of the sole may indicate foot drop, excessive wear at the heels may often be the result of foot shuffling while sitting for long periods. Similarly uneven wear on the sole or the heel may indicate an uneven weight alignment and the need for modification. Mis-shapen items can suggest a contributory factor to recent falls as can cut upper.

Assessing Under Plantar Pressure by Dynamic Footprint

Under plantar pressure is measured using a two plate system, each plate measures $630 \times 325 \times 32$ mm. The position of plates can be adjusted to accommodate length of individual stride. This system provides 2048 sensors in a matrix 64×32 cm. The footprint data is displayed as coloured squares, each square corresponding to the sensor on the plate. The colour of each square represents the pressure against time applied to that sensor; different colours correspond to different pressure values, with the pressure values being displayed at the right hand side of the window. The pressure is recorded in kg/cm^2. This system also provides coloured dynamic footprints that can be obtained in three dimensions.

Figure 4   Small goniometer used to measure deviation of the first toe.

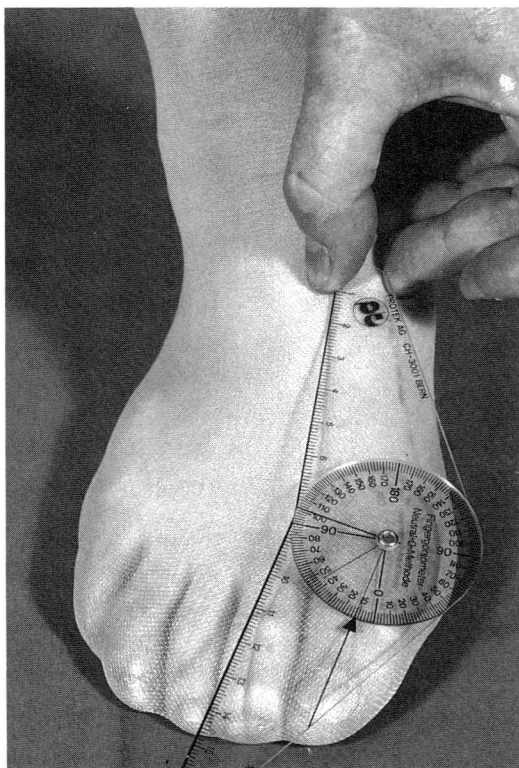

The client data is first recorded, and this includes the client's weight in kilograms. If independent, the client walks across the plates (if minimal support is required, the plates are placed between the parallel bars for safety). The printout superimposes the line of weight transference from heel-strike to toe-off. The computer scans the footplate and gives qualitative and quantative measurements of the pressure of each weight bearing area of the foot.

This equipment quantifies and supports sound clinical judgement. It can also be used to provide bio-feedback for the client by demonstrating and recording change.

Goal-setting

After the assessment, the care plan and goals must be clarified, with the client and any carers being involved in the discussions of options and in making decisions. This process can be facilitated by photographs, catalogues, easy to understand handouts, wall charts and most importantly by encouraging the client to try on several pairs of the indicated shoe size as well as some slightly larger or smaller. However, should the advice given prove unacceptable, the physiotherapist should then ensure the safety of the shoes the person prefers to wear, as far as it is possible to do so. The client and any relatives or other carers should be provided with sufficient written information to be able to make an informed decision about future purchases. A record should be made of the advice given and any action taken.

Factors to be Considered when Recommending Footwear

Weight

Shoes should be light-weight yet supportive, heavy products will be particularly disadvantageous to frail older clients. Slippy soles, together with excessive length, hazardous heels, unsupportive uppers and inadequate fastening may all contribute to feelings of insecurity.

Soles

These should be non-slip. If they are very smooth, such as leather or non-ribbed plastic, they may slide on wet surfaces and contribute to falls whereas deeply cleated soles, i.e. with high ridges may increase the likelihood of tripping and even immobilize an apraxic person. Soles should be of adequate thickness for protection. Robbins *et al.* (1992) suggested that shoes with thin, hard soles are preferable for optimal stability among older individuals, but some people find that thin flexible soles aggravate under-sole problems (Rose, 1981). A person suffering from Parkinsonism may find that the slight slippage from leather soles facilitates movement, however.

Shoes fitted to artificial limbs are easier to apply if they have flexible soles. Flexibility also permits the artificial foot, itself flexible, to be used in as normal a manner as possible with good 'toe-off'. Stick-on rubber soles should be avoided as they reduce flexibility. Robbins *et al.* (1992) found that shoes with thick yielding midsoles, such as running shoes, tend to increase the risk of falling among unstable older men.

Heels

The upright body is basically unstable, relative to height. This instability will be increased by tapered or high heels, and increases upon movement. Thus, heel height is critical, and should not exceed 3.6 cm, providing as stable a base as possible. Balance problems may increase with high heels or sling backs. The metatarsophalangeal joints are most likely to be affected (about 77%), when a person with rheumatoid arthritis develops joint erosion (Brook and Corbett, 1977). Because as much protection as possible is needed for these vulnerable small joints, heels should not exceed 2.5 cm.

An obese person will find a wedge heel more supportive than the conventional heel as extreme weight can put excessive pressure on the midsole, destroying the shape of the shoe's upper.

Metal protectors or edging can be treacherous on wet pavements, or on stairs with metal nosing, and should be avoided.

Heel counters are the stiffener at the back of a shoe running around the heel inside the shoe. They should be firm to ensure that adequate support is provided, in slippers as well as in shoes. The manufacturing construction is important. Counters should lie between the lining and the shoe upper leaving no rough surfaces exposed to traumatize vulnerable skin. The physiotherapist should ensure that the edges are properly bound. Heel cradles are the part of the insole on which the heel rests inside the shoe. They should be supportive, and preferably of some shock absorbing material. The depth of this insock is highly critical, as excessive thickness can inhibit proprioception.

When a person uses a cane its height should be adjusted when the person is wearing flat shoes. They should be warned that should they alter the height of their heels, they may alter the effectiveness of their appliance. If an above-knee limb has been fitted, the heel height should not be altered without contacting the limb centre, as it may affect the alignment of the limb.

Uppers

Traditionally, leather uppers were claimed to be best, but this is not necessarily true today. An important factor is that in order to minimize foot odours, they should be permeable, and provide adequate foot support. Plastic or non-permeable footwear can exacerbate problems of foot hygiene, and increase the risk of lesions developing which in turn can affect gait. Seams and stitching on the uppers can cause roughness, especially in canvas styles. Unlined products should be dye-fast and checked for seam finishes. Hardened and discoloured leather or suede may indicate incontinence; in this case, man-made uppers are often preferable. Shoes should be comfortable from the start; it is inadvisable to recommend that a shoe will stretch with wear.

Linings

Smooth linings of absorbent material are recommended if a person suffers from excessive sweating or has lower limbs that slough or weep with excessive fluid exudation. Sweating can be aggravated by nylon linings.

Vamp openings and fastenings

Easy access for the feet into shoes is essential, especially for old people who may not be able to reach their feet easily and for those who wear an orthosis. A six-eyelet style or velcro fastened style that allows easy access to the toe box is usually the most satisfactory. Excessive swelling on the dorsum of the foot can often be accommodated by this style.

Laces should hold the foot secure, maximum effect is achieved if sited over the instep. Elastic laces should be avoided, as often sufficient support is not achieved. Heavy duty velcro fastenings are helpful for stroke clients or those who have lost fine finger movement. Zip fastenings are satisfactory in slippers or boots, and strapped styles are acceptable if they hold the foot in a stable position. Loose or overlong fastenings can lead to a shuffling gait. Slip-on footwear, not equipped with fastenings, may increase the tendency to claw or hammer toes.

Toe box

This area should provide sufficient room to ensure that the under surface is not in contact or causing friction on the toes. A hardened or stiffened toe-cap is unsuitable when a person's toes are painful or deformed. Extra depth will be required if swelling, clawed or hammer toes are present.

Length

There should be at least 1.2 cm gap between the end of the longest toe and the interior front surface. Slip-on styles are often too short with the foot being compressed between the heel counter and the toe box, often resultng in swelling being forced upwards onto the dorsum of the foot. Slip-on shoes, mules or slippers often encourage clawing of the toes in order to increase ground contact and improve stability.

Width

Insufficient width is often compensated by the purchase of unnecessarily large sizes. Ideally there must be adequate space across the ball of the foot and the toes, yet not too excessive otherwise the foot will slip forward and cause instability.

Depth

Usually forefoot depths of less than 4.0 cm can be accommodated from the commercial market. Depths 4.0–5.5 cm will require a semi-bespoke style. Should the depth exceed 5.5 cm then bespoke footwear is usually required with a longer delivery time which can mean that the client has often gone home before final fitment.

Modifying Footwear

Modifications to commercial footwear can play a crucial part in keeping older people on their feet and maximizing their function. Modifications or adaptations may be either temporary or permanent. Temporary alterations can help people to come to terms with the need for modifications to their shoes and to appreciate the benefit to be gained. Physiotherapists use them to evaluate potential benefit and acceptability prior to making or ordering permanent changes, thereby avoiding waste in terms of time and materials. An added advantage of the adaptations being made within the department is that the modified footwear can often be completed on the same day or even within a single treatment.

The cost of all modifications in the UK is the responsibility of the hospital but making them in the physiotherapy department can lead to considerable savings to the hospital budget.

Raises

Raises are applied under the heel of a shoe and usually under the sole as well, to add length to that leg. They are most commonly used to correct true shortening leading to differences in leg length, especially when the difference is greater than 1.5 cm. Quite apart from the effect on balance, such differences require the body to make large adjustments that may prove harmful in the longer term. Among the various problems that might arise are: an unstable waddling or Trendelberg gait, back pain, compensatory scoliolis.

Usually, the body can compensate for differences of less than 1.5 cm but people with marked uncorrected leg shortening often adopt hazardous compensatory postures. The foot may be held in the equino varus position when walking, thereby reducing the area of support dramatically and increasing the pressure exerted per square centimetre. Alternatively, they may try to equalize leg length by walking with a flexed knee on the contralateral side.

When correcting large differences, it is advisable to keep the raise as light as possible. To this end the height of the raise can be 1.5 cm less than the true difference, as the body will usually accommodate to this small difference. A raise is usually applied to the whole length of the shoe and tapered at the toe to facilitate swing through during gait. When the raise is less than 1.5 cm, a taper of 0.5 cm is sufficient but when the raise is greater than 2.5 cm the tapering can be as much as 1.5 cm, to ensure a smooth heel-to-toe transference of weight.

Material coloured to match the shoes renders raises, wedges and floats less conspicuous. Contact adhesive is satisfactory for the majority of composition rubber modifications, but very occasionally it slides off. Physiotherapists should check the manufacturer's specifications to verify the suitability of the product and the precautions to be taken. It is essential to use these adhesives in well ventilated areas and some manufacturers recommend the use of odour masks.

Trials using temporary raises should always precede permanent application. Some people who present with long-standing leg shortening may have compensated adequately, so the temporary raise makes little improvement in symptoms or function indicating that a permanent one is unnecessary. Clients often have difficulty accepting the need for a shoe raise, so it is advisable to apply a temporary raise at first to allow them to get used to the idea.

Light-weight slippers will rarely support raises. Occasionally when a raise is indicated but the person adamantly refuses to wear shoes then certain types of heavy duty soled slippers can be used and often if a raise is required then it may help frail older people with very low levels of function to transfer or to walk a few steps. To be modified successfully, the slipper should have a fastening rather than being a slip-on model and it should have a heavy duty sole; nevertheless, such a slipper will rarely provide adequate support if the person is obese.

Various materials can be used to make raises. High density polyethelene foam splinting material is satisfactory for short-term, temporary raises but it is not ideal for permanent ones due to its lack of flexibility. However it can be satisfactory if applied in two pieces on the sole and heel with a 'waist' between. Micro rubber or a synthetic composition are usually more satisfactory, especially for raises greater than 2.5 cm. For such high raises, lighter but more expensive cork is best.

Sandals are available which can be strapped temporarily over normal shoes to provide a raise. They allow cork or plastazote raises of different heights to be inserted under the sole of the client's shoe. Unfortunately they can make walking difficult. It is more satisfactory to use strapping to fix the raise directly onto the outside of the heel. Care has to be taken not to put any strapping directly onto leather uppers as it can damage the surface.

Wedges

A wedge is used for stabilization and can be applied to heels or soles or both. Various gait problems can be alleviated by wedging:

- A person with rheumatoid arthritis who, when viewed from behind, has an angle greater than 50% between the line of the tibial shaft and the calcaneum, may find that an inner heel wedge is sufficient to relieve symptoms (Thomas 1989).
- After a stroke resulting in flaccid paralysis, a person may require re-alignment of body-weight to prevent the ankle ligaments being stretched through abnormal stresses when weight bearing.
- Genu valgum can usually be improved when the distance between the malleoli is less than 7.5 cm. Wedges can rarely effectively alter weight alignment when malleoar separation is greater.
- Clients suffering from antropulsion should have heels wedged from 1.5 cm at the front to 0 cm at the back to counteract the forward thrust.
- Clients suffering from retropulsion should wear heels as low as possible, to bring their body-weight forward. Occasionally further alteration in posture will be achieved by adding a wedge at the back of the heel tapering to nothing at the front.

The severity and type of deformity dictates the size, degree of slope and position of the wedge. It is tapered towards the middle or the opposite side of the shoe depending on the amount of re-alignment and weight remodification required and usually increases the area of ground contact. Commercially available self-adhesive trial wedges can be used to assess the angle of slope required. Besides wedging, exercises to improve strength and co-ordination of the muscles working over the foot and ankle may be recommended.

Floats

Floats are added to the outside of the shoe's heel to provide added support and to prevent the breakdown of the heel or counter when excessive weight or abnormal stresses are present. They also increase the area of floor contact.

Floats and wedges may be used in conjunction

with each other to improve stability. It is possible at times to widen heels (i.e. floats at both sides) for people where height of the heel exceeds safety levels and who refuse to change to safe footwear. This procedure should diminish the risks. A float should not protrude excessively as clients with narrow based gait may catch their other foot on it.

Insoles

Insoles are extra soles placed inside shoes. A wide variety is available and they can be used for several purposes. They can be helpful to people with painful or tender feet and to relieve pressure on vulnerable areas under the feet. The depth of the shoe must be deep enough to accommodate the insert and if the client suffers from periodic swelling a removable insole may be advisable.

The deeper and softer the insole the greater the risk of falling due to the reduction of propioception. Therefore the additional comfort for painful feet with greater depth of insole must be considered in relation to safety. A young person with very tender feet due to rheumatoid arthritis can cope with soft insoles 1.0 cm or even 1.5 cm deep but an older person may find that such insoles decrease postural stability. Polyethelene foam insoles are more suitable for old people. They may be more comfortable covered with either pig skin, shiver skin, chamois leather or a similar product. When longitudinal or transverse arch supports are required, it is helpful to place these between the two layers of polyethelene foam or the insock, ensuring the support maintains its correct position in the shoe.

Toe Fillers

Toe fillers may provide the answer when it is not possible nor desirable to obtain two shoes of the same style but in different sizes, for example following partial amputation of the forefoot. The filler is inserted into the toe box to fill-up the extra space in the larger shoe. A potential danger is the tendency for the tip of the shoe to crease and add to the risk of tripping.

A cast is made of the shorter foot and a polyethelene foam filler fashioned to occupy the space left in the toe-box, but it should not fully occupy it. Besides polyethelene foam, microcellular latex may be used, or the fillers faced with this type of latex or a similar substance to prevent friction with the foot. In addition, tongue pads should be used to hold the foot well back and to afford extra protection.

Tongue Pads

A tongue pad is useful if the person's foot tends to slip forward in the shoe, as may happen when the shoe is too long. This heel slippage causes pressure on the forefoot. The pad is made of adhesive orthopaedic felt or microcellular latex or similar material which is shaped and stuck in place on the under surface of the tongue. It will keep the foot back in the heel cup and make some extra space under the toe box so helping to prevent excessive pressure on the toes.

Temporary Footwear

Occasionally when clients are admitted to hospital with grossly swollen feet, or a contagious condition, footwear must be supplied urgently if they are not to be left to walk about barefoot. There are numerous commercial products available for this, many of which are unsupportive and far from ideal. Foam and towelling slippers provide little or no heel support and are often difficult to put on, although they do have excellent non-slip, ribbed rubber soles. Foam styles are unsuitable for smokers or for use close to open fires, even if fire retardant. Rigid sole designs with adjustable straps provide ground protection but little support and are generally unsatisfactory. A physiotherapist involved in footwear management should be able to produce a well fitting, cosmetically acceptable, temporary, made-to-measure product, within hours of referral. They should be reasonably supportive, have non-slip soles, be cosmetically acceptable and cater for the needs of the individual client in the short-term. Various designs have been developed (Harrison, 1984; Kinsman, 1980) and the choice depends upon the condition and the shape of the foot and ankle. Composition rubber may be used to make the soles and heels. Clients may find the pink uppers unacceptable when the shoes are made of plastazote. This problem can be avoided if upholstery tweed is applied over the plastazote; this also facilitates aeration.

Heavy duty velcro for the fastening can be sewn in place with a household sewing machine, providing very inconspicuous and satisfactory fastenings.

Gross or enlarged ankles can be accommodated best in the two piece 'Kaffir' design which can be moulded under the oedematous tissue, thus providing a neater fit. It is easier to reduce the height of the heel cup in this model. Care must be taken to ensure the sole is sufficiently supportive otherwise it tends to disintegrate at the midtarsal area. Should the forefoot swelling exceed 7–9 cm in depth, when measured at the metatarsophalangeal joint with a bridge, then the wrap-round pattern is the more comfortable and robust.

Advice to Clients

Physiotherapists advise on footcare and to improve retention of the information, supplement this with user-friendly leaflets. Although there are many commercially available, the advice they give may seem patronizing and even banal. It may be advisable for a service to draw up its own to reflect local needs. In some areas it may be thought necessary to remind people to 'Clean your feet daily using warm water and a soft cloth', or always to wear socks or stockings and 'change them daily'. All leaflets should warn clients to 'Regularly use moisturising cream to condition your feet' (if they can reach their feet), not to walk barefoot especially if they suffer from diabetes or reduced sensation as they may be unaware of injury from sharp objects, that if they wear modified shoes they should also wear modified slippers, that antislip overshoes are necessary in icy weather, and to wear low heeled shoes and not reduce walking speeds or safety by wearing hazardous products outdoors, as this will increase the risk of road traffic accidents (Finlay, 1993).

Summary

Foot problems of the older client present the physiotherapist with many challenges. Incorporating footwear management into the programme of care results in an inexpensive approach that improves the quality of life of older people. This simple method can minimize the risk of accidents, reduce pain, improve function, in some instances reduce the task of carers and bring pleasure into the life of those who required help and advice.

Knowledge of footwear is surprisingly low amongst professionals and the public alike. There is a need

- to establish more cost effective schemes to

provide easier provision of footwear to frail and elderly people,

- to ensure a speedy response to need,
- to encourage manufacturers to produce satisfactory products for older people, to ensure comfort, reduce accidents and improve mobility,
- for more education for health care professionals in this complex subject,
- for the undergraduate curriculum to include 'footwear and associated problems',
- to educate people to care about their feet.

References

Brook, A., Corbett, M (1977) Radiographic changes in early rheumatoid disease. *Annals of the Rheumatic Diseases* 36: 71–73.

Dieppe, P, Cooper, C, Kirwan, J, Mcgill, N (1990) *Arthritis and Rheumatism. The Foot and Ankle* pp. 3.44–3.49. London, New York: Gower Medical Publishing.

Disabled Living Foundation (1990) *Footwear – A Quality Issue.* London: Disabled Living Foundation.

Evanski, PM (1982) The geriatric foot. In Jahss, MH (ed) *Disorders of the Foot and Ankle* 2nd edn, pp. 964–978. Philadelphia: WB Saunders.

Finlay, O (1986) Footwear management in the elderly care programme. *Physiotherapy Journal* 72: 4.

Finlay, O (1993) Exercise training and walking speeds in elderly woman following hip surgery: 'Beating the Little Man'. *Physiotherapy Journal* 79: 12.

Hart, FD (1983) *Practical Problems in Rheumatogy: The Foot*, p. 48. London: Dunitz.

Harrison, RA (1984) A simple pattern for plastazote boots. *Physiotherapy Journal* 70: 114–115.

Herold, DC, Palmar, RG (1992) Questionnaire study of the use of surgical shoes prescribed in a rheumatology outpatient clinic. *Journal of Rheumatology* 19: 1542–1554.

Kelihian, H (1982) The adult foot, the hallux. In Jahss, MH (ed) *Disorders of the Foot and Ankle* 2nd edn, p. 589–621. Philadelphia: WB Saunders.

Kinsman, R (1980) Do it yourself shoe. *Physiotherapy* 66: 304–305.

Kwok, T (1994) A survey of in-patients footwear. *Care of the Elderly Journal* March: 118.

Neale, D, Boyd, PM, Whiting, MF (1989) The adult foot. In Neale, D. Adams, IM (eds) *Common Foot Disorders*, pp. 53–59. London: Churchill Livingstone.

Robbins, S, Gouw, GJ, McClaren, J (1992) Shoe sole thickness and hardness influence balance in older men. *Journal of the American Geriatric Society* 40: 1089–1094.

Roggero, P, Blanc, Y, Krupp, S (1993) Foot reconstruction in weight bearing areas. Long term results and gait analysis. *European Journal of Plastic Surgery* 16: 186–192.

Rose, GK (1981) The geriatric foot. *Geriatric Medicine* December: 17–20.

Thomas, WH (1989) The ankle and foot. In Kelly, WN *et al.* (eds) *Textbook of Rheumatology* 3rd edn, p. 2072. Philadelphia: WB Saunders.

27

Ethical and Legal Issues

SARITA VERMA

Introduction

Mr G. is a 98-year-old man who has had a long history of heart problems and had a major stroke two days ago which left his right arm and leg paralysed. He is also unable to speak or swallow solid foods. He is found on the ward late at night with a significantly increased respiratory rate and fast heartbeat. It is likely that he will need a respirator and may never recover. The health care team struggles with the decision to provide aggressive interven-tion. The nurse A wants to call the 'intensive care team'; Dr B suggests someone call the family and ask them what to do; the physiotherapist thinks that comfort measures would be best; the medical student wonders what Mr G would say; the hospital administrator is worried that Mr G.'s son, a lawyer, might sue if he dies.

This case illustrates many of the ethical and legal issues confronting health care professionals, including physiotherapists, in contemporary society — especially relating to older and chronically ill adults (see Chapter 3). Older people and their interaction within the health care system can raise several clinical issues, which may require the skill and expertise of an ethicist or a lawyer to solve. Such services are not always available or accessible at crucial times, so one is well advised to be learned in some basic ethical and legal principles (see also Chapters 3 and 23).

> The branch of philosophy concerned with principles that allow us to make decisions about what is right and wrong is called ethics or moral philosophy. Medical ethics is specifically concerned with moral principles and decisions in the context of medical practice, policy and research. (Munson, 1992)

Moral rights are difficult to quantify but commonsense allows most people in developed countries to expect an internationally accepted standard of human behaviour. Although the concept of moral rights has its origins in religious and secular philosophy, it has been undeniably influenced by the international community, and includes the right:

- to be treated with respect and dignity,
- to freedom from slavery; unjust imprisonment or discrimination,
- to food, shelter and health care,
- to freedom of expression or religious persuasion,
- to counsel or legal representation,
- to freedom from persecution, risk of death and war,
- to vote.

While ethical principles form the basis for clinical decisions in health care, legal precepts and legislation govern a country and regulate application of these principles in a manner the community believes to be consistent with social and public policy. For example, euthanasia may be considered ethical by some people, but active euthanasia may be illegal according to the law of the state. Ethics exert a strong influence on the development of the law and in the evolution of public policy. People are always bound by the law but statutes and court decisions are constantly challenged by differing opinions on what a community may consider to be ethical. The current debate about assisted suicide exemplifies conflicting legal, ethical and religious views.

Health care technology has expanded considerably duing the last 25 years. With the continued demand for excellent and contemporary care, health care professionals face growing challenges in clinical decision-making. The shortages of health care finances put a strain on the allocation of services and the delivery of up-to-date resources to all people. Terms such as 'rationing' and 'fair distribution' are commonplace in countries where budget constraints necessitate difficult moral and ethical choices on services for infirm, chronically ill and poor people. These issues have become especially germane to the elderly. The 'greying' of our population has led to the reality that we are living longer (Chapter 2), but in a prolonged survival, a large proportion of health-care dollars are being spent on care during the last months of life. One out of seven health care dollars per year in the USA is spent on providing care during the final 6 months of someone's life. Older people comprise 70% of those who die each year and are therefore the most intensive consumers of end-of-life care monies (Carton and Brown, 1993). The equitable distribution of health care services among various generations raises a variety of ethical and legal concerns.

The health care professional is called upon to be the gatekeeper for these decisions, many of which have social and fiscal ramifications. Well-informed patients may demand the latest technology or medication for their condition.

Despite the recent proliferation of academic literature in medical ethics on this topic there continues to be a dearth of training or guidelines on how health care professionals should make these decisions, or how they should counsel patients in making their choices. Many of the ethical quandaries about old people arise in situations where the allocation of resources is judged inappropriate for reasons relating to the 'quality of life'. Is quality of life to be judged on the basis of age alone? Does this entitle the refusal of sophisticated health care such as heart surgery or dialysis to anyone say, over the age of 70, merely on the basis of their age? In countries like Canada one must ask whether it is constitutionally permissible to deny equal access to universal health care on the basis of age.

In providing health care to an ageing population one encounters a variety of ethical and legal issues. In many ways, the fields of ethics and law merge in this population, more than in any other group. Issues about competency and decision-making capacity have become very relevant. Health-care workers must meet the expected standard of care, avoid negligent actions and maintain confidentiality. The values of society and as individuals are put to a test with contemporary questions about the older people, relating to advance directives, euthanasia, assisted suicide, clinical experimentation, sexual impropriety, elder abuse, the use of aggressive interventions, and issues concerning confidentiality and consent.

This chapter will address many of these topics in relation to the older people. The emphasis of discussion will be on general principles. Although many of the legal examples are taken from Canadian sources, the essential principles are globally accepted. Specific statutory requirements differ between countries and so do their criminal laws. It is essential to consult the laws of each jurisdiction when confronted with a difficult legal problem. It is also prudent for all health care professionals to be versed in the standards of care and code of ethics laid down by their peers.

Ethical Considerations and Age-related Limits to Health Care

Over the last century, life expectancy at birth in developed countries has risen by 25 years. It is predicted that the number of people over the age of 100 in Canada, the USA, UK and Australia will triple. Much of the debate over health care resources stems from the fear that a 'demographic time bomb' will cause an unsustainable explosion of costs unless reasonable steps are taken to defuse it by setting limits to the utilization of services.

Age alone should not be a criterion to deny health care. However, in appropriate circumstances it may be ethical and legal to withhold certain interventions, such as cardiopulmonary resuscitation (CPR) or end-stage renal dialysis, from a patient. The elderly are generally considered to be persons aged 65 and older. Yet, functional age is quite different from chronological age and because people age at a different pace, there is little homogeneity in this group. Diseases, social conditions and financial status can have an influence on the natural progression of ageing changes in the human body. Thus, it is not appropriate to set rules for the care of older people by chronological age. This practice is commonly called 'ageism' (Chapter 3) and is generally regarded as being taboo in health care. Age itself may be a contributing factor, but it is the extent of co-existing chronic or debilitating illness alone which should influence clinical decision-making.

The accepted practice is to limit certain interventions to those circumstances where the benefit outweighs the risk and the outcome is more likely to be a favourable one. Thus, CPR, dialysis or intubation with the installation of a respirator may be withheld in situations where it is 'not clinically indicated' or considered to be 'futile'. Before the decision to do so, each case must be considered individually and all circumstances including the patient's wishes should be reviewed, preferably by the entire health care team. In the case of Mr G, in the scenario outlined at the beginning of this chapter, the team should investigate whether he had left directions or expressed wishes regarding the extent of intervention, or whether someone had been designated to make the decision in his place. They should look at the likelihood of a favourable outcome in his case if resuscitation or intubation should be offered and be prepared to justify their decisions based on scientific evidence and hospital practice. In any event, the patient's wishes will prevail in most jurisdictions.

In situations where clinical decisions must be made whether to offer or to withhold interventions such as CPR, dialysis, surgery, anticoagulation or transplantation, advanced age itself should not be the determining factor. Each case must be considered on its merits taking into account co-existing conditions, the individual's wishes, the common practice at the hospital or in the community and the availability of resources and funding. It is essential to know the legal requirements governing this area including constitutional law and criminal law.

Negligence and The Health Care Professional

Each health care profession has standards of practice and ethical codes. It is incumbent on every member of the profession to abide by these professional standards. With only rare exceptions, in medicine and other health care professions, the 'best interests' of the patient are paramount. Claims of negligence may arise against any health care professional and serve as the basis for malpractice lawsuits. In most countries, especially in the common law, liability for malpractice is established when four elements of negligence have been proved:

1. *Duty*: the clinician/health care professional had a legal duty to the patient or client as a consequence of an established relationship.
2. *Breach of the standard of care*: the clinician has broken (breached) that legal duty by failing to meet the standard of care.
3. *Damage*: the patient or client has sustained damage.
4. *Causation*: the damage was sustained in fact as a result of the clinician's breach of duty. It is necessary to prove a causal link between the breach of duty and the actual damage.

Health care professionals are expected to meet the reasonable standard of care which other members of the same profession would exercise in the same circumstances. A failure to meet these professional standards is a breach of duty and is subject to charges of negligence and disciplinary action by governing bodies of that health care profession in most countries. Many allegations of unprofessional conduct or negligence arise out of miscommunication. The maintenance of open communication and a good relationship between the patient and the clinician are crucial to the dynamics of health care.

> *Negligence arises when a health care professional has breached a legal duty of care and there are damages to the patient as a foreseeable result. All members must meet the standards of care laid down by the profession.*

Confidentiality

All health care workers have a legal and an ethical obligation to their patients to maintain the highest standards of confidentiality. Confidentiality is the practice of keeping all the information that is entrusted to them within the proper boundaries of their professional role. The principle of confidentiality has strong ethical underpinnings in the professional relationship of dependence and trust between a clinician and a patient. A person who has put him- or herself in the hands of a health care professional is entitled to expect that sensitive information will be kept in the highest regard and that control will be maintained over its dissemination. There are exceptions to the rule in special situations. When caring for older people, circumstances may arise where it is necessary to break confidentiality in the best interests of the patient, e.g. to discuss treatment options or changes in status with members of the family or when seeking the expert opinion of other health care professionals. But even in these circumstances it is prudent to obtain consent in advance.

It is very important to maintain the confidentiality of medical and other clinical records. In most countries, access to these records is allowed only to those persons who have obtained the patient's consent.

In certain cases, however, confidential information may be shared with others. This is potentially possible in:

1. a life-threatening emergency,
2. if the patient is incompetent or incapacitated and is unable to give consent,
3. if it is in the best interest of the patient's welfare,
4. to protect the public i.e. in outbreaks of infectious disease or imminent peril, such as in elder abuse, meningitis or dangerous psychiatric illness

> *Health care professionals have a special duty to keep information about their patients confidential. There are few exceptions to this. As a general rule, obtain the patient's consent to release information before sharing it with others.*

Consent

The laws on consent to treatment are very complex in most industrialized countries. Consent is an area where standards vary considerably from jurisdiction to jurisdiction. For example, the British standard continues to be professionally based, while the American States are divided, and in Canada the standard is more patient-centred. Consent must always be obtained from the patient for any health care intervention. Proper consent requires that:

1. the person giving consent is competent to do so and has mental capacity to make the decision,

2. there has been reasonable disclosure of the subject about which consent is sought and this has been free of misrepresentation or coercion,
3. the patient has had the opportunity to ask questions and to receive answers,
4. the person giving consent is able to demonstrate an understanding of the matter for which consent is sought and appreciate the consequences of giving or withholding consent.

If the patient is judged to be 'competent' to give consent, and it is a decision made after a reasonable disclosure of the facts, their decision must be honoured by the health care professional, even though it may seem to be unreasonable. For example, a person refusing extensive chemotherapy for disseminated breast cancer may choose to do so though others may believe that even the slightest chance of life-sustaining treatment should be vigorously pursued. In many countries, the wishes of Jehovah's Witnesses to refuse transfusions of blood or blood products have been upheld in court despite the fact that death was imminent without such transfusions.

If the person is not competent or capable to make the decision, the health care professional must look for a substitute-decision maker (usually the next-of-kin) or evidence that the patient expressed their wishes prior to the onset of the incapacity (i.e. in a living will or advance directive) before proceeding with treatment.

Always get consent from the patient. There are a few exceptions to this i.e. in an emergency. If there is doubt over the person's capacity to give consent, get a second opinion or look for a substitute decision-maker. Although a signed document is clear evidence of consent, consent may also be implied or expressed by the patient; consent must be specific to a particular treatment.

Competency and Decision-making Capacity

In the law of most countries, all adults are presumed to be competent, that is to say, to have decision-making capacity, unless proven otherwise. This presumption comes from the acknowledgement of an individual's right to liberty and autonomy. The responsibility to displace this presumption lies on the person alleging the incompetence. Society recognizes that an individual's liberty must be preserved, but it can be limited in situations where the individual's welfare or the public good are perceived as more important. This leads to the determination of incompetence in certain circumstances such as coma, significant dementia or mental illness, and the need for appointment of a guardian or substitute decision-maker.

Older people rarely refer themselves to a professional for the assessment of their competency. They are more often assessed for suspected mental losses after an event has occurred such as a fall (see Chapters 3 and 8), an illness or an episode of 'wandering'. The assessment of competency becomes particularly important when an older person is 'at risk of harm'. This can arise where there is concern that the person is unable to care for himself, i.e. prone to accidents with the stove, the iron or the car; shows poor personal hygiene, declining nutrition, wandering or delusional behaviour; is frequently lost or locked out of their home; or is showing an inability to take medications properly, pay bills on time or attend appointments (see Chapter 8).

Competency is a measure of an individual's ability to function in society, to make decisions for him or herself and to perform the tasks expected by society. A person may be competent for some tasks i.e. to feed and clean himself, but incompetent for others such as managing stocks, bonds and investments. A person may have a temporary loss of capacity while in a coma, and then regain it when medically stable. In the determination of competency, age is not a criterion; rather, it is an individual's ability to demonstrate an understanding and an appreciation of the facts and the ability to make a reasoned decision.

Professionals make informal determinations of a person's competence on a daily basis, i.e. when a person is too ill to get out of bed a health care worker may decide to feed and clean them. However, if there is doubt regarding a person's competence, such as in dementia or delirious states, a formal assessment of competence is desirable, even if this precipitates a legal or medical crisis.

Such an assessment is usually done by a physician or lawyer, and should always serve the 'best interests' of the patient. An assessment is always justified when a person is at risk of harming themsleves or the public and will not voluntarily accept help. An assessment is never justified where behaviour is merely eccentric or unusual.

> An older person's 'competency' is often called into question when it comes to financial or legal decisions such as managing finances or making a will . . . or the ability to drive. This issue also arises in situations where there is evidence that there is a loss of mental ability such as failing memory or an inability to manage at home. Rather than assume incompetence, a person should be formally assessed for a specific task and for a specific reason.

Euthanasia

The term 'euthanasia' comes from Greek meaning *eu*=well and *thanatos*=death. Literally translated the word means a painless or good death. Active euthanasia describes an actual act of doing something to end a life such as injecting poison, while passive euthanasia refers to inaction — by not doing something to save a life which could be saved i.e. by withholding CPR. Assisted suicide means helping someone to take the necessary steps to kill themselves i.e. to provide the means to take lethal doses of medication.

The controversy over euthanasia is one of the oldest and most difficult subjects in medical ethics, dating back to Greco-Roman times. In those days, it was acceptable, even honourable, for a person to commit suicide. Over the course of history, these attitudes have changed and have been significantly swayed by social, religious and moral influences. This has led to laws that prohibit suicide, or helping someone commit suicide in North America, while resulting in an acceptance in case law (but not in statute) of active euthanasia in parts of Europe. In the Netherlands 85% of assisted suicides occur in people over the age of 50 with medical illness (Koenig, 1993). This raises questions about the perceived value of life in later years.

The topic of euthanasia arises with older people in many clinical situations and the debate regarding its morality and legality continues to concern health care workers. When a patient is in unbearable pain, has an incurable or terminal illness or has a wretched quality of life due to infirmity and disability it is not infrequent to encounter expressed wishes for death and to 'put an end to it all', by a person who is cognitively intact and seems logical and rational. In these trying circumstances, a health care professional must show compassion and make reasonable efforts to ease suffering. Advocates for the legalization of euthanasia and assisted suicide maintain that such patients should be allowed to end their own lives and provided with assistance to do so. Opponents argue that legalization would open the doors for the abuse of older people, would not account for depression (which is common in this age group and with the chronically ill) and would send a message to both the old and the young that 'old age can have no meaning ... if accompanied by decline, pain and despair' (Callahan, 1987).

Active euthanasia and assisted suicide have not been legalized in most jurisdiction, although, in a case where a person requests to die or asks for assistance to commit suicide, a health care professional must exercise caution and compassion. There are situations where it is right to deny heroic medical intervention and treatment but this must be done in accordance with the law, in the best interests of the patient and taking into account the patient's wishes.

Other Challenges

Research Needs

Although most older people keep good health into old age, they have a higher prevalence of illness and disability, a greater utilization of prescription and non-prescription medications and a conspicuous use of hospital and health care services (Chapters 6 and 22). There is a clear need for more research and clinical experimentation on the diagnosis, management and treatment of sickness in older people. However, there is also controversy regarding the type of research which can be done on the 'incompetent' elderly. Some diseases, especially the ones of dementia such as Alzheimer's disease, can cause devastating problems for the patient and their families. Research into the natural history of the disease requires studying the human subject whose dementia interferes with their ability to give informed consent to research protocols. One must be careful to preserve individual autonomy while doing research for the public good. Any studies which involve demented patients must be scrutinized especially thoroughly by ethics committees and only approved after the most rigorous consideration.

Elder Abuse

In recent years the subject of elder abuse has emerged from the shadows as an important and disturbing societal problem. A recent Canadian survey estimated that 4% of elderly persons had experienced some form of abuse, either verbal or physical (Patterson and Podnieks, 1993). Health care workers should be alert to recognize signs of abuse and be prepared to intervene where necessary. To date, there is no legal requirement to report in any country 'elder abuse' as is required in 'child abuse', but discussions in the USA point in this direction.

Older people are no different from any other vulnerable group. Frail, poor and infirm older people can be victims of neglect or physical, sexual, psychological and financial abuse. Unfortunately elder abuse is underreported. The victim is often in a situation of dependency to the abuser. Older adults who are afraid of abandonment, reprisal or embarrassment will deny the problem. The scarcity of financial and community resources, family stress and a history of family violence are all related to elder abuse. Sexual abuse is also not uncommon especially where the abuser lives with the victim. A history of 'doctor shopping' or an 'accident-prone' parent, or a story that does not match the extent or type of injury should be suspect. On physical examination health care professionals should be alert to bruises, burns, bite marks, injuries around the mouth, face and eyes; poor nutrition and dehydration; ulcers in the skin caused by areas of pressure; and unusual behaviour such as depression, fear, withdrawal, paranoia or over-sedation. It is very important to recognize warning signs in a stressed caregiver such as fatigue, frustration and irritability, and to intervene to prevent a potentially abusive situation.

Patients' Rights (see also Chapters 5 and 23)

It is not uncommon to run into the assertion of rights by many groups – the rights of one gender versus the other, the rights of the unborn, the right to life and the right to die. During the past quarter of a century, the rights of patients have also taken on increasing importance; the most

pertinent are 'legal rights' and 'ethical rights'. The former are easier to enforce as they are rights laid down by a court, by a law or by a legally constituted authority. In Canada, some rights of the person or patient are raised by the Constitution and the Charter of Rights. In many countries there is equivalent legislation or a Code of Civil Liberties. Some 'essential' rights are accepted by the international community as a matter of entitlement of every human being, such as the right to life, liberty, food, shelter and freedom. In health care systems in most industrialized countries certain rights are inalienable (Storch, 1982). These can include:

- the right to treatment in an emergency room,
- the right to an appropriate standard of care,
- the rights to voluntary, informed consent and to refuse health care treatment,
- the right to decide whether or not to be used for research or teaching purposes,
- the right to confidentiality,
- the right to health care free from discrimination,
- the right to protection of personal and private property,
- the right to make your own decisions

There are situations where the patients' rights can be suspended or overruled. The laws of society and the rights of the individual sometimes conflict. In many countries, children, legal minors and the mentally handicapped are protected by the law.

Legal Issues in Community Health Care – The Rights of the Health Care Provider

The health care of older people is becoming increasingly centred in the patient's home or in community health care institutions. Health care providers need to be aware of their own rights, and opportunities for redress for any losses that may be sustained to their person or property during the delivery of their services in these settings.

This is a large and cumbersome area of law which differs in various states, provinces and countries. This chapter will outline some general principles but it should be understood that each situation must be addressed according to the laws which apply in a specific community especially those on Occupational Health and Safety, Employment Contracts and Criminal Laws.

SAFETY

Every person is entitled to safe conditions in their place of work. This means that a health care provider must have the opportunity to work in premises, private or public, which are free from harm. Health care institutions, especially those which are funded or controlled by the government, are subject to the health and safety regulations of the country. A failure to provide such premises at the standard of safety prescribed by the law, may give rise to claims for damages sustained by the worker under Worker's Compensation, Occupational Health and Safety or Occupier's Liability Legislation. An injury sustained as a result of the employer's or the property owner's negligence may also give rise to a cause of action.

A loss or injury may also be sustained as a result of a breach of contract. Each health care provider should be well-versed in their terms of employment and any benefits which arise out of his or her contract of employment. Government contracts and institutional contracts may provide compensation or access to state welfare or dis-ability benefits (Chapter 5). These options must be explored when injury is sustained at work.

There are also possible avenues for financial compensation and personal redress through civil actions. This means that the general principles of employer's liability, occupiers liability or contract law may permit an injured worker to sue the employer, owner or contractor for damages. Again, the rules governing negligence and contract law will apply to these circumstances.

Community health practitioners may encounter: violent neighbourhoods where street crime predominates; angry animals or unprovoked attacks by household pets; unsafe electrical devices or plumbing; poor health conditions such as extremely dirty and cluttered homes; violent patients or violent family members; poorly shovelled driveways or icy steps causing falls; infectious illness or virulent disease such as hepatitis or meningitis.

Conclusion

This chapter has highlighted some common ethical and legal issues which arise in the care of older persons. Health care professionals who work with chronically ill or frail elderly persons will face many difficult problems regarding the extent of treatment, the allocation of financial resources, mental competency and standards of care. Older people who utilize health services usually employ a variety of workers in their care. Interdisciplinary teamwork has become fundamental in the delivery of effective and comprehensive health services to older people. We are faced with many new challenges as health care extends from the hospital into the home or community. The rights of the individual and the dignity of the incompetent must be respected. Older people have the same rights as younger patients.

These encompass both constitutional legal rights and internationally recognized human and moral rights. Movements for the protection of these rights and advocacy for older persons are beginning to rise in many countries. All health care professionals working with older people should be knowledgeable about the ethical and legal principles which apply in the community in which they work, especially those on euthanasia, living wills, negligence, competency, informed consent, elder abuse and occupational safety.

References

Callahan, D (1987) *Setting Limits.* New York: Simon and Schuster.

Carton, RW, Brown, MD (1993) Ethical considerations and CPR in the elderly patient *Clinics in Chest Medicine* 14: 596.

Cassel, CK (1992) Issues of age and chronic care: another argument for health care reform. *Journal of the American Geriatrics Society* 40: 404–409.

Kluge, EW (1993) *Readings in Biomedical Ethics.* Scarborough: Prentice Hall Canada Inc.

Koenig, HG (1993) Legalizing physician — assisted suicide: some thoughts and concerns. *The Journal of Family Practice* 37: 171.

Levinsky, NG (1990) Age as a criterion for rationing health care. *The New England Journal of Medicine* 322: 1813–1815.

Munson, R (1992) *Intervention and Reflection: Basic Issues in Medical Ethics,* 4th edn. California: Wadsworth Inc.

Patterson, C, Podnieks, E. (1993) A guide to the diagnosis and treatment of elder abuse. *Ontario Medical Review* January issue: 11–17.

Pawlson, LG, Glover, JJ, Murphy, DJ (1993) An overview of allocation and rationing: implications for geriatrics. *The Journal of the American Geriatrics Society* 40: 628–634.

Seedhouse, D, Lovett, L (1992) *Practical Medical Ethics.* Chichester: Little, Brown and Company.

Sneiderman, B, Irvine, J, Osborne, P (1989) *Canada Medical Law.* Toronto: Carswell.

Storch, J (1982) *Patients' rights,* p. 249. Toronto: McGraw-Hill Ryerson Limited.

F

Integrated Case Management

SECTION EDITORS: CHERYL A COTT, ANN COMPTON

28

Health Care Teamwork

CHERYL A COTT

External Factors that affect Team Function
•
Internal Factors that influence Team Function
•
Team Performance

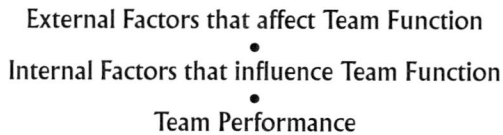

Physiotherapy with older persons is usually delivered in a team context. It is generally accepted that no single health care professional can meet the diverse needs of the older person who is frail and has multiple problems. The team approach is not unique to geriatrics. It is pervasive throughout health care. Acceptance of the value of teamwork is taken for granted by health professionals, despite the lack of a systematic analysis of its effectiveness.

One of the first challenges we meet when trying to understand teams is to identify a consistent definition of a team. The terms interdisciplinary, multidisciplinary, intradisciplinary, transdisciplinary, intraprofessional and interprofessional are all used interchangeably in the literature, although

some attempts have been made to differentiate between them. Campbell and Cole (1987) define a multidisciplinary team as a group of professionals who work independently in the same setting and interact informally. An interdisciplinary team, on the other hand, consists of a blend of different professionals who work interdependently in the same setting and interact both formally and informally.

Payne (1982) differentiates between the team as a work group and collaborative teamwork. In work groups, people are brought together by virtue of working together in the same setting, but they do not necessarily share work tasks or responsibility, nor do they work together to enhance the work that they are doing. Work groups correspond with the multidisciplinary team approach. The collaborative team has common goals, and divides up the work so as to make the best of each individual member's activities and to ensure that the goals are met. Collaborative teamwork corresponds to the interdisciplinary teamwork approach.

In practice, most teams probably fall on a continuum somewhere from work group to collaborative team.

Trute and Macpherson (1977) proposed an interesting typology of health care teams based on analogies to sport teams. Many health care teams resemble a curling team with the skip calling all the shots with the rest of the team members in a rigid hierarchy, i.e. lead, second, vice-skip; usually, the skip is the physician. The structure of other health care teams resembles a volleyball team in which each member plays every position in turn. Although some of the mental health teams of the 1960s operated on this basis, this model is no longer considered sound for mental health service delivery.

Between these two extremes, we have highly structured team sports like baseball, where initially the catcher calls the signals but after the ball has been hit, players improvise on virtually every play. All players share basic skills in hitting and catching the ball and have more specialized skills as well; pitcher, infield and outfield. Some geriatric outreach assessment teams fit very closely with this model. Any member of the team can do an initial assessment, but after that point, other team members are involved according to their specialized skills. Less structured are hockey and soccer teams, where people have more or less assigned positions but may play all over the field as circumstances warrant. Macpherson and Trute concluded that the hockey model was the most desirable one for health care teams.

Teams consist of members of many health disciplines, with diverse knowledge and skills, who share an integrated set of goals, and who utilize interdependent collaboration that involves communication, sharing of knowledge and coordination of services to provide services to patients and their caregiving system (modified from Drinka, 1990).

This composite definition underlines some of the basic assumptions of the concept of interdisciplinary team care. Although not explicitly stated, most literature on health care teams subscribes to three basic assumptions: 1) that team members have a shared understanding of roles, norms and values; 2) that the team functions in an egalitarian, cooperative, interdependent manner; and 3) that the combined effects of shared, cooperative decision making are of greater benefit to the patient than the individual effects of the disciplines on their own.

A review of the few studies that have been done of teams suggests that a shared understanding of roles and egalitarian decision making are not always confirmed by the research, but when these conditions are present greater benefits to the patient can be expected.

If teams are more effective when their members work collaboratively, why are there problems in the way that many teams function?

Figure 1 contains a framework of the external and internal factors that have been identified as important in understanding teamwork (Cott, 1995).

External Factors that affect Team Function

The team does not exist in a vacuum. There are

Figure 1   A framework of the external and internal factors that have been identified as important in understanding teamwork.

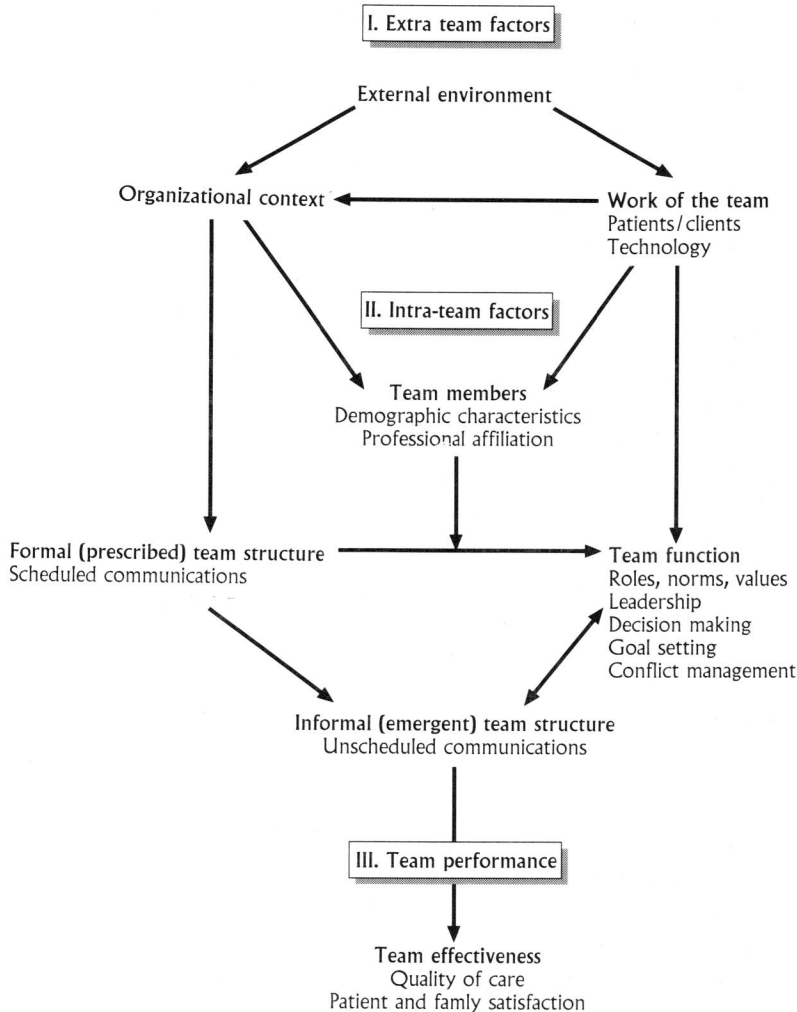

many levels of influence on a team (see Chapter 5). The team usually exists within a health care organization which itself has broad social and political influences that determine organizational goals and priorities. Within the organizational hierarchy the team has influences from the 'top down', such as from administrative and medical lines of authority, and from the 'bottom up' from clients and their families.

Every organization exists in a specific physical, technological, cultural and social environment to which it must adapt and within which it must survive (Hasenfeld, 1983). The general environment defines the range of resources available to the organization, the range and types of human problems and needs that it will face, the value system within which it functions, the political and legal constraints it will need to adapt to and the human services technology available to it (Hasenfeld, 1983).

The work that the team is doing has an important influence on how the team functions. The patients or clients are the recipients of the service, the human beings who form the clientele of the organization and therefore the team. The nature of the clients' problems and the human services technology available to the team determine the nature of the work to be done and how it will be structured. For example, if a surgical team and a rehabilitation team are compared, the work they do is very different and will lead to different team structures. In a surgical situation, all of the team members are working on the patient at the same time in a carefully coordinated series of moves. The implementation and outcome of the technology require a hierarchical structure with clear differentiation of roles.

In the rehabilitation setting, team members work individually, but coordinate their actions through written plans, team meetings, and informal communication. Assessment, treatment and evaluation are coordinated along physical, psychosocial and vocational lines. The structure of the rehabilitation team therefore needs to be less hierarchical, with more sharing of decision making and reaching consensus about work plans.

The organization itself influences the way that a team functions. The organization's goals are important influences on the team's structure and function. What the organization is attempting to do with its clients will determine team composition and availability of resources. For example, in the long-term care setting, whether the organization sees itself primarily as warehousing older clients or rehabilitating them will have an impact on the mix of professionals that are hired to compose the team. Similarly, if the organization values teamwork as a means for achieving its goals,

certain aspects of teamwork such as team rounds may be prescribed.

The structure of the organization itself is an important consideration. Typically, health services organizations consist of a large number of professional staff who are organized along departmental lines, but are brought together to work as teams. This matrix type of organization results in a dual reporting structure of team members; administratively, staff may report through a departmental hierarchy, while clinically they may report through a medical hierarchy. This dual reporting structure can lead to conflicting demands and loyalties for team members, as well as different perspectives on individual team members in terms of the perceived goals of the team.

This traditional type of structure is changing dramatically with recent changes to clinical units or programme management. In these situations the teams in specific clinical areas may exist independently of professional departments. Physiotherapists may no longer be hired by a central physiotherapy department that determines staff allocation throughout the organization; rather they are hired by a particular clinical unit.

The external environment, the organizational context, the clients and human services technology are extra-team influences. Each has an influence on how the work group or team will be structured. However, 'It is naive to bring together a highly diverse group of people and expect that, by calling them a team, they will in fact behave as a team' (Wise et al., 1974, p. xviii). These extra-team influences help explain some influences on team structure and function, but they only go so far in determining the extent to which the team functions in an interdisciplinary manner.

Internal Factors that influence Team Function

The team is not a homogenous unit, within each team there are also a number of intra-team considerations. A number of characteristics of the individual team members influence the team process and how members interact. These include gender, ethnicity, age and professional affiliation; each of these are linked to status differentiation within the group, and have many implications for interaction.

Not only does professional affiliation create status differentials, it also influences the perceptions that team members will have of teamwork. Although both physicians and nurses advocate the use of teamwork, they do so for different reasons (Temkin-Greener, 1983; Campbell-Heider and Pollock, 1987). Physicians tend to see nurses as helpers and extenders of their role and encourage a form of teamwork in which nurses are subordinate. In contrast, nurses view teamwork as providing access to direct patient care and as a means to gain status and seek a form of teamwork that encourages mutual collegiality with physicians.

Health care professionals differ in how they view themselves and other professions, and how they think other professions view them. There is the potential for disagreement amongst health care providers in understanding the capabilities of other professions, encroaching on professional territory, defensiveness about professional prerogatives and not utilizing fully the capabilities of other professions (Ducanis and Golin, 1979).

In addition, each person comes to the team with a different set of notions and values about teamwork and patient care, based on their professional socialization and personal experience and beliefs. Not all health professionals view the world the same way. Different professional groups may define problems differently and value different behaviours and goals. For example, some team members may focus on ruling out problems until a single problem is identified, while others may focus on ruling in problems, developing lengthy problem lists that cover a broad range of social, psychological and medical issues. Team members may also differ on which problems or issues they feel the team should address. These and other differences in professional perspectives, are addressed in an article by Qualls and Czirr (1988) in which a number of professional models of good health care and of team functioning are identified.

The major strength of teamwork is the collaboration of multiple health disciplines with diverse knowledge and skills, but at the same time this creates some difficulties for understanding each other and working together. Professionals who do not recognize that others may not share their perceptions, may judge others within their own framework, and may make erroneous conclusions about the others' willingness to cooperate or behave in an appropriate manner.

There are also some worker characteristics that are thought to ensure team solidarity. These include: 1) the team members' attitudes to their work, such as their willingness to share a client, their flexibility, their willingness to learn and their willingness to accept decisions by consensus; 2) the team member's attitude towards colleagues, such as having respect for their colleagues and having confidence in their colleagues' good will and competence; and, 3) the team members' personal qualities, such as having an outreaching personality, self-confidence, high level communication skills, and professional self-respect and competence (Sampson and Marthas, 1981).

Team process refers to the way that the team actually performs its work. Factors deemed universally important in the study of team process include roles, norms and values; leadership; decision-making and goal setting. Most studies of teams have focussed on some aspect of team process such as communication or decision making, or power within teams.

Roles are the specific forms of behaviour associated with a given task. Much time and energy in the literature has been devoted to the notion of roles on teams, with very little systematic analysis. Much of what we know is still at the theoretical stage. The importance of clearly defined roles is argued in the literature, with some authors saying they are essential and others saying they are not as important (Ducanis and Golin, 1979).

Many authors identify role ambiguity as a potential source of team conflict, particularly when there are inappropriate or undefined expectations of the roles of other team members (Ducanis and Golin, 1979). A person's role in a team may be considered from two directions: the expectations of the other team members as to what that person's role should be; and the person's own expectations and how he or she interprets the expectations of others (Katz and Kahn, 1966). Clearly, within a team composed of a number of individuals with different educational backgrounds and differing extents of understanding of the function of other disciplines, the potential for conflict in terms of role expectations of others as well as for misinterpretation of others' expectations of oneself is considerable.

Studies on interprofessional perceptions suggest the potential for disagreement exists between professionals in terms of understanding each other's capabilities, encroaching on each other's professional territory, being defensive about professional prerogatives, and not fully utilizing the capabilities of other professions (Ducanis and Golin, 1979).

Whether teams function better if their roles are very clearly defined depends on the team and the nature of the work to be done. In an interdisciplinary geriatric team, there is a need to tolerate role blurring — to be flexible enough to take on some of the other roles of other disciplines and yet confident enough to tolerate someone else taking on part of your role, without becoming defensive. Roles in an interdisciplinary team can be related only in the broadest outline to activities and relationships typical of one or another profession in some other operational context. Role relationships in interdisciplinary teams are usually the outcome of ongoing negotiation and bargaining.

The discussion so far has focussed on roles based on professional affiliation. There is also a considerable literature on roles within groups that enhance or impede group function. These 'group roles' refer to roles assumed by group members within the team such as energizer, information seeker, opinion-giver, evaluator-critic and harmonizer (Sampson and Marthas, 1981). These roles may be performed by separate individuals or shared by team members at different points in time. The combination of professional and group roles that a team member takes influences their relative status and prestige in the team.

Norms serve important functions for task performance and team maintenance (Katz and Kahn, 1966). Norms can be thought of as a shared understanding of 'the way that we do things around here'. These implicit rules direct how the team functions, and as well guide a team's decision as to which problems it will consider appropriate for action. The presence of shared norms increases the likelihood of team members responding in predictable ways. Norms of flexibility, support and openness of communication are important for avoiding team dysfunction (Wise *et al.*, 1974). Becoming aware of and understanding group norms is important to the socialization and incorporation of new team members.

Values are generalized ideological justifications and aspirations (Katz and Kahn, 1966). The values of the team are influenced both by the values of the overall organization within which the team functions and by the individual values of the team members. These sets of values are interactive in that the task performance of the team reflects the outlook and beliefs of individuals, while at the same time, the team influences individual values. Again, different team members will have different values, but in order for the team to function well, members will have to share key values such as the importance of independence or of living in one's own home.

Leadership is another key consideration in team functioning. Although there may be disagreement over who should assume the leadership function within teams, there is consensus that the function of leadership is necessary for effective team function (Sampson and Marthas, 1981; Ducanis and Golin, 1979). These leadership functions include helping the group decide on its purpose and goals; facilitating the achievement of common goals; helping the group evaluate its progress and development; and allocation of work (Sampson and Marthas, 1981).

Leaders may have formal authority from the institution, but teams have some of the characteristics of informal groups, so an individual's status is dependent in part on the quality of their relationships with other team members. In interdisciplinary teams, it is often appropriate for

leadership to rotate among group members. Rarely within a group is one individual capable of fulfilling all leadership functions; depending on the situation, different individuals within the group may assume leadership functions (Sampson and Marthas, 1981; Ducanis and Golin, 1979). For example, in one situation it may be more appropriate for the physiotherapist to take leadership or initiative, while in another situation, the nurse may be the more appropriate leader. This model has been formalized in certain organizations that use case management.

In many teams, the leadership role tends to be given to the individual whose profession dominates the organization within which the team practices. Medical dominance of health care has led to the physician often being considered the leader of the team quite automatically for both legal and traditional reasons. However, the acceptance of medicine's power and right to leadership on the health care team is not universally accepted by other health professionals and is one of the potential sources of conflict in the team (Temkin-Greener, 1983). Numerous studies of power in teams underscore medicine's dominance (Dingwall, 1980; Fried, 1989; Fiorelli, 1988). Factors identified as reinforcing medical dominance include gender and class differences between physicians and other team members, an ideology of exclusivity and assumed monopoly of medical knowledge, and authoritarian decision making styles.

Goal setting and decision making represent major functions of the interdisciplinary team (Ducanis and Golin, 1979). Team goals give direction to the team's actions and define its overall purpose. Determinants of team goals include the client's goals, the professional's goals, and the organization's goals. The way that teams actually set goals can reflect on the way that they function. For example, if team members set their own professional goals independently without collaborating with each other, they may end up working at cross-purposes. In contrast, if the overall team goals are developed by team members in collaboration with each other and with clients and their families, individual team members will find it easier to set their own, professional goals, while keeping the overall team goals in mind.

Team goals are either task-related (usually related to patient care) or team maintenance goals (related to the smooth functioning of the group). Many teams focus solely on patient-related issues and spend little time addressing issues of team functioning. However, a failure to deal openly with team maintenance goals can lead to problems in team interaction, since issues such as conflict and communication are never addressed openly. Well-functioning teams, while focussing on patient-related goals, also spend a portion of their time on team maintenance.

There are three types of decision-making, each of which is appropriate in different circumstances (Qualls and Czirr, 1988). Executive decision making occurs when one person makes all the decisions; this is appropriate and necessary in a situation such as a medical emergency. Consensus decision making occurs when all team members have an equal voice and no decision is made until all members agree; this is time and effort consuming, but is appropriate when major decisions about team policy are being made. Collaborative decision making occurs when all team members who have information or expertise relevant to the issue contribute to the decision; this is most appropriate when routine team decisions are being made.

Decision making and goal setting are related to

power and leadership in the team. Evers (1982) examined the way goal definition and decision making occurred in multidisciplinary teams working with older people, and concluded that although decisions about patients and work with patients sometimes looks like teamwork, often it is not, particularly in situations where patients do not entirely fit the clinical-medical 'cure' approach to illness and when consensus about goals has not been reached. In these situations, the imposition of the medical view on the rest of the 'team' was observed to occur.

Although involvement of the patient and their families in goal setting and decision making is deemed to be of importance, it does not appear to occur. Rintala et al. (1986) examined patient contributions in team meetings and found that patients contributed minimally to the discussion. Further, team professionals tended to over-emphasize the physical content area and under-emphasize psychosocial issues, when compared with the patients' perceptions of their needs.

The move towards client-centred practice that acknowledges the importance of involving older people and their families in deciding treatment goals is relatively new. In order to make this involvement meaningful, team members will need to be sensitive to the difficulties that older clients and their families face when interacting with a large, varied group of health professionals. This can be particularly challenging in the team meeting when clients and families may feel outnumbered and intimidated by the presence of health professionals.

The prescribed structure refers to the formal definitions of how the team should be structured and function. It consists of formal definitions of status and function such as job descriptions, and the rules and regulations laid down by the organization as to how the team should work. In contrast, the emergent structure refers to the informal relations amongst workers that develop as they go about their work. Although never entirely independent, the formal and informal structures can be clearly differentiated. The informal interaction structure seldom parallels exactly the formal structure of positions in the group or the channels of communication that the formal organization defines or specifies.

Structurally, one team may be a pyramid, its members sorted by professions into successive levels, with a chief from some traditionally authoritative discipline at the top; another way may be a clearly defined discussion circle with no senior person (Sampson and Marthas, 1981; Ducanis and Golin, 1979). However, this relationship changes as relationships within a group evolve over a period of time. The way the work may actually get done may prove on close examination to be quite different from the processes outlined in an organization chart.

Informal relationships that develop amongst team members affect the pattern of work itself, through the formation of norms about how much work to do, the division of work groups into subgroups, and the emergence of a status hierarchy not recognized by management. The informal structure of a team can strongly influence how the team does its work. One of the challenges for new team members trying to gain acceptance to the team is to understand the informal structure of the team.

Team Performance

The final concept in the model is team performance. The assumption in geriatric rehabilitation is that more collaborative teamwork results in better client outcomes. It is thought that, by working cooperatively, team members arrive at solutions that are better than the sum of their individual efforts. However, few studies have directly addressed the issue of the effectiveness of a team versus a non-team approach. Most studies of geriatric team effectiveness have treated the team as a 'black box', without simultaneously measuring the processes and outcomes of teamwork.

The lack of studies examining the effectiveness of teams and quality of care is probably due to the complexity of both the independent variable (team functioning) and the dependent variable (quality of care), as well as to the difficulties inherent in using a rigorous research design in field settings (Schmitt et al., 1988). However, there are other indicators of quality such as client and family satisfaction with care. The literature on satisfaction with health care is vast and not without methodological difficulties, however, client satisfaction with care is certainly a legitimate indicator of quality.

References

Campbell, LJ, Cole, KD (1987) Geriatric assessment teams. *Clinics in Geriatric Medicine* 3: 99.

Campbell-Heider, N, Pollock, D (1987) Barriers to physician-nurse collegiality: an anthropological perspective. *Social Science and Medicine* 25: 421–425

Cott, C (1995) *The Structure of Multidisciplinary Long-term Care Teams.* University of Toronto; unpublished Doctoral Dissertation.

Dingwall, R (1985) Problems of teamwork in primary care. In Lonsdale, S, Webb, A, Briggs, TL (eds) *Social Services and Health Care*, pp. 111–137. Syracuse, NY: Syracuse University School of Social Work.

Drinka, T (1990) A Case Study of Leadership on a Long-Term Care Interdisciplinary Health Care Team. Unpublished doctoral dissertation, University of Wisconsin, Madison.

Ducanis AJ, Golin, AK (1979) *The Interdisciplinary Health Care Team: A Handbook.* London: Aspen.

Evers, H (1982) Professional practice and patient care: multidisciplinary teamwork in geriatric wards. *Ageing and Society* 2: 57–75.

Fiorelli, JS (1988) Power in work groups: team member's perspectives. *Human Relations* 41: 1–12.

Fried, BJ (1989) Power acquisition in a health care setting: an application of strategic contingencies theory. *Human Relations* **41**: 915–927.

Hasenfeld, Y (1983) *Human Services Organizations.* New Jersey: Prentice-Hall.

Katz, D, Kahn, RL (1966) *The Social Psychology of Organizations.* New York: Wiley & Son.

Payne, M (1982) *Working in Teams.* London: MacMillan Press.

Qualls, SH, Czirr, R (1988) Geriatric health teams: classifying models of professional and team functioning. *The Gerontologist* **28**: 372–376.

Rintala, DH, Hanover, D, Alexander, JL *et al.* (1986) Team care: an analysis of verbal behavior during patient rounds in a rehabilitation hospital. *Archives of Physical Medicine and Rehabilitation* **67**: 118–122.

Sampson, EE, Marthas, M (1981) *Group Process for the Health Professions,* 2nd edn. Toronto: Wiley & Sons.

Schmitt, MH, Farrell, MP, Heineman, GD (1988) Conceptual and methodological problems in studying the effects of interdisciplinary geriatric teams. *The Gerontologist* **28**: 753–764.

Temkin-Greener, H (1983) Interprofessional perspectives on teamwork in health care: A case study. *Millbank Memorial Fund Quarterly* **61**: 641–658.

Trute, B, Macpherson, AS (1977) Psychiatric teams, sports and mental health practice. *Canada's Mental Health* **25**: 4.

Wise, H, Beckhard, R, Rubin, I, Kyte, AL (1974) *Making Health Teams Work.* Cambridge: Ballinger.

29

Interdisciplinary Assessment

DOROTHY HAMMOND, JOHN AH PUXTY

The Context of Assessment
•
The Goals of Assessment
•
The Assessment Process
•
The Geriatric Assessment Team
•
The Assessment Site
•
Standardized Tools of Assessment
•
Evaluation of Geriatric Assessment

Interdisciplinary assessment is a dynamic process that involves a comprehensive, multidimensional evaluation of an older person's, social, physical, psychological (see Chapters 2, 6 and 8), and functional status using diverse tools. It may be carried out in variety of settings; hospital, day hospitals, long-term care institutions, and in the community. Due to the multidimensional aspect of the assessment the input of a variety of professionals is desirable, and is achieved by the use of various kinds of teams. The goals of interdiscplinary assessment vary widely depending on the individual situation.

The Context of Assessment

Assessment services for older people are best targeted towards the 'frail elderly' who may live in a variety of settings. These are older individuals who have multiple, complex, interacting physical and psychological problems that are brought on by the interaction of disease and ageing, often with the result of functional impairment and dependency. Social factors often compound these problems. Therefore, the need for interdisciplinary assessment is not determined by virtue of age alone, but rather by the complexity of the individual's problems. Those who require multidimensional assessment are generally 65 years or over, frail or ill, with multiple complex biomedical and psychosocial problems. They usually present with a cluster of some of the following characteristics: presence of complex multifactorial illness, resulting in escalating use of community support; polypharmacy; multiple interacting chronic pathologies; frequent visits to emergency and/or multiple hospital admissions; illness that presents atypically; potentially reversible functional disabilities requiring a multidimensional assessment; recent unexpected increases in functional dependency and potential need for placement; need for advice regarding investigation, diagnosis, and management of specific diseases commonly seen in older people.

In contrast to the younger adult, two sets of factors have a significant impact on the approach to assessment of older people – pathophysiological changes with ageing and social factors. The pathophysiological changes of ageing modify the body's internal environment (see Chapter 6) and the body's reaction to disease. With increasing age, there may be an increased diversity of presentation of disease and reaction to stress which has come to be known as the 'geriatric presentation' or 'atypical presentation'. Coupled with this is a loss of functional reserve of organs and systems that may only become apparent when an acute illness occurs. Persons who experience these ageing changes often present with confusion, loss of mobility (confinement to a chair or bed), postural instability with falls, incontinence of urine, bowel dysfunction, and social crisis. The onset of one or more of these symptoms may be the first signs of illness and systemic disease. Ageing can make the elderly extremely susceptible to iatrogenic disease from a variety of sources including: polypharmacy, inactivity and failure to apply appropriate preventive and restorative rehabilitation principles.

When pre-existing chronic disease, disability and dependency are present, the onset of an additional problem may be associated with the atypical signs and symptoms. The exact reasons for this are not fully understood, but are related to changes in homeostatic mechanisms, waning inflammatory response, decreases in visceral sensation and decreased pain appreciation. Although the usual phenomena of acute disease may be masked, functional impairment becomes an increasingly common feature.

When dealing with any atypical presentation, especially careful assessment to identify remedial components and avoid premature 'labelling' is essential. When dealing with confusion and memory failure it is imperative to obtain the history from a third party; this should also be done for most other older patients since many tend to underplay their problems. According to Robertson (1984), older people tend not to report problems such as mental (see Chapter 8), urinary (see Chapter 16), foot (see Chapter 26) or locomotor problems (see Chapter 7), all of which potentially have a great impact on their ability to function.

Social factors have an important influence on the ability of the older person to deal with the impact of disease and disability. Many elderly are in fact relatively isolated, without immediate caregivers (Chapter 2). Approximately 40% of women over 65 years of age and 20% of men have no spouse. Nearly 20% have no immediate family and a further 20% have family more than 90 minutes away by car. Financial barriers are also common with nearly 20% living on or below the poverty line.

The functionally impaired or disabled older patient is often dependent upon others for various aspects of their care. With the 'geriatric presentation' there usually comes an increase in dependency. For example, much more care is required for the patient who becomes immobile or incontinent, or mildly forgetful and is now awake disturbing the household throughout the night. The care providers, finding the increased demands for care an unacceptable strain, seek help due to this 'social crisis'. In other instances, there may be no appropriate care provider. It is best to avoid the use of terms such as 'social problem' or 'social admission' in this situation; these terms are prejudicial and do not encourage a careful diagnostic approach to identify remedial conditions which are often present.

The Goals of Assessment

Many health providers share the overall goal of good quality of life for older people, through promoting wellness and encouraging optimal functioning, thereby preventing inappropriate or unnecessary utilization of long-term care resources. Comprehensive assessment contributes to this overall goal by improving diagnostic accuracy, and providing better guidance in the selection of interventions to restore or preserve health, recommending an optimal environment for care, predicting outcomes, and monitoring clinical change over time. Assessment goals vary depending on the individual situation, the individual's own goals and, in some cases, the goals of the caregiver and the setting (see also Chapter 14).

The goals for hospitalized older patients are to treat the illness and to prevent or reverse the clinical decline that frequently accompanies acute illness and hospitalization (see also Chapter 21). Treatment of the patient's illness requires identification of the risks and benefits of drug regimens, therapies and interventions. The possible impact of various treatments on the patient's quality of life should be assessed in advance, to prevent iatrogenic problems, such as polypharmacy or decreased mobility, that may result from hospitalization.

In hospitalized patients, overall functional prognosis is best estimated by considering not only the patient's age and severity of illness, but also the premorbid level of function and the rate of functional decline that precipitated hospitalization. In general, the higher the level of pre-illness function and the steeper the slope of decline, the better the prognosis for recovery. For example, a fully mobile, independent person who falls and fractures a hip and subsequently develops pneumonia has a good chance of regaining health, whereas a person of the same age with Alzheimer's disease who suffers the same hip fracture and pnuemonia will probably not regain functional ability. This general rule would not apply to such catastrophic illnesses as massive cerebrovascular accidents or myocardial infarctions.

For community-based older people (see Chapter 31), the main goals are to identify and treat reversible illness, improve function, avoid iatrogenic conditions and minimize psychosocial stress. In addition to medical treatments and other therapies, interventions include educating caregivers about management of the patient's condition, training them in environmental and behavioural management techniques, and providing them with information about available resources. Access to information and referral services is especially important for those who live alone.

The goal of assessment in long-term care facilities (see Chapter 30) differs depending on the expected length of stay. For those patients expected to improve and be discharged (e.g. patients with hip fractures), aggressive rehabilitation is indicated. Patients who have progressive diseases, such as severe arthritis, congestive heart failure, or chronic pulmonary disease, require stabilization and ongoing care. The goals of treatment for these patients are to improve or preserve function and to minimize the use of medications.

When living arrangements are a concern, assessment can help to identify the level in the continuum of care at which the patient will function best. For hospitalized patients returning home, the prehospitalization living situation may require adjustment, ranging from temporary home assistance or augmentation of existing home services to full-time nursing care in the home. Some may need to be placed in an assisted living facility or in a nursing home.

The Assessment Process

Assessment is a process that can take a variable length of time to complete, depending upon the nature of the patient's problems. Assessment often continues over a period of time until optimal function is attained; that is, the process begins with the initial consultation and determination of the problems that need treatment and ends with the patient having attained a plateau of optimal function. The assessment is multidimensional in order to identify and consider the complex, diverse problems and disabilities in their full social context and requires a team of health care professionals to collect and organize a variety of clinically relevant information. This process is referred to as the 'comprehensive assessment'.

Each individual professional discipline brings its own orientation and perceptions to the method of assessment, interpretation and treatment of problems. Collaboration is necessary when two or more health professionals are involved in com-

mon assessment and treatment. The Geriatric Assessment Team or Assessment Team for Older People is the mechanism by which communication and coordination between health professionals is achieved in order to share and interpret information, and to produce a consensus of how to respond.

The Geriatric Assessment Team

A variety of geriatric assessment team models exist, each with its own merits depending on the situation. Teams may be unidisciplinary, multidisciplinary, intradisciplinary or transdisciplinary.

All members of a unidisciplinary or intradisciplinary team are from the same discipline. The approach of such a team reflects the sub-specialization within a discipline. The generalist seeks advice regarding a component of the care process from another of the same discipline. The interaction may not be comprehensive or prolonged. Indeed the individuals may function independently approaching the issue from their own perspective and addressing care within the context of their own speciality.

A multidisciplinary team comprises various professions or disciplines. Individual professionals conduct assessments and interpretations independently, develop care regimens and evaluate outcomes from the perspective of their discipline. Communication occurs, but it remains within their professional boundaries. The approach has the merit of recognizing the complex, multidimensional nature of the needs of older people and enabling multiple skills to be utilized in resolving these. Inherent in this approach is the potential for duplication, the use of diverse and possibly contradictory approaches and the likelihood of conflict.

When functioning in an interdisciplinary team, members work on common problems, communicating freely and pooling their expertise to resolve issues. Cross referral, and the type and extent of direct involvement, is based on the patient's problem profile, not on an administrative requirement. Necessarily, the team must achieve consensus on individual roles, assessment interpretations, problem definition and goals of further assessments and treatments.

Transdisciplinary teams are made up of differing disciplines. Wtihin this team, no firm boundaries exist between the disciplines. A portion of knowledge and skills that traditionally lies within the domains of each of the disciplines is internalized by each member of the transdisciplinary team allowing one member to perform an assessment that is the synthesis of the perspectives of the various disciplines.

The different models of team functioning have applications to health care responses towards older people (Chapter 28). A transdisciplinary team approach would be appropriate for a first-contact in any setting, where a multidimensional screening assessment might be desired for purposes of problem identification and triage. Individuals within the same team may function in an interdisciplinary manner by cross-referring to each other in specific instances. Contact by this team may be sufficient to meet the goals of assessment. However where further assessment is required, referrals from the initial assessment may be made to services utilizing a multidisciplinary/interdisciplinary approach where, although common goals are established, specific discipline assessment and treatment skills may be needed. The results of such assessment within a discipline may indicate the need for more refined assessment resulting in an intradisciplinary referral. The assessment of older people therefore often

requires the use of a selective approach of different team models if service uses are to be rationalized. As the patient situation dictates, membership of the teams varies as does the method of functioning.

The Assessment Site

The initial assessment can occur in various places; the patient's home, a nursing home, a hospital ward or an outpatient setting. The site is determined by the needs of the patient and the purpose of the assessment.

It has been claimed that all elderly patients should be seen in their own home prior to admission for the purpose of developing a baseline of information, adding context to the situation seen in hospital and assisting in the development of appropriate goals for treatment. This would usually be done by an interdisciplinary team that would conduct a multidimensional assessment during a home visit. Occasionally, a physician may also make a home visit when it is impossible for the patient to visit the doctor's office or hospital department.

Another purpose of assessment in the home by an interdisciplinary or transdisciplinary team is to identify factors concerning a recent increase in caregiver stress or factors of mobility and environmental safety. This initial assessment may provide sufficient information to yield preliminary recommendations. However, an in-depth assessment may be necessary at which time other disciplines would become involved by cross-referral between interdisciplinary team members, still within the home. If the in-depth assessment requires several extended periods of time, a number of visits to a day hospital setting would be appropriate, if a multidisciplinary team is available there. Assessments in nursing homes are often for purposes similar to those noted above for home visits, but may also be for the purpose of providing advice for the staff regarding the management of the patient.

If the purpose of the assessment is to clarify a complex diagnosis which requires a number of discipline specific assessments and diagnostic tests, it is probable that this would best be done in day hospital, outpatient clinic or in hospital. If the purpose of assessment is primarily to sort out a problem of polypharmacy and intensive monitoring of medications and the patient's condition is required, then admission to hospital would be desirable.

It is not uncommon for the goal of assessment to include a comprehensive evaluation that requires intensive review and monitoring by a number of disciplines. The geriatric day hospital and the geriatric inpatient assessment unit (GAU) are two major sites that are usually available for assessment by a team which has representation from a broad spectrum of health professionals.

Other factors that determine which of these is the appropriate site, include the degree of functional impairment, the extent of the support network within the community and the accessibility of the service to the patient. Accessibility and transportation are the common determinants of whether a day hospital is a practical option. Otherwise patients need to be admitted to the inpatient unit.

Standardized Tools of Assessment

For some of the areas of assessment, standardized tools have been developed and are useful in bringing objectivity into clinical practice. Categories of such tools include psychological (mental status, depression, quality of life), social (caregiver burden), and functional (activities of daily living).

The Folstein Mini-Mental State Examination (1975) is an appropriate short mental status tool routinely used in assessment programmes for older people. It is reported as having excellent sensitivity and specificity, when used with geriatric populations in a variety of settings. Although recognizing the relative wealth of literature concerning its use with Canadian and American populations, some concerns can be expressed about the brevity of instructions particularly in relating to scoring of the assessments. The instrument is criticized for missing mild cases.

Another useful screening tool for cognitive function is the 10 point Kahn Mental Status Questionnaire (1960) which has been validated in Europe and North America and is a popular tool in the UK. This is a useful and sensitive screening tool, and takes only a few moments to perform.

A variety of instruments have been described and used in the assessment of depression in the elderly. The Yesavage Geriatric Depression Scale (1983) is one such instrument, that has been validated for North American populations.

Assessment of quality of life has been relatively neglected. Two possible instruments for consideration are Lawton's Philadelphia Geriatric Centre Morale Scale (1975) and the Quality of Life Index developed by Spitzer (1980). The Lawton scale measures dimensions of emotional adjustment in persons aged 70–90; it is reliable and valid when used with either community residents or people in institutions. The Spitzer Quality of Life Index (1980) measures the general well being of patients with cancer and other chronic disease. It was originally intended to evaluate the effects of treatment and supporter programmes. The instrument is practical, brief and easy to administer yet broad in scope. It has been acceptable to clinicians and clients and used in a wide range of populations and cultures. It seems particularly relevant for use with an ill elderly population and its advantage over the Lawton instrument is its relative brevity (only 5 items compared with 22).

Scales assessing function concentrate on Activities of Daily Living (ADL) and Instrumental Activities of Daily Living (IADL); ADLs include self-care (feeding, bathing, grooming, dressing of upper and lower body), mobility (transfers from sitting to standing, bed to chair, toilet and bathtub, walking on the level and negotiating stairs) and continence. The parameters commonly measured under IADLs commonly include food preparation, grocery shopping, housekeeping, laundry, telephone use, administration of medications and finance, and the use of public transport.

A large number of ADL Scales have been described. The three commonly used are the modified Barthel Index (Mahoney and Barthel, 1965), Rapid Disability Rating Scale (Linn, 1967), and the Philadelphia Geriatric Physical Centre Maintenance and Instrumental Activities of Daily Living Scale (Lawton, 1982). Each instrument has different merit depending upon the actual need. The Barthel Index is brief and has been shown to be predictive of prognosis in stroke rehabilitation, but has the disadvantage of insensitivity to change on some ADL parameters. The Rapid Disability Scale is simple and includes several additional parameters, but its main use is in measuring care level needs in the stable situation. The Lawton ADL Scale, although taking longer and requiring more standardization, is more use-ful in measuring functional change within a rehabilitation programme.

Standardized tools for assessing social aspects mainly revolve about assessing caregiver burden and suffer from similar problems to quality of life indexes. The Zarit Family Burden Scale (1982) was developed for use of caregivers of clients with Alzheimer type dementia; it measures feelings about health, psychological well being, financial and social life and relationships with the patient. Validation against a caregiver's perceptions has been attempted. The Robinson's Caregiver Training Index (1983) measures the impact of caring for seniors in the community after hospitalization.

Standardized tools are incorporated into the overall guide for assessment that is used in the clinical setting. No one set of tools for assessment is ideal. The assessment package should remain dynamic and continue to evolve as team members develop expertise, increase in their understanding of the professional orientation of other team members, new knowledge emerges and team members come and go. The assessment tool used by the interdisciplinary team in the Southeastern Regional Geriatric Programme in Kingston, Canada is going through another revision as the team which has developed it continues to refine their practice. It is included at the end of this chapter as a sample of such tools and represents the outline of the assessment. It does not include the detailed glossary that determines its use and interpretation. Embedded in this tool is the Folstein Mini-Mental State examination, the Yesavage Geriatric Depression Scale and a modified Lawton ADL scale.

The content and process of an assessment is tailored to the individual being assessed. Clinical judgement on the part of the professional during the assessment determines the emphasis of the various components of assessment. Depending on the individual situation, such as how frail and tired the patient is, the presenting concerns, the physical and psychological status at the time of the assessment, the availability of a significant other person to provide additional insights and the goal of the assessment, the professional selects the areas on which assessment should concentrate.

Evaluation of Geriatric Assessment

Comprehensive assessment is a worthwhile process, quite apart from any effect it may have on length of hospital stay or functional status. According to Campion (1987), older people may appreciate the focused attention, multidimensional approach that includes a sensitivity to areas significant to their well-being, and the coordinated approach of a team. However, there have been a number of problems in demonstrating efficacy due to the variety in the 'what', 'who', 'why', 'when', 'how', and 'where' of the assessment. The varying types of patients to be assessed, goals identified, composition of teams involved, when assessment begins and ends, the length of follow-up, differing sites for assessment, and the variety of pertinent outcome measures, provide challenges to researchers.

Assessments in Ambulatory Settings

In a classic study, Williamson et al. (1964) demonstrated a high prevalence of unreported illness and disability (50–60%) in a random sample of older people from three Scottish general practices. Studies of geriatric screening programmes (Hendricksen et al., 1984; Puxty, 1989) have shown significant reduction in hospitalization, morality, institutionalization and community services utilization.

An Australian study conducted by Smith and O'Malley (1993) examined the effectiveness of the geriatric assessment team providing services to clients who were referred for nursing home placement. After a 12-month follow-up, the researchers found that some of these clients could be maintained in the community, and this resulted in a substantial cost benefit ($89 per week compared with $449 to $776 per week). This supports earlier work done by Williams et al. (1973) and Brocklehurst et al. (1978).

Geriatric Consultation Service

Parameters of outcome such as length of stay, survival rate, discharge rate, use of services and measure of function at discharge have been evaluated in the various studies of geriatric consultation services.

In a retrospective comparative report (Burley et al., 1979) found that geriatric consultation teams providing service to acute medical wards resulted in reduced lengths of stay and increased percentages of persons discharged home, particularly for women.

Hogan et al. (1987) reported that although length of stay was not significantly different, the intervention group had a lower death rate, used significantly more physiotherapy and occupational therapy, had a significantly better mental status, received fewer medications at discharge, and significantly more referrals to community services at discharge. In contrast, other studies (Gayton et al., 1987; Campion et al., 1987) have reported no significant difference in controlled experimental studies. These two studies did not target referrals and had possible 'contamination' as the controls and intervention groups were cared for by the same medical and non-medical staff.

Saltz et al. (1988) found no significant differences between the control and intervention groups regarding discharge location nor in re-hospitalization or re-institutionalization rates within 6 months of discharge for patients who received geriatric consultation. Interpretation of this is limited since Saltz's population was principally males (96%) with a high proportion of involved caregivers (71%). There is a lack of research that examines the readmission rate and functional level at discharge for seniors who received inpatient consultation services.

The available evidence would suggest that geriatric inpatient consultations may have some positive effects in reducing length of stay, improving survival and making home discharge more likely. The effect is less clear in studies where the population is principally male, where good caregiver support exists and no targeting of referrals is used. The effects of inpatient consultation on functional status, readmission rate and long-term maintenance in the community have not been adequately examined.

In-hospital Assessment and Treatment Units

The literature related to these assessment/treatment units is less equivocal, although randomized clinical trials are few. Descriptive studies suggest that these units reduce institutionalization, promote an increase in ambulation, ADL, mental status and continence (Applegate et al., 1983; Lefton et al., 1983).

In the first randomized clinical trial, Rubenstein et al. (1984) found several benefits of the inpatient unit approach. When frail acute care older patients with a high probability of nursing home placement were given specialized assessment, therapy, rehabilitation and follow-up, they experienced a significantly lower mortality rate at one year and had significantly lower nursing home admissions, either at discharge or during the next year. On the other hand, the controls had significantly more days in hospital and nursing home and higher acute care readmission rates.

Collard et al. (1985) using a randomized control study method found a significant reduction in mortality, length of stay and costs in one of the two units studied. Similar findings were reported by Liem et al. (1986).

Applegate et al. (1990) conducted a randomized study of the value of an assessment unit for functionally impaired elderly patients recovering from medical or surgical illness who were considered to be at risk of nursing home placement. Treatment within this assessment unit was demonstrated to result in improved functional outcome and reduced likelihood of nursing home placement.

Meta-analysis of Research on Geriatric Assessment

Despite the complexity of programme diversity which prevents the drawing of firm conclusions, the vast majority of studies report positive, if not uniformly significant results (Rubenstein et al., 1991). In addition, these authors undertook a meta-analysis to evaluate the effect of geriatric programmes on mortality. All published controlled trials were grouped into four major service categories: inpatient consultation services; inpatient geriatric evaluation and management units; home assessment services; and outpatient geriatric evaluation and management programmes. All except the last of these demonstrated a reduction in mortality after 6 months. Generally, programmes linking geriatric evaluation with strong long-term management are effective for improving survival and function in older persons (Stuck *et al.*, 1993).

Several recurring themes may be drawn from the literature on inpatient and ambulatory geriatric programmes. Reported benefits such as improved diagnostic accuracy, reduced use of medications, reduced use of institutionalization, are variable and appear to be more effective when early, accurate assessment results in patients being directed towards other assessments, therapies and support systems which are combined into a comprehensive programme that utilizes sound rehabilitation principles, and which features careful early discharge planning.

Regional Geriatric Assessment Programme
St Mary's of the Lake Hospital

OUTREACH/CONSULT ASSESSMENT

1. **KEY**

C	Comment below
–	Asked, but not notable
	Not assessed

2. Information can be collected through:

> client
> family/friends
> family practitioner/specialists
> chart/staff
> health care professionals

3. WHEN COLLECTING DATA: Explore an identified problem

> –onset, duration
> –factors that improve or worsen
> –treatment
> –interfere with daily function
> –assets/resources

4. Order of tool

> = MEDICAL/PROBLEMS
> = SOCIAL SETTING
> = PHYSICAL
> = PSYCHOLOGICAL HEALTH-GDS-MMSE
> = FUNCTIONAL-IADL-ADL
> = MEDICATIONS
> = PROBLEM LIST, RECOMMENDATIONS, PROGRESS NOTES

5. IF IT IS A COMMUNITY VISIT REMEMBER TO HAVE THE CONSENT FORM SIGNED

OUTREACH/CONSULT ASSESSMENT FORM

Client's name: _____

Assessment date: _____ Assessor's signature: _____

Present at interview: _____

Facility	Room	Date of Admission

1. CLIENTS RECENT CHANGE (PROBLEMS AND GOALS)

_____

_____

_____

_____

_____

_____

_____

2. FAMILY'S PERCEPTION

_____

_____

3. HEALTH (SURGERY, HOSPITALIZATION, DIAGNOSIS)

_____

_____

_____

_____

_____

_____

4. HEALTH APPOINTMENTS/REFERRALS

_____

_____

_____

NAME:	DOB:	Page

Social

1. LIVING ARRANGEMENT		5. SOCIAL/LEISURE	
2. FAMILY DYNAMICS		6. PLACEMENT ISSUES	
3. CAREGIVER SUPPORT		7. LEGAL/FINANCIAL	
4. SUPPORT SERVICES		8. OTHER	

Physical

1. HEARING		7. FOOT CARE		13. RANGE OF MOTION	
2. VISION		8. SKIN CARE		14. MOVEMENT DISORDER	
3. COMMUNICATION/SPEECH		9. URINARY FUNCTION		15. PARALYSIS/SENSATION	
4. DENTAL		10. BOWEL FUNCTION		16. CIRCULATORY SYSTEM	
5. NUTRITION/SWALLOWING		11. PAIN/DISCOMFORT		17. RESPIRATORY SYSTEM	
6. WEIGHT		12. JOINT PROBLEM		18. OTHER	

NAME:	DOB:	Page

G D S

		YES	NO
1.	Are you basically satisfied with your life?	___	___
2.	Have you dropped many of your activities and interests?	___	___
3.	Do you feel that your life is empty?	___	___
4.	Do you often get bored?	___	___
5.	Are you hopeful about the future?	___	___
6.	Are you bothered by thoughts you can't get out of your head?	___	___
7.	Are you in good spirits most of the time?	___	___
8.	Are you afraid that something bad is going to happen to you?	___	___
9.	Do you feel happy most of the time?	___	___
10.	Do you often feel helpless?	___	___
11.	Do you often get restless and fidgety?	___	___
12.	Do you prefer to stay at home rather than going out and doing new things?	___	___
13.	Do you frequently worry about the future?	___	___
14.	Do you feel you have more problems with memory than most?	___	___
15.	Do you think it is wonderful to be alive now?	___	___
16.	Do you often feel downhearted and blue?	___	___
17.	Do you feel pretty worthless the way you are now?	___	___
18.	Do you worry a lot about the past?	___	___
19.	Do you find life very exciting?	___	___
20.	Is it hard for you to get started on new projects?	___	___
21.	Do you feel full of energy?	___	___
22.	Do you feel that your situation is hopeless?	___	___
23.	Do you think that most people are better off than you?	___	___
24.	Do you frequently get upset over little things?	___	___
25.	Do you frequently feel like crying?	___	___
26.	Do you have trouble concentrating?	___	___
27.	Do you enjoy getting up in the morning?	___	___
28.	Do you prefer to avoid social gatherings?	___	___
29.	Is it easy for you to make decisions?	___	___
30.	Is your mind as clear as it used to be?	___	___

Have you been feeling sad or blue lately [or]
How have your spirits been lately?

THE FOLSTEIN MINI-MENTAL STATE EXAMINATION

Ask client his:

Name _____ Date of Birth ____(YY) ____(MM) ____(DD)

Occupation _____

Education _____

Maximum Correct Score	Client's Score	

ORIENTATION

1) 5   ( )   What is the   - date_____, day of week_____, month_____

                              - season_____, year_____?

2) 5   ( )   Where are we - name of province_____, town_____

                            - street_____, place_____, floor____?

3) 3   ( )   REGISTRATION

Name 3 objects (APPLE, TABLE, PENNY). Take 1 second to say each. Then ask the patient all 3 after you have said them. Give 1 point for each correct answer. Then repeat them until he learns all 3. Count trials and record TRIALS___

4) 5   ( )   CALCULATION

Serial 7's. 100-7=( ) 93=( ) 86=( ) 79=( ) 72=( ) 65.

5) 3   ( )   RECALL

Ask for 3 objects - APPLE ( ), TABLE ( ), PENNY ( ).

6) 5   ( )   ATTENTION

Spell "WORLD" backwards.

7) 9   ( )   LANGUAGE

Name a pencil and watch (.   )   2 points
Repeat the following - "NO IFS, ANDS OR BUTS"   1 point
Follow a 3-stage command:
"Take the paper in your right hand, fold it in
half and put it on the floor." (   )   3 points
Read and obey command on reverse (CLOSE YOUR EYES)   1 point
Write a sentence.   1 point
Copy design shown on reverse.   1 point

Assess level of consciousness: [ ]   [ ]   [ ]   [ ]
                                 Alert Drowsy Stupor Coma

SCORE: 30 ( ) - MENTAL STATUS SUBSCORE (Minus ATTENTION score)

        35 ( ) - MENTAL STATUS TOTAL SCORE (Including ATTENTION score)

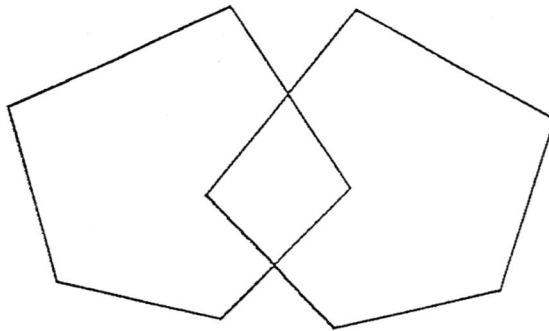

NAME:	DOB:	Page

Psychological Health

1. ORIENTATION	5. SIGNIFICANT LOSS/CHANGE
2. COGNITION	6. BEHAVIOUR
3. MOOD\AFFECT	7. THOUGHT DISTURBANCES
4. SLEEP	8. OTHER

Preceded by the GDS and MMSE...

Client Profile: Functional
ACTIVITIES OF DAILY LIVING

Skill Performance Score (S)	.	Resource Score (R)

1. Independent.
2. Needs supervision, cuing or set up.
3. Needs some physical assistance and contributes to the task.
4. Dependent.

YES Has resources necessary to safely and effectively overcome deficit on a consistent basis.

NO Safe and effective resource is not constantly available.

SKILL PERFORMANCE	S	RESOURCE	R
TOILET			
FEEDING			
DRESSING			
GROOMING			
BATHING			
MOBILITY			
a) bed mobility			
b) transfers			
c) ambulation			
d) stairs			

N/A – Not Assessed. Please record the reason.

NAME:	DOB:	Page

Client Profile
Functional
ACTIVITIES OF DAILY LIVING

Skill Performance Score (S)	Resource Score (R)

1. Independent.

2. Needs supervision, cuing or set up.

3. Needs some physical assistance and contributes to the task.

4. Dependent.

YES Has resources necessary to safely and effectively overcome deficit on a consistent basis.

NO Safe and effective resource is not constantly available.

SKILL PERFORMANCE	S	RESOURCE	R
TELEPHONE			
SHOPPING			
FOOD PREPARATION			
HOUSEKEEPING			
LAUNDRY			
TRANSPORTATION			
RESPONSIBILITY FOR OWN MEDICATIONS			
FINANCIAL MANAGEMENT			

N/A – Not Assessed. Please record the reason.

Functional

1. FALLS	5. ACCESSIBILITY/PHYSICAL/ENVIRONMENT
2. BALANCE	6. HOME MAINTENANCE
3. SAFETY ISSUES/HAZARDS	7. DAILY ROUTINE
4. ACTIVITY TOLERANCE	8. OTHER

Medications

1. MEDICATION	4. TOBACCO USE
2. ALLERGIES/INTOLERANCE	5. ALCOHOL USE
3. MANAGEMENT	6. OTHER

PHARMACY USED:

NAME:	DOB:	Page

Problem List

....
....
....
....
....
....
....
....
....
....
....
....

Recommendations

....
....
....
....
....
....
....
....
....
....
....
....
....

NAME:	DOB:	Page

443

Progress Note

Client Name:		Date of Birth:
Date of Progress Note:	Assessor:	

References

Applegate, WB, Akins, D, Vander Zwagg, R et al. (1983) A geriatric rehabilitation and assessment unit in a community hospital. *Journal of American Geriatric Society* 31: 206–210.

Applegate, WB, Miller, ST, Graney, MJ et al. (1990) A randomized, controlled trial of a geriatric assessment unit in a community rehabilitation hospital. *New England Journal of Medicine* 322: 1572–1578.

Brocklehurst, JC, Carty, MH, Leeming, JT et al. (1978) Medical screening of old people accepted for residential care. *Lancet* 2: 141.

Burley, LE, Currie, CT, Smith, RG et al. (1979) Contribution from geriatric medicine within acute medical wards. *British Medical Journal* 2: 90.

Campion, EW (1987) The merits of geriatric consultation. *Journal of the American Medical Association* 257: 2336.

Collard, AF, Bachman, SS, Beatrice, DF (1985) Acute care delivery for the geriatric patient: an innovative approach. *Quality Review Bulletin* 6: 180–185.

Folstein, MF, Folstein, S, McHugh, PR (1975) Mini-mental state: A practical method for grading the cognitive state of patients for the clinician. *Journal of Psychiatric Research* 12: 189–198.

Gayton, D, Wood-Dauphinee, S, de Lorimer, M et al. (1987) Trial of a geriatric consultation team in an acute care hospital. *Journal of American Geriatric Society* 35: 726–736.

Hendrickson, C, Lund, E, Stromgard, E (1984) Consequences of assessment and intervention among elderly people: a three year randomized controlled trial. *British Medical Journal* 289: 1522–1524.

Hogan, DB, Fox, FA, Badley, FWD et al. (1987) Effect of a geriatric consultation service on management of patients in an acute care hospital. *Canadian Medical Association Journal* 136: 713–717.

Kahn, RL, Goldfarb, AI, Pollack, M, Peck, A (1960) Brief Objective Measures for the determination of mental status in the aged. *American Journal of Psychiatry* 117: 326–328.

Lawton, MP (1975) The Philadelphia geriatric better morale scale: A revision. *Journal of Gerontology* 30: 85–89.

Lawton, MP, Moss, H. et al. (1982) A research and service-oriented multilevel assessment instrument. *Journal of Gerontology* 17: 91–99.

Lefton, E, Bonstelle, S, Frengley, JD (1983) Success with an inpatient geriatric unit: A controlled study. *Journal of American Geriatric Society* 31: 149–155.

Liem, PH, Chernoff, R, Carter, WJ (1986) Geriatric Rehabilitation Unit: A three-year outcome evaluation. *Journal of Gerontology* 41: 44–50.

Linn, MW (1967) A rapid disability rating scale. *Journal of the American Geriatric Society* 15: 211–214.

Mahoney, FI, Barthel, DW (1965) Functional evaluation: the Barthel Index. *Rehabilitation* 14: 61–65.

Puxty, JAH (1989) Geriatric assessment tools. In *Writings in Gerontology*. Ottawa: National Advisory Council on Ageing.

Robertson, C (1984) Old people in the community: Screening for Health. *Nursing Times* 80 (33): 44–45.

Robinson, B (1983) Valediction of a caregivers strain index. *Journal of Gerontology* 38: 344–348.

Rubenstein, LZ, Josephson, KR, Wieland, GD et al. (1984) Effectiveness of a geriatric evaluation unit: A randomized clinical trial. *New England Journal of Medicine* 311: 1664–1670.

Rubenstein, Z, Stuck, A, Siu, A et al. (1991) Impacts of geriatric evaluation and management programs on defined outcomes: overview of the evidence. *Journal of American Geriatrics Society (Supp.)* 39: S8–S16.

Saltz, CC, McVey, LJ, Becker, PM et al. (1988) Impact of a geriatric consultation team on discharge placement and repeat hospitalization. *Gerontologist* 28: 344–350.

Smith, B, O'Malley, S (1993) The costs and experiences of caring for sick and disabled geriatric patients: Australian observations. *Australian Journal of Public Health* 17: 131–134.

Stuck, AE, Siu, SL, Wieland, GD et al. (1993) Comprehensive geriatric assessment: a meta-analysis of controlled trials. *Lancet* 342: 1032–1036.

Williams, TF, Hill, JG, Fairbank, ME et al. (1973) Appropriate placement of the chronically ill and aged: A successful approach by evaluation. *Journal of the American Medical Association* 226: 1332–1335.

Williamson, MB, Stokoc, IH, Gray, S et al. (1964) Old people at home: their unreported needs. *Lancet* 1: 1117–1120.

Yesavage, HA, Brink, RL (1983) Development and validation of a geriatric depression screening scale: A preliminary report. *Journal of Psychiatric Research* 17: 37–49.

Zarit, S, Reever, K, Bach-Peterson, J (1982) Relatives of the impaired elderly: correlates of feelings of burden. *Gerontologist* 20: 649–655.

30

Institutional Health Services

KELLI O'BRIEN, ANGELA U TOPPING

Introduction
•
Institutional-based Long-term Care Services
•
Out-of-Pocket Cost for Institutional-based Long-term Care
•
Reasons for Admission: A Client Profile
•
Role of Physiotherapy Services

Introduction

The objective of this chapter is to provide a general overview of institutional-based long-term care services available to seniors. After reading this chapter the student will be able to describe four common institutional-based long-term services, the reasons for admission and the role of physiotherapy in each of these settings. A general client profile for each long-term care setting will clarify the differences between each of the services.

Institutional-based Long-term Care Services

Long-term care services refer to a variety of health, psychosocial, support and maintenance services that can be provided on a prolonged basis to individuals with chronic functional impairments or who are at risk of developing such impairments. Long-term care services promote independence and improved quality of life by improving and/or maintaining an individual's physical, social, and psychological function. Long-term care services can be provided in a variety of institutional-based settings such as rehabilitation hospitals, day hospitals, and nursing homes.

Rehabilitation Hospitals / Geriatric Assessment Units

Rehabilitation hospitals / Geriatric Assessment Units (GAU) are specialized units within a hospital that provide comprehensive geriatric assessment that includes an evaluation of medical, functional, psychosocial and environmental problems and a range of therapeutic interventions on an in-patient basis. The general goals of this type of facility are to provide improved diagnosis and treatment, to improve an individual's level of function, to reduce inappropriate use of health care, and to avoid inappropriate placement. An older adult whose independent living has become compromised by a mixture of medical, functional, or psychosocial problems, such as geriatric conditions (e.g. falls, incontinence, polypharmacy), physical disorders (e.g. chronic illnesses, CVA) (see Section D) and psychosocial disorders (e.g. unstable or abusive home situation, perceived need for service) are appropriate for this type of facility (Rubenstein *et al.*, 1991). Cognitively impaired or terminally ill individuals are usually not targeted by this type of facility. Older adults can be referred to this type of service by a geriatrician, family doctor, family member or caregiver from home, acute care ward, or nursing home settings (Rubenstein *et al.*, 1991).

The specialized services available in this type of institution include diagnostic testing, nursing care, medical management, physiotherapy, occupational therapy, speech language pathology, psychology, social and recreational services, nutritional services, mechanical aids, medications, and medical supplies (Rubenstein *et al.*, 1991). Intensive multidisciplinary rehabilitation programmes are developed for individuals who have severe impairments or disabilities that are amenable to intervention. Rapid significant functional gains are anticipated by clients undergoing this type of rehabilitation programme. The length of stay in a rehabilitation hospital or GAU is dependent upon an individual's condition, his/her response to therapeutic intervention, and his/her future living accommodations.

Geriatric Day Hospitals

Most geriatric day hospitals (GDH) provide a similar comprehensive assessment and therapeutic intervention programme for older adults, without requiring hospital admission (see Chapter 29). Structurally, GDHs are often located within a district hospital or a rehabilitation hospital. Most GDHs operate only on weekdays. Clients attend for full or half-day programmes as appropriate and for any combination of rehabilitation, assessment, maintenance treatment, medical or nursing investigation and/or social care. Nearly 75% of day hospital clients attend for rehabilitation and/or functional assessment (Brocklehurst, 1992).

Rehabilitation refers to the acquisition of skills needed for independent life, and the restoration of an individual to his/her former or another environment (Ebrahim, 1992). Any functional assessment is used to determine rehabilitation potential and long-term accommodation plans. Maintenance programmes allow a client to sustain his/her functional level achieved through rehabilitation. Occasionally, clients discharged from a rehabilitation programme are at risk of functional deterioration when contact from health professionals is lost. Some clients may continue to attend GDH once or twice a week after discharge from the hospital for maintenance of function.

Most clients attending GDHs are referred from inpatient geriatric wards or outpatient geriatric clinics. The major diagnostic categories of GDH clients include stroke and arthritis. The frequency and length of attendance is dictated by the severity of the disability functional level, programme objectives and familial choice.

Specialized services provided through GDHs include medical supervision, nursing care and supervision, physiotherapy, occupational therapy, speech language pathology, social work, health education, nutritional care, personal care, chiropody and referral services. This type of institutional-based care is appropriate for older adults who require extensive assessment and treatment but who are well enough to continue to live with these services that cannot be given at home (Kolleck, 1989). Gradual, significant gains in function can be expected from rehabilitation programmes offered by day hospitals.

Nursing Homes

Nursing homes provide long-term accommodation, personal care and a variety of social and recreation activities for individuals who cannot continue to safely live in their own homes. The length of stay in a nursing home is unpredictable, and usually involves months to years. From country to country, nursing homes acquire slightly different definitions; consequently, the type of client served by these institutions varies considerably between countries.

The objectives of most nursing homes are to restore/maintain the health status and functional capabilities of residents, as well as providing for their psychosocial needs. Considerable assistance is provided by nursing staff with personal care for things such as toileting, dressing and mobility. Recreational and social programmes maintain residents' activity levels and social contacts. Rehabilitation specialists are employed by some nursing

homes or appropriate referrals may be made to private agencies. Physiotherapists service many roles when working in a nursing home, such as assessment, maintenance, rehabilitation and consultation to staff. Nursing home residents are expected to show limited or slow functional gains. As well, some nursing homes offer multidisciplinary, geriatric assessments that are performed upon admission and when a significant, unexpected change in functional or clinical status occurs, such as an unexplained change in cognitive status, or repeated falls (Rubenstein et al., 1991). In an effort to control inappropriate placement Australia has established the aged care assessment teams (ACATs) to screen all nursing home applicants.

Rest Homes/Retirement Homes

Rest homes provide temporary or long-term accommodation for older adults. Retirement homes are referred to as hostels in Australia (Moss, 1989). The length of stay in a rest/retirement home is usually prolonged. The services provided by a rest home include meal preparation, social and recreational activities and intermittent nursing supervision. Older adults who require assistance with meals and home activities such as cleaning, but who are independent or require minimal assistance with daily living activities such as feeding, dressing and toileting, are suitable for rest homes. Residents of rest homes do not require regular nursing or medical assistance. Residents who require more nursing or personal care services can hire additional assistance from home carers, district nurses, or, if this is insufficient, residents may choose to relocate to a nursing home. As well, residents who require the services of rehabilitation specialists may receive private or government provided home care by referral only. Intervention would be determined by individual needs. For these individuals, a rapid, significant gain to premorbid functioning is anticipated through intervention.

Out-of-Pocket Cost for Institutional-based Long-term Care

The cost of institutional-based long-term care services for the recipient varies according to country. In Canada, hospital-based long-term care services are provided free of charge on a universal and comprehensive basis (Datta, 1993). There are user fees for provincially regulated nursing homes and for those individuals who occupy a chronic care hospital bed. The Old Age Security and Guaranteed Income Supplement are the standards against which user fees are regulated. The rate is about 85% of the maximum OAS and GIS rate for single persons. The daily user fee is about $25.00 Canadian in most provinces. A minimum guaranteed disposable income ($83.00–$105.00/month) is available for all residents after paying out-of-pocket costs, even for those with only federal income support. There are also for-profit nursing homes in various provinces in which residents must cover the full cost of their stay.

In the UK, where hospitals are the major setting for long-term care services, the National Health Service covers all long-term care hospital costs without charge to the client. Nursing homes are operated by for-profit or non-profit agencies. Private nursing homes charge residents for the full cost of their care; in 1993 fees ranged from £240 pounds to £300 per week. Income support is available to assist individuals with private nursing home costs. The maximum amount of public support available is insufficient to cover private nursing home costs. Charitable foundations may help to make up the difference (Datta, 1993).

In Australia, long-term care services are provided by public, private and volunteer sectors (Moss, 1989). The Commonwealth government provides funding to geriatric programmes such as regional geriatric assessment programmes and public nursing homes. Nursing homes can also be funded by private or volunteer agencies. The private sector controls for-profit nursing homes and hostels (Moss, 1989). Information regarding fees for these services is not available because the funding system of these programmes is currently under review.

Reasons for Admission: A Client Profile

Clients are referred to institutional facilities when their medical, functional and psychosocial problems are serious enough to impair independent living. The presence of two or more chronic disorders can guarantee referral to any long-term care service. These chronic disorders include visual and auditory deficits, CVA, Parkinson's disease, cardiovascular disease, lower extremity amputation, cognitive impairment and psychiatric problems (e.g. depression and reactive disorders) (see Chapters 8 and 19). Decreased performance in activities of daily living and mobility are also factors that contribute to institutionalization (Jette et al., 1992). Living alone is a psychosocial factor that has been associated with early institutionalization (chronic care or nursing home care) (Steinbach, 1992).

The type of institutional service that a geriatric

Table 1
Client Profile

	Rehabilitation hospital/geratric assessment unit	Day hospital	Nursing homes	Rest homes/ retirement homes
Applied self-care	Minimally effective in bladder and bowel management and in skin care	Function at nearly premorbid levels in bowel and bladder management and skin care. May still be dependent in their use of medications	Completely dependent for all nursing and medication-related activities	Independent in personal self-care with some difficulty in home management tasks such as meal preparation and shopping
Physical	Require minimal assistance in feeding, moderate assistance in hygiene, position changes, and dressing and maximum assistance in all transfer, mobility, and home management tasks	Nearly normal levels of functioning in feeding and personal hygiene and largely independent functioning in most transfer and mobility tasks. May be dependent on others in home management skills.	Dependent for all physical mobility tasks and activities of daily living	Normal level of functioning with some difficulty in home management skills
Cognitive	Normal alertness and orientation. Linguistic processing, abstraction skills, reading and writing, visual-spatial processing, and short-term memory were likely to be moderately impaired.	Nearly normal levels of alertness and orientation, with mild impairment of linguistic processing and verbal abstraction. Reading and writing, visual-spatial processing, and short-term memory likely to be mildly to moderately impaired	Mild impairment in alertness and responsiveness to stimuli, marked impairment in orientation and severe impairment in verbal abstraction and linguistic processing, reading, writing skills, short-term verbal memory and visual/ spatial processing	Normal levels of alertness and orientation. May have mild but functional impairments in linguistic processing and verbal abstraction. Reading and writing, visual-spatial processing and short-term memory were likely to be normal or mild impaired with little functional effect
Social	Intense rehabilitation programming allows continuous social contracts	Dependent on the individual whether living alone or with family	Social isolation a possibility because programming intermittent	Social contacts, programmes and activities usually a strong part of the rest home milieu

Adapted from: Harvey *et al.* (1992).

client receives depends largely upon their functional level and rehabilitation potential. Table 1 provides a brief overview of the four institutional-based long-term care services, and how the clients in each institution differ along four functional domains: applied self-care, physical, cognitive and social. Rehabilitation/GAU hospital clients receive the most intense rehabilitation while clients in retirement homes/rest homes receive the least intense services. In general, nursing home clients have the lowest level of function, while retirement home residents appear to have the highest. Clients of rehabilitation hospitals have a fairly low level of function, while day hospital clients have a slightly greater functional level. This is logical because day hospitals are usually the next step for many discharged rehabilitation hospital clients.

Role of Physiotherapy Services

The general goals of physiotherapy in institutional-based care for the elderly are to restore/improve function and to prevent further declines in function.

Physiotherapists working in institutions providing health services for the elderly must collaborate with other rehabilitation professionals (see Chapter 28) such as occupational therapists, speech-language therapists and rehabilitation nurses. Each profession offers a unique perspective that can complement physiotherapy. There are generally seven areas in geriatric care where physiotherapists can provide expertise (Lewis and Bottomley, 1993):

1. Exercise prescription such as range of motion, strengthening, co-ordination and relaxation exercises.

2. Functional mobility such as balance, transfer and gait retraining.

3. Assistive devices such as provision of ambulation aids (e.g. canes, walkers) and joint protection devices (e.g. ankle foot orthosis, heel lifts).

4. Modalities such as functional electrical stimulation, ultrasound, laser or diathermy.

5. Pain management, either acute or chronic pain.

6. Cardiorespiratory function such as conditioning or endurance training, and respiratory techniques such as postural drainage and breathing control exercises.

7. Education (client/family/staff) regarding safe transfers, positioning, health promotion and prevention activities.

Exercise programming at the individual or group level is probably the most commonly prescribed maintenance activity but its benefits can be dramatic particularly to the very old. Reduction in cardiovascular risk, improvements in functional capacity, and improvements in semantically cued memory are positively related to physical activity with general well-being and lower levels of anxiety and depression especially in women over 40.

Older persons can experience problems in gait and wheelchair mobility that are often correctable by improving functional capacity or by developing compensation strategies (Nelson and Stucky, 1992). Gait re-training with assistive devices such as a walker or cane often improves the ability of individuals to ambulate safely without physical assistance of staff or family. Education can be provided regarding the importance of proper footwear to effectively stabilize the foot during ambulation. Wheelchair prescription may be needed for longer distances or when it is no longer physically possible or safe for an individual to ambulate (for example late stages of multiple sclerosis) (Lewis and Bottomley, 1993). Assistive devices, such as bedrails or grab bars, can facilitate safe transfers in the bedroom or bathroom. Bathrooms can also be equipped with raised toilet seats and shower chairs. There are numerous devices that can make the environment safe and accessible for the disabled older adult.

Various modalities, such as laser and ultrasound, can be used for short-term restorative treatment of ulcers and contractures. Transcutaneous electrical stimulation and moist heat may be used for the treatment of chronic arthritic pain. Respiratory techniques, such as percussion and deep breathing exercises, can be employed during certain acute illnesses such as pneumonia. The client, family and staff can benefit from educational sessions designed to improve transfer safety, suggest proper positioning in lying and sitting and encourage increased mobility.

These seven treatment areas provide a general outline of the services provided by physiotherapists in geriatric rehabilitation hospitals / units, geriatric day hospitals, nursing homes and retirement homes. Programme intensity is determined by the individual client needs and the focus of the institution to which the physiotherapist is affiliated. Rehabilitation and geriatric day hospitals employ staff to provide comprehensive assessment and restorative programmes in a therapeutic milieu that uses multidisciplinary interviews and cooperative discharge planning. The client enters these programmes with specific time-limited goals that are designed to maximize function, and which take into consideration the physical and social demands of the client's home environment. Discharge plans are based on the interdisciplinary assessment of the client's rehabilitation potential. Decisions to discharge are based on many factors (Table 2).

Clients who receive assessment, treatment, and rehabilitation in a GAU are more likely to experience functional gains, and reduced risk of nursing home placement, when compared with clients not receiving this specialized care. Applegate et al. (1990) reported larger improvements in bathing, dressing and transfer ability among elderly clients who attended a GAU for a mean length of stay of 24 days (sd = 13 days) when compared with controls. Clients at low risk of nursing home

Table 2
Before Discharging to Long-term Care Services Ask Yourself:

1. What is the client's functional level?
2. Is there a caregiver? What is the capacity of the caregiver to meet the needs of the client?
3. How much and what type of care do they require (medical, nursing or / and rehabilitation)?
4. What is the client's rehabilitation potential?
5. Are the rehabilitation goals restorative, maintenance or monitoring?
6. What intensity of rehabilitation would most benefit the client given their rehabilitation potential?
7. What are the client's goals? Are those goals realistic given the client's functional abilities, rehabilitation potential and available resources (social and financial)?
8. Get an accurate description of the original living situation. Would the client function effectively in that environment? If the answer is no, what is the level of functional the individual would need to function safely in that environment? Or what type of assistance would be necessary to maintain that person in their home environment? (e.g. assistive devices, community supports, therapeutic services)

placement improved in seven of eight activities of daily living.

It is difficult to examine the effectiveness of geriatric day hospitals due to the multiple functions which they serve. A randomized, controlled study by Tucker *et al.* (1984) reported greater improvements in ADL in GDH group when compared with controls after 6 weeks. This difference was no longer significant after 5 months. A more recent study by Young and Forster (1992) illustrated improvements in Barthel index and motor assessment scores in a group of GDH clients. However, a comparison between improvements in GDH and home care groups indicated more favourable results for clients receiving home care therapy.

The primary focus of nursing homes is to provide for the client's medical and nursing needs, while residents of retirement/rest homes require only intermittent nursing and medical supervision. For these two levels of care, physiotherapy is usually provided on a referral basis only, although some nursing homes do hire their own physiotherapist, whose role is to prevent functional impairments and to maintain the mobility level of residents for the maximum length of time possible. These services are often provided by rehabilitation assistants who are supervized by the physiotherapist. Restorative physiotherapy is sometimes provided in both facilities, on an intermittent basis, when a problem amenable to active intervention is identified.

A recent study by Fiatrone *et al.* (1994) examined the benefits of a 10-week period of exercise in frail nursing home residents. A control group of nursing home residents received nutritional supplements during the same 10-week period. The exercise group exhibited improved muscle strength, increased gait velocity, improved stair climbing power and increased spontaneous physical activity.

McMurdo and Rennie (1993) had previously evaluated the benefits of seated, low-intensity, bi-weekly exercise sessions in residents of a local authority home. This programme resulted in increased grip strength, increased spinal flexion range of motion, improved ADL scores, and decreased the time required to transfer from chair to standing. Preliminary evidence has also been reported on the effectiveness of physiotherapy in nursing homes, even when provided for cognitively impaired and functionally dependent older adults (Chlodo *et al.*, 1992).

Providing rehabilitation services in skilled nursing facilities is challenging for two reasons: clients have complex multiple impairments and disabilities; and staff often have limited knowledge and understanding of rehabilitation goals and benefits. Nursing home clients lack the endurance or cognitive function to fully participate in and/or benefit from intense interdisciplinary therapy. Consequently, rehabilitation efforts are oriented toward maintaining rather than restoring function, although there are some clinical situations where restorative therapy is appropriate. Generally, in rehabilitation and day hospitals, there is solid respect for the contribution of rehabilitation professionals in helping to improve client function and mobility. This translates into better implementation of therapy recommendations and more appropriate referrals. In some nursing homes, therapeutic intervention may still be devalued or misunderstood, decreasing the likelihood of compliance (Mann, 1990).

Physiotherapists working in skilled nursing facilities must deal with these issues constructively. Christensen (1987) and Mann (1990) both recommend following an education/consultative process, that involves creating a system of physiotherapist consultation and documented review. Written communication of the goals and treatment plan is not enough. Effective implementation of treatment goals requires communicating with supervisors and hands-on staff so that therapeutic initiatives are understood and supported. Providing opportunities for follow-up visits after completion of direct treatment allows the physiotherapist and staff to review the client's progress, to correct errors and to praise accomplishments. Adherence to an educative/consultative process with rigorous review benefits the client, physiotherapist and staff.

References

Applegate, WB, Miller, ST, Graney, MJ et al. (1990) A randomized, controlled trial of a geriatric assessment unit in a community rehabilitation hospital. *The New England Journal of Medicine* **322**: 1572–1578.

Brocklehurst, JC (1992) The geriatric service and the day hospital in the United Kingdom. In Brocklehurst, JC, Tallis, RC, Fillit, HM (eds) *Textbook of Geriatric Medicine and Gerontology*, pp. 1005–1016. New York: Churchill Livingstone.

Chlodo, LK, Gerety, MB, Mulrow, CD et al. (1992) The impact of physical therapy on nursing home patients outcomes. *Physical Therapy* **72**: 168–175.

Christensen, MA (1987) The therapist as geriatric environmental consultant. *Topics in Geriatric Rehabilitation* **3**: 79–83.

Datta, S (1993) Out-of-pocket costs for long-term care. *Aging International* **20**: 55–59.

Ebrahim (1992) Rehabilitation. In Brocklehurst, JC, Tallis, RC, Fillit, HM (eds) *Textbook of Geriatric Medicine and Gerontology*, pp. 1038–1054. New York: Churchill Livingstone.

Fiatrone, MA, O'Neill, EF, Ryan, ND et al. (1994) Exercise training and nutritional supplementation for physical frailty in very elderly people. *The New England Journal of Medicine* **330**: 1769–1775.

Harvey, RF, Silverstein, B, Venzon, MA et al. (1992) Applying psychometric criteria to functional assessment in medical rehabilitation: III. Construct validity and predicting level of care. *Archives of Physical Medicine and Rehabilitation* **73**: 887–892.

Jette, AM, Branch, LG, Sleeper, LA et al. (1992) High-risk profiles for nursing home admission. *The Gerontologist* **32**: 634–640.

Kolleck, D (1989) Geriatric stepped care. *Canadian Family Physician* **35**: 613–616.

Lewis, CB, Bottomley, JM (1993) *Geriatric Physical Therapy: A Clinical Approach*. Norwalk, Connecticut: Appleton & Lange.

Mann, WC (1990) Improving care for nursing home patients: A model for therapist consultation. *Physical and Occupational Therapy in Geriatrics* **9**: 65–72.

McMurdo, MET, Rennie, L (1993) A controlled trial of exercise by residents of old people's homes. *Age & Ageing* **22**: 11–15.

Moss, B (1989) Long-term care for the elderly in Australia. In Schwab T (ed.) *Caring for an Aging World: International Models for Long-Term Care, Financing, and Delivery*, pp. 212–244. New York: McGraw-Hill Book Company.

Nelson, DL, Stucky, C (1992) The roles of occupational therapy in preventing further disability of elderly persons in long-term care facilities. In Rothmann, J, Levine, R (eds) *Prevention Practice: Strategies for Physical and Occupational Therapists*, pp. 19–35. Philadelphia: WB Saunders.

Rubenstein, LZ, Goodwin, M, Hadley, E et al. (1991) Working group recommendations: targeting criteria for geriatric evaluation and management research. *Journal of the American Geriatrics Society* **39**: 37S–41S.

Steinbach, U (1992). Social networks, institutionalization and mortality among elderly people in the United States. *Journal of Gerontology* **47**: S183–S190.

Tucker, MA, Davison, JG, Ogle, SJ (1984) Day hospital rehabilitation — effectiveness and cost in the elderly: a randomised controlled trial. *British Medical Journal* **289**: 1209–1213.

Young, JB, Forster, A (1992) The Bradford community stroke trial: results at six months. *British Medical Journal* **304**: 1085–1089.

31

Community Services

ROBIN L STADNYK, ANN COMPTON, SUSAN M JOHNSON

Links Between Institutions and Community
•
Community Services
•
The Role of Physiotherapy in Community Services

Community health and support services exist in order to enable older persons and their caregivers — family members and friends who care for them — to function as independently as possible in their home communities. While older persons are heavy users of hospitals, government statistics show that the majority of them live in their own homes or in the homes of family members (see Chapters 2 and 5). Numerous studies have indicated that older persons wish to receive health services, whenever possible, in or near their own homes.

Community services must not only enable peo-ple to stay in their own homes, but to participate in the life of their communities. Physiotherapy is only one of these services; other needs include physician care, nursing, other therapies, personal care, help with housework, transportation, meals, recreation, respite care, and caregiver support.

This chapter will explore (1) how community services link with hospital services; (2) how com-munity services meet rehabilitation and long-term care needs of older persons; and (3) the role of the physiotherapist in community services.

Links Between Institutions and Community

Some older persons needing community services are identified during a hospital stay, whether it be for an acute illness or for rehabilitation. Therefore, it is important for institutions to be able to communicate easily with community services about client needs, so that services can be planned and the transition from institution to community is smooth. This is accomplished through discharge planning and case finding. Hospitals have discharge planners or community liaison officers whose job is to anticipate client needs in the community and enable the client and family to obtain the services they need. Case finding is performed by various professionals in hospitals, including those working with geriatric assessment programmes and disease-specific support programmes. The client's needs are not necessarily directly related to professional involvement. Using this approach clients are assessed by the appropriate agents, total care needs identified and services are mobilized in advance of hospital discharge.

Optimally, discharge planning and case finding strategies are coordinated. Clients are monitored while in hospital to ensure that needed services and supports are in place before discharge. After discharge, a community case coordinator may continue to monitor and adjust services in partnership with the client and family and can communicate with the hospital in the event of a subsequent hospitalization.

Many industrialized nations, such as the UK and Canada, are grappling with health care systems in which all costs, particularly hospital costs, are rising dramatically. As a result, hospitals and community services are working together in many communities to develop ways to reduce length of stay, or avoid admissions altogether.

Older persons use hospitals far more than younger people; approximately 55% of all hospital days are used by elderly persons, with an average stay of over 7 days compared with under 2 days for persons under the age of 65 (Statistics Canada, 1994). As older persons have a longer average stay they are particularly targeted for new programmes to reduce or eliminate hospitalization by more effective use of community services.

Examples of such initiatives include:

Early discharge programmes Increasingly, hospital patients are being discharged earlier after procedures such as joint replacement, with the bulk of their follow-up therapy being carried out at home.

Same day surgery programmes Clients undergo surgical procedures as outpatients, receiving follow-up care at home.

Pre–admission teaching/assessment programmes As part of pre-admission teaching about hospital procedures, clients' home needs are discussed and planned in advance of hospitalization to ensure smooth transition from institution back to community.

Quick response programmes Intensive in-home services are arranged for persons with emergency needs so that hospital admission is not necessary. Clients are assessed at home or in emergency rooms of hospitals as an alternative to an emergency admission.

Day hospital Medical investigations and intensive therapy are carried out in a day unit preventing overnight admissions. In all of these initiatives, it is vital that the link between hospital and community services be strong and formally structured.

It is also important to recognize that an increasing number of older persons access community services without having contact with a health care institution. For this reason, communities increasingly rely on public and health worker education and streamlined access to ensure that all older persons have access to services they need.

Public and health worker education   Services in each community are usually numerous and have varying eligibility criteria; therefore, increasing community awareness of services and entitlements is crucial. Such information needs to be targeted not only to older patients but to those who care for them, particularly their relatives. People who work in the health care system need this knowledge in order to refer older persons to appropriate services.

Streamlined access   Many communities are developing a 'one-stop' telephone number to access all community health and support services. One of the main target groups for this initiative are older persons. The telephone is answered by an intake coordinator who can assist the client to access needed services. In UK the social support is accessed directly through the Social Services' Office and medical support through the general practitioner.

Long-term care systems have been recently reorganized to try to increase ease of access, improve service coordination, flexibility and responsiveness, reduce duplication of assessments and treatment, enhance consumer choice and provide more support to caregivers. This should result in systems which are more understandable to clients and to those who refer them for services, such as hospital workers and physicians.

In the UK, in response to the Community Care Act 1990, considerable efforts have been made to restrict long-term care within hospital facilities to those with acute medical needs. Other patients, after comprehensive assessment, have returned to suitable care placements, either to family care with community service support, to rest homes or nursing homes in their local communities.

The links between institutions and community described above focus on communication at the systems level, although many valuable linkages occur on a person-to-person basis. It is important that physiotherapists working in institutions and community service agencies communicate clearly with each other about the client's status, goals and abilities, through the appropriate channels. Physiotherapists, whether they work in the community or in institutions, must respect each other's work with the clients and endeavour to maintain good communication, in order to ensure optimum care for the client.

Community Services

Many similarities exist between community services in different industrialized countries since there is a common wish to enable an older person to remain within the community with an acceptable quality of life by maintaining health, function and social contact. The different service funding systems from government and private health insurance alter the administrative procedures rather than the practice.

Mobile Specialist Teams

Specialist teams provide services to communities which have limited services of their own. This type of service varies in its organization, but typically it is a multidisciplinary team of specialized health professionals which originates from an institutional rehabilitation centre. Some teams have mobile units so that they may transport equipment and supplies with them to the outreach site. The focus of such teams may be geriatric assessment or rehabilitation. Some teams focus on a specific disease such as arthritis, or provide a specific service such as prosthetics and orthotics.

Specialist teams usually have the following roles:

Assessment Specialist teams often focus on comprehensive and interdisciplinary assessment of the elderly person.

Treatment/intervention Usually, except for very specialized treatment such as fitting for personalized equipment, travelling teams make treatment recommendations which can be carried out by identified people in the local community.

Education Education is a major function for most mobile teams. Education may be directed at the client or those responsible for implementing a client programme, at health care workers in the community to improve their skills and knowledge, or towards the public, to raise awareness of disability/ageing issues.

Advocacy Many travelling teams actively advocate for the development and improvement of relevant services in the communities they visit (Lavallee and Crupi, 1992).

Specialist teams are not meant to supplant local resources, but rather to enhance and develop them. Because of their limited involvement with clients (perhaps one or two visits per year) they rely heavily on local resources to implement their recommendations.

Private Practice

Private practice is a quickly growing area of employment for physiotherapists in Canada and the UK, and is perhaps the largest sector of practice in Australia. In Britain this has been precipitated by recent changes within the National Health Service, whereby the provider units purchase the services required. With the advent of self-governing Trusts and General Practitioner fundholding practices, private physiotherapists are eligible to negotiate contracts with these organisations. Such arrangements are negotiated individually and are independent of NHS employment (Whitley Council) conditions.

A sample agreement is shown in Figure 1. The actual fee per session and number of sessions to be provided would be agreed between the physiotherapy provider and the Practice or Trust, and is usually renegotiated annually. In the event of a private practitioner providing service to an NHS Trust or to a Private Hospital fees per unit may be applied.

Trusts and GP Practices will have limited budgets for physiotherapy care. It is important for them to understand the types of patient conditon that will benefit most from physiotherapy. They are then able to prioritize their referrals for NHS treatment. The patients still have the option of choosing private physiotherapy.

Private physiotherapy practice has three components: in-home care, office-based practice and consultation practice, although some physiotherapists combine two or more of these.

Figure 1   A sample fundholder service agreement.

TRUST / G P FUNDHOLDER SERVICE AGREEMENT

BETWEEN: Physiotherapy Provider Name   PROVIDER CODE: . . . .

AND: Trust or GP Fundholding Practice Name   PRACTICE CODE: . . . .

1. *Objectives*

    1.1   The objective of this service agreement is to reduce the administrative burden on both the Physiotherapy Provider and the Practice / Trust.

    1.2   The agreement is for the period of 1 April 1994 to 31 March 1995, with the potential for renewal in subsequent years.

2.   *Contractual Arrangements*

    2.1   Outpatient referrals are made to the Physiotherapy Provider for funded appointments. These may include surgery, home or nursing home visits.

    2.2   The Physiotherapy Provider will invoice the practice on completion of the physiotherapy course of treatment.

    2.3   The Physiotherapy Provider will provide a clinical report with the invoice, together with a summary of the number and dates of treatments. Patient name, date of birth and costs will be included.

    2.4   The prices will be as per agreement between the Practice and the Physiotherapy Provider. This will be reviewed annually.

    2.5   On receipt of the invoice, the Practice will authorise payment and pass the invoice to their FHSA within 2 weeks.

    2.6   Questions with regard to patient care will be discussed with the referring GP by the Physiotherapy Provider.

    2.7   Questions related to invoices will be discussed between the Practice Manager and the Physiotherapy Provider.

Signed: The P.T. Provider: . . . .   Date: . . . .

Signed: The Practice / Trust: . . . .   Date: . . . .

IN-HOME PRIVATE PRACTICE

Many private practitioners provide in-home therapy as described below. They may contract their services to a home care programme, or provide such services privately. This affords the therapist the opportunity to specialize.

OFFICE-BASED PRIVATE PRACTICE

Most office-based practices are based on an area of specialization, such as pain management, injury management, or orthopaedics. The rules governing the eligibility of private practice therapists to be funded through public health insurance have varied over time and by location; typically most services are paid for privately or through supplementary health insurance (which is often paid for by the employer). Therefore development in this field has been very uneven between jurisdictions. There is no data available about the utilization of such services by older persons. Office-based services often have the advantage of being closer to the client's home community, having a shorter or non-existent waiting list, and having fewer bureaucratic constraints. On the other hand there are some disadvantages, in that most private services are concentrated in urban areas, transportation to and from the office may be a problem for an older client, and the costs of the services may not be funded through an insurance plan. For the relatively mobile client who needs rehabilitation rather than long-term care, office-based practices may offer a timely alternative to institutional outpatient services. For the physiotherapist, office-based practice often offers the opportunity to practise in a specialized area of interest. Many private practitioners report that they feel that they can offer a service which is more responsive to client demands.

CONSULTATION PRACTICE

Increasingly, private practice physiotherapists are being asked to consult with a variety of organizations about the needs of older persons. Some examples of such consultations might be:

Consulting to fitness centres, seniors' centres or other leisure organizations to increase staff awareness of the needs of older clients, or to develop specialized physical activity programmes for older clients or clients with specific disabilities such as arthritis.

Consulting to staff of nursing homes, housing projects or home support workers about safe ambulation, use of ambulation aids, transfer techniques, safe lifting.

Reviewing educational content of voluntary agency brochures.

Consulting to government about therapy needs of communities.

Community Health Centres

The Community Health Centre concept represents many similar models of ambulatory care which are growing in popularity both in Canada and UK. Community Health Centres are characterized by

- Globlal or capitation funding; non-profit status.
- Multidisciplinary team approach including physician care.
- Holistic orientation.
- Single access to health and social services, including primary physician care, health promotion, rehabilitation, counselling and education and perhaps including in-home services.

- Community-control by a Board or Council that determines the services to be offered.
- Emphasis on coordination and continuity of care (Fulton, 1993; Sutherland and Fulton 1988).

A physiotherapist employed in or seconded to a community health centre might be involved in a wide variety of activities at the community level including community development, health promotion and health education. When working with individual clients or client groups, the therapist may be involved in primary care, rehabilitation, or long-term care of older persons at the centre or in the home.

Home Care

Most communities have some form of organized home care available to older persons. The greatest number of physiotherapists employed in community services for older persons are working in home care.

Home care programmes exist in order to substitute for hospitalization, provide follow-up care from hospitals, and delay or prevent the need for institutional care (such as care in nursing homes). In-home services available in a community may include the following:

- Treatment services (wound care, dressings, intravenous therapy, etc.).
- Health maintenance services (occupational therapy, physical therapy, nutrition counselling, speech therapy, foot care).
- Personal hygiene and care.
- Household maintenance.
- Individual and family social services.
- Community liaison services.
- Facility care liaison services (i.e. referral to nursing homes, chronic care hospital beds, respite care, etc).
- Home aids and adaptations.

Many agencies are involved in the provision of in-home care. These might include (Sutherland and Fulton, 1988):

- Provincially-organized home-care programmes, which usually offer some form of case coordination and may also directly provide some of the services listed immediately above.
- Public health organizations.
- Mental health organizations.
- Community support service and volunteer organizations, which may be involved in professional or support service provision.
- Not-for-profit and for-profit service provision agencies.
- Community health centres.

Home care services in a community typically develop strong liaisons with each other and with local institutions.

ROLE OF THE PHYSIOTHERAPIST

Because of the rather broad mandate of home care and the increasing emphasis on community versus institutional services for older persons, the role of the home-care physiotherapist can be extremely varied. The therapist might be involved in:

Acute care Intensive, short-term therapy, post-surgical care, or care related to an acute illness.

Rehabilitation Rehabilitation for conditions such as cerebral vascular accidents (CVA), and orthopaedic procedures are increasingly being carried out in the home.

Long–term care Maintenance of functional abilities, mobility, and safety (particularly fall prevention) of older persons with disabilities is crucial if they are to remain in their own homes (see also Chapter 21).

Good results have been reported from intensive in-home exercise and education programmes targeted to people with chronic illnesses or disabilities such as ankylosing spondylitis. Generally, these programmes have resulted in both functional gains and reduction in the rate of institutionalization.

Palliative care   Increasingly, palliative care occurs in the home setting. The physiotherapist is an important team member in the areas of pain control, positioning and maintenance and promotion of physical function (Chapter 21).

Support to caregivers   Many older persons with disabilities require help from a family or friend in the area of personal care. It is generally recognized that 75–85% of the assistance provided to older persons is by family or friends, rather than other health professionals (Pruchno, 1990). Most caregivers are spouses or children and are female (Brody, 1981; Kaden and McDaniel, 1990). The unrelenting burden of caregiving frequently results in burnout, illness or injury of caregivers (Marcus and Jaeger, 1984; Zarit *et al.* 1980). Physiotherapists can assist caregivers in maintaining client mobility, transfer training, maintenance of range of motion (to make transfers and dressing easier). Because family caregivers are the true 'experts' in day-to-day care, the physiotherapist must work in a collaborative fashion with caregivers to identify and solve problems.

Health promotion   The caregivers, who may not have good health themselves, often need some input, such as safe handling and transfer techniques, to maintain their health and cope with the physical stress. Home care may be extended to input to local seniors' groups or day centres which the older clients attend to assist staff and other members with individual client needs or to promote members' general health needs.

Community Support Services Liaison

Community support services are those services which support older persons to live in and interact with their community, excluding treatment, health maintenance, and personal care services (Ministry of Health *et al.*, 1991). The importance of community support services is underscored by an examination of the needs reported by older persons in the Health and Activity Limitation Survey in 1986. In this survey 33% of older people expressed the need for help with outdoor maintenance, 31.3% with heavy housework, and 19.9% with groceries. In contrast, only 3.8% expressed the need for assistance with personal care (Hamilton, 1989). Similar surveys in the UK have produced comparable results.

Community support services are characterized by a volunteer or non-profit orientation; many systems rely on volunteers for the bulk of their client services. Most services are based on needs identified in their communities. A great number of older persons are maintained in their homes solely through the provision of such services. The types of services provided include:

- Heavy housework: e.g. provision of heavy house-cleaning, gardening or snow shovelling.
- Visiting: a volunteer visits regularly with an older person.
- Security checks and call-in services: the older person has a daily telephone contact with a volunteer; there are follow-up services if the

older person fails to make contact on a particular day.

- Meals-on-wheels or community dining programmes: hot meals are provided for clients in their own homes – or clients are transported on a weekly basis or more frequently to a community centre for a hot meal.
- Foot care clinics.
- Transportation.
- Social events.
- Peer support networks for older persons and/or caregivers, often based on specific health problems.
- Health promotion programmes, including information sessions and physical activities (Ministry of Health *et al.* 1991).

Community support services may be provided by seniors' groups (in which the activities are organized by and for older persons), church groups, organizations related to specific health problems, and many other community groups.

It is very important that strong liaisons exist between community support services and other services providing health care for older persons.

The Role of Physiotherapy in Community Services

While different involvements of physiotherapy have been described in some sections above, it is important to consider the role of physiotherapy in community services for older persons. Is community practice different? Does it require different skills and expertise than institutional practice?

In order to try to understand how community therapists practised, a survey of physiotherapists and occupational therapists practising in the community was undertaken in Ontario by Queen's University School of Rehabilitation Therapy (1992). Responding to the survey, physiotherapists identified the skills and expertise which they felt were most required for successful community practice as follows.

CLIENT ASSESSMENT, EDUCATION, TREATMENT

Solid clinical skills are demanded of community physiotherapists, who tend to practise quite independently. The need to be a generalist rather than a specialist is much greater in community than in institutional practice; therefore good overall knowledge, and the ability to keep abreast of changes in all areas of physiotherapy are important. Physiotherapists must also be able to adapt their interventions to the space and materials at hand, particularly if treatment occurs in the client's home.

CONSIDERATION OF THE CLIENT IN THE CONTEXT OF HIS/HER ENVIRONMENT

Assessment, goal setting and treatment are all activities undertaken in collaboration with the client in community practice. The client's values and interests often determine the success of intervention. The goals of treatment must be valued by the client, as well as being functional in terms of his or her needs. For example, a reasonable goal for physiotherapy might be to enable the client to ambulate independently and safely using a quadriped walker for a distance of 10 metres, while what the client really wants to be able to do is to walk the short distance down the hallway to his bathroom!

The cultural, physical and social environment of the client must always be most carefully considered in community practice. The physiotherapist must consider the ethos and value system of the client; the natural and man-made surroundings in their home and community; and the client's relationships with other people (Canadian Association of Occupational Therapists, 1991).

HEALTH PROMOTION APPROACH

Using a health promotion approach (see also Chapter 13) means helping clients to take measures to improve their own health. Physiotherapists recognize the need to take this approach to any intervention on either an individual or a community consultant basis. The health promotion approach involves an attitude shift from 'doing for' individuals to 'working with' individuals and groups to develop strategies to improve health in areas identified as important by them.

CONSULTATION APPROACH

Increasingly, physiotherapists working in the community use a consultation model. This may appear fairly straightforward in the case of travelling specialist teams. However, it is pervading all practice. For example, those working in home-based care must strive to educate the client to carry out his or her own exercise programme. If this is not possible, the physiotherapist often teaches a family member or support person to assist in treatment. The emphasis on consulting ensures that the physiotherapist's time is used more efficiently, and that those persons most appropriately involved in the client's life carry out ongoing therapy needs whenever possible. Physiotherapists must be comfortable with transferring their skills to other people.

SKILLS IN EDUCATING OTHERS

With the emphasis on consultation comes the realization that physiotherapists must possess good teaching skills. While involvement of physiotherapists in client education has been widely recognized, it is time to expand this education to also include caregivers and relevant community workers, and for greater involvement in the in-service education of other health professionals.

COMMUNICATION SKILLS

Related to skills in educating others are communication skills (see also Chapter 10). The need to communicate clearly with others, verbally, in writing and in documentation is well recognized. It is important to consider both the technical background and the literacy level of clients, family members, and community health care workers in these communications.

NETWORKING AND KNOWLEDGE OF COMMUNITY RESOURCES

In many communities people lack information about the health and support services that are available. Community physiotherapists understand how these services are organized in their community and can speak knowledgeably to clients about what is available and how to access it. They must be open to learning about resources from others, and to teaching others what those services have to offer.

One physiotherapist who responded to the survey summarized the uniqueness of community practice:

> The environment modifies the relationship between the therapist and client; it shapes the treatment goals and outcomes and it limits the therapeutic tools available. Therapists must be sensitive to the client's lifestyle and cultural values. Clients often present differently at home, focusing on their functional needs and limitations which can make them more anxious, difficult, manipulative, or dependent than was anticipated on the discharge from hospital. We

have the opportunity to view the global picture – the problems they face, their isolation, unreliable support systems, lack of financial resources, inadequacy of their coping mechanisms. The therapist therefore has to be creative in problem-solving, resourceful, independent and self-reliant and adept at being able to tap into many community resources. The 'global picture' enables the therapist to identify the essential elements and focus the intervention to meet the client's needs. The partnership formed with the clients (and family) enables the therapist to be effective in helping them reach this goal.

The results of this survey are borne out by other surveys carried out between 1981 and 1986 for the Association of Chartered Physiotherapists in the Community before planning postgraduate education in the UK to assist staff in the transition from institutional to community care.

References

Brody, EM (1981) Women in the middle and family help to older people. *The Gerontologist* 18: 471–480.

Canadian Association of Occupational Therapists (1991). Occupational Therapy Guidelines for Client Centred Practice. Toronto: CAOT.

Fulton, J (1993) *Canada's Health Care System: Bordering on the Possible.* New York: Faulkner & Gray.

Hamilton, MK (1989) The health and activity limitation survey. *Health Reports* 1: 175–188.

Kaden, J, McDaniel, SA (1990). Caregiving and care receiving: a double bind for women in Canada's ageing society. *Journal of Women and Aging* 2: 3–26.

Lavallee, DJ, Crupi, CD (1992) Rehabilitation takes to the road. *Holistic Nursing Practice* 6: 60–66.

Marcus, I, Jaeger, V (1984) The elderly as family caregivers. *Canadian Journal on Aging* 13: 33–43.

Ministry of Health, Ministry of Community and Social Services, Ministry of Citizenship (Ontario) (1991) *Redirection of Long Term Care and Support Services in Ontario:* a Public Consultation Paper, 72 pp. Toronto.

Pruchno, R (1990) The effects of help patterns on the mental health of spouse caregivers. *Research on Aging* 12: 57–71.

Queen's University School of Rehabilitation Therapy (1992) Community practice in rehabilitation: development and evaluation of an undergraduate multidisciplinary course and training materials for community fieldwork supervisors. Final report to Ministry of Health, Queen's University.

Statistics Canada (1994) *Profile of Canada's Seniors*, 112 pp. Ottawa: Statistics Canada.

Sutherland, RW, Fulton, MJ (1988) *Health Care in Canada: A Description and Analysis of Canadian Health Services.* Ottawa: The Health Group.

Zarit, SH, Reever, KE, Bach-Paterson, J (1980) Relatives of the impaired elderly: correlates of feeling of burden. *The Gerontologist* 20: 649–655.

G

Future Directions

SECTION EDITOR: BARRIE PICKLES

32

Future Directions

AMANDA SQUIRES

Introduction

Throughout history, societies have always undergone change. The cumulative effect has influenced world change through agricultural, industrial and now technological eras. What is unique about the twentieth and twenty-first centuries is the increasing pace of this change as technological developments accelerate the recurring cycles of disaster and recovery (Chirot, 1994). Such change is inevitable, and affects all sectors of society. Those sectors driving the economy (e.g. money markets), or which are focus funded (e.g. defence), have responded to change faster than non-competitive public services. The influencers of change are usually categorized under the acronym STEP –

the social, technological, economic and political factors (Toffler, 1971, 1981; Handy, 1990) (see Chapters 2, 4 and 5).

SOCIAL (SEE ALSO CHAPTERS 4 AND 5)

Occupation and promotion are increasingly based on merit rather than influence, widening opportunities and aspirations. Travel has expanded expectations and promoted tolerance through experience and understanding of other cultures. Equality for women, largely as a consequence of planned fertility, has resulted in greater employment opportunity, confidence and consumer power. This has resulted in demand for products with inherent qualities to meet the newly emerging lifestyle needs. Employment of women in developed countries is accelerating, with the consequent decrease in time available for traditional caregiving roles, with job demands requiring travel and resulting in physical separation from families. In addition the changes in patterns of marriage, divorce, partnerships, single parenting and family size also alter responsibilities for, and expectations of, informal care provision. Where such responsibilities are able to be retained, stress and its subsequent effect on paid work must be considered. Some employers provide a 24-hour care facility on site where employees can bring dependents, for the benefit of employer, carer and dependent.

TECHNOLOGICAL

Advances in traditional technologies have enabled the convenience, leisure and travel described above. Medical technology has facilitated survival at all ages by decreasing birthrate and increasing longevity. Information technology (IT) is enabling the handling and comparison of vast amounts of data — faster, further and in more detail than ever before — facilitating consultation, monitoring and communication over almost infinite geographic distances. Also it facilitates the development of appropriate 'quality tools' from the already quality conscious manufacturing sector to service industries and will therefore become integral to the work of all staff — at all levels.

ECONOMIC

Consumerism has increased demand for more, better, cheaper and unique products. The environmental consequences of overpopulation, and in many cases consumerism beyond need (Cordon et al., 1992), has focused public attention on the environmental consequences of extravagance in all its forms. This public scrutiny is added to

that of governments who are already increasing their demands for cost-effective use of those resources for which they are accountable.

POLITICAL

The move from the industrial to the technological era has also changed the political balance. The move to the right which occurs with blue collar ascendancy, is anticipated to change the welfare focus of a society to a more personal focus, with increasing reluctance of tax payers to fund societies' dependents — the old, ill, disabled and poor (see also Chapter 23).

MANAGEMENT OF CHANGE

How such change is managed is crucial to its success. For example fluctuations in demand and pressure for efficiency are indicating a 'portfolio' style of career rather than a 'job for life' which will require considerable staff counselling as roles, job security and opportunities change. The organizations of the future are described by Handy as 'shamrock', with the three leaves depicting a central core, competitively contracted out-work and flexible labour to meet the variations in quality, quantity and content.

OVERALL FUTURE OF HEALTH CARE IN A CHANGING WORLD

From the preceding overview, certain key factors will have the greatest impact on health care and each is addressed. To put the health care industry in perspective, its history can be described as beginning with self care, followed by the use of traditional remedies by lay specialists, and leading to professionalization and power supported by secrecy and autonomy. Centralization of services in hospitals has only occurred since the nineteenth century when the development of technology required accommodation and attendant staff (see Chapters 30 and 31).

Social

Whatever the service, expectations for its improvement abound. Some health services which have evolved from limited 'charitable' provision, such as the UK National Health Service (NHS), have historically had 'grateful' recipients. Users have come to realize that even in a welfare health service, their income is being taxed to provide the benefits and users are therefore customers — with perhaps constrained choices. The more that competition is introduced to stimulate efficiency in the health care market, the more demand there will be for choice of a health service provider who can deliver the expected qualities demanded.

Women, with their new confidence and consumerism, have traditionally been the largest providers, informal carers and escorts of the sick. Their increasing responsibilities at work will decrease their availability for these traditional roles. Women have also been the main users of health care — mostly when 'non-ill' such as when child bearing. Their personal knowledge of 'hotel services' is compared with what they observe — and is questioned by them. They may also question the discharge plan for a relative that assumes 'home care by the family'. Their own care is increasingly demanded within an environment of choice, control and empowerment. These concerns of women users are unlikely to change as they cross the patient/provider divide at 9 am and 5 pm wearing the signs of clinical authority as health care providers. This influence from within health care provision will be increasingly valued.

Ovretveit (1992) has described quality in health care as dependent on the views of patient, potential patient, provider and purchaser — all having different perspectives. For instance the potential patient has expectations of service availability, its purpose and how to access it. These assumptions may be based on information of varying accuracy. Much public information on health care is obtained from women's magazines where contributions are unlikely to have been submitted for peer review as in academic journals.

The patient's expectations are similar to those for other services and have been summed up for health care by Maxwell (1992): Accessibility — can people get it when they need it; Acceptability — what do people think of it; Effectiveness — what is the result; Efficiency — how does it compare with other approaches, and how are funds used; Equity — are people treated fairly relative to others; and Relevance — are services balanced to meet the needs and wants of the population.

The service provider will have particular concerns about professional standards, whilst the service funder (insurance or public funds) will seek cost effectiveness, equity and assurances on professional standards.

There will therefore remain a tension within and between providers, funders and users on the quality of service that is expected and provided. The narrower the gap the greater the all round satisfaction. Informed communication between all stakeholders, resulting in greater agreement on definitions; the standards to be set; the monitoring methods to be used, and systems for continuous improvement to be employed, will combine to form the Quality Cycle. Technical aspects which can only be credibly evaluated by peer review, should none the less be publicly reported. Professional bodies will need to increase their roles in accreditation and audit if they are to retain a credible position, and thereby encourage continuous improvement in the work of their members.

The area of greatest concern will continue to be effectiveness of services — its meaning differing between patients as well as their carers and funders. Elimination of unproven or ineffective treatments will need to be made.

Medical Technology

The ability to extend life between the cradle and the grave by early and intensive intervention in a crisis, or replacement parts during life, has built on the dramatic improvement in survival through public health measures introduced in previous generations (McKeown, 1986). Infections as the major killers, have now been largely dealt with although some organisms are now adapting and proving to be drug resistant. Malignancy, accidents (often from new found leisure pursuits), and simply wearing out are now the major causes of death. The resource consequences of high technology, the growing personal and social care problems resulting from imperfect outcomes and opportunity costs of public expectation that 'all that can be done, should be done' are seldom calculated. Health economists debate the value of Quality Adjusted Life Years (QUALYs) in prioritizing such care for older people, while the actual short- and long-term outcomes of much medical care remains unevaluated. It is a strange irony that traditional medicine, so ineffective in dealing with the acute infections of its day has been replaced by scientific medicine, so often ineffective in dealing with the chronic health problems of today. The growing resurgence of interest in some aspects of traditional medicine,

revived by travel experiences and immigration, is timely. Its accessibility and acceptability, especially the personal and holistic approach, are particularly valued by users.

This imbalance between need and supply in health care in developed countries demands a reorganization of services, facilities and resources, to ensure that changing needs are met. Such changes will increasingly focus on care in, and by, the community for its dependents. Institutions are generally inappropriate for non-acute health care, but are convenient for staff and economies of scale. The success of reprovision of services in the community requires education and appropriate — not necessarily the same — funding. For example a UK study of comparative physiotherapy input between hospital and home for the same size and type of case mix found the latter to require at least twice the input to cover travel, single handed tasks, and the expected social skills of the visitor role (Williams, 1993). The additional responsibilities of working in unexpected, and sometimes threatening, circumstances should not be underestimated.

The opportunity to use technology in its widest sense to facilitate independence of people with disabilities has yet to be fully realized. The costs are viewed as high, but should be seen as a necessary consequence of the investment in survival and repair. Home based medical technology such as dialysis; environmental systems to run a home from a keyboard; and pavement scooter mobility, will all extend opportunities for independence.

Economic and Political

The costs of increased technology, increased survival and increased expectations have to be understood and borne by the society that supports these principles. The options are increased income (tax / insurance), decreased expenditure (salaries — which make up around 70% of all health expenditure) or changes in demand (health promotion, priorities and alternatives). This will require education — 'encouraged' by funders through sanctions where necessary.

These cost and benefit calculations will be made against a backdrop of the changing dependency ratio — as fewer people work and more people seek benefits. The most cost-effective use of staffing, with use of trained assistants for unskilled care will be expected. Dynamic skill mix reviews will become a daily occurrence to meet the comprehensive changing needs of clients identified through objective multidisciplinary functional assessment. Artificial barriers and protectionism between professions will naturally decrease in the fight for group survival as the demand for cost-effective services increases.

Use of facilities, the next highest cost to a service after salaries, will continue to need review. Usage of hotels for recovery, home care, hospital at home programmes and community care will all increase. Reduced duration of institutional stay through changes in medical technology, especially anaesthetics and keyhole surgery, can be expected. More appropriate community placement for continuing care, as a result of public concern at the consequences of institutionalization, will reduce the need for health care bricks and mortar. Unfortunately, in a time of change, attachment to a solid visible structure is a natural human reaction, resulting in public outcry at the loss of a local building, as opposed to questioning what service might replace it. Such reactions could be lessened by improved communication and genuine assurances, although intangible services are a less convincing and a less attractive

focus for voluntary effort. The threat of change to the dependent and the institutionalized, including long-serving staff of all disciplines, requires particular understanding and appropriate action.

Management of chronic disability is a major clinical cost to health care. Some national and international initiatives, e.g. the 1974 Lalonde Report in Canada, Health for All 2000 by the World Health Organization in 1978, and Health of the Nation in the UK in 1992 all promote the prevention and management of disabilities. Where such chronic disabilities do ultimately surface, traditional medicine may have much more to offer, both in effectiveness, efficiency and acceptability. Colleagues in developing countries, using such traditional techniques may offer alternative approaches to other countries when evidence of effectiveness is secured (see also Chapter 28).

Management of Change

The acceptance of the inevitability of change must be the first step. Management of health care, as opposed to past 'administration' will be influential. Seeking opportunities, rather than anticipating threats, will facilitate personal and professional survival. The method of communicating the reasons for change and consequences for health care must be consistent to all stakeholders. Wide consultation on change will do much to smooth the way, engendering an atmosphere of co-operation rather than conflict. Training in these skills is essential for all staff (Plant, 1987), and should be valued equally with the development of technical skills. Up-to-date political awareness and understanding of the issues will be the bedrock on which to move forward.

Opportunities for Physiotherapy

Demographic and Epidemiological Opportunity

There will be no shortage of older people seeking help from physiotherapists – but will older people of the future be different? An increasing number will have retired earlier, probably be fitter, and expect to have a long and active retirement. For this group, compression of disability into a shorter proportion of the life span by preventative measures has been suggested by Fries (1980); death would be by wearing out rather than wearing down. Other older people will survive illness and injury to which their parents would have succumbed, although they may be left to face multiple and progressive disabilities as a result. Chronic disease will be increasingly prevalent – a challenge for which physiotherapists are uniquely placed to respond.

The increasing assertiveness of successive generations has led to expectations of 'informed partnerships' in care – not grateful, passive receipt. When illness is acute and the person dependent on care, the term of patient is appropriate. The disabilities and handicaps of chronic disease change the role of patient to that of client – one who seeks advice and then makes informed choices. It is essential that physiotherapists accept and adapt to this power change.

Physiotherapists have a long-term perspective, developed from their goal setting expertise. This will be invaluable in developing a vision for the future. Advice on development or contraction of physiotherapy services as the needs of society change must be objective and supported by relevant research. If the demand for services from older people exceeds that of other age groups an obvious need for reorganization to meet this demand exists. Physiotherapists and their managers must move in the direction of demand, acquiring the appropriate skills en route, or the financial incentive of the 'health care market' may be needed to achieve the result.

Accurate and comprehensive assessment will be a key task (see also Chapter 14). It will determine the use of resources to achieve agreed outcomes. The identification and cost-effective matching of needs and skills will be a sought after ability. Such treatment should address the full breadth of need – in many cases we have yet to be sure what is cost effective, or how society will wish to make informed decisions to prioritize the use of its resources. Until this has been achieved intuition will continue to be the guide, and much energy expended in its defence.

The need for organization and interpretation of information, gained from assessment and other activities, will make the use of Information Technology essential for all health care professionals, but evidence indicates a void to be overcome. For example, a survey in the UK of 42 incoming physiotherapy students showed 40% had no computer knowledge, 52% had limited knowledge, while only 7% considered themselves experienced in this area (Lipscombe, 1994).

Following assessment, a comprehensive treatment programme with goals leading to maximum self-sufficiency will be developed. Such treatment will be undertaken by the patient where possible, with unskilled assistance where needed, and the physiotherapist involved only where essential. Self operated equipment will be used increasingly by patients to enhance personal skills or replace those of less available carers (Concar, 1993). Monitoring of progress with regular re-assessment of needs will remain a therapy consultant task. Physiotherapists will become teachers in different circumstances, and will need to be clear about what they will need to 'teach or treat'. Less time will be spent on individual treatment sessions.

The success of rehabilitation programmes will be dependent on increasing the older person's functional ability. The aims should be understandable to all stakeholders. The functions needed by older people in the future may differ from those required today. The 'convenience' lifestyle may not only reduce joint damage, but also exercise tolerance. Will walking remain the essential function of today, or will posture and the ability to manipulate the environment through technology become more important for older people? Physiotherapists already use their skills to initiate designs for independence, they must market their knowledge based innovations more aggressively in the future.

Assessment should also lead to advice regarding health promotion. Despite the relatively short life expectancy of people of advanced age, health promotion can still be valuable, especially physical activity (Govindasamy and Paterson, 1994). Opportunities exist here for physiotherapists to teach the skills of exercise to representatives of the group, and monitor progress, rather than necessarily carrying out group work personally. There remains a void waiting to be filled in providing education, through all media opportunities, on a variety of topics for older people. For instance group exercise could be by two way video link up from the polyclinic to individual homes. There is no restriction on authorship of such work – all comers can bid for a place, which will be won largely by marketing ability.

The key worker principle, whereby the most appropriate member of the team takes responsibility for co-ordinating a package of care to maximize independence in the community, is increasingly falling to physiotherapists because of their clinical, managerial and social skills. Such a reputation is welcome, but training and support must also be available to enable the role to be carried out successfully without the risk of 'burnout' in such dedicated professionals, the preventative strategy being realistic goal setting and appropriate supervision (Squires and Livesley, 1984).

Whatever the style and content of future physiotherapy, the need for information on the service must be available, and its acceptability to the client determined and assured. How new generations of older people will balance their own needs with those of others in society has yet to be revealed, but indications are that the criteria on which this will be judged will be more objective, equitable and cost effective than in the past. Such intelligence is reliant on acquiring information from clients, using it and evaluating the impact. Older people have been shown to be very responsive to such surveys – having more likelihood of time, and the anticipation of considerable personal benefit from any changes. Older people have demonstrated that from their vast experience of life they have well considered, practical ideas for change.

Portfolio Careers and Brain Power

The whims of the market, as well as changes in actual demand, require a flexible workforce for maximum efficiency. Facilities and programmes for older people have traditionally employed mature, part time staff, who bring to the job clinical experience, life skills and hours convenient to the user. Many of these established staff may be threatened by an increasing need for change. Sensitivity to the reaction to change by such stalwarts needs careful preparation.

Greater brain power to undertake more technical

and fewer labour intensive tasks will be sought — we now have equipment, much self-operated, to help lift, bath, get up after a fall, call for help, reduce swelling and pain etc. There are infinite technical opportunities for development of such devices, limited only by encouragement and funds. The refinement of this equipment, and the availability of timely repair and maintenance facilities, will become crucial. Again physiotherapists are ideally placed to meet this challenge.

The responsibilities of the new style of community based health care will require physiotherapists to have experience in all specialties to cope with what they may find. Older people present with a mixture of pathologies and overlapping symptoms which require considerable clinical experience to assess. Once the acute medical issues have been dealt with, the resulting handicaps have to be addressed — the answers to such complex and unique problems are seldom found in any text book, requiring knowledge from many past experiences. The skills required also extend to social and cultural knowledge, magnified in importance when in the role of 'visitor' to the patient's home.

Labour intensive work will be called upon only as and when needed — staff will no longer be employed on a 'just in case' or historical basis. Documented standards, protocols and records will enable responsible transfer of tasks between individuals.

Consequences for Physiotherapy Education

As the foundations for the future of individuals as well as professions is established during training, undergraduate programmes have an opportunity to address anticipated future issues within their curriculum. Such topics include an understanding of change, its consequences and management; the different clinical and social needs of successive generations; appropriate clinical skills; and particularly the ability to evaluate the consequences of interventions and make appropriate changes. These needs will never be fully met in a changing world, and will form the basis of a self led programme for continuing education.

Conclusion

It is crucial for physiotherapists to appreciate the need for change, accept an expanded role in working with older clients and undertake this colaboratively with all stake holders. Above all physiotherapists must decide what to teach or treat, how to evaluate the results and market their potential. Others are waiting impatiently to seize the opportunity.

References

Chirot, D (1994) *How Societies Change*. California: Pine Forge Press.

Concar, D (1993) Can robots come to care for us? *New Scientist* 140: 40–42.

Cordon, A, Robertson, E, Tolley, K (1992) *Meeting Need in an Affluent Society.* Aldershot UK: Avebury.

Fries, JF (1980) Ageing, natural death and the compression of morbidity. *New England Journal of Medicine* 303: 130–135.

Govindasamy, D, Paterson, DH (1994) *Physical Activity and the Older Adult: A knowledge base for managing exercise programmes*. Illinois US: Stipes Publishing.

Handy, C (1990) *The Age of Unreason*. London: Arrow.

Lipscombe, H (1994) The computer generation. *Physiotherapy Journal* 80: 88.

Maxwell, RJ (1992) Dimensions of quality revisited: From thought to action. *Quality in Health Care* 1: 171–177.

McKeown, T (1986) *The Role of Medicine*. Oxford: Blackwell.

Ovretveit, J (1992) *Health Service Quality*. Oxford: Blackwell.

Plant, R (1987) *Managing Change and Making it Stick*. London: Fontana.

Schneider, El, Brody, JA (1983) Ageing, natural death and the compression of morbidity: Another view. *New England Journal of Medicine* **309**: 854–856.

Squires, A, Livesley, B (1984) Beware of burnout. *Physiotherapy* **70**: 235–238.

Toffler, A (1971) *Future Shock*. London: Pan.

Toffler, A (1981) *Third Wave*. London: Pan.

Williams, R (1993) *Health Advisory Service: Directors' Annual Report*. London: HMSO.

33

A Review Case

BARRIE PICKLES, ANN COMPTON

Case Study
•
A Summary of the General Issues to be Considered
•
Questions

Case Study

Now that you have completed this book why not try to deal with the problems identified in the following case?

Mrs Smith is a 72-year-old married woman who was admitted 4 weeks ago to the general hospital in the medium-sized manufacturing town in which she has lived for the past 45 years, for removal of a herniated intervertebral disc at the L5-S1 level. She had complained of back pain periodically during the past 5 years, but had not been incapa-

citated by this until just prior to her current admission, when, after a stumble, she had a sudden onset of intense pain in her low back area and radiating down her right leg. A myelogram performed soon after admission revealed extrusion of the disc; surgical removal was perfomed later that same week.

Since her surgery Mrs Smith reports no real relief from her discomfort. She continues to have more or less continuous pain, which is aggravated by movement, and especially intensified by sitting or standing for more than 15 minutes. The pain is greatest on the right side of the lumbar area, and is accompanied by marked spasm of the paravertebral muscles, especially on the right side. There is some left lumbar pain and spasm as well, plus pain radiating down the right leg into the buttock, posterior thigh and calf.

The neurologist's report on her following an examination 2 weeks after her surgery mentioned some reduction in the triceps surae reflex on the right side, and slight numbness over the sole and lateral border of the right foot. There appears to be little or no reduction in strength in the right limb, although this is difficult to assess because of the discomfort elicited by her attempts to perform resisted movements. The right leg is somewhat cooler to touch than the left; there is no noticeable oedema.

For many years Mrs Smith has been a slight underweight woman, with very poor abdominal muscle tone, and generally poor posture. She says she has never enjoyed being physically active. Since her operation she has been very anxious about her discomfort and the failure of surgery to provide immediate relief for her symptoms. She has tended to sleep poorly and has had little appetite. She is often bad-tempered and excitable.

Last week, 3 weeks after her operation Mrs Smith suffered a slight stroke. She woke during the middle of the night and complained initially of a severe headache. Later that night the nurse noticed that Mrs Smith appeared somewhat confused, and was not responding to questions or instructions in her usual manner. The Surgical Resident was called; he discovered that Mrs Smith was not able to move her left leg at all, and that all movements in the left arm were considerably weakened. Both skin sensibility and proprioceptive capacity in the left leg were severely impaired. However, most of these symptoms disappeared within a couple of days, although Mrs Smith is now left with a mild degree of spasticity in her left leg, and some loss of grip strength and fine motor control in her left hand. Since her stroke, Mrs Smith has experienced urinary incontinence on a number of occasions, much to her embarassment.

Mrs Smith lives with her husband in the family home they have rented for the past 45 years. Their two daughters, who are both married and have grownup children of their own, continue to reside in the same neighbourhood close to their parents. Family ties appear to continue to remain strong.

Mr Smith is now 75 years of age. He retired from his job as a railroad brakeman 10 years ago. At the time of his retirement he was in good health, but for the past 6 years has had problems resulting from chronic bronchitis and emphysema. He now has a persistent cough, which is productive of considerable sputum especially in the morning, and he complains of shortness of breath and fatigue on exertion. These symptoms have become significantly worse recently.

He is tense and anxious in appearance, pale but without marked cyanosis around the lips or in the nail beds. He coughs frequently and appears to find this exhausting, expecially since his coughing is often prolonged and not always productive. He sits down whenever possible, walks very slowly, and becomes anxious and very much out of breath on even moderate exertion. He appears to breathe largely using the upper chest. When he is out of breath, Mr Smith occasionally uses a pursed lips pattern of breathing. Last year he rejected the advice of his doctor regarding the desirability of oxygen supplementation when his dyspnoea was particularly bad. Although he was once a heavy smoker, he has not smoked for almost 3 years.

Since the onset of his respiratory problems Mr Smith has become increasingly discouraged about his health and his wife had complained to their family physician that he spends most of the day sitting in his favourite chair in their living room dozing and watching television. Until 2 years ago he used to go out in the afternoon or evening quite regularly to meet his friends and play cards at the Elks Club to which he still belongs. He used to enjoy attending baseball games but it is now more than 2 years since he last attended one of the games, although he still enjoys watching sports on television. During the 6-month period prior to his wife's surgery he had only occasionally left the house to take a short walk outdoors; on other occasions one of his daughters had driven him to medical appointments, and irregular visits with his wife to the church in which they had been married and which they used to attend regularly together. Until her recent admission to hospital for surgery Mrs Smith made a special point to attend her church at least once every Sunday.

The Smiths have a small nest-egg of around $5000 tucked away in a savings account. In addition to their government pensions Mr Smith receives a small pension from his previous employment as a railway brakeman; while they have found these pensions adequate for their needs, there is little left over for luxuries.

Contact with their two married daughters is very regular — one daughter assists Mrs Smith with her weekly shopping, while the second, who lives just down the street, calls in to see her mother every day. Both have continued to see their mother regularly since she was admitted to hospital, taking it in turns to bring Mr Smith by car each day, and also provide him with an evening meal. The two sons-in-law have undertaken responsibiliy for maintenance and repair work to the Smith's property, and, for the past 2 years, have paid one of the local teenagers to keep the yard tidy during the summer and the driveway clear of snow and ice in the winter. Most of the Smiths present neighbours are young families with school age children who have only recently come to live in the area; they have had no meaningful contact with the Smiths who have always given the impression that they wanted only a casual acquaintance with their younger neighbours.

The question of the long-term management of the Smith's family problems is now under consideration. You, as the Senior Physiotherapist on the Regional Geriatric Assessment Team have been asked to review Mrs Smith's case, and offer your suggestions, not only for her immediate and longer-term treatment programme, but also for ongoing support to the family.

A Summary of the General Issues to be Considered

1. What are the cultural norms of society regarding participation in the kind of programme? Do the perspectives of the group reflect these norms? Is the group culturally homogeneous? (Chapter 4, 5).

2. What attitude(s) of individual members of this group of older people might affect their willingness to participate in this kind of activity? (Chapter 3).

3. What ethical and/or legal issues have to be considered in developing and implementing this type of programme with older people? (Chapter 27).

4. How can you communicate more effectively with older people? (Chapter 10).

5. Taking into account how older people learn, what teaching strategies are most likely to be successful to assist cognitive learning (Chapter 8), and motor learning (Chapter 9).

6. How can you increase the possibility that ongoing changes in the lifestyle of older people may result from participation in your programme? (Chapter 13).

7. Do you have a knowledge and understanding of the biological and physiological changes of both ageing and inactivity? (Chapters 6, 7).

8. Are you familiar with the principles of design of exercise and activity programmes for older people, and how these principles may differ from those designed for younger persons? (Chapter 12).

9. What treatment goals need to be set for each of the impairments, disabilities and handicaps that are identified in this older patient? (Chapter 14).

10. Is there any evidence of unusual presentation of signs and symptoms in this older patient that might lead to an expectation of altered response to any treatment you might consider? (Chapter 1).

11. Do any special considerations need to be given to the fact that in this older patient some problems are of long duration? (Chapter 22).

12. What adjustments are necessary to treatment programmes for older people, to take into account that changes resulting from ageing and disuse are always superimposed on the impairments of disease and injury, and increase the resulting disabilities? (Chapter 12).

13. Is any assistive device likely to help the older person decrease or overcome a disability or handicap that may be present? (Chapter 25, 26).

14. Would a referral to any other health care professional be in the best interests of the patient? (Chapter 28).

15. When multiple impairments and disabilities are present in older persons, their reduced energy capacity may make it necessary to prioritize these in order of precedence for attention. What priorities would you set, and how would you establish these? (Chapter 14).

16. In situations where more than one problem exists it may not always be possible to provide comprehensive treatment for each. The presence of one problem may mean that some aspects of treatment for another may not be possible, or may be contraindicated. Is this a difficulty in the case under review? (There can be no general reference given to this question. Each case is different, and the physiotherapist will need to decide each situation on its individual merits.)

17. Are any of the problems that have been

identified likely to be iatrogenic i.e. created or worsened by the physiotherapy, or by drugs the older patient may be taking? (Consult standard texts about these various possibilities.)

18. To what extent is it appropriate for the older person to make their own decisions regarding the physiotherapy interventions, and their rehabilitation? (Chapter 11). Is the older person a patient, client or consumer? (Chapter 1). What is the importance of independence to older people with disabilities? (Chapters 22, 23).

19. Severe, multiple, and long-standing problems in older persons often place severe strain and hardship on their primary caregiver. Is there any evidence of this, and if so, what forms of support that are available might be appropriate? (Chapter 31).

20. Are the present housing arrangements the most satisfactory? What alternatives might be considered? (Chapter 24).

21. How can the efforts of the physiotherapist be linked most effectively with those of other members of the Day Hospital team? (Chapter 28).

22. How should a comprehensive assessment be done to identify and prioritize the medical, rehabilitative, economic and social needs of an older person with multiple problems? (Chapter 29).

23. What range of services is available in the community that enable older people with multiple problems to continue to live in their own homes? (Chapter 31).

24. In those cases where it is no longer feasible for older persons to remain in their own home, what alternative type of institutional care would be most appropriate? (Chapter 30).

Questions

1. From the Case Study, identify each of the impairments, disabilities and handicaps that are reported. Classify these problems into medical, psychological, psychosocial, environmental, economic, rehabilitation and/or other categories as you see fit. Recognize that a problem may overlap between these categories.

2. What other disabilities and handicaps that have not been identified in the Case Study might you expect to find in clients with this collection of impairments?

3. From your lists, identify the order of priorities for the different items you have placed in each category. What factors need to be considered when determining these priorities?

4. From your knowledge of clinical conditions, are any unusual or unexpected signs and symptoms reported, or is there no mention of any important features that you would expect to be present? Is there any indication that the responses of this patient to treatment might differ from those normally expected?

5. List an optimal set of specific treatment goals that deal with the many problems reported, and indicate which physiotherapy procedures might be used to achieve each of these goals. Is it feasible to address each of these objectives at the start of the programme, or must attention to some that have a lower priority be delayed until some higher priority goals have been achieved?

6. Outline what you believe will be the maximum functional status that this patient could achieve eventually, and also within the next month.

7. Plan a detailed, progressive physiotherapy programme for this patient, which you believe to have the greatest potential for achieving your selected

goals. Be specific in terms of dosage (intensity, duration, frequency etc). Develop this plan in terms of what you might do in each contact with the patient, rather than stating how each problem might be approached if it were the only one. Pay particular attention to how the existence of a second (or third) set of problems might require a modification of the way in which you might have preferred to deal with the primary difficulty. Take into account how the responses of an older person may differ from those of a younger patient. How might you help improve the motivation of an older client?

8. What measurement tools do you consider will give you the best information on the patient's problems? How will you use this information to determine when and how to progress each aspect of the patient's treatment?

9. Identify those assistive devices that would be useful in helping to reduce the severity of any of the disabilities that have been identified.

10. Suggest the medium and long-term prospects in this case. Will the patient return home? Would any modifications to the home be appropriate? Which community health and social services will be needed to maintain this person in her own home? If return home is not considered to be practical, what form of institutional care would be most appropriate.

These questions cannot be answered fully without considerable knowledge and experience in a wide range of areas. The issues are complex. It is not always easy for the physiotherapist to differentiate the treatable symptoms of disease, the remediable features of disablement and the reversible aspects of disuse from those age-related changes for which nothing can be done. Yet, the capability to make this distinction is a vital first step in the design of a realistic rehabilitation programme. The results may take longer to achieve, and may be less dramatic, and perhaps more variable, than in younger people. It would be difficult, however, to identify another area of practice where the physiotherapist makes such a difference to the lives of their clients. We must not forget the Hippocratic principles 'to cure sometimes, to relieve often, and to comfort always', but we should add to these a commitment to do what we can to help improve the quality of life for older people.

Index